MODERN PACEMAKERS - PRESENT AND FUTURE

Edited by **Mithilesh Kumar Das**

Modern Pacemakers - Present and Future
Edited by Mithilesh Kumar Das

Published by InTech

Janeza Trdine 9, 51000 Rijeka, Croatia

Publishing Process Manager Jelena Marusic

Technical Editor Teodora Smiljanic

Cover Designer InTech Design Team

Additional hard copies can be obtained from orders@intechopen.com

Modern Pacemakers - Present and Future, Edited by Mithilesh Kumar Das
p. cm.
ISBN 978-953-307-214-2

For EU product safety concerns:
IN TECH d.o.o., Prolaz Marije Krucifikse Kozulić 3, 51000 Rijeka, Croatia,
info@intechopen.com or visit our website at intechopen.com.

Meet the editor

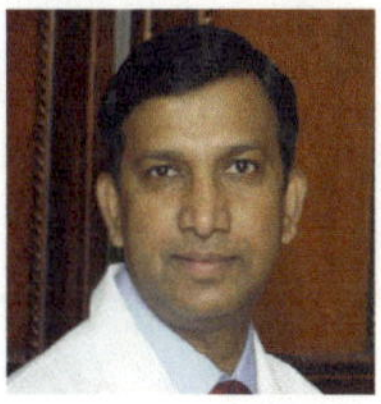

Dr. Mithilesh Kumar Das
Associate Professor of Clinical Medicine
Krannert Institute of Cardiology, Indiana University School of Medicine Director, Cardiac Electrophysiology Service, Roudebush VA Medical Center Program Director of Cardiac Electrophysiology Fellowship, VA Medical Center

Contents

Preface

Cardiac pacing has been one of the greatest inventions of 20th Century. Since the first pacing system was implanted in 1958, pacemakers have evolved into very sophisticated machines. Conduction system disease being more prevalent in elderly, however, it can effect younger population. At present pacemaker is the only definitive treatment for symptomatic conduction system disease. It is implanted by cardiologists, electrophysiologists, and surgeons. Patients with pacemakers are primarily managed by electrophysiologists and cardiologists but many emergency physicians and general physicians encounter these patients. In addition, many pacemaker clinics are managed by nurses who often have more contact with patients than physicians. Therefore, understanding of modern pacemaker functions is necessary for many people in medical science who manage patients.

The first edition of this book emphasizes the science, implantation techniques and management of cardiac pacing. This book also covers the lead related issues, interference with magnetic resonance imaging, device related complications and utility of remote monitoring. Future of pacemaker may ley in understanding the mechanisms of pacemaker currents and conduction system physiology. Therefore, we have incorporated chapters related to these topics along with a chapter discussing the status of bio-pacemakers. I have tried to integrate every aspect of modern pacemaker function important for managing patients and help to understand the mechanism and future of cardiac pacing.

I hope that this textbook will meet the needs of clinicians, nurses, scientists, engineers and also patients. I sincerely believe that being accessible on the web, many patients may be able to visit the book will get acquainted with modern pacemaker functions and complications. The book will make them aware the present status and future of their device. Therefore, I am excited about the opportunity to present the whole spectrum of cardiac pacing in a comprehensive scientific manner that will not only be helpful to electrophysiologists but also benefit a large spectrum of people in medical science. We have also included chapters regarding gut pacemakers as well as pacemaker mechanisms of neural network.

I greatly acknowledge the valuable assistance of Mrs. Jelena Marusic of Intech, an Open Access publisher for all the help in compiling this comprehensive book of 32 chapters. I sincerely thank all the contributors for their excellent efforts in making their book chapters very elaborate and useful. It was only possible by taking out time form their family, busy schedules and other scientific assignments. Therefore, all contributors deserve a great credit and thanks in making the book comprehensive. I would also like to thank my wife Rekha and our sons, Awaneesh and Mohineesh, for being impetus in my continued effort to practice medicine at a highest level and contribute to medical science.

I hope that this book will provide valuable information to all the medical and paramedical personnel who take care of our patients with pacemaker. I hope that this book will provide the basic knowledge and comprehensive reference for clinicians to help improve their lives of our patients.

Mithilesh Kumar Das, MD, MRCP, FACC
Associate Professor of Clinical Medicine
Krannert Institute of Cardiology
Indiana University School of Medicine,
USA

Part 1

Pacemaker Basic Information

1

Information Technology Aspects of Integrated Cardiac Rhythm Disease Management

Dieter Hayn, Hannes Kumpusch, Rene Labenbacher,
Robert Modre-Osprian and Günter Schreier
AIT Austrian Institute of Technology GmbH
Austria

1. Introduction

Since several decades pacemakers and *implantable cardioverter defibrillators* (ICDs) are a common therapy for patients with cardiac rhythm abnormalities. More recently developed devices like *implantable cardiac resynchronization therapy devices* (CRTs) (Anand et al. 2009) or *implantable loop recorders* (ILRs) (Boersma et al. 2003) are implanted with increasing frequency and provide promising results.

Selection and implantation of devices are only first steps in cardiac rhythm disease management. Continuous adaptation of device settings to patient's needs, monitoring of device's battery status, revision of devices and several other issues need to be considered. Additionally, the functionality of devices is closely related to other therapeutic aspects, such as medication or the patient's health parameters - assessed either by general practitioners or by the patient him/herself (e.g. blood pressure).

In many cases a given patient needs more than one therapy: e.g. pacemaker therapy is closely related to medication monitoring; or an increasing number of remotely monitored congestive heart failure patients also have an implanted CRT device. Therefore, a system is needed which is able to handle data from various sources (from implanted devices, from patient's home, from general practitioners, from hospitals, etc.) and provide the physician with all information necessary for an optimal therapy.

While from the patient's view it is primarily essential that all data from various sources are combined in one single system, from the physician's view it is also important to have one single system for all the patients she/he is responsible for. There are several manufacturers for each of the therapeutic tools used in cardiac rhythm disease management. Each of those provides the physician with its own proprietary data interface. And, of course, one physician's patients are not all equipped with devices of one and the same manufacturer. Therefore, it is not only necessary to combine devices supporting different therapies (pacemakers, remote monitoring, etc.), but also to combine systems from different manufacturers within one single platform.

Additionally, eHealth infrastructures with electronic health records are currently envisaged, conceived or already established in many environments (single healthcare institutions, health management organisations, whole healthcare systems, or even nation-wide) (Pfeiffer

2009). The relevance of such developments for integrated cardiac rhythm disease management also has to be considered.
A similar complex situation can be found in the field of radiology, picture archiving and communication. Though this field is rather defined by the devices used than – as for cardiac rhythm disease management – by the physiological system concerned, many aspects are very similar. Anyway, while *picture archiving and communication systems* (PACS) are nowadays state of the art, a similar system approach has not been established for the domain of cardiac rhythm disease management. While a state-of-the-art PACS can communicate with various devices (e.g. CT, NMR, PET, ultrasound, etc.) from several manufacturers, by the use of one single review station, current cardiac rhythm disease management systems are mostly isolated solutions for single applications (e.g. remote CHF monitoring) and/or for single manufacturers.
This chapter describes the current state of the art in cardiac rhythm disease management and the theoretical requirements for an integrated solution in terms of involved information technology aspects. Finally, a ***P****latform for* ***I****ntegrated* ***CA****rdiac* ***R****hythm* ***D****isease management* (PICARD) combining the functionality of heterogeneous systems is proposed. An overview of the information ecosystem influencing PICARD is shown in Fig. 1.

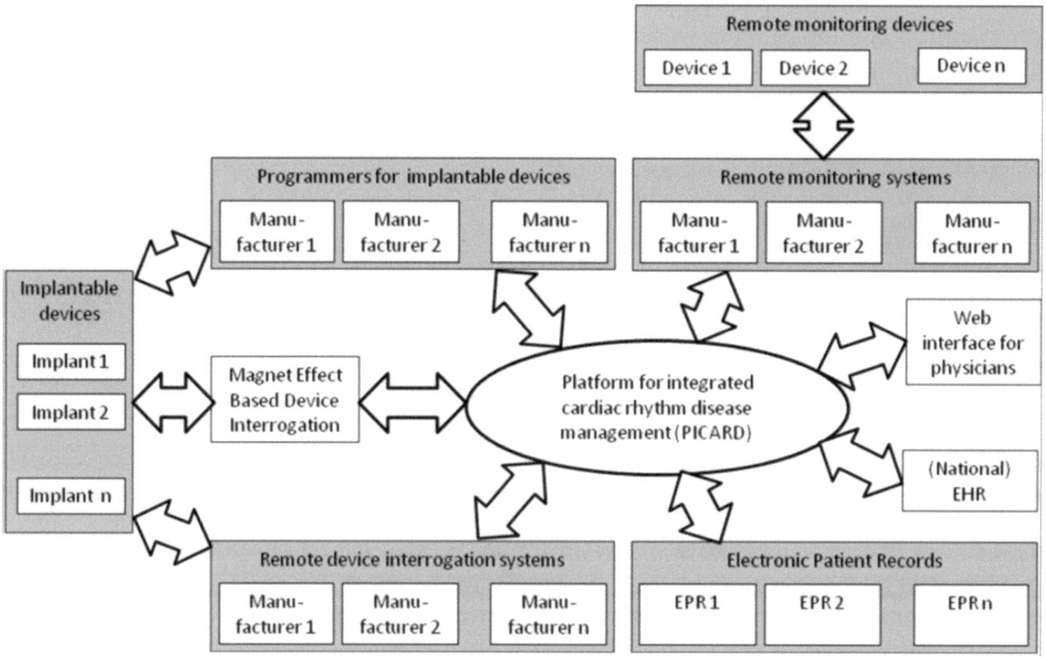

Fig. 1. Information ecosystem where a platform for integrated cardiac rhythm disease management (PICARD) is embedded. EPR...electronic patient record. EHR...electronic health record.

2. The data path

There are several data sources in cardiac rhythm disease management. Some of the sources are implanted devices (pacemakers, ICDs, ILRs, CRTs). Others are located at the patient's home, such as devices used for remote monitoring of *congestive heart failure* (CHF) – e.g. utilising body weight scales, blood pressure meter, etc.

From these distributed, local sources, data are transmitted to more and more global systems. The data path from local data sources to a centralized electronic health record is summarized in Fig. 2. It contains the following components:

- Multiple measurement devices may be linked to each other via a *body area network* (BAN). Measurement devices can be:
  - implanted devices (pacemakers, ICDs, CRTs, ILRs, etc.)
  - monitoring devices (blood pressure meter, body weight scales, etc.)
- Aggregators are devices that collect data from several measurement devices. Aggregators are located at the patient's vicinity. Data are exchanged between measurement devices and aggregators via a so called *personal / local area network* (PAN/LAN).
- Within an electronic patient record (often also called electronic medical record), data from different dislocated sources of information can be stored – linked via a *wide area network* (WAN). Electronic patient records can be parts of *hospital information systems* (HISs), telemonitoring platforms of single device manufacturers or disease management platforms such as PICARD, etc.
- Data from different electronic patient records may finally be linked to each other on the level of an *electronic health record* (EHR), which summarizes all health information e.g. on a national level.

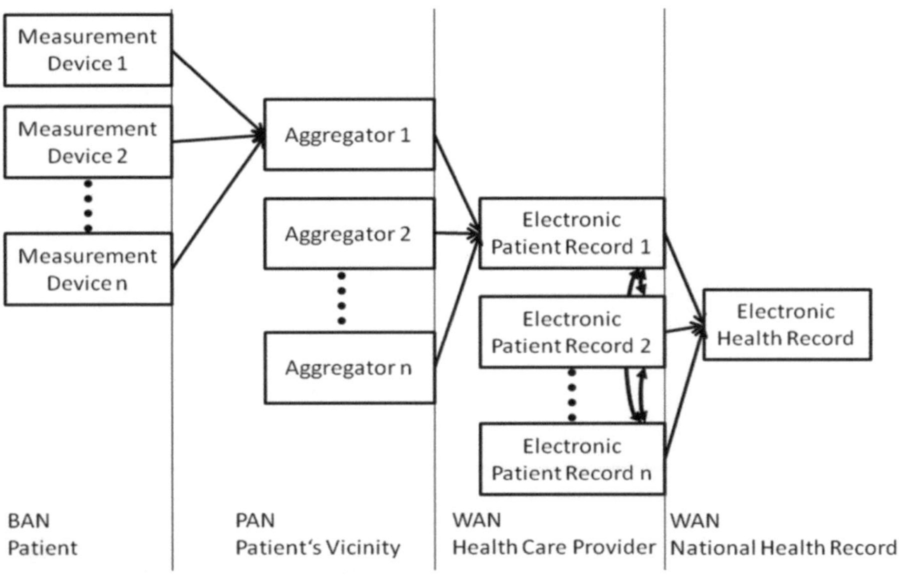

Fig. 2. Data path for cardiac rhythm disease management.

Aggregators need to be in the patient's "vicinity", a term covering several locations such as:

- Operating room – right after or even during implanting a measurement device
- Operating room – after surgeries that may influence the device's functionality (American Society of Anesthesiologists Task Force on Perioperative Management of Patients with Cardiac Rhythm Management Devices, 2005)

- Follow-up centre during regular follow-ups of a measurement device (e.g. programmers)
- Doctor's practice
- Patient's home (e.g. remote monitoring)
- Acute day wards in case of emergency situations (e.g. myocardial infarction).
- Anywhere in case of emergency situations

Some of the most common data acquisition situations which are currently used in cardiac rhythm disease management are described in the following chapter. Each of those is typically associated with a particular data source.

3. Data sources

3.1 Data source 1 – In-clinic follow-up with manufacturer-specific programmers

The aim of a follow-up is to optimise the condition of the patient and of the implanted device, to identify abnormal system function as well as lead problems, and to detect critical battery depletion (Sutton, 2006). According to international guidelines, patients with implanted pacemakers are usually requested for follow-up every 6 to 12 months, depending on patients' general condition and type and configuration of the pacing system (Task Force on Practice Guidelines, 2002 ; Kainz 1999, European Society of Cardiology & European Heart Rhythm Association, 2007). After first signs of battery depletion, the follow-up interval is decreased to every 3 months until the device is replaced.

There are two types of in-clinic follow-ups:

a. Basic follow-ups (sensing, pacing, battery, patient contentedness)

b. Extended follow-ups (additional check and optimization of pacemaker parameters)

All pacemakers provide a bidirectional telemetric interface that enables the implant to communicate with a special vendor-specific programmer. For this purpose, a so-called "wand" is connected to the programmer and placed above the implanted device. Using this wand, pacemaker data can be read out (e.g. electrode impedance) and settings of the pacemaker can be updated (e.g. pacing pulse amplitude) if necessary.

Since up to now each manufacturer provides a proprietary interface in between his implanted devices and his programmer, programmers from all manufacturers need to be available at in-clinic follow-up centres (see Fig. 3, left). Today, data read out by the programmers are usually printed out and archived in paper based patient records (Fig. 3, right). If an electronic patient record is available, manual data input is required and the data recorded electronically are mainly restricted to administrative aspects (Niederlag, 2001).

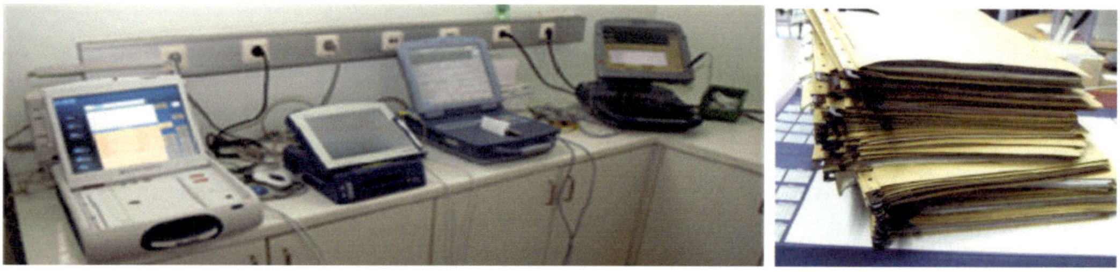

Fig. 3. Current state of in-clinic follow-ups using various programmer devices from different manufacturers (left) and paper based patient records (right).

3.2 Data source 2 – Remote device interrogation

The initial telemedical concept of so-called *Transtelephonic Monitoring* (TTM), is widely used in the US and Canada to evaluate battery depletion of pacemakers remotely (Calisto et al., 1993; Dreifus et al., 1986). Patients are asked to record an ECG in predefined intervals and to transmit the data via the standard telephone line to a service centre where the ECG is analysed by a cardiologist (Platt et al., 1996). If patients put a magnet close to their pacemaker simultaneously, the ECG will be recorded while their pacemaker is in magnet mode. This ensures that the pacemaker paces in a predefined way that can later on be analyzed by a specialist. The patient is requested for an in-clinic follow-up only in case of detected abnormalities.

New generations of implantable pacemakers available from various manufacturers support data transmission from the device to a remote monitoring centre automatically, e.g.:

- Home Monitoring (Biotronik, Berlin, Deutschland) (Nielsen et al, 2008)
- CareLink Network (Medtronic, Inc., MN, USA) (Raatikainen et al., 2008)
- Latitude Patient Management system (Boston Scientific, St Paul, USA) (Saxon et al., 2007)
- Merlin.net (St. Jude Medical, Sylmar, USA)

Depending on the particular system, the pacemaker may send diagnostic, therapeutic and technical information wirelessly to an external aggregator using a proprietary protocol. The aggregator forwards the data to the manufacturer's database using different transfer methods (SMS, https, FAX, etc.). At the monitoring centre the incoming data are analyzed and filtered. Pre-processed data are provided to the physician via a web-interface.

The data flow of such a remote device interrogation system is shown in Fig. 4.

Using such systems, remote follow-ups can be performed and/or remote monitoring can be realized: For remote follow-ups the interrogation can be triggered by a physician or by the patient him/herself whenever a follow-up seems necessary. During remote monitoring, device interrogation is done automatically according to a predefined schedule - usually once per day in the night time. Additionally, in case of arrhythmic episodes *intracardiac electrograms* (IEGMs) can be recorded and transmitted to the monitoring centre.

Up to now, remote device interrogation is used for reading out data only, and not for remote system updating or re-programming.

An overview over the properties of remote device interrogation systems from four manufacturers is given in Table 1.

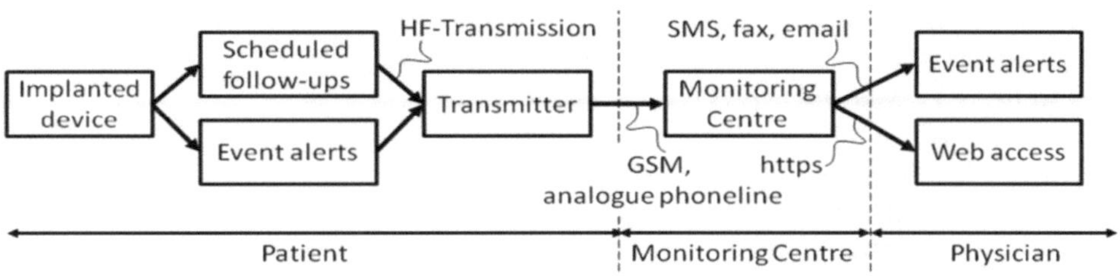

Fig. 4. Remote device interrogation system. Data from the implanted device are sent to an aggregator (transmitter) at the patient's home either regularly (scheduled follow-up) or event triggered (event alerts). The transmitter sends the data via GSM or analogue phone line to a monitoring centre where the data are analyzed. If necessary, an alarm is sent to the physician via SMS, fax or email. All data can also be accessed via a web interface.

	Biotronik Home Monitoring	Medtronic CareLink	Boston Scientific Latitude	St. Jude Merlin.net
Transmitter	GSM network	Analogue phoneline	Analogue phoneline	Analogue phoneline
FUs	Daily	Scheduled	Scheduled	Scheduled
Physician notification	SMS, e-mail, fax	SMS, e-mail	Fax, phone	Fax, e-mail, SMS
Feedback to patient via transmitter	LED indicating normal status or call to clinic	LED indicating normal status or call to clinic	Colored lights and indications	LED indicating call to clinic, automated phone calls
IEGM (real-time at remote FU)	30 s (monthly periodic EGMs)	10 s	10 s	30 s
Configurable alerts	All	Red and yellow	Red and yellow	All
Threshold adaptation	Automatic RV and LV thresholds (only Lumax 500/540)	Automatic RA, RV and LV (only Consulta) pacing thresholds	-	Automatic RA, RV and LV pacing thresholds (next generation of ICDs)
Heart failure monitoring support		Optivol lung fluid status alert	Weight scales and blood pressure cuffs	
Special features	GSM network - mobile transmitter		Configurable data transmission to associated caregivers Data export to electronic health records	Possibility of sending automated phone calls to patients Events visible on the transmitter's display

Table 1. Comparison of the remote device interrogation systems of Biotronik, Medtronic, Boston Scientific and St. Judes – based on (Burri et al., 2009). FU...follow-up.

3.3 Data source 3 – Magnet effect based device checks

An "intermediate" solution in between in-clinic follow-ups and telemedical device interrogation was presented in (Kollmann et al., 2005) using the pacemaker's magnet effect: To be compliant with international standards, battery depletion level and basic pacing function of any pacemaker must be accessible by applying a magnet to the pacemaker, which forces the pacemaker to switch to magnet mode (Task Force on Practice Guidelines, 2002). One motivation for this feature is to ensure that a physician can easily check - without any special equipment - whether the pacemaker is still working properly. In magnet mode, a predefined sequence of pacing pulses is applied to the patient's heart. These stimulation patterns depend on the manufacturer and the type of the pacemaker, as well as on the depletion level of the pacemaker's battery (Lampadius, 2010).

Hence, the basic working status and the depletion level of the battery can be determined by the means of a surface ECG recording during magnet application and looking for specific stimulation patterns within the signal. Additionally, possible lead malfunctions with respect to sensing and pacing or arrhythmias can be detected (Schreier et al., 2004; Kollmann et al., 2007a; Kollmann et al., 2005).

For magnet effect based device checks, the following units are necessary (Fig. 5):

- A mobile ECG recording unit, that can e.g. be situated at a general practitioner
- A monitoring centre that receives the data from the mobile ECG recording units. The monitoring centre needs access to a pacemaker database containing the properties of all pacemakers currently available.
- An ECG analysis unit comparing the received ECGs with all possible magnet mode pacing patterns of the implanted device - as stored in the pacemaker database.

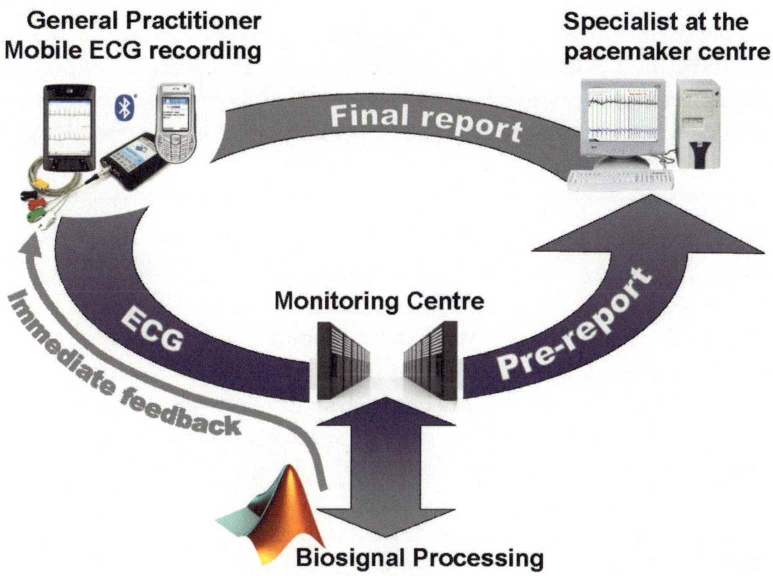

Fig. 5. Magnet effect based device checks consisting of mobile ECG recording units at the general practitioner, a monitoring centre with biosignal processing units and reviewing units for specialists at the pacemaker centre.

Depending on the results of the biosignal analysis, a preliminary report is generated and provided to a physician at the pacemaker centre. The ECG is shown to the physician, including data from the pacemaker database and the result of the ECG analysis (Fig. 6). The physician uses the ECG and all data entered by the general practitioner to review the preliminary report and finalize it. The final report is then returned to the general practitioner. In case of detected malfunctions, battery depletion, uncertainties, or if the patient reports any problems possibly related to the pacemaker, the patient is assigned to the specialized follow-up centre. If no such problems are detected, no additional actions are necessary.

Advantages of this method compared to in-clinic follow-ups and remote device interrogation are:

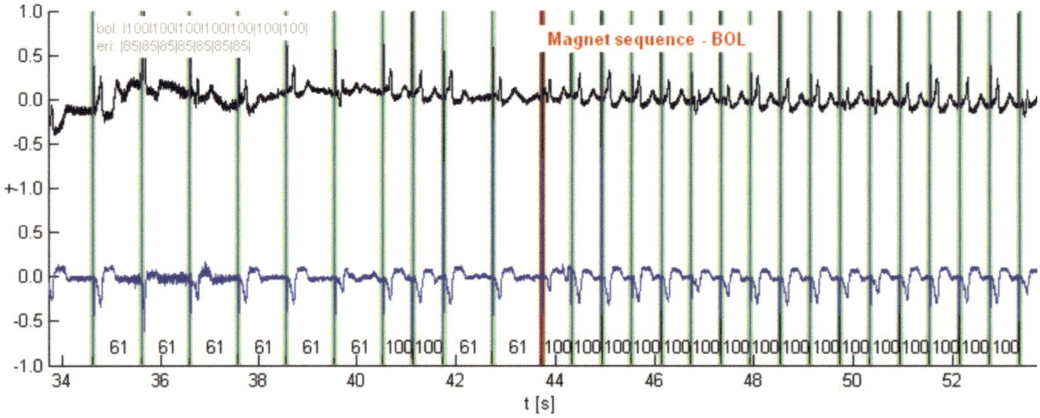

Fig. 6. ECG with magnet pattern (starting at second 44) as presented to the specialist. Possible magnet patterns for the present pacemaker in Begin-Of-Life (BOL) and Elective Replacement Indication (ERI) state are shown (upper left). Pacemaker spikes as detected by the biosignal analysis unit are marked with green lines. The beat-to-beat pacing rate [bpm] is written in between each two spikes. The suggested pacemaker state ('Magnet Sequence - BOL') is shown in red.

- Part of the in-clinic pacemaker follow-ups can be moved from specialized in-clinic follow-up centres to extramural physicians such as cardiologists or general practitioners, who a) do not need various programmers and b) need not to be pacemaker specialists.
- Specialized follow-up centres can be disburdened
- Travel costs and burden for patients can be reduced
- This method can be used for all pacemakers currently available on the market with no need for special transmitters, programmers, adaptations of the pacemaker etc. All that is needed is a magnet, an ECG recorder with an interface to a PC and Web-access.

Drawbacks of this method are:

- Device parameters cannot be adapted (equal to remote device interrogation)
- ICDs and complex device features cannot be assessed

3.4 Data source 4 – Remote monitoring systems

In recent years several systematic reviews indicate that remote monitoring concepts may be a valuable tool to optimize therapy of patients with several diseases such as CHF with respect to mortality, morbidity, quality of life, and costs (Schmidt et al. 2010; Inglis et al. 2010). Remote monitoring is already used in several scientific studies (e.g. Scherr et al. 2009) as well as in routine care (e.g. Kastner et al. 2010), and its importance is likely to increase within the next years. During remote monitoring, patients need to collect relevant data of their therapy, such as medication, blood pressure, body weight, well-being etc. and transmit them to a monitoring centre where they are accessible for the physicians.

An overview over a typical system for telemonitoring of CHF is given in Fig. 7. Measurement devices used during remote monitoring are either real devices like blood pressure meters etc. or "virtual" devices, representing data entry by the patient, such as well-being or medication intake. Mobile phones, PCs, laptops, and special devices are used as aggregators. The telemonitoring service centre provides an electronic patient record.

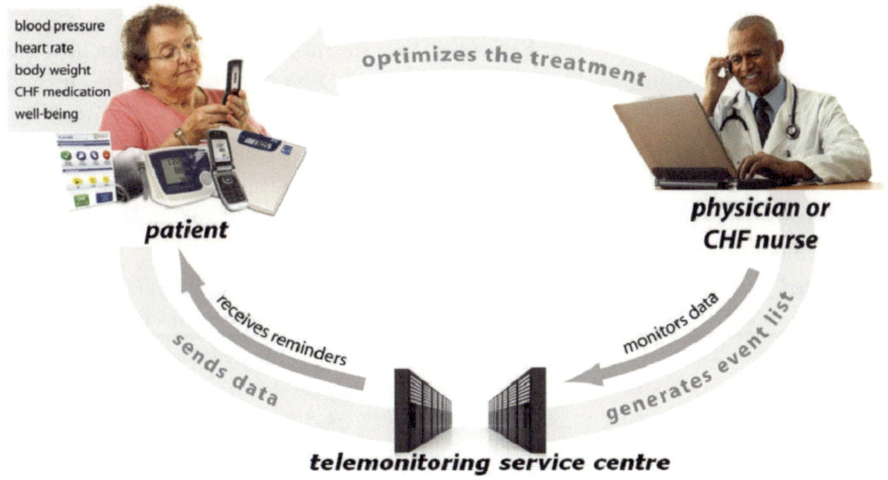

Fig. 7. Typical remote monitoring system as used for the monitoring of congestive heart failure. Several health parameters (e.g. blood pressure, heart rate, body weight, medication and well being) are recorded at the patient's home and sent to a data centre, over which the physician has access to the data (Kastner et al., 2010).

Boston Scientific has already introduced the system "Latitude" (Saxon et al., 2007). It combines telemedical device interrogation with a remote monitoring system for congestive heart failure. The system is expected to improve congestive heart failure therapy and help physicians in getting more of the information necessary for therapy optimization provided by different measurement devices at the patient site. Due to proprietary interfaces at the physician's site, however, no combination with similar systems of other manufacturers is possible - forcing the physicians to deal with several different systems.

4. Standardization aspects

Due to these heterogeneous data sources and since there are various systems data are stored in, standardized interfaces in between all partners concerned in cardiac rhythm disease management are essential. There are several standards that deal with a) information exchange in between heterogeneous information systems and b) structured information archiving. Many aspects need to be considered, such as a consistent nomenclature, data access, data transmission, data formats, where to save which data, safety and security, etc. Several consortia such as the *Continua Health Alliance* (Piniewski et al., 2010) or *Integrating the Healthcare Enterprise* (IHE) (IHE, 2010) aim to improve interoperability by forcing standardization in different health environments.
In the following, selected standards will be presented, which play an important role in cardiac rhythm disease management.

4.1 Standardized nomenclatures

Standardization begins with the vocabulary used for describing the thing one is talking about. For example, "breathing frequency", "breathing rate", "respiratory frequency" or "respiratory rate" may all mean one and the same observation term but are often labelled differently by different manufacturers. The nomenclature concerns all aspects of cardiac rhythm disease management - measurement devices, aggregators, electronic patient records, electronic health records, etc. Examples for common medical nomenclatures are:

- *Logical Observation Identifiers Names and Codes* (LOINC) is a database and universal standard for identifying medical laboratory observations. It is widely used, especially (but not only) for laboratory values. A formal, distinct and unique 6-part numerical name is given to each term for test or observation identity. Currently, over 58,000 observation terms (e.g. blood oxygen saturation, systolic blood pressure, etc.) can be accessed and understood universally.
- *Systematized Nomenclature of Medicine - Clinical Terms* (SNOMED CT) is similar to LOINC but covers a larger area of terms - currently there are more than a million terms available. SNOMED CT is the most comprehensive and complex clinical vocabulary available today. It crossmaps to other terminologies such as LOINC.
- *ISO/IEEE X73* nomenclature was especially developed for remote monitoring.

4.2 Messaging standards

Soon as terms (words) are found that describe medical findings, a standard for how to combine these words (to sentences) is needed. These aspects are covered by messaging standards. Messages are sent in between all partners of cardiac rhythm disease management (from measurement devices to aggregators and back, from aggregators to electronic patient records and back, and from electronic patient records to electronic health records and back).
The most common messaging standard is *Health Level Seven* (HL7).
HL7 v2.x is the most commonly used medical messaging standard worldwide. It has the aim to support hospital workflows by enabling different systems to communicate with each another. HL7 v2.x messages use a textual, non-XML based syntax based on delimiter.
HL7 v3 was introduced in 1995 to upgrade HL7 v2.x. HL7 v3 messages are XML-based.
XML (Extensible Markup Language) is a general open standard for encoding documents in a format which is readable by both machines and humans.

4.3 Communication standards

Of course, communication is more than just expressing a sentence. Communication starts with some kind of indicating that one has something to tell. Next, someone else has to acknowledge she/he is ready to listen. Only then the transmission of information can begin and every now and then the speaker will expect some kind of confirmation that the receiver is still listening. Finally, the speaker will indicate the end of data transmission and the communication is terminated.
Communication standards concern these and similar aspects of communication in between different systems or devices. Since the requirements for communication standards depend on their application, there are different standards for different applications.

- The *ISO/IEEE X73* standard consists of different ISO, IEEE and CEN joint standards addressing the interoperability of medical devices. It defines parts of a system, with which it is possible to exchange and evaluate vital signs data between different medical devices, as well as remote control of devices. E.g., by the use of this standard, data can be sent from a measurement device such as a blood pressure meter to an aggregator such as a mobile phone. Data transfer can be done via different media, such as USB or Bluetooth and either wired or wireless.

- The *IHE Implantable Device Cardiac Observation* (IHE IDCO) profile is used for the communication of programmers with their environment. It defines a standard based translation and transfer of summary device interrogation information from the interrogation system to the information management system. It specifies a mechanism for the creation, transmission, processing, and storage of discrete data elements and report attachments associated with cardiac device interrogations.
- *IHE Patient Care Device Domain* (IHE PCD) was developed for use cases in intensive care units and also concerns remote monitoring workflows. Due to these applications alarm management or patient identity binding are important topics of this standard.
- The *Health Informatics - Electronic Health Record Communication standard EN 13606* is a standard especially designed for accessing, transferring, adding or modifying EHRs.

4.3 Document standards

Medical information is often transferred from one location to another via medical reports, laboratory reports, etc. In the past such reports were usually printed out or sent as PDF files. Since content within PDF files does not have a standardized format, automated analyses of the data within PDF documents is not possible. It is the aim of document standards to structure the data stored within a document in a way that specific content can automatically be found, analyzed, visualized and so on.

Unlike HL7 v2.x, HL7 v3 is not only a messaging standard, but - among others - also contains a standardized format for storing documents: *Clinical Document Architecture* (CDA) is a commonly used document standard that is part of HL7 v3. For each examination a CDA document can be generated within which the information of that examination is stored in a structured way. The CDA document consists of a header containing patient data, author and document type, and a body within which the medical data is stored.

There are three levels of CDA documents:

- Level 1 can easily be implemented. Only the document header needs to be coded as specified in the standard, while the body contains the data as free text. Parsing and automated processing of the data themselves is not possible.
- Level 2 structures the body in sections such as anamnesis, diagnostic findings, laboratory values etc. The different sections can be defined using a coding system, such as LOINC, SNOMED CT or IEEE/ISO X73.
- Level 3 is used for storing each single parameter in a standardized way and therefore enables automated algorithms to parse the whole document and further analyze the data stored in the document. That way, e.g. the evolution of parameters over time can be visualized etc.

4.4 EHR standards

Apart from interfaces to various aggregators and due to the involvement of several healthcare actors, a platform for integrated cardiac rhythm disease management may have the need to be connected to storage systems with a wider scope in terms of health data management aspects like an electronic health records (EHR). It is the aim of EHRs to systematically collect health information about individual patients or populations over a longer period of time - so as to facilitate continuity of care. The data can be stored centrally within the record itself, or they can only be referenced in a registry while the data themselves are stored elsewhere - e.g. in distributed electronic patient records. Therefore, specification of an EHR not only considers the way data are stored, but also which data are stored within which record. Additionally, privacy and security concerns as well as authorization and encryption issues are an important part of each EHR as well.

Two common EHR concepts are described in the following:

- *IHE Cross-Enterprise Document Sharing* (IHE XDS) (IHE, 2010) is an integration profile which facilitates the registration, distribution and access across health enterprises of electronic patient records. It focuses on standardized sharing of documents in between healthcare enterprises, ranging from a private physician office to clinic to an acute care patient facility and personal health record system. This is managed through federated document repositories and a document registry to create a longitudinal record for information about a patient within a given clinical affinity domain. Among others, IHE XDS makes use of HL7 CDA documents which has the advantage, that all medical documents can easily be shared and read among different systems. Anyway, due to CDA's rather undefined data structure, information may be hidden within the vast amount of documents belonging to each patient.
- *openEHR* (Heard & Beale 2010) is an open standard that describes management and storage, retrieval and exchange of health data in an EHR. EN 13606 is used for exchanging data in between different openEHR-compliant EHRs. While IHE XDS stores data as CDA documents, openEHR is based on so called *archetypes*, computable expressions of a domain content model in the form of structured constraint statements, based on the openEHR reference model. That way, data can easier be accessed, processed, visualized etc. Anyway, implementation of such a system and - probably more important - adaptation of existing systems to the openEHR standard are more complex than for the IHE XDS standard.

4.5 Standards – Overview

Fig. 8. summarizes standards mentioned in this chapter and the environments they concern.

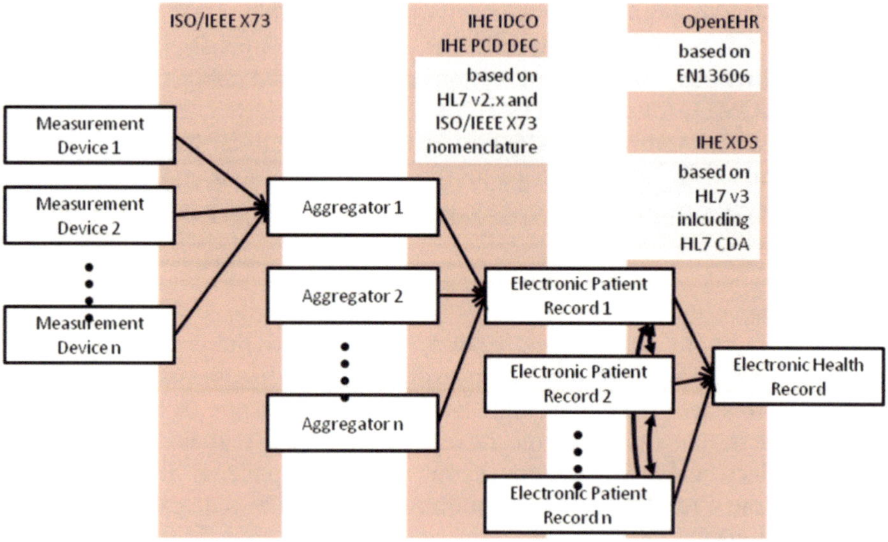

Fig. 8. Standards in cardiac rhythm disease management and environment they concern.

5. Platform for Integrated Cardiac Rhythm Disease Management (PICARD)

There are many different data sources from many different manufacturers available on the market, transmitting data to many different data storage systems like HIS or EHRs from which all data should be accessible by authorized caregivers. Additionally, there are many different standards involved, each of them developed for different sub-aspects of cardiac rhythm disease management, partly complementing, partly contradicting one another. And there are devices and systems that support the standards mentioned while others don't.

Within this complex environment, we have developed a web-based platform for integrated cardiac rhythm disease management (PICARD). Throughout the last years we have implemented several interfaces to different devices and systems involved in cardiac rhythm disease management. Some of these interfaces were standard conform, others were not. Some of the solutions were implemented prototypically, others were used in clinical studies, and some were used in routine care already.

In the following, the current state of implementation is described in details.

5.1 PICARD – Architecture

A three-tier client-server architecture was designed (Fig. 9), which consisted of a web/application server, application specific services, data management and data storage components, a database adapter, an FTP server, an SMS gateway, data security components, and various clients.

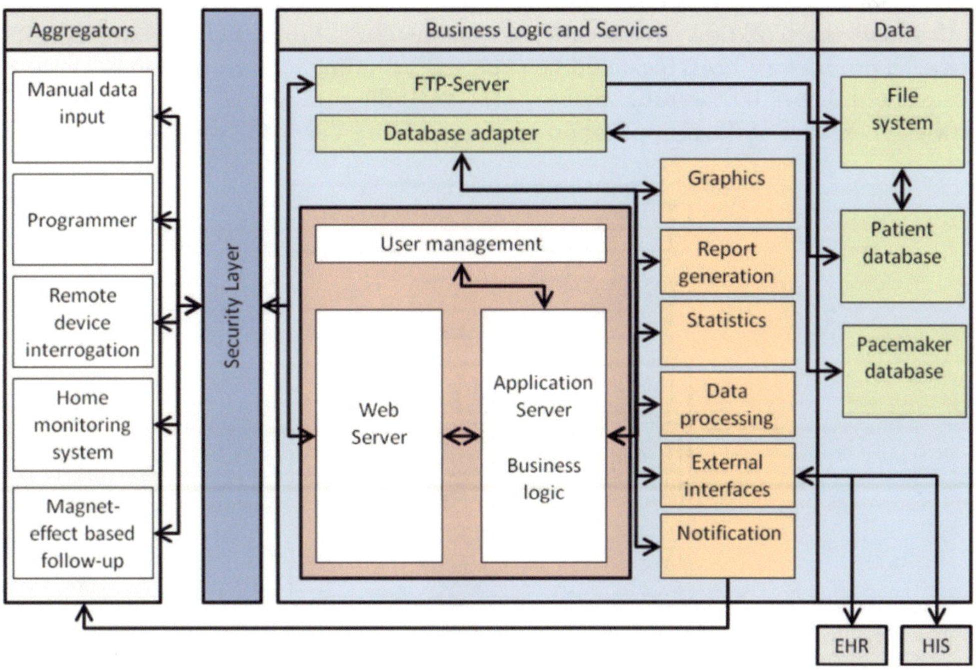

Fig. 9. Three-tier client-server architecture comprising web/application server (red box), special services (orange boxes), interfaces to electronic health records (EHR) and hospital information systems (HIS), data management and data storage components, database adapter, FTP server, security layer and communication capabilities to various aggregators.

5.2 Web interface

Via a Web-interface physicians were able to

a. inspect data of their patients and

b. enter data relevant for the patient's rhythm disease management.

Therefore, the physician had to login to the Web-server using username and password. Personal data about the patient, about his/her anamnesis, diagnosis, and medication etc. could be entered, as well as data read out from the patient's implanted device via a programmer. Several services were used for supporting the physician in inspecting the data as well as optimizing and documenting the therapy, such as graphical representations, report generation, statistics, data processing (e.g. ECG analysis) or notification services.

5.3 Programmer integration

The physician had the possibility to manually enter data read out from an implanted device by a programmer. Since programmers usually interrogate a large amount of data from the implanted device, the physician either had to spend lots of time on entering all these data via the web-interface, or she/he decided only to enter selected data. We found that usually a few parameters were entered via the Web-interface and additionally, reports from the programmers were printed out and stored in a paper based patient record.

In order to simplify the process of entering data read out by the programmer into PICARD, a standardized interface to a pacemaker programming device (Biotronik ICS 3000 DS, Biotronik SE & Co. KG, Berlin, Germany) was implemented, which allowed for automated integration of the data read out by the programmer into PICARD.

Fig. 10 shows the workflow of the programmer interface. From the programmer's RS232 interface, a proprietary XML file could be exported including all information read out from the implanted device by the programmer. This XML file was sent to the client-PC's RS232 interface. Thereafter, a Java application running on the client-PC received the data and

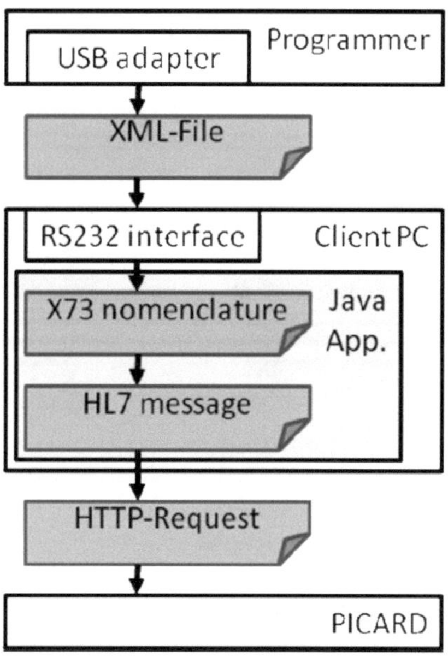

Fig. 10. Programmer integration as realized prototypically for the Biotronik programmer.

processed it. The proprietary data structure of the programmer's XML file was mapped to a standardized data format according to the *ISO/IEEE* X73 nomenclature. A mapping table was generated that translated each parameter of the programmer to a standardized *ISO/IEEE* X73 parameter. In the next step, the standardized data were included into an HL7 v2.5 message and sent to PICARD via HTTP.

The interface was prototypically implemented and its functionality was tested in the course of an interoperability showcase at the eHealth2008 conference (Sabutsch et al., 2008).

5.4 Upload of data form magnet effect based remote device checks

In the course of a clinical study (Kollmann et al., 2007a) PICARD was used for managing data achieved during magnet effect based remote device checks as described in chapter 3.3. It could be shown that integration of magnet effect based device checks to PICARD is feasible and that the proposed follow-up concept has the potential to work as an efficient screening method. It may also spare a significant number of patients the burden of having to travel to specialized follow-up centres.

5.5 Interface to remote device interrogation systems

Up to now, no electronic interface to remote device interrogation systems has been implemented. Parameters transmittable by the system of one manufacturer have been included to PICARD's database and to the Web-interface. However, only manual input of the data was possible so far.

5.6 Upload of data from remote monitoring systems

PICARD was designed so as to be able to receive data from remote monitoring systems and was already used in several studies concerning heart failure (Scherr et al., 2009), psoriasis (Hayn et al., 2009), diabetes (Kollmann et al., 2007c), and adipositas (Morak et al., 2008). Currently it is also used in a routine remote monitoring scenario (Kastner et al., 2010).

5.7 Interface to hospital information systems (HISs)

Interfaces to HISs are necessary for two basic purposes:

- To read out selected patient data from the HIS
- To write back selected data (reports) to the HIS

So far, we implemented an interface to a single HIS. Since this HIS was not completely standard based, the following proprietary workflow was used (Fig. 11).

In the course of patient registration, patient's demographic data and unique PID were requested from the HIS. For this purpose, a unique case ID generated by the HIS was entered to PICARD and sent to the HIS using an HL7 v2.3 Admission Discharge and Transfer (ADT) query (1). The communication server mapped the case ID to the corresponding patient ID (2), which was returned to PICARD in addition to patient demographic data (3). Via several sources (e.g. Web-portal, ECG upload, etc.) data from different aggregators were uploaded to PICARD (4). Consequently, data were reviewed (5) and a PDF report was generated (6). Besides the PDF file, a description file was generated that contained metadata including the patient ID. The FTP server fetched both files (7) and stored the report to the file archive of the HIS (8). The description file provided information for the registration of the document in the HIS database.

According to the proposed concept, the PDF report summarised the most important findings of a particular follow-up session, whereas source data remained in PICARD. The layout of the report and its content was designed in cooperation with our clinical partners and was structured as following:

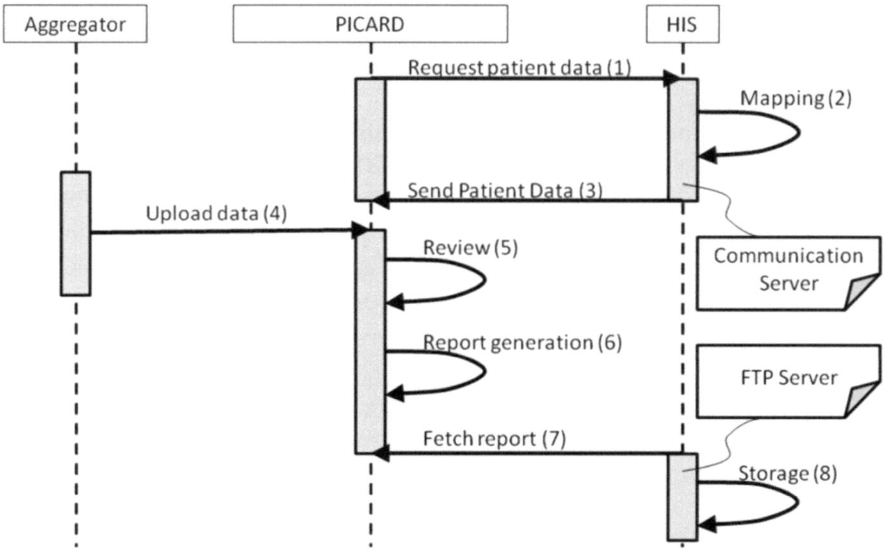

Fig. 11. Information exchange between aggregator (e.g. programmer), PICARD, and Hospital Information System (HIS).

- *1st Page:* A header provided information about the document itself, information about the patient, and information about the responsible physician and the responsible institution. Additionally, important data and crucial clinical observations were summarised on the first page including information about the implanted device, its functional status, and therapy regimen. In general, the first page contained observation data that was applicable for the primary care physician.
- *2nd Page:* Additional observation data (e.g. specific interrogation data, device settings, etc.) were summarised on the second page. This information was important for documentation and advanced therapy management. Data summarised on the second page was targeted primarily to the cardiologist.
- *3rd Page (optional):* Here, a list of current medication was provided.

5.8 Integration of PICARD into an IHE XDS conform EHR

In Austria, a national EHR is currently developed. It will be based on the IHE profile XDS and the content itself is stored as HL7 CDA documents (ARGE ELGA, 2009).

Fig. 12 shows the concept of Austria's IHR XDS based EHR. The patient index provides a unique identifier for each patient. Several case IDs can exist, and each case ID refers to several document IDs for a given patient. These IDs together with a small set of meta-data are stored within the national EHR document registry. The data itself (CDA documents) are stored in decentralized document repositories within electronic patient records. Only data that are registered in the central document registry can be found in the national EHR, while all other data are visible to the decentralized electronic patient records only.

Integration of PICARD into an IHE XDS conform EHR required a) patient cross identification and b) document registration. While only a basic version of patient cross identification has been implemented so far, document registration was implemented comprehensively. Since Austria's future EHR will use HL7 CDA documents, an HL7 CDA document was generated whenever an examination was registered within PICARD.

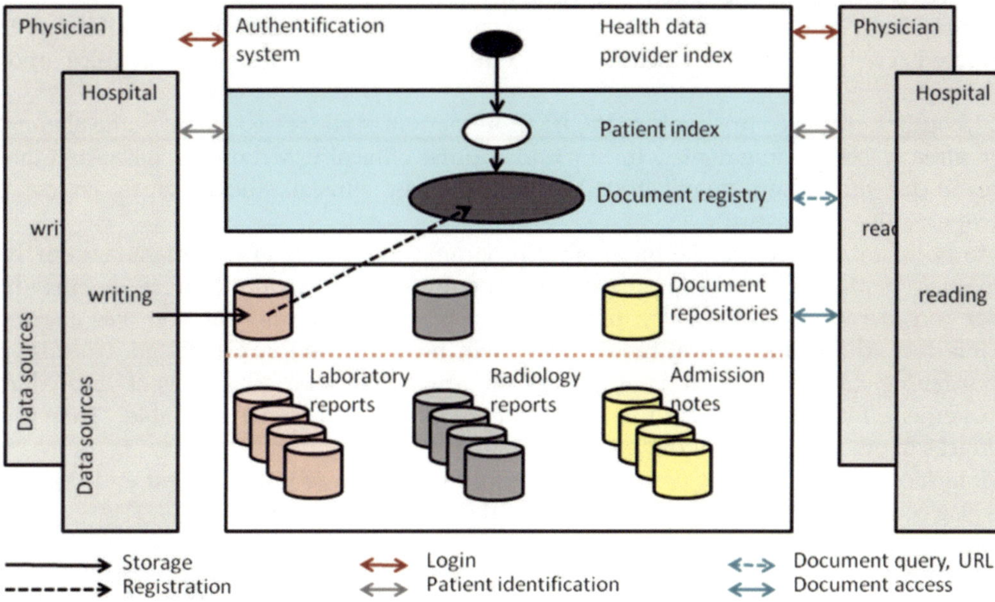

Fig. 12. Concept of the Austria's future IHR XDS based EHR (based on ARGE ELGA, 2007). The upper most two boxes build up Austria's EHR. The lower box represents electronic patient records that can be adapted to the EHR. The red dotted line represents the border in between data that can be seen from out of the EHR and data that are only visible within each single electronic patient record.

CDA level 2 was used for most of the data, and additionally, selected parameters were included in CDA level 3. Within PICARD's document repository, all the CDA reports were stored and meta-information about these reports was registered to the EHR's document registry.

Integration of PICARD into an IHE conform EHR infrastructure such as Austria's future national electronic health record has been demonstrated in a virtual environment (Kollmann et al. 2007b).

6. Discussion

Cardiac rhythm disease management represents a complex medical domain with many requirements concerning information management. A variety of systems must be handled by the cardiologist and telemedical aspects are rapidly gaining importance.

Healthcare manufacturers in this domain have focused on the devices, since, up to now, those were the most complex elements in the whole ecosystem. With constantly evolving new devices and systems for diagnosing, treating and monitoring of cardiac rhythm disorders new concepts for more integrated approaches are desperately in need. Information and communication technologies are important enablers of telemedicine-based new ways to re-organise the care of cardiac patients and to move from a predominately device-centred follow-up concept to a patient centred system (Boriani 2008).

6.1 PICARD – State of implementation and outlook

Resulting from the analysis of the involved sub-domains we presented a platform for integrated cardiac rhythm disease management (PICARD) designed to fulfil those requirement.

Fig. 13 outlines those components of PICARD our activities addressed so far. Some elements have already been implemented to work in routine clinical environment whereas others have so far only been demonstrated in the lab, in clinical studies or in course of interoperability showcases:

Up to now, an interface to the pacemaker programming device of one manufacturer has been implemented. Interfaces to programming devices of other manufacturers are currently under consideration. Additionally, magnet effect based device interrogation was enabled. An interface to one telemedical follow-up system has also been implemented. In order to disburdening cardiologists, it is necessary to implement one single event and alarm management for all telemedical and remote monitoring systems available. Therefore, interfaces to other home-monitoring systems will be needed.

An interface to the electronic patient record of a local HIS was implemented and PICARD was also connected to an IHE XDS conform EHR.

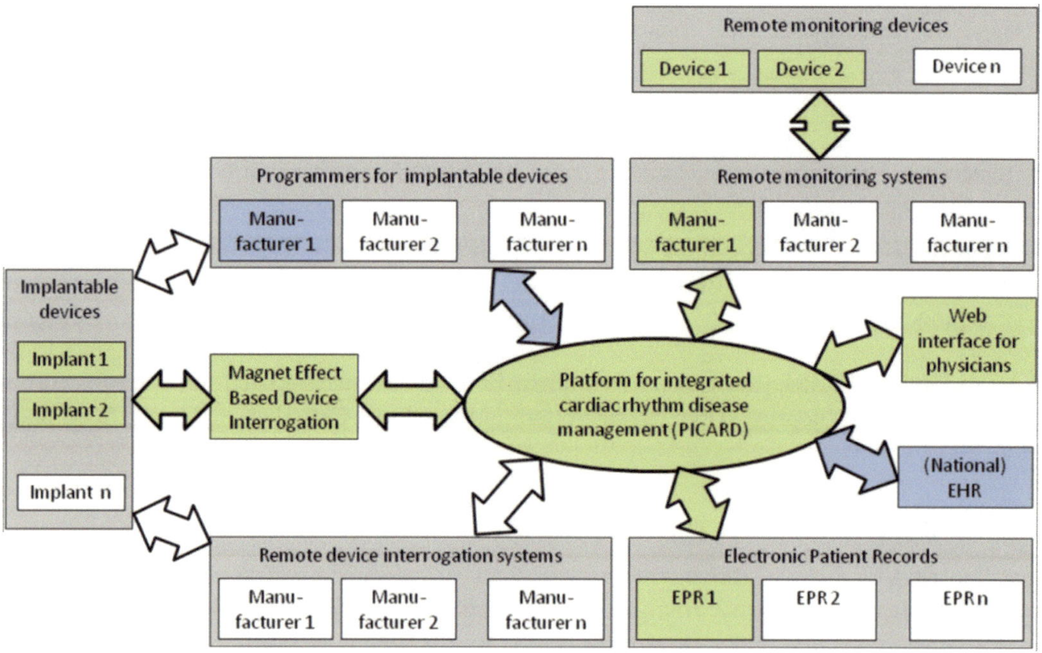

Fig. 13. Information ecosystem of PICARD. Interfaces, that have already been implemented, are plotted in green. Interfaces that have been implemented in a prototypical way are plotted blue.

The solutions developed so far have been implemented and operated in different scenarios. For most of these scenarios a separate clone of PICARD was developed. Though the same core components were used in all these clones, none of the implementations combined all modules described in chapter 5. Rather, most specialized modules were used in one single cone of PICARD only. Therefore, implementation of a clone that contains all modules is still outstanding.

6.2 State of standardization

In the future it is likely that all (or at least most) interfaces in between the various partners of the data chain will be standardized.

The most promising standard for connecting measurement devices to aggregators is currently specified by the Continua Health Alliance. Standardized communication from programmers to electronic patient records is defined in the IHE IDCO standard. And standardized communication from remote monitoring systems to electronic patient records can be implemented using the IHE PCD profile (Kumpusch, 2009). Upcoming standards for communication in between different EHRs and electronic patient record are openEHR and IHE XDS.

However, up to now only very view devices and systems fully support these upcoming standards. Therefore, proprietary interfaces are needed in the meantime.

6.3 Outlook

As Niederlag stated in (Niederlag, 2010), cardiac rhythm disease management is a fast moving topic. 1958 the first pacemaker was implanted and initially each patient received one and the same type of device. The next step was selection of the most suitable pacemaker for a patient out of four different groups. Thereafter, programmable pacemakers were developed and the same type of pacemaker could be implanted for each patient, while after implantation the device was programmed for optimally fit to the patient. The next step was rate adaptive pacemakers, where the pacemaker itself was able to adapt to the patients momentary needs. Remote monitoring of pacemakers followed, enabling the physician to check pacemaker status, no matter where she/he is or where the patient is. Since 2005, pacemakers can individually and automatically adapt their parameters to the patient's current state.

While even modern devices currently only react on changes affecting themselves or their "direct contact" to the patient, in future it is likely that implanted devices will also consider other information - received from external sources. By that way, the devices will become more and more integrated into the whole rhythm disease management process.

Therefore, a future system for cardiac rhythm disease management needs to be able to handle data from various sources (from implanted devices, from patient's home, from general practitioners, from hospitals, etc.) and from different manufacturers - all of them communicating with one another.

7. Conclusion

Since cardiology in general and cardiac rhythm disease management in particular is still a field with a strong innovation process, new methods and devices are entering the scene all the time. Doing things in a different and better way is part of this innovation process and standardisation will always be one step behind. As far as basic and routine procedures and follow-ups are concerned, however, for the sake of safety and efficiency, neither the patient nor the physician should be forced to deal with multiple systems and multiple interfaces that are not related to one another. Information and communication technologies can help to bridge the gap between both standardisation and innovation and will increasingly become a key technology for cardiac rhythm disease management.

8. References

American Society of Anesthesiologists Task Force on Perioperative Management of Patients with Cardiac Rhythm Management Devices (2005). Practice advisory for the perioperative management of patients with cardiac rhythm management devices: pacemakers and implantable cardioverter-defibrillators. *Anesthesiology* 103:186:198

Anand, I.S., Carson, P., Galle, E., Song, R., Boehmer, J., Ghali, J.K., Jaski, B., Lindenfeld, J., O'Connor, C., Steinberg, J.S., Leigh, J., Yong, P., Kosorok, M.R., Feldman, A.M., DeMets, D. & Bristow, M.R. (2009). Cardiac Resynchronization Therapy Reduces the Risk of Hospitalizations in Patients With Advanced Heart Failure. Results From the Comparison of Medical Therapy, Pacing and Defibrillation in Heart Failure (COMPANION) Trial. *Circulation*. 119 :969-977, 1524-4539

ARGE ELGA - Arbeitsgemeinschaft elektronische Gesundheitsakte (2009). ELGA Kernanwendungen - CDA Dokumente für das österreichische Gesundheitswesen - Implementierungsleitfaden. Available from : http://www.arge-elga.at/fileadmin/user_upload/uploads/download_Papers/Harmonisierungsarbeit/Leitfaden/Leitfaden_ELGA_CDA_Dokumente_1.00.pdf. Last Accessed July 2010.

ARGE ELGA - Arbeitsgemeinschaft elektronische Gesundheitsakte (2007). Die elektronische Gesundheitsakte - Ausblick auf die erste Umsetzungsphase. Available from http://www.arge-elga.at/fileadmin/user_upload/uploads/download_Papers/Arge_Papers/ELGA_Umsetzung_Phase1__V2.0.pdf. Last accessed July 2010.

Boersma, L., Mont, L., Soinis, A., García, E. & Brugada, J. (2003). Value of the implantable loop recorder for the management of patients with unexplained syncope. Europace 6(1):70-6, 1099-5129

Boriani, G., Diemberger, I., Martignani, C., Biffi, M., Valzania, C., Bertini, M., Domenichini, G., Saporito, D., Ziacchi, M. & Branzi, A. (2008). Telecardiology and remote monitoring of implanted electrical devices: the potential for fresh clinical care perspectives. *J Gen Intern Med*. 2008 Jan;23 Suppl 1:73-7.

Burri, H. & Senouf, D. (2009). Remote monitoring and follow-up of pacemakers and implantable cardioverter defibrillators. *Europace*. 11(6) :701-9, 1099-5129

Calisto J, Faria H, Pego G, Angelo FA, Rufino E, Raposo A, Paisana, F., Goncalves, T., Lucete, M. & Providencia, L.A. (1993). A follow-up by telephone of patients wearing a pacemaker-the experience of the Cardiac Pacing Center of the Hospitais de Universidade de Coimbra. *Rev Port Cardiol*. 12(6):551–5, 510. 0870-2551

Dreifus, L., Zinberg, A., Hurzeler, P., Puziak, A., Pennock, R., Feldman, M. & Morse, D.P. (1986). Transtelephonic monitoring of 25,919 implanted pacemakers. *Pacing Clin Electrophysiol*. 9(3):371–8. 0147-8389

European Society of Cardiology; European Heart Rhythm Association. (2007). Guidelines for cardiac pacing and cardiac resynchronization therapy: the task force for cardiac pacing and cardiac resynchronization therapy of the European Society of Cardiology. Developed in collaboration with the European Heart Rhythm Association. *Eur Heart J*. Sep;28(18):2256–95. 0195-668X

Hayn, D., Koller, S., Wellenhof, R.H.; Salmhofer, W.; Kastner, P. & Schreier, G. (2009), Mobile Phone-Based Teledermatologic Compliance Management - Preliminary Results of the TELECOMP Study, *Stud Health Technol Inform* 150, 468--472. 0926-9630

Heard, S. & Beale, T. (eds.) (2007). openEHR Architecture Overview. Available from http://www.openehr.org/svn/specification/BRANCHES/Release-1.0.2-candidate/publishing/architecture/overview.pdf. Last accessed Augutst 2010.

IHE - Integrating the Healthcare Enterprise (2010). Available from : http://www.ihe.net. Last Accessed: July 2010.

Inglis, S.C., Clark, R.A., McAlister, F.A., Ball, J., Lewinter, C., Cullington, D., Stewart, S., Cleland, J.G.F. 2010. Structured telephone support or telemonitoring programmes for patients with chronic heart failure (Review). *The Cochrane Library 2010, Issue 8.*

Kainz W.(1999). Richtlinien zur Nachsorge antibradykarder Schrittmachersystem. *J Kardiol Suppl.* 15–18.

Kastner, P., Morak, J., Kollmann, A., Ebner, C., Fruhwald, F.M. & Schreier, G. (2010), Innovative telemonitoring systems for cardiology: from science to routine operation, *Applied Clinical Informatics* 1(2), 165-176. 1869-0327

Kollmann, A., Hayn, D., Garcia, J., Rotman, B., Kastner, P. & Schreier, G. (2005). Telemedicine framework for manufacturer independent remote pacemaker follow-up. *Comput Cardiol.* 49–52. 0276-6574

Kollmann, A., Hayn, D., García, J., Trigo, J.D., Kastner,P., Rotman, B., Tscheliessnigg, K. & Schreier, G.. (2007a). Feasibility of a telemedicine framework for collaborative pacemaker follow-up. *J Telemed Telecare,* 13(7) 341-347. 1357-633X

Kollmann, A., Hayn, D., Rotman, B., Tscheliessnigg, K. & Schreier, G. (2007b). H.ELGA - Herzschrittmacher . Elektronische Gesundheitsakte - Erste Ergebnisse aus der Steiermark. *Tagungsband der eHealth2007: Medical Informatics meets eHealth,* pp. 93-96, 978-3-85403-227-4, Wien, Austria, Jun 2007, OCG, Vienna

Kollmann, A.; Ried, M.; Kastner, P.; Schreier, G. & Ludvik, B. (2007c), Feasibility of a mobile phone based data service for functional insulin treatment of type 1 diabetes mellitus patients, *J Med Internet Res,* 9(5), 36. 1438-8871

Kumpusch, H., Kollmann, A., Sabutsch, S. & Schreier, G. (2009). Evaluierung des IHE PCD Technical Frameworks für mobiltelefonbasiertes Telemonitoring. *Tagungsband der eHealth2009 & eHealth Benchmarking 2009 – Health Informatics meets eHealth.* pp 61-67, 978-3-85403-250-2, Wien, Austria, Mai 2009, OCG.

Lampadius, M.S. (2010). Typenkartei Herzschrittmacher - Defibrillator - CRT. FGS-Forschungsgesellschaft Elektrostimulation mbH. Available from http://www.fgs-mbh.de/leistungen/typenkartei/index.html. Last accessed July 2010.

Morak, J., Schindler, K., Goerzer, E., Kastner, P., Toplak, H., Ludvik, B., Schreier, G. (2008). A pilot study of mobile phone-based therapy for obese patients. *J Telemed Telecare.* 14(3):147-9.

Niederlag, W. (2001). Communication technologies for improvement of pacemaker therapy. *Prog Biomed Res.* 6:6–12.

Niederlag, W. (2010) Personalisierte Medizin. *E-HEALTH-COM.* Available from http://www.e-health-com.eu/details-news/personalisierte-medizin/. Last Accessed July 2010.

Nielsen, J. C., Kottkamp, H., Zabel, M., Aliot, E., Kreutzer, U., Bauer, A., Schuchtert, A., Neuser, H., Schumacher, B., Schmidinger, H., Stix, G., Clementy, J. & Danilovic, D. (2008). Automatic home monitoring of implantable cardioverter. *Europace.* 10(6) :729-35, 1099-5129

Pfeiffer, K. P. (2009). Future development of medical informatics from the viewpoint of health telematics. Methods Inf Med. 48(1):55-61.

Piniewski, B., Muskens, J., Estevez, L., Carroll, R. & Cnossen, R. (2010). Empowering healthcare patients with smart technology. *Computer.* 43/7 :27-45. 0018-9162

Platt, S., Furman, S., Gross, J., Andrews, C. & Benedek, M. (1996). Transtelephone monitoring for pacemaker follow-up 1981–1994. *Pacing Clin Electrophysiol.* 19(12 Pt 1):2089–98, 0147-8389.

Raatikainen, M. P., Uusimaa, P., van Ginneken, M. M. E., Janssen, J. P. G., & Linnaluoto, M. (2008). Remote monitoring of implantable cardioverter defibrillator patients: a safe, time-saving, and cost-effective means for follow. *Europace.* 10(10) :1145-51, 1099-5129

Sabutsch, S., Csuk, D., Kumpusch, H., Oberbacher, A., Storer, A., Kollmann, A. & Schreier, G. (2008). Interoperability-Framework zur automatisierten Integration von Herzschrittmacher-Daten in die H.ELGA (Herzschrittmacher . Elektronische Gesundheitsakte). *Tagungsband der eHealth2008 – Medical Inforamtics meets eHealth,* pp. 191-194, 978-3-85403-235-9, Vösendorf bei Wien, Austria, OCG, Vienna

Saxon L.A., Boehmer J.P., Neuman S. & Mullin C.M. (2007). Remote Active Monitoring in Patients with Heart Failure (RAPID-RF): design and rationale. *J Card Fail.* 13,4 (May 2007):241-6. 1071-9164

Scherr, D., Kastner, P., Kollmann, A., Hallas, A., Auer, J., Krappinger, H., Schuchlenz, H., Stark, G., Grander, W., Jakl, G., Schreier, G., Fruhwald, F.M. & the MOBITEL investigators (2009). Effect of Home-Based Telemonitoring Using Mobile Phone Technology on the Outcome of Heart Failure Patients After an Episode of Acute Decompensation: Randomized Controlled Trial, *J Med Internet Res.* 11(3):e34, 1438-8871

Schmidt, S., Schuchert, A., Krieg, T., Oeff, M. (2010). Home telemonitoring in patients with chronic heart failure: a chance to improve patient care? *Dtsch Arztebl Int.*(Feb 2010) :107(8):131-8.

Schreier, G., Hay, D., Kollmann, A., Scherr, D., Lercher, P., Rotman, B., Klein, W. (2004) Automated and manufacturer independent assessment of the battery status of implanted cardiac pacemakers by electrocardiogram analysis. *Conf Proc IEEE Eng Med Biol Soc.* 2004;1:76-9.

Sutton, R. (1996). Guidelines for pacemaker follow-up: report of a British pacing & electrophysiology group (BPEG) policy conference on pacemaker follow-up. *Br Heart J.* 1–11. 0007-0769

Task Force on Practice Guidelines American College of Cardiology/American Heart Association/North American Society for Pacing, American College & Committee, Electrophysiology (2002). ACC/AHA/NASPE 2002 guideline update for implantation of cardiac pacemakers and antiarrhythmia devices: summary article. A report of the American College of Cardiology/American Heart Association Task Force on Practice Guidelines (ACC/AHA/NASPE Committee to Update the 1998 Pacemaker Guidelines). *J Cardiovasc Electrophysiol.* 13(11):1183–99. 1045-3873

2

Different Automatic Mode Switching in DDDR Pacemakers

Maurizio Santomauro MD[1], Carlo Duilio MD[1], Carla Riganti MD[1], Paolo Di Mauro MD[1], Gennaro Iapicca MD[1], Luca Auricchio Eng[2], Alessio Borrelli MD[3] and Pasquale Perrone Filardi MD[1]
[1]Department of Medicine, Cardiology and Immunology. Federico II School of Medicine University of Naples, Naples
[2]Boston Scientific, CRM Department, Milan,
[3]Department of Cardiology, Humanitas Hospital, Bergamo, Italy

1. Introduction

Mode-switching algorithms are designed to alleviate symptoms related to tracking of atrial arrhythmias, that may result in inappropriately rapid or irregular ventricular pacing[1-19]. The ideal mode-switching algorithm should discriminate sinus tachycardia, a rhythm that should be tracked, from pathological atrial arrhythmias,
rhythms that generally should not be tracked. In order to minimize symptoms related to the occurrence of atrial arrhythmias, the mode-switching algorithm should change quickly from a tracking to a non-tracking mode at the onset of the pathological atrial rhythm and remains in this mode until the arrhythmia terminates. Once sinus rhythm has been restored, the pacemaker should revert quickly to the normal atrial tracking mode.
There are several potential causes of symptoms that relate to mode switching. First, an irregular paced ventricular intervals at the onset of an atrial arrhythmia before conversion to a non-tracking mode. Second, failure of the device to convert to a
non-tracking mode because of intermittent undersensing of the atrial electrocardiogram may result in continued irregular or rapid ventricular pacing [20]. Third, inappropriate reversion to a tracking mode despite persistence of an atrial arrhythmia may also be caused by intermittent undersensing of the atrial electrocardiogram. Fourth, an overly sensitive mode-switching algorithm may result in loss of atrio-ventricular (AV) synchrony in sinus rhythm [2,11,17,19]. Finally, intrinsic AV conduction of an atrial arrhythmia may produce symptoms that are unrelated to the pacemaker [21]. Although all manufacturers of dual chamber pacemakers offer devices that provide mechanisms for managing the occurrence of atrial arrhythmias, the mode-switching algorithms that are available differ significantly in their sensitivity, specificity, and speed of mode conversion at the onset and termination of atrial arrhythmias. There are potential compromises between sensitivity and specificity with these algorithms, the balance of which may determine the frequency of arrhythmia-related symptoms. Atrial-based pacing is associated with a risk of developing atrial fibrillation lower than ventricular-based pacing for patients with sinus node dysfunction [22-25].

Although AAI(R) pacing provides AV synchrony without tracking of atrial arrhythmias, this mode is not appropriate for patients with impaired AV conduction. For individuals in whom AV conduction is unreliable, atrial-based pacing requires a dual chamber pacemaker to be implanted. Although the physiological benefits of atrio-ventricular synchrony are well documented in these patients, tracking of atrial tachy-arrhythmias can lead to rapid ventricular pacing and the occurrence of palpitation, dyspnea, chest pain, or lightheadedness. Although reprogramming to a non-tracking mode (such as DVI, DDI or DDIR) prevents this clinical event, these modes do not provide appropriate AV synchrony if the sinus rate exceeds the programmed lower rate. (26-37) Limitation of the upper tracking rate only partly addresses this problem and may compromise exercise capacity or lead to symptoms from pacemaker Wenckebach behaviour at relatively slow rates. In response to this clinical dilemma, a variety of mode-switching algorithms has been devised that are meant to prevent tracking of pathological atrial tachy-arrhythmias while allowing ventricular pacing that is synchronous with the atrial electrocardiogram during sinus rhythm [17-19]. These algorithms differ in the criteria that must be satisfied at the onset of a tachy-arrhythmia to trigger a change from a tracking to a non-tracking mode as well as the conditions for return to a normal tracking operation upon arrhythmia termination. As a result, each algorithm provides its own balance in terms of sensitivity and specificity for the accurate detection of atrial arrhythmias. If the criteria that must be satisfied to initiate mode switching are too strict, inappropriate tracking of atrial arrhythmias may occur. In contrast, if the criteria are too sensitive, mode switching may occur in response to single atrial extrasystoles, myopotentials, or far-field signals (26).

The hemodynamic and clinical usefulness of automatic mode switching (AMS) to control the ventricular pacing rate of dual chamber pacemakers was reviewed previously (38-63). The clinical behavior and programmability of the various types of AMS algorithms are reviewed in this part of the manuscript. Current AMS algorithms can be classified according to the way atrial tachy-arrhythmias are detected:

1. "Rate cut-off" criterion: the sensed atrial (As) rate exceeds a programmable value;
2. "Running average rate" criterion: the atrial rate exceeds a mean atrial rate calculated by the pacemaker from the duration of the preceding atrial rate;
3. "Sensor-determined" physiological rate to distinguish sinus rhythm from atrial tachy-arrhythmia;
4. Complex algorithms that combine one or more of the above criteria, with or without additional methods such as examining the atrio-ventricular (AV) relationship.

2. Types of AMS

This discussion focuses mainly on atrial tachy-arrhythmia detection by algorithms developed by several major pacemaker companies to illustrate their complexity and evaluation. Different device behaviors in switching mode are shown in Table I while different algorithm mode termination are shown in Table II.

2.1 Boston scientific / guidant - Atrial Tachy Response (ATR)

The Boston Scientific devices offer two methods of handling atrial tachyarrhythmia, a true automatic mode switch (ATR) that switches mode when consecutive atrial cycles fall below a programmable cutoff and a fast-switch algorithm (AFR) that responded rapidly to the onset of atrial tachyarrhythmia for example in case of atrial flutter.

The ATR function in the Altrua (Boston Scientific Natick, MA, USA) and Insignia pacemakers (Guidant Inc., St. Paul, MN, USA) uses a rate cutoff and counter-based algorithm. Atrial events above the atrial tachyarrhythmia detection rate start the algorithm.
When the entry count (programmable number of cycles above the trigger rate) has been satisfied (+1 beat for beats above the trigger rate, and -1 beat for beats below the trigger rate until the entry count is met), Duration (programmable number of ventricular beats at MTR) will begin.
During Duration the device counts atrial intervals (for the atrial trigger rate) and V-V cycles (for number of Duration beats). If counter is still above zero at the end of Duration, device will go in fallback mode (DDI(R) or VDI(R)) and mode switch.
After fallback rate decrease to LRL or sensor indicated rate for the fallback time (programmable) until end of the ATR episode that occurs when atrial exit count (programmable number of cycles below the trigger rate) goes zero.
The AFR algorithm is designed to prevent pacing in to the atrial vulnerable period and provide immediate dissociation to the atrium and ventricle for atrial rates higher than the AFR trigger rate. When an atrial event is detected inside the PVARP a programmable interval will be set and atrial events inside the AFR interval will be classified as refractory sensed and will not be tracked.
If ATR is programmed ON with AFR, an ATR episode may also be initiated if the atrial tachy is fast and sustained enough to fulfill the ART criteria.
Normal dual-chamber operation resumes immediately when both the PVARP and AFR windows have expired without P-waves being sensed within them.

2.2 Medtronic - Auto Mode Switching algorithm

Mode Switch has a programmable Detect Rate that specifies when to switch modes and a Detect Duration setting to screen out short tachycardia episodes. It also has a Programmable Blanked Flutter Search setting to switch modes if 2:1 blanking of a rapid atrial arrhythmia is detected. The pacemaker defines an atrial tachyarrhythmia based on the programmable Detect Rate and Detect Duration:
Detect Rate – The rates above which pacemaker-defined atrial tachyarrhythmia starts. Note that ventricular tracking is limited by the Upper Tracking Rate or the total atrial refractory period, even when the atrial rate rises above the Detect Rate.
Detect Duration – The minimum duration (in seconds) that the atrial tachyarrhythmia must persist above the Detect Rate before the rate is considered tachyarrhythmic.
When the A–A rate exceeds the Detect Rate and is sustained for the Detect Duration, the pacemaker assumes that atrial tachyarrhythmia is in progress.
The pacemaker first monitors for any four of the last seven consecutive A–A intervals that are shorter than the detect rate interval.
If these criteria are met, the pacemaker will extend PVARP and the VA interval to uncover any blanked AS events. If an A-A interval shorter than the detect rate interval is detected, 2:1 sensing of an atrial tachyarrhythmia is assumed. Otherwise, the pacemaker resumes monitoring for 2:1 sensing of atrial tachyarrhythmias in 90 seconds.
When an atrial tachyarrhythmia is detected, the pacemaker switches to the appropriate non-atrial tracking mode. To avoid an abrupt drop in the ventricular rate, it smoothly reduces the pacing rate from the atrial synchronous rate to the sensor-indicated rate over several pacing cycles.

After the rate transition is completed, the pacemaker continues sensor-driven pacing in the ventricle, operating in the non-atrial tracking mode until the atrial tachyarrhythmia ceases. When the last seven A-A intervals are longer than the upper tracking rate interval or when five consecutive atrial paces occur, the pacemaker assumes atrial tachyarrhythmia has ceased and begins to switch back to the programmed atrial tracking mode (DDDR, DDD, or VDD).

2.3 S Jude Medical - AMS

The St. Jude Medical (St. Paul, MN, USA) Auto Mode Switch (AMS) parameter prevents atrial-based timing modes from tracking atrial tachycardias and causing pacemaker-mediated tachycardia (PMT). The Auto Mode Switch algorithm switches the mode from DDD(R) to a ventricular-timing mode (DDI, DDIR, DDT, DDTR, VVT, VVTR, VVI, or VVIR)5 when the atrial rate surpasses the Atrial Tachycardia Detection Rate (ATDR) setting. At mode-switch, the device paces in the ventricle at the AMS Base Rate setting.
Rather than use the actual atrial rate, which cannot always distinguish between sustained tachycardia and intermittent fast cycles, AMS uses the Filtered Atrial Rate Interval (FARI), which is based on a comparison of the current atrial rate to a continually updated average rate. When the tachyarrhythmia subsides and the FARI falls below the AF Suppression™ Algorithm pacing-driven rate setting, Max Track Rate setting, or the Sensor-indicated rate (whichever is faster), the device switches back to the DDD(R) or VDD(R) mode.
Diagnostic data on mode switching can be found in the Mode Switch and AT/AF diagnostic.
The Atrial Tachycardia Detection Rate (ATDR) parameter sets the atrial rate at which the device mode-switches when the Auto Mode Switch parameter is enabled. A mode-switch occurs when the Filtered Atrial Rate Interval (FARI) exceeds the programmed ATDR setting. The device switches back to DDD(R) pacing when the FARI falls below the AF Suppression™ Algorithm pacing-driven rate, Max Track Rate setting, or the Sensor-indicated rate.The ATDR parameter is always available because it is also used to classify events in atrial tachycardia and trigger EGM storage.

2.4 Ela Medical Algorithm

AMS function in the Ela Medical pacemakers (ELA Medical, Montrouge, France) combines an initial UR switch at the onset of atrial tachyarrhythmias, followed by AMS based on the detection of a sustained atrial rate above a preset atrial tachyarrhythmias detection rate. The atrial tachyarrhythmia detection interval is termed the "diagnosis of atrial rhythm acceleration period." This varies from 62.5% (for sinus rate 80 beats/min) to 75% of the preceding PP interval (for sinus rate 80 beats/min). At the onset of atrial tachyarrhythmia, only events outside the atrial tachyarrhythmia detection rate will be sensed and ventricular pacing triggered. This in effect switches the URI to the atrial tachyarrhythmia detection interval (termed "temporary mode switch" in the device). When 28 of 32 or 36 of 64 consecutive beats above the atrial tachyarrhythmia detection rate are detected, AMS will be initiated termed "permanent mode switch" in the device). A further refinement during AMS allows the pacer to function in the DDIR mode for spontaneous ventricular rate 100 beats/min, and VVIR mode when this rate. 100 beats/min to avoid atrial competitive pacing. Resynchronization to sinus rhythm occurs if 24 consecutive atrial cycles are, 110 beats/min. This counter will be reset if premature beats are sensed within this confirmation period until the 24 atrial/ventricular cycles, 110 beats/min are satisfied.

2.5 Vitatron algorithm

The Vitatron (Vitatron Medical BV, Dieren, the Netherlands) pacemakers have a different AMS algorithm that use a physiological band to define normal versus pathological atrial rate. A physiological atrial rate is calculated from the running average of the actual As or Ap atrial beats and the rate change in this moving average is limited to 2 beats/min. The physiological band is defined by an upper boundary equal to the physiological rate plus 15 beats/min (minimum value of 100 beats/min) and the lower boundary by the physiological rate minus 15 beats/min (or the sensor indicated rate if it is higher). As the physiological rate during sensordriven pacing will be determined by the sensor, it follows that atrial tachyarrhythmia detection is sensor-based when the sensor is active. If an atrial event occurs above the upper boundary of the physiological band, AMS to DDIR mode will immediately occur. The ventricular escape rate is the sensor indicated rate or lower boundary of the the pacemaker detects a P wave in the TARP, an AV interval is not initiated and the atrial refractory period is extended by an amount equal to the TARP. If further atrial events are sensed within the new TARP (outside the atrial blanking period), the TARP is further extended, causing the pacemaker to function in the DVIR mode with ventricular- based LR timing. Instantaneous resynchronization occurs when an atrial event occurs outside the TARP, or when the LR has been reached and an Ap event is initiated. Although this algorithm functions effectively in a different mode (DVIR), it provides a sensitive and fast reacting response to onset and termination of atrial tachyarrhythmia. However, it has a low specificity and may result in frequent switching to DVIR pacing during noise and atrial ectopics. In addition, competitive (aysnchronous) atrial pacing occurs during tachycardia, and may paradoxically reinduce AF should AF terminate spontaneously.

2.6 Biotronik algorithm

The Biotronik algorithm offers a choice of two algorithms that effectively repress the conduction of an atrial tachycardia in the ventricle. At the start of a tachycardic episode, the pacemaker automatically switches from an atrial-controlled to a ventricular-controlled mode.

The following functions are available:

- Automatic Mode Conversion
- X/Z-out-of-8 Mode Switching

3. Automatic mode conversion

This option is available in the atrial modes DDD(R) and VDD(R) as well as in DDT(R)/A and DDT(R)/V modes. In the case of tachycardias -- when the P-P interval is shorter than the ARP (atrial refractory period) -- this activates an automatic switch to a mode without atrial control. If the pacemaker is in DDD(R), DDT(R)/A, or DDT(R)/V mode, it switches to DVI(R); if it is operating in VDD(R) mode, it switches to VVI(R). This procedure prevents P-wave-triggered ventricular pacing during tachycardia.

When mode conversion is disabled, an atrial sensed event within the refractory period does not trigger an interval. In activated mode conversion, however, an atrial sensed event within the refractory period triggers a restart of the refractory period. The basic interval and the AV delay are not restarted. If the coupling interval between the consecutive P-waves becomes shorter than the atrial refractory period, the atrial refractory period will be continuously restarted. This means that the pacemaker remains refractory in the atrium during the entire basic interval.
This leads to non-P-wave-triggered AV sequential pacing with the basic rate for the duration of the atrial tachycardia.

3.1 Mode switching with X/Z-out-of-8 algorithm

This X/Z-out-of-8 algorithm can be used to program activation and deactivation criteria. This prevents unnecessary mode oscillations in the case of atrial extrasystoles or instable atrial signals. In addition, this algorithm can be employed to determine the speed at which a de- and resynchronization with ventricular depolarization ensues. This intervention rate can be programmed within a range from 100… (10)... (10)... 250 ppm.
In addition, the postventricular atrial blanking time (PVAB) after a ventricular event can be programmed in a range from 50 - 200 ms. This prevents any ventricular events in the atrial channel from being registered.
When an atrial tachycardia is detected, the pacemaker automatically switches to a non-atrial-controlled mode: from DDD(R) to DDI(R), from DDD(R)+ to DDI(R), or from VDD(R) to VDI(R) as well as from DDT(R)/A and DDT(R)/V to DDI(R).
The mode switch can be programmed so that you can switch from a non-rate-adaptive mode to a rate-adaptive mode, and vice versa. This serves to prevent an undesirable rate drop to the basic rate in case of physical stress.
An atrial tachycardia is considered sensed when the so-called Xout- of-8 conversion criterion has been fulfilled. The X value can be programmed in the value range (X = 3... (1)...8). Detection is based on the continual evaluation of the last 8 atrial intervals. When X out of 8 intervals reveal an atrial rate which lies above the programmed intervention rate, then the conversion criterion is fulfilled and mode switching automatically follows.
The pacemaker works in the programmed non-atrial mode until the switch-off criterion (Z-out-of-8) has been fulfilled. The Z value can be programmed in the value range (Z = 3... (1)...8). Likewise, the last 8 consecutive atrial intervals are continuously evaluated. When Z out of 8 intervals lie below the programmed intervention rate, the atrial tachycardia is considered to be over, and the pacemaker automatically switches to the originally programmed atrial-controlled mode.
The X or Z counter is reset to zero after every completed switching.

3.2 Sorin algorithm

The Sorin (Saluggia, Italy) pacemakers measure the "peak endocardial acceleration" with an implantable acceleration sensor at the tip of the right ventricular pacing lead. In addition, it also has a gravitational type of activity sensor. Atrial tachyarrhythmia is defined as atrial events at a rate exceeding the UR. In the DDD mode, on detection of atrial tachyarrhythmia, the pacemaker will mode switch to the VVI mode at the UR for 1,000 cycles before it falls back gradually to a nonprogrammable ventricular pacing rate of 77 beats/min. In the DDDR mode using the activity sensor, the device will temporarily mode switch to the VVI mode at the UR for 250 cycles. Should the sinus rate fall below the UR during this period, AMS will not occur. This is designed to avoid AMS during nonexercise related sinus tachycardia. If the atrial rate remains above UR for 250 cycles, the sensor indicated interval is then checked. If there is a discrepancy between it and the As rate, the pacing rate will fall back to the sensor indicated rate. When the peak endocardial acceleration sensor DDDR mode is activated, the As rate above the UR will be compared with the sensor indicated rate. When the atrial rate is above the sensor indicated rate, the pacemaker will immediately mode switch to VVIR mode and the pacing rate will fall back to the sensor indicated rate. In activity and peak endocardial acceleration DDDR mode, atrial tracking resumes when three As cycles are at a rate lower than the UR.

3.3 AMS in VDD pacemakers

Stable long-term atrial sensing and ventricular stimulation have been demonstrated single-lead for VDD pacing with "floating" atrial electrodes. Many VDD pacemakers have AMS algorithms similar to their DDD counterparts. However, the absence of atrial pacing in VDD pacemakers prevents AV synchrony during atrial asystole after atrial tachy-arrhythmia termination or when the atrial rate drops below LR. Inadequate AV asynchrony may paradoxically predispose to AF. However, the absence of atrial pacing, particularly during atrial undersensing, may prevent inappropriate atrial pacing during AF as may occur with a DDDR pacemaker. Indeed, a recent short-term study in 23 patients with second- or third-degree AV block and paroxysmal AF showed that in the DDDR mode, inappropriate atrial pacing occurred in 50% patients despite mode switching. (27) In patients with AV block implanted with DDD pacemakers, 9.8% developed AF at a mean of 23 months.28 In a report on patients with a singlelead VDD pacemaker, 9% developed AF over a follow- up of 5.5 years. (28-29). Thus, the incidence of AF between DDD and VDD appears comparable. Further studies will be required to compare the incidence of VDD versus DDD pacing in suppressing AF. (30)

4. Conclusions

Overall experience with AMS has been satisfactory so far. Barring economic considerations, all pacemakers should possess an AMS function as one of its programmable options. AMS allows the benefits of AV synchrony to be extended to a population with existing or threatened AF. These devices are indicated in all patients with the brady-tachy syndrome. They should also be considered in patients with sinus node disease without paroxysmal AF, obstructive hypertrophic cardiomyopathy, or any condition that predisposes patients to paroxysmal AF. Indeed, like the rate adaptive function (R), it could be argued that all patients should receive a device with AMS capability because one cannot predict which patients will eventually develop AF (or atrial chronotropic incompetence in the case of the rate-adaptive function). Many algorithms have been used by different manufacturers, and they do not behave similarly. Optimal care of the pacemaker patient requires a thorough knowledge of his or her arrhythmia history, atrial electrocardiogram amplitude (in sinus rhythm and atrial tachy-arrhythmia), basic timing cycles required for all AMS algorithms, and the characteristics of the various available algorithms.

Devices	*Pacing During AMS*
BOSTON SCIENTIFIC ALTRUA®	DDD(R) → DDI(R), VDI(R)
GUIDANT INSIGNIA® / PULSAR® / MERIDIAN® / DISCOVERY®	DDD(R) → DDI(R), VDI(R)
MEDTRONIC ENRHYTHM® / RELIA® / SENSIA® / VERSA® / ADAPTA®	DDD(R) → DDI(R) - VDD(R)→VDIR
VITATRON SERIE T / SERIE C	DDD(R) → DDI(R), VDI(R)
S.JUDE MEDICAL IDENTITY® / VICTORY® / INTEGRITY® / ACCENT® /VERITY®	DDDR → DDIR - DDD→ DDI
BIOTRONIK EVIA®	DDD(R) → DDI(R), VDI(R)
BIOTRONIK CYLOS® / PHILOS®	DDD(R) → DDI(R), VDI(R), VVI(R), DVI(R)
SORIN GROUP NEWLIVING® / ESPRIT® / NEWAY®	DDD(R) → DDI(R)
ELA MEDICAL REPLY® / RHAPSODY® / SYMPHONY® / TALENT®	DDD(R) → DDI(R)
MEDICO SOPHOS®	DDD(R) → DDI(R), VDI(R)

Table I. Pacing Mode During Mode Switching

Devices	*Mode*
BOSTON / GUIDANT	PROGRAMMABLE NUMBER OF ATRIAL EVENTS < ATR
MEDTRONIC	(PROGRAMMABLE) NUMBER OF ATRIAL INTERVALS > PROGRAMMABLE SLOW INTERVAL
S.JUDE MEDICAL	FARI < MTR or MSR
BIOTRONIK	X/Z ON 8. PROGRAMMABLE NUMBER OF INTERVALS (X e Z) ON 8 WITH RATE < ATR
SORIN GROUP	ATRIAL RATE=FV
ELA MEDICAL	18/32 ATRIAL EVENTS OUT OF WARAD
MEDICO	PROGRAMMABLE NUMBER OF ATRIAL EVENTS < ATR

MTR= MAXIMUM TRACKING RATE; MSR= MAXIMUM SENSOR RATE ; ATR= ATRIAL TRACKING RATE, CUTOFF OF FAST ATRIAL RATE (PROGRAMMABLE); FARI= FILTERED ATRIAL RATE INTERVALS, based on current atrial rate confronted with average atrial rate ; WARAD= WINDOW OF ATRIAL RATE ACCELERATION DETECTgbvION ; FV= MAXIMUM ATRIAL VARIATION RANGE STILL CONSIDERED SINUSAL VARIATION

Table II. Mode Switching Termination

5. References

[1] Goethals M, TimmermansW, Geelen P, et al. (2003). Mode switching failure during atrial flutter: The '2:1. lock-in' phenomenon. *Europace*. 5:95-102.

[2] Barold SS, Israel CW, Stroobandt R, et al. Diagnosis of supraventricular tachyarrhythmias by automatic mode switching algorithms of dual chamber pacemakers. In Barold SS, Mugica J (2004) (eds.): *The Fifth Decade of Cardiac Pacing*. Elmsford, NY, Blackwell-Futura, 161–177.

[3] Israel CW. (2002) Analysis of mode switching algorithms in dual chamber pacemakers. *PACE*; 25:380-393.

[4] Kolb C, Aratma S, Zrenner B, et al. (2004) Preventricular far-field sensing in the atrial channel of dual chamber pacemakers—An occasional cause of inappropriate mode switch. *J Interv Card Electrophysiol*; 10:231–235.

[5] Barold SS. (2003). Far-field Rwave sensing causing prolongation of the atrial escape interval of DDD pacemakers with atrial-based lower rate timing. *PACE*; 26:2188-2191.

[6] Stroobandt RX, Barold SS, Vandenbulcke FD, et al. (2001) A reappraisal of pacemaker timing cycles pertaining to automatic mode switching. *J Interv Card Electrophysiol*; 5:417–429.

[7] Israel CW, Neubauer H, Ossowski A, et al. (2000). Why did mode switching occur? *PACE*; 23:1422–1424.

[8] Dodinot B. (2000). Effondrement de la frequence de stimulation a l'effort. Stimucoeur; 28:89–92.

[9] Lau CP, Leung SK, Tse HF, et al. (2002). Automatic mode switching of implantable pacemakers. I: Principle of instrumentation, and clinical and hemodynamic consideration. *PACE*; 25:967–983.

[10] Lau CP, Tai YT, Fong PC, et al. (1992). Atrial arrhythmia management with sensor controlled atrial refractory period and automatic mode switching in patients with minute ventilation sensing dual chamber rate adaptive pacemakers. *PACE*; 15:1504–1514.

[11] Pitney MR, May CD, Davis MJ. (1993). Undesirable mode switching with a dual chamber rate responsive pacemaker. *PACE* 1993; 16:729–737.

[12] Lau CP. (1991). Sensor and pacemaker mediated tachycardias. (editorial) *PACE*; 14:495–498.

[13] Provenier F, Jordaens L, Verstraeten T, et al. (1994). The "automatic mode switch" function in successive generations of minute ventilation sensing dual chamber rate responsive pacemakers. *PACE*; 17:1913–1919.

[14] Ricci R, Puglisi A, Azzolini P, et al. (1996). Reliability of a new algorithm for automatic mode switching from DDDR to DDIR pacing mode in sinus node disease patients with chronotropic incompetence and recurrent paroxysmal atrial fibrillation. *PACE*; 19:1719–1723.

[15] Ovsyscher IE, Ketz A, Bondy C. (1994). Initial experience with a new algorithm for automatic mode switching from DDDR to DDIR mode. *PACE* ; 17:1908–1912.

[17] Seidl K, Meisel E, Van Agt E, et al. (1998). Is the high rate episode diagnostic feature reliable in detecting paroxysmal episodes of atrial tachyarrhythmias? *PACE*; 21:694–700.

[16] Levine PA, Bornzin GA, Barlow J, et al. (1994). A new automode switch algorithm for supraventricular tachycardias. PACE; 17:1895–1899.
[17] Leung SK, Lau CP, Lam CT, et. al. (2000). Is automatic mode switching effective for atrial arrhythmias occurring at different rates? A study on efficacy of automatic mode and rate switching to simulated atrial arrhythmias by chest wall stimulation. *PACE*; 23:823–831.
[18] Lee MT, Adkins A, Woodson D, et al. (1990). A new feature for control of inappropriate high rate tracking in DDDR pacemakers. *PACE*; 13:1852–1855.
[19] Lau CP, Tai YT, Fong PC, et al. (1992). Clinical experience with an activity sensing DDDR pacemaker using an accelerometer sensor. *PACE*; 15:334–343.
[20] Lau CP, Tai YT, Fong PC, et al. (1992). The use of implantable sensors for the control of pacemaker medicated tachycardias: A comparative evaluation between minute ventilation sensing and acceleration sensing dual chamber rate adaptive pacemakers. *PACE*; 15:34–44.
[21] Mahaux V, Verboven Y, Waleffe A, et al. (1992). Clinical interest of a sensor driven algorithm limiting ventricular pacing rate during supraventricular tachycardia in dual chamber pacing. *PACE*; 15:1862–1866.
[22] Gencel L, Geroux L, Clementy J, et al. (1996). Ventricular protection against atrial arrhythmias in DDD pacing based on a statistical approach: Clinical results. *PACE*; 19:1729–1734.
[23] Geroux L, Limousin M, Cazeau S. (1999). Clinical performance of a new mode switch function based on a statistical analysis of the atrial rhythm. *Herzchr Elektrophys*; 10(Suppl. 1):15–21.
[24] Begemann MJ, Thijssen WA, Haaksma J. (1992). The influence of test window width on atrial rhythm classification in dual chamber pacemakers. *PACE*; 15:2158–2163.
[25] den Dulk K, Dijkman B, Pieterse M, et al. (1994). Initial experience with mode switching in a dual sensor, dual chamber pacemaker in patients with paroxysmal atrial tachyarrhythmias. *PACE*; 17:1900–1907.
[26] Brignole M, Gianfranchi L, Menozzi C, et al. (1994). A new pacemaker for paroxysmal atrial fibrillation treated with radiofrequency ablation of the AV junction. *PACE*; 17:1889–1894.
[27] Jayaprakash S, Sparks PB, Kalman JM, et al. (2000). Dual demand pacing using retriggerable refractory periods for ventricular rate control during paroxysmal supraventricular tachyarrhythmias in patients with dual chamber pacemakers. PACE; 23:1156–1163.
[28] Rickards AF, Bombardinin T, Corbucci G, et al. (1996). An implantable intracardiac accelerometer for monitoring myocardial contractility. The Multicenter PEA Study Group. *PACE*; 19(Pt. I):2066–2071.
[29] Leung SK, Lau CP, Lam C, et al. (2000). Automatic optimization of resting and exercise atrioventricular interval using a peak endocardial acceleration sensor: Validation with Doppler echocardiography and direct cardiac output measurements. *PACE*; 23(Pt. II):1762–1766.
[30] Lau CP, Leung SK, Lee IS. (1996). Comparative evaluation of acute and long-term clinical performance of two single-lead atrial synchronous ventricular (VDD) pacemakers: Diagonally arranged bipolar versus closely spaced bipolar ring electrodes. *PACE*;19:1574–1581.

[31] Schuchert A, van Langen H, Michels K, et al. (1997). Frequency of atrial pacing in patients with intermittent atrial fibrillation and 2nd or 3rd degree atrioventricular block. Thera DR Pacemaker Study Group. *Zeitschrift fur Kardiologie*; 86:81–84.

[32] Gross J, Moser S, Benedek ZM, et al. (1990). Clinical predictors and natural history of atrial fibrillation in patients with DDD pacemakers. *PACE*; 13:1828–1831.

[33] Folino AF, Buja G, Corso LD, et al. (1998). Incidence of atrial fibrillation in patients with different mode of pacing. Long-term follow-up. *PACE*; 21:260–263.

[34] Schuchert A, Meinertz T. (1998). Pacemaker therapy in patients with atrial fibrillation. (review) *Herz*; 23:260–268.

[35] Leung SK, Lau CP, Lam CT, et al. (2000). A comparative study on the behavior of three different automatic mode switching dual chamber pacemakers to intracardiac recordings of clinical atrial fibrillation. *PACE*; 23:2086–2096.

[36] Wood MA, Ellenbogen KA, Dinsmoor D, et al. (2000). Influence of autothreshold sensing and sinus rate on mode switching algorithm behavior. *PACE*; 23:1473–1478.

[37] Kamalvand K, Tam K, Kotsakis K, et al. (1997). Is mode switching beneficial? A randomized study in patients with paroxysmal atrial tachyarrhythmias. *J Am Coll Cardiol*; 30:496–504.

[38] Marshall HJ, Kay GN, Hess M, et al. (1999). Mode switching in dual chamber pacemakers: Effect of onset criteria on arrhythmia - related symptoms. *Europace*; 1:49–54.

[39] Leung SK, Lau CP, Lam CT, et al. (1998). Programmed atrial sensitivity: A critical determinant in atrial fibrillation detection and optimal automatic mode switching. *PACE* 1998; 21:2214–2219.

[40] Walfridsson H, Aunes M, Capocci M, et al. (2000). Sensing of atrial fibrillation by a dual chamber pacemaker: How should atrial sensing be programmed to ensure adequate mode shift? *PACE*; 23:1089–1093.

[41] Ellenbogen KA, Mond HG, Wood MA, et al. (1997). Failure of automatic mode switching: Recognition and management. *PACE*; 20:268–275.

[46] Palma EC, Kedarnath V, Vankawalla V, et al. (1996). Effect of varying atrial sensitivity, AV interval, and detection algorithm on automatic mode switching. *PACE*; 19:1734–1739.

[42] Lam CT, Lau CP, Leung SK, et al. (1999). Improved efficacy of mode switching during atrial fibrillation using automatic atrial sensitivity adjustment. *PACE*; 22:17–25.

[48] Garrigue S, Barold SS, Cazeau S, et al. (1998). Prevention of atrial arrhythmias during DDD pacing by atrial overdrive. *PACE*; 21:1751–1759.

[43] Tse HF, Lau CP, Ayers GM. (1999). The incidence and modes of onset of spontaneous re-initiation of atrial fibrillation following successful internal cardioversion and its prevention by intravenous sotalol. *Heart*; 82:319–324.

[44] Tse HF, Lau CP, Ayers GM. (2000). Atrial pacing for suppression of early re-initiation of atrial fibrillation after successful internal cardioversion. *Eur Heart J*; 21:1167–1176.

[45] Chauvin M, Brechenmacher C. (1989). Atrial refractory periods after atrial premature beats in patients with paroxysmal atrial fibrillation. *PACE*; 12:1018–1026.

[46] Murgatroyd FD, Nitzsche R, Slade AK, et al. (1994). A new pacing algorithm for overdrive suppression of atrial fibrillation. Chorus Multicentre Study Group. *PACE*; 17:1966–1973.

[47] Swerdlow CD, Schsls W, Dijkman B, et al. (2000). Detection of atrial fibrillation and flutter by a dual-chamber implantable cardioverterdefibrillator. *Circulation;* 101:878–885.
[48] Tse HF, Lau CP, Sra JS, et al. (1999). Atrial fibrillation detection and R wave synchronization by Metrix implantable atrial defibrillator: Implication for long term efficacy and safety. *Circulation;* 99:1446–1451.
[49] Wang Q, Lau CP, Tse HF, et al. (2000). Is there a role for back-up atrial defibrillating in patients with sick sinus syndrome undergoing implantation of DDDR pacemaker? (abstract) *Europace;* 1:D276.
[50] Lau C.P, Leung S.K., TSE H.F., Barold S.S. (2002). Automatic Mode Switching of Implantable Pacemakers: II. Clinical Performance of Current Algorithms and Their Programming *PACE;* 25:1094-1113
[51] Santomauro M, Ottaiano L., Borrelli A. et al. (2008). Efficacy of automatic mode switching in DDDR mode pacemakers: The most 2 study J. *Interv Card Electrophysiol;* 21:13-17
[52] Ishikawa T, Sumita S, Kikuchi M, et al (2000). Incidence of atrial flutter and atrial fibrillation in patients with implanted physiological pacemakers. *Jpn Circ J.;* 64: 505-9.
[53] Cheung J.W., Keating R.J., Stein K.M. et al. (2006). Newly detected atrial fibrillation following dual chamber pacemaker implantation *J Cardiovasc Electrophysiol,;* 17, 1323-1328.
[54] Lau C.P., Mascia F., Corbucci G., Padeletti L. (2004). Methods for testing automatic mode switching in patients implanted with DDD (R) pacemakers. *Ital Heart J.* 5:11-15.
[55] Padeletti L., Gasparini M., Porciani M.C., et al. (2002). How to test mode switching in pacemakers implanted in patients: the MOST study *Pacing Clin Electrophysiol.;*25 :156-60.
[56] Stabile G., De Simone A., Romano E. (2005). Automatic mode switching in atrial fibrillation *Indian Pacing Electrophysiol J.;* 5: 186–196.
[57] Tronconi F., Porciani M.C., Gianfranchi L., et al. (2004). A Device and a Method for Simulating Supraventricular Arrhythmias in Pacemakers Implanted in Patients: Assessment of Safety and Reliability *Cardiov Engineering* ; 4 : 219-227.

Address for corrispondance:
Maurizio Santomauro, MD, FESC,FHRS
Department of Medicine, Cardiology and Immunology
Federico II School of Medicine, University of Naples
Via Sergio Pansini 5
80131 Naples, Italy
santomau@unina.it

3

Advanced Techniques for CRT Implantations

Béla Merkely, Levente Molnár, Szabolcs Szilágyi and László Gellér
Heart Center, Semmelweis University
Hungary

1. Introduction

Cardiac resynchronization therapy (CRT) is an important breakthrough for the drug-refractory heart failure patients with reduced left ventrical ejection fraction (LVEF: <35%) and wide QRS (>120 ms). The primary objective of CRT is the coordination of the myocardial contraction with a right atrial (RA), right ventrical (RV) and a left ventrical (LV) lead and a biventricular device. The standard approach for implantation of the LV lead is transvenous epicardial approach through the subclavian vein to the lateral or posterolateral sidebranch of the coronary sinus. The average implantation time of CRT in high volume centers is under 120 minutes. Nowadays the procedural success ranges between 87% and 96% (Alonso, 2009). Early complications were seen in 10% and late complications were reported in further 5.5% (Khan et al., 2009). However we do not have all the evidence based predicting criterias to select the CRT responders and the different definitions of responders are numerous (Paul et al., 2009), the basics of all comparison is the successful left and right ventricular lead implantation. The growing numbers of heart failure patients recieving CRT and the limitation of the first line transvenous approach enhanced the evolution of alternative techniques. In this chapter we focus on the advanced CRT techniques which might help to reach the optimal lead positions and increase the success rate of implantations.

The standard transvenous approach unfortunately has significant drawbacks as it is totally dependent on the inconsistent venous anatomy. The tributaries of the coronary sinus is usually visualised by the late phase of left coronarography, direct contrast injecion or by inserting an occlusion balloon into the coronary sinus (CS). Several reasons can cause the inabilty to reach the desired sidebrach and to insert the LV lead. The main reasons are: inability to cannulate the CS caused by dilatated right atrium, atypical orifice of CS, prominent Thebesian valve, small vessel size of the CS, severe kinking of the vein or venous valve in the CS. The secondary reasons are the high pacing threshold or phrenic nerve stimulation at the optimal site, inability to fixate the lead at the desired position and the insuffitient experience of the implanters. Stenosis or occlusion of the subclavian vein, or presence of a persistent left superior vena cava might be the cause for alternative LV implantations. Small or occluded sidebranches or tortuous branches and CS dissection or perforations might overcome with advanced transvenous techniques.

The selection of the optimal site is an unsettled debate. Several noninvasiv and invasive techniques were investigated to confirm the optimal site, but no clear proven evidence is shown for the selection. However there is a consesus that the lateral and posterolateral veins are preferable rather than the anterior or apical veins. The anterolateral vein might be selected as a last resort in the absence of lateral and posterolateral veins. The identification of the veins

and their course can be followed by multiple flouroscopic views 30-60° LAO. Finding the individual optimal site and the access to that region is the task for the implanters.
The alternative approaches may be classified in terms of access: open chest or percutaneous, the lead insertion can be transvenous or transatrial. The lead tip site can be differentiated as epicaridal or endocardial.

2. Transvenous epicardial approach – LV lead in the tributaries of coronary sinus

The first line approach for LV lead implantation is transvenous epicardial access, through the coronary sinus to the tributaries. It is less invasive, can be performed in local anaesthesia and therefore preferable. The most challenging part of the implantation is the positioning of the left ventricular electrode through the coronary sinus (CS). The standard technique is well known and widely used in CRT implanting centers. In this section we emphasize the advaced alternative techniques which might help to overcome difficulties and failure components during the standard technique.

2.1 Cannulation of the coronary sinus

The main reason for failure in CRT is the inability to canulate the CS. The first essential step is to get clear view of the coronary venogram. Preprocedural venography can be visualized at the late phase of left coronarography performed as the part of the rule out of ischaemic heart disease of the heart failure patient. The position of the orifice, the angle of the beginning of CS, tortuousity and diameter of the vein are valuable informations for the selection of target vessel and the implantation approach. With the known unique limitation of the vascular venous anatomy and the reachability of the desired optimal site, the selection of the CRT techniqe is the implanters responsibility.
Additional help can be to position and fixate the RV lead into final place at the beginning of the procedure. The movement of the lead might show the tricuspid valve as a landmark. After fixation and threshold test RV lead ensures the further procedure by the ability to pace the ventricle.
Beacuse of interindividual differences of the geometry of the right atrium and CS variatons, several fixed shaped and deflectable sheaths are used to cannulate the orifice. (Fig. 1.)

2.2 Atypical orifice of CS, prominent Thebesian valve, small vessel size of the CS

In cases of unsuccessful cannulation of CS with the fix or flexible catheters, coronary angiography catheter can be inserted into the guiding catheter to create individual curves. Regularly Amplatz II curved catheters advanced 1-5 cm distally of the tip of the guiding catheter give help to manipulate with a new curve. By changing the length of advancement and small rotations of the angiographic catheter in the guiding catheter a great variety of shaped curves can be created. Depending on the atrial anatomy Amplatz I or III, Judkins Right or Multi-Purpose angiography catheter might find the orifice more easily. Contrast is injected through the catheters to identify the orifice. After cannulation, inserting a guidewire through the catheter helps to advance the catheter deep into the coronary sinus safely. The CS sheath is then forwarded over the coronary catheter. Contrast injection through the guide catheter shows the coronary sinus venogram. In some cases occlusion balloon inflated in the main branch and injection of contrast into the other lumen can prove smaller distal sidebranches (Fig.2.).

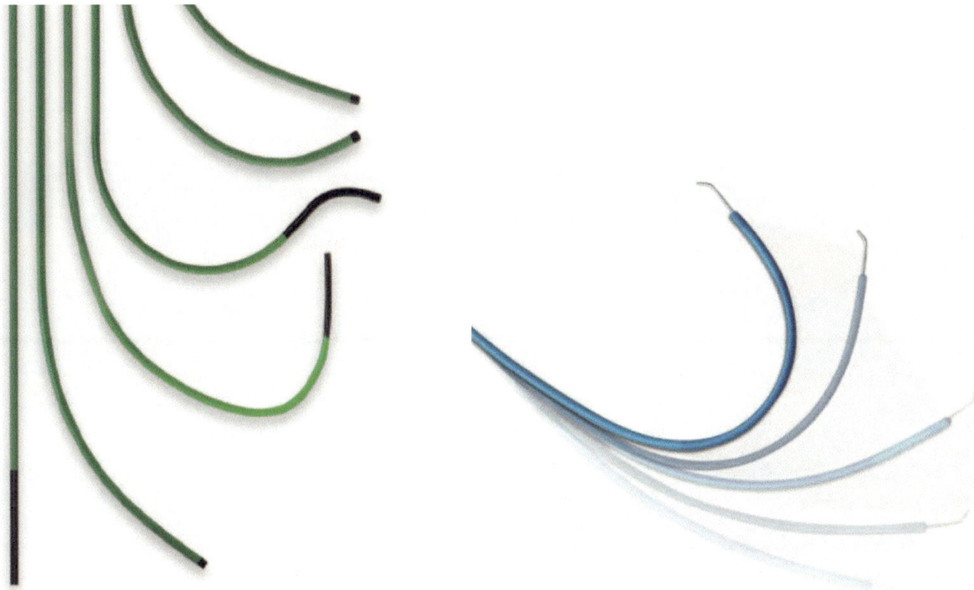

Fig. 1. Fixed curved and flexible guiding catheters (Courtesy of Medtronic Hungary)

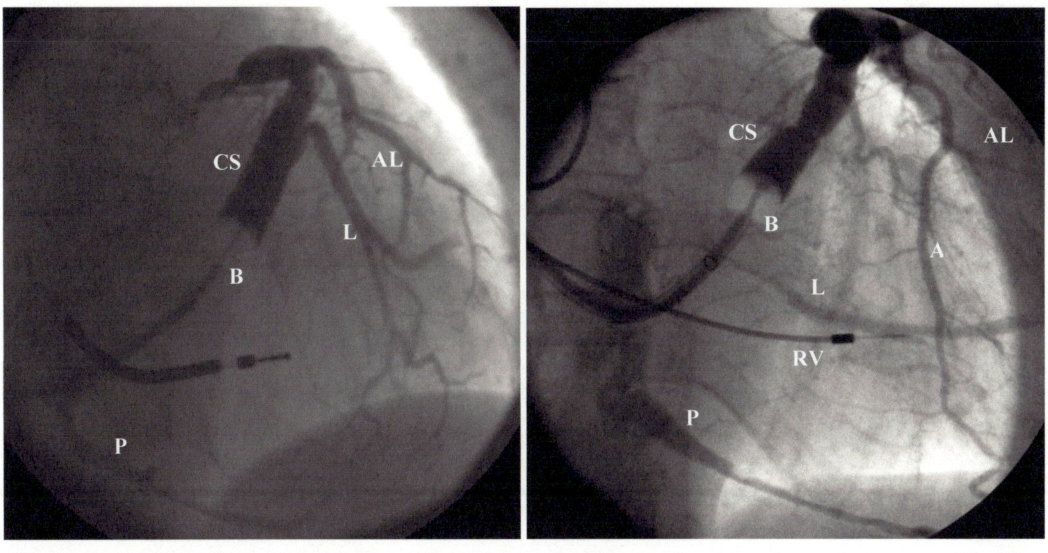

Fig. 2. Various coronary anatomies CS - coronary sinus, AL- anterolateral, A - anterior, L - lateral, P- posterior, RV - right ventricular lead, B - balloon

In patients with atypical anatomic variations or prominent Thebesian valve the use of a curved or steerable electrophysiology catheter inserted into the guiding catheter helps to cannulate the CS (Fig.3.). Intracardiac signals of the catheter help the orientation within the cavitiy of the atrium. Obligate atrial signals on the CS 1, 2 (distal electrode) show the proximity of the orifice. The catheter is advanced by simultaneous counterclockwise rotation and straightening of the catheter. The concurrent signals on the other CS electrodes prove the achieved CS position (Fig.4). After the EP catheter is in the CS, the sheat is advanced until the tip of the catheter.

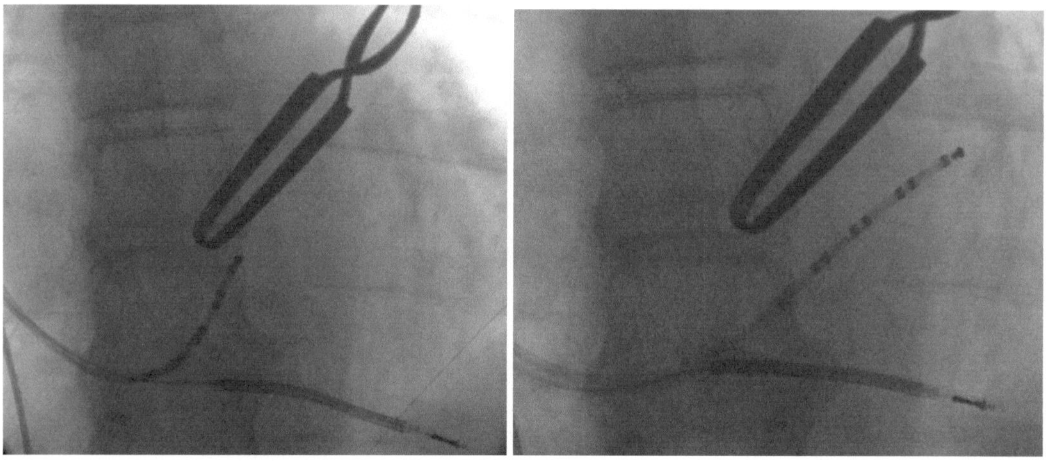

Fig. 3. EP catheter in the orifice of CS (left) and in the middle CS (right)

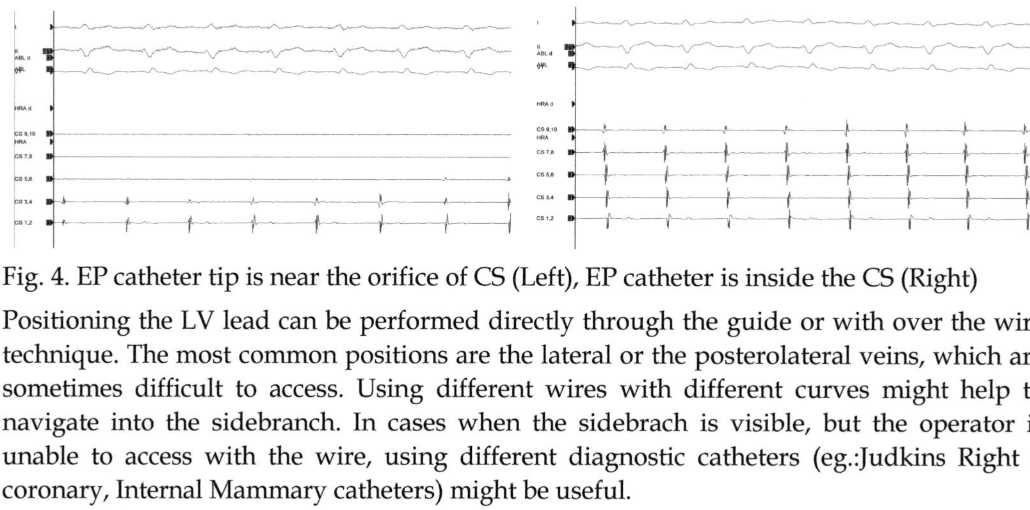

Fig. 4. EP catheter tip is near the orifice of CS (Left), EP catheter is inside the CS (Right)

Positioning the LV lead can be performed directly through the guide or with over the wire technique. The most common positions are the lateral or the posterolateral veins, which are sometimes difficult to access. Using different wires with different curves might help to navigate into the sidebranch. In cases when the sidebrach is visible, but the operator is unable to access with the wire, using different diagnostic catheters (eg.:Judkins Right 4 coronary, Internal Mammary catheters) might be useful.

2.3 Absence of lateral branch

The absence of visible lateral branch can occur when the inflated ballon is positioned distally in the CS. Pulling back and inflating the balloon at the orifice might show the origin of a posterior vein or sometimes separatly originating vein can be found (Fig.5.). A different preshaped fixed or a steerable catheter can find access to the vein. If the orifice is too wide for the occlusion balloon, advancing the balloon to the middle of CS and by givining contrast retrograde filling of the posterior vein can visualise the orifice of the vein.

If the sidebranches are not visible after reinflations of the balloon, the small vessel size tributaries deny the transvenous implantation, the transseptal approach can be continued immediatly or surigcal approach can be considered.

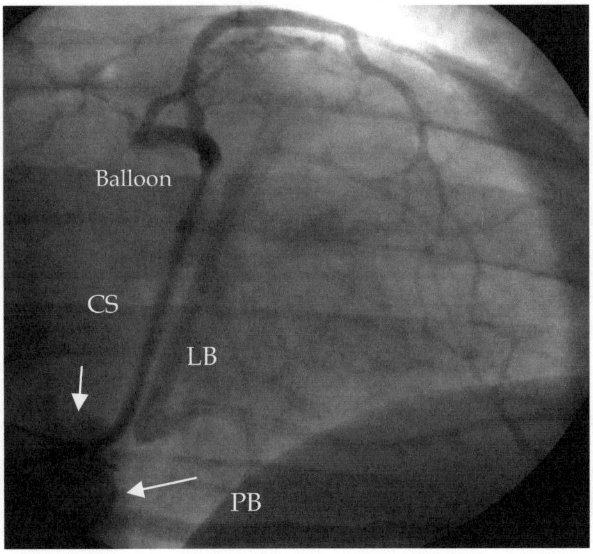

Fig. 5. Separatly originating vein: CS - coronary sinus, LB -lateral branch, PB- posterior branch, upper arrow - CS orifice, lowwer arrow - seperate posterior vein orifice

2.4 Intervention of the vein - Stenosis, sharp angulations, small vessel size or occluded sidebranches

Stenosis, sharp angulation, small vessel diameter of the sidebranch can be solved by predilatation of the branch with a balloon or stenting the proximal part of the branch using a coronary stent. After succesful balloon dilatation the venogram may confirm patent target vein. However the visual success is almost reached, in some cases the vessel is still not accessible. Often tortuous veins can be the cause of unsuccessful LV implantation (Fig.6.). Stiffer, more dangerous wires PT-2 and PT Graphix Extra Support (Boston Scientific, Natick, Massachusetts), *Jindo* and SV8 (*Cordis* Corporation, Miami, Florida) are recommended for experienced operators. Advancing the wires as far as possible around the veins anchores the system (Fig.6.). If the distal soft part of the wire is advanced through the stenosis or the angulation, the stiffer middle segment of the wire straightens the vessel and the lead can be inserted (Fig.7.). Pull-push maneuver, pulling the wire and simultaneously pushing the lead can also help to andvance the lead. The buddy wire is also an alternative technique to facilitate the lead positioning.

2.5 Venous valve in the sidebranch

Valves at the beginning of the tributaries can also present unexpected difficulties. In case of only one lateral sidebranch the delivery of the wire and the lead is the key to the success of CRT. The standard coronary interventional procedure ensures the performance. After crossing the leasion with a coronary guiding wire, a 2.0-2.5 mm diameter balloon is positioned and inflated between the valves (Fig.8.).

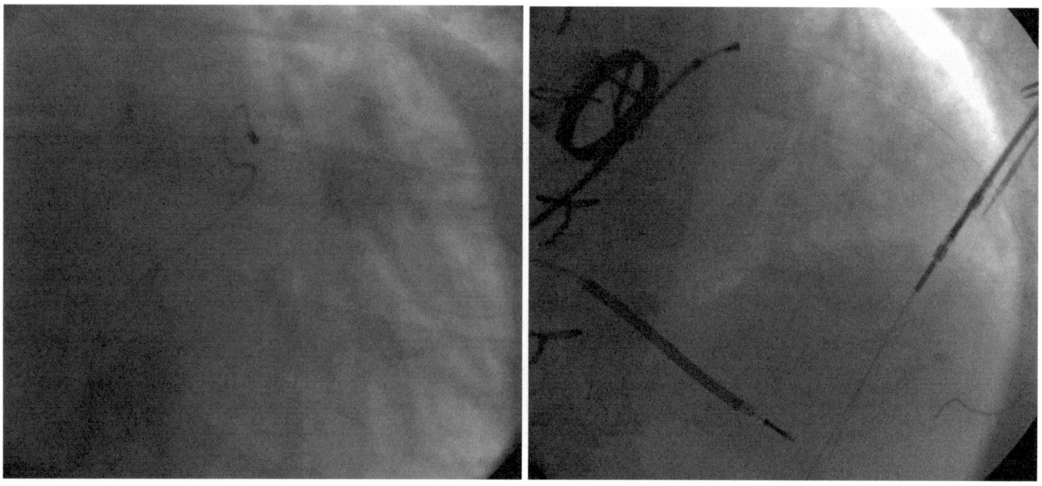

Fig. 6. Tortuous sidebranch (left), anchoring the wire, advancing over the apex (right)

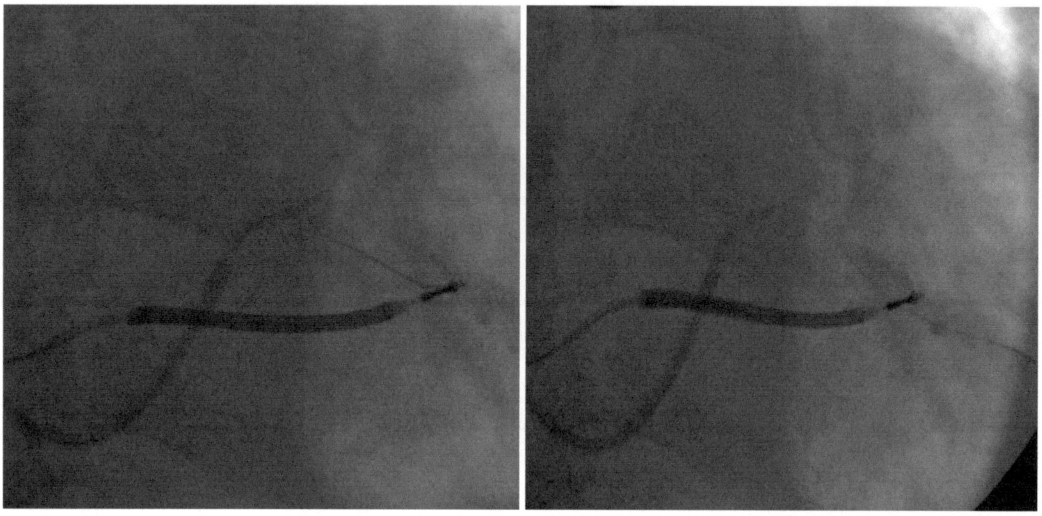

Fig. 7. Proximal kinking straighted with the advancement of the wire.

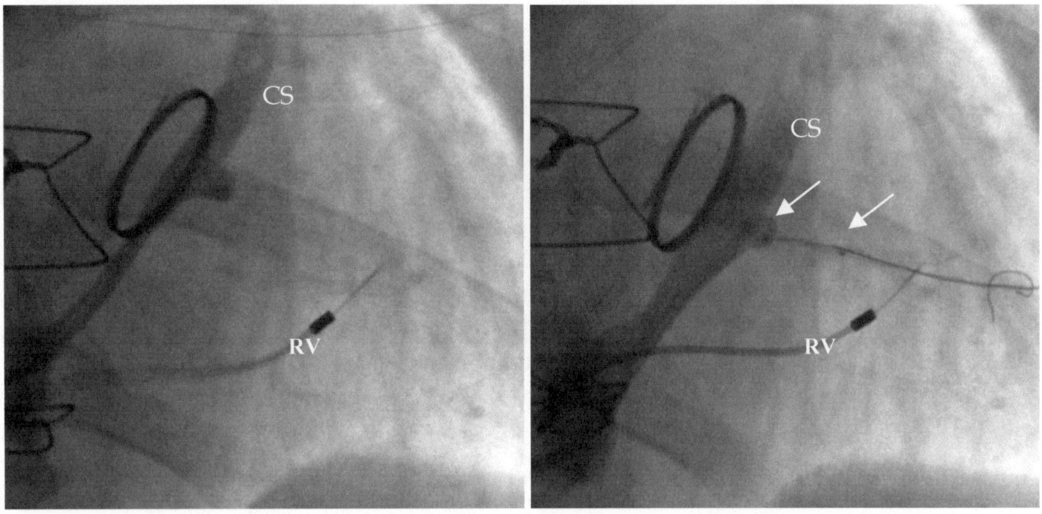

Fig. 8. Valve at the origin of sidebranch (left), Positioning the balloon with the help of buddywire; CS - coronary sinus, LB -lateral branch, RV - right ventricular lead, arrows - proximal and distal marker of the balloon)

Insuffitient results need further intervention, coronary stent deployment may be useful. The selection of the length is adjusted to cover the valves entirely. Moderatly oversized stent can ensure the free retrograde access over the valve (Fig.9.). Undersized or malappositioned stents cause difficult wire and lead delivery.

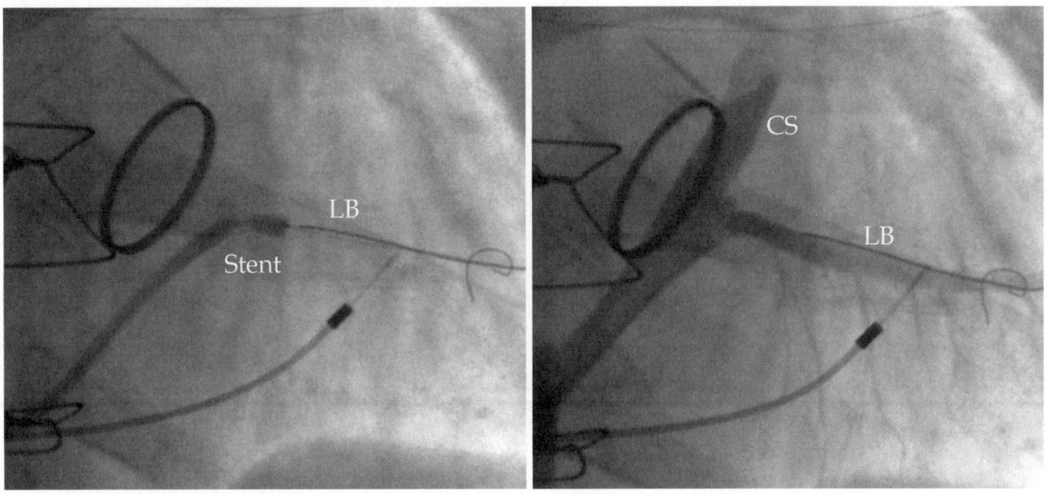

Fig. 9. Stent deployment (left), Contol venogram of the sidebranch (right); CS - coronary sinus, LB - lateral branch, RV - right ventricular lead

2.6 High ventricular pacing threshold or phrenic nerve stimulating, inability to fixate the lead

Finding the individual optimal site is always a task. After accessing the lateral vein with the LV lead, pacing threshold is measured. Scarred myocardial tissue and abundant fat between the vessel wall and epicardium may increase the capture threshold. Chronic heart failure originates often from ischeamic heart disease, therefore scarred tissue is relavant component in high pacing threshold. When insuffitient pacing thresholds are measured in the target vein, sidebranches should be explored with a 0.014 inch coronary guidewire, and advancing the lead to the wedge position can bring success. Ultimately alternate vein should be searched. To reach everyones goal, the successful resynchronisation, higher thresholds are accepted at LV lead in case of effective resynchronisation. The phrenic nerve stimulation is the other limiting factor to reach the optimal site. Occurence of phrenic nerve stimulation while stimulating at the target position yields for alternative sidebranch. Minimal movements of the lead should be considered after implantation in stand up position. The optimal site for the individual is the latest contracting, optimal capture threshold site without phrenic nerve stimulation. Inability to fixate a passive fixation lead in this position can result in changing the lead to active fixation lead or stenting the lead (Fig.10.). Stenting during the first implantation (Szilagyi et al., 2007) can be a choice when macroscopic or microscopic dislocation occurs and there is no other suitable vein accessible or phrenic nerve stimulation is seen in stable anatomical position in the distal part of the side-branch and the lead needs to be fixed in the more proximal, wider, otherwise unstable parts of the target vein.

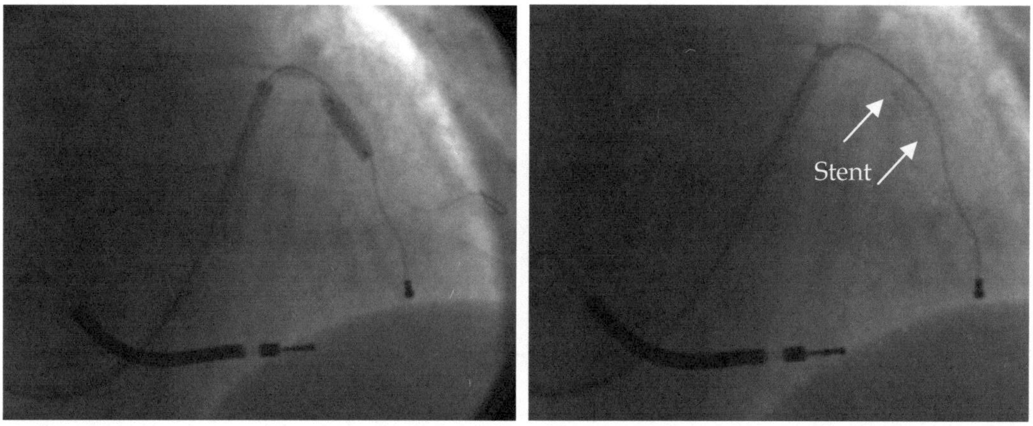

Fig. 10. Stenting of the lead (left), CS lead with the stent (right)

2.7 Recurrent dislodgement of LV lead - stenting

Despite continous technical development in the last few years, in the large CRT trials 5-10 % of patients required reoperation during follow up because of CS lead dysfunction. The stenting of the LV lead in cases of postoperative dislocation may be an effective and feasible alternative stabilising technique. Convetional wires, balloons and stents are used as in coronary artery interventions. The wall of the veins are thinner and more expansive, therefore the size of the stents are oversized with 20-30% of the vessel size and dilatation pressures are fit to reach the desired size. In our 5 years experience no rupture or any serious complications of the veins due to the stenting of the LV lead has been observed. Though it seems to be effective procedure, indiscriminate, reagular use is not recommended. Long term results are needed to prove the safety of this method.

2.8 Left ventricular leads

Unipolar and bipolar LV leads are available in different angeled, curved shape (Fig. 11., 12.). The industry is continously developing new designs to enhance the delivery and the stability of the leads. The operators selection is to find the best lead desing for the individual coronary sinus anatomy. Most of the leads have over-the-wire desings and the steroid-eluting distal tip provide better long term pacing parameters. Passive fixation leads have single or double angulations, helical shapes or silicon anchors, diameters range between 4-6 Fr. Deployable lobes of the active fixation leads can expand up to 24 Fr allowing stable lead positions. The biggest advantage of the active fixation lead is the 0% chronic dislodgement rate. This secure stabilization of the lead might only be disadvantageous in case of need of extraction.

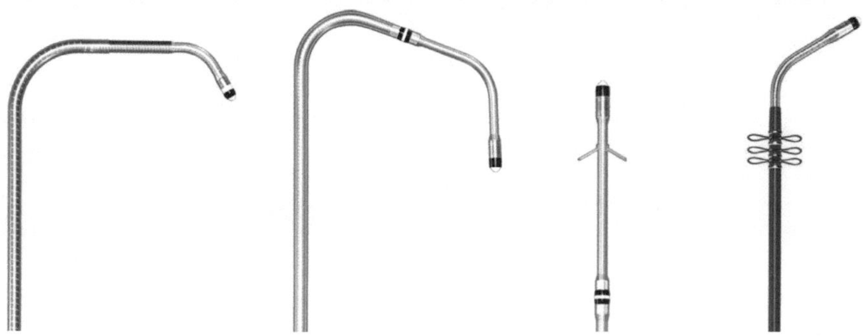

Fig. 11. Unipolar, Bipolar, passive and active fixation leads (courtesy of Medtronic Hungary Ltd.)

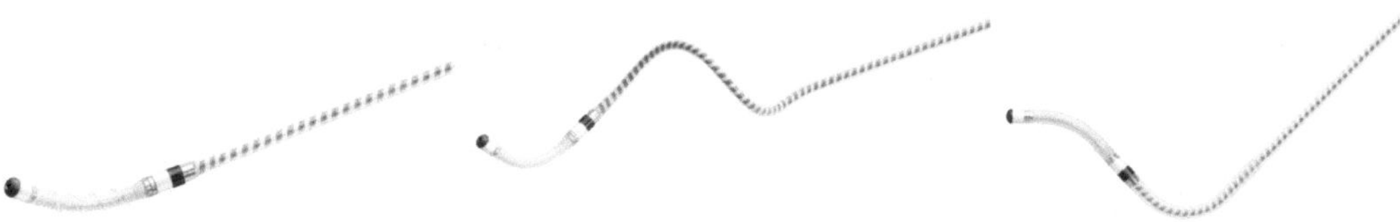

Fig. 12. Bipolar, passive fixation leads (courtesy of Biotronik Hungary Ltd.)

2.10 Venous valve in the CS or severe kinking of the vein

Valves are commonly present in the main CS, but they are usually not recognized. We realize this as a problem, when crossing the valve with the sheath or the LV lead is very difficult (Fig. 13.). Severe tortuousity of the proximal CS can inhibit the advancement of the guiding sheat. Withdrawal of the tip of the guiding sheath more proximal from the valve enhance to find the way over the valve with a 0,014-inch guidewire. Individual formation of the tip of the wire might be necessary. After crossing the valve with a 0,014-inch guidewire, a second 0,035- inch wire should be advanced paralelly. If the second wire is able to cross the valve, predilatation of the valve on the 0,014-inch wire can secure the crossing. The outer diameters of the valves are similar to the main CS, therefore coronary interventional balloons similar to the size of the sheath will not harm the vessel. The purpose is to open the valve for retrograde wiring. If the valves still prevent the advancement, a second and third 0,035- inch guidewire should be inserted into the sheath to the distal CS. This will keep the valve open to the size of the sheath and the three identical wire anchores the system. Using the push-pull technique, pushing the guiding sheath and pulling the wire, crossing can be achieved. This method is useful in case of tortuous and stenotic proximal CS (Fig. 13.).

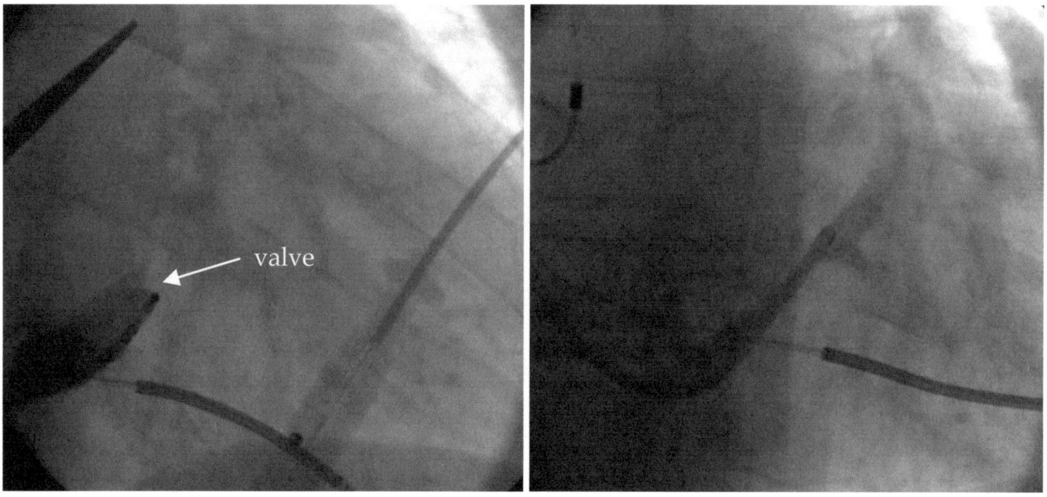

Fig. 13. Upsream occlusion of CS caused by valve in the proximal CS (left), Stenosis of the proximal CS (right)

2.11 How to avoid CS dissection, when to stop the procedure?

A rare, but potentially dangerous complication of the manipulation is the dissection of the CS (Fig.14.). Pericardial tamponade can be lifethreatening, though on the venous, low pressure side of the circulation contrast clouds seem to diminish between the epicardial space without any symptoms. Small amount of persistent contrast in the pericardium or in the myocardium can be followed with X-ray without clinical relevance.

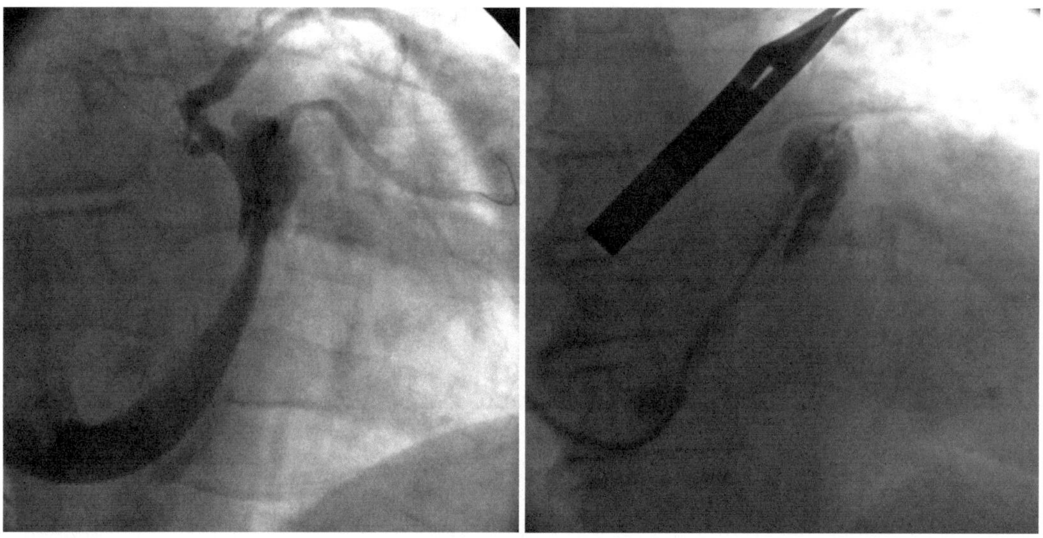

Fig. 14. Dissection of the CS by advancent of the sheath (left), Contrast cloud after positioning the occlusion balloon without a wire (right)

The availability of an intraoperative ultrasound is essential to provide the safety of the patient and to help the decision of discontinuation of the procedure. The completion of the implantation should be contiued as this might be the last chance of the LV lead positioning in the CS if there is no sign of tamponade and there is any chance of finding the CS lumen with a wire. In case of dissection over the wire lead insertion is recommended, after the wire ensures the intraluminal position of the tributary. The most often causes are the forceful or not paralel advancement of the guiding sheath or the occlusion balloon. Using a J guidewire during advancement of the manipulating devices can avoid this complication. The pullback technique of the sheath can help to reach the desired site and injection of small contrast confirms the size and relation between the vein and the balloon as well as the proper position of the sheath in the CS.

2.12 CS myocardial bridge

Myocardial bridge is rare and caueses minor difficulty. This can be suspected when the lumen of the vein filled with contrast varies during the systolic and diastolic phase of the heart (Fig.15.). The problem can overcome by the advancement of the guiding catheter during diastolic phase of the heart cycle. The importance of using guiding wire is increased, because of the higher probability of dissection. The advancement should be in the diastolic phase. The use of occlusion balloon is discouraged, direct contrast filling can prove the tributaries.

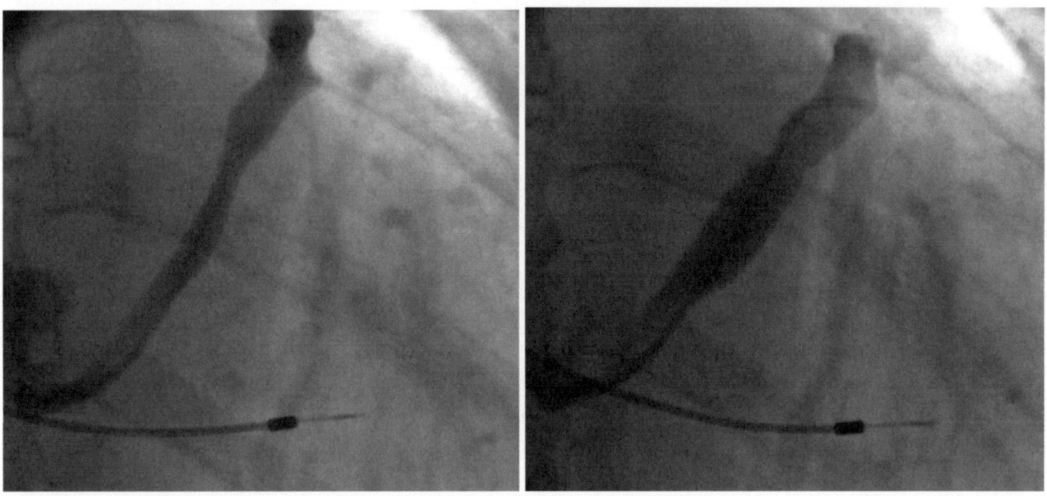

Fig. 15. Muscular bridge in systolic (left) and diastolic phase (right)

3. Reintervention of the LV lead

In a long term follow up 7 % of the transvenous LV leads needed reintervention (Borleffs et al., 2009). These median follow-up of 645 day data are not comparable with others usually terminated at 6 month. In this series 33% of the reinterventions were indicated after 6 months. Reoperation is an other surgical trauma for the patient and might have higher infection rates. Minimal invasive femoral approach technique is feasible and effective for the retraction of the LV lead from distal dislocation (Szilagyi et al., 2008). At reoperation original LV leads might need to be extracted. Passive fixation leads are usually extracted easily, no fibrosus adhesion complication occurs in the coronary sinus. No considerable data are available for the extraction of the active fixation leads. In our limited experience in stented leads series, leads were always extractable when needed and minimal invasive retraction was able to perform in cases of phrenic nerve stimulation. At reoperation the original lead can be inserted to other sidebranch, or new passive or a new active fication lead can be delivered. At surgical approach where irreversible fixation of the lead was performed, reintervention can be solved only with implantation of a new lead. The surgical reoperation carries out further difficulties due to the adhesions, therefore in some surgical techniques at the first implanatation a second back-up lead is applied.

4. Transvenous endocardial pacing - Transseptal approach

Patients who are ineligible for surgical epicardial implantation and have no contraindication for lifelong oral anticoagulation can be selected for this approach. Advantage of this second line option is the same setting used for transvenous epicardial implantation, which makes it easy to convert the unsuccesful CS lead implantation to this rescue approach. The procedure does not require general anaesthesia and minimal postoperative recovery is needed. The significant physiological benefit of endocardial pacing compared to epicardial pacing during CRT was described in a series of 23 patients (Garrigue et al., 2001). The transseptal approach has been used for over 40 years for haemodynamic measurements, mitral and aortic valve angioplasty and in invasive cardiac electrophysiology for left sided accessory pathway ablations as well as for the isolation of the pulmonary veins. Therefore, there is little debate about the risks of the procedure with well experienced operators. However the major concern is about the long term risks of thromboembolic complication and mitral valve disruption or endocarditis related to permanent presence of the LV lead. The first case report was originally described using femoral transseptal puncture and a snare technique via the right jugular vein (Jais et al., 1998). The lead tunneled over the clavicle increases the risk for lead damage and skin erosion. Small modificatons were described until the recently applied techique was clarified (van Gelder et al., 2007).

The transseptal implantation begins with a standard transseptal puncture via the right femoral vein. After the successful puncture, controlled by the left atrial pressure curve, iv. 5000 IU of heparin is administered. The 0,035-inch guidewire is administered to one of the pulmonary veins and then the dilator and the sheath are removed. A 6-8mm wide balloon is inserted and dilated at the septal puncture site. In the guiding sheath a steerable electrophysiological catheter is avanced from the subclavian area towards the septum of the right atrium (Fig.16.).

The balloon is deflated and the EP catheter is advanced transseptally into the left atrium and then to the left ventrical. Holding the EP catheter in position the guiding sheath is forwarded to the left atrium (Fig.17.). The invasive pressures prove the proper localisation of the sheath. The optimal activation site is measured with the EP catheter. Standard bipolar leads are screwed into the desired location of the postero-lateral wall of the LV. Keeping a suffient slack in the lead, the proximal end is sutured in the pectoral region after pacing and sensing threshold tests and then the generator is connected (Fig.18.).

Postoperatively subcutaneous heparin is administered until the target (3,5-4,5) INR is accomplished with oral anticoagulant. Theoretically this might increas the risk of pocket haematoma.

In our practice we supplemented the transseptal technique with the recording of an electroanatomical map during the procedure (CARTO group, Biosense Webster, Diamond

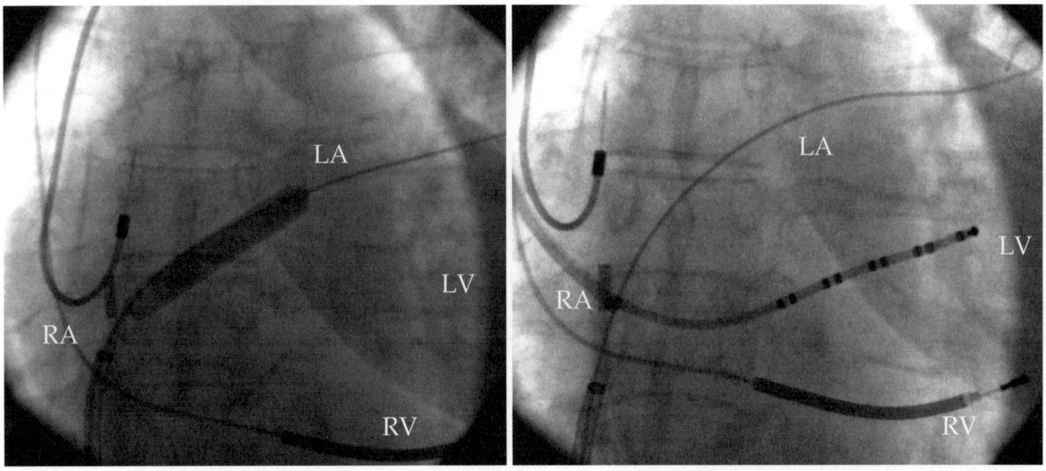

Fig. 16. Transseptal ballon dilatation (left), Advancement of the EP catheter to the left atrium (right)

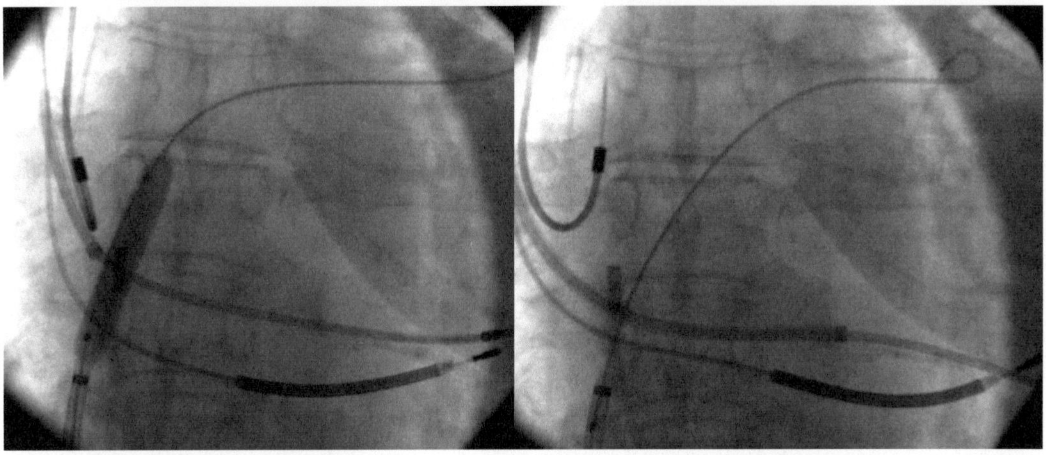

Fig. 17. After balloon deflation (left), the sheath is advanced transapically into the LV (right)

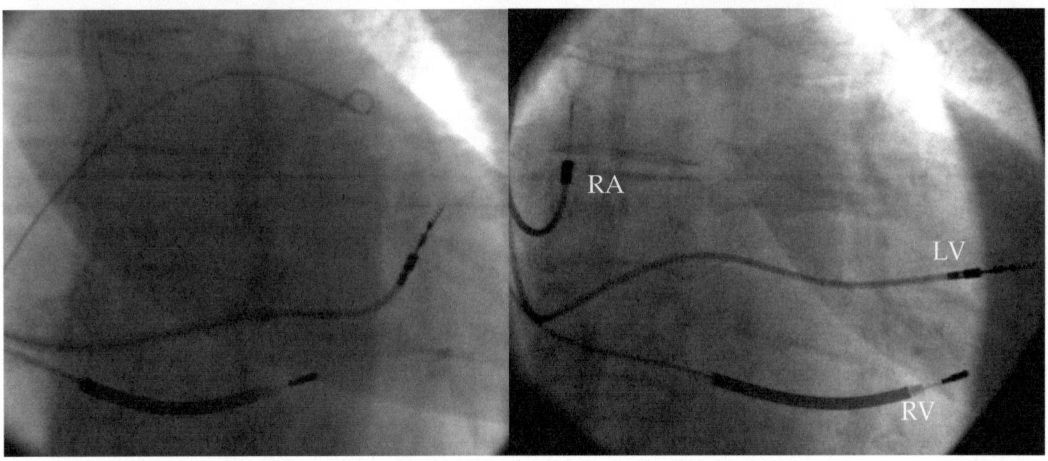

Fig. 18. Active fixation lead is positioned (left), Final position of RA, RVand LV leads (right)

Bar, CA, USA) to identify precisely the latest activated endocardial site of the lateral LV wall, concerning, that in our cases these were the last options for CRT. We used additionally intracardiac echocardiography (ICE) during the puncture and the dilatation of the atrial septum for safety reasons.
The main disadvantage of this technique is the unknown long term thromboembolic risk. While there are only small numbers of patients with endocardial LV pacing lead, we might accept that the risk similar as after mechanical valve implantation. Over an 85±5 month follow up of 6 patients, one patient had LV dislodgment at 3 months necessitating reintervention, later on no significant change in LV electrical parameters was observed. Five patients had thromboembolic event free period, however one patient had transient ischaemic attack whose anticoagulation was accidently interrupted (Pasquie et al., 2007).
This technique seems to be a feasible and safe second option with a benefit of endocardial pacing site. The possible disadvantage is the lifelong antiocagulation, the lead crossing the mitral valve and is inserted into the lateral wall, though no major complications due to this phenomena were published yet.

5. Open chest and percutaneous surgical epicardial approach

The fundamental invention, the first reported CRT implantation case (Cazeau et al., 1994) was described with epicardial LV lead and transvenous insertion of the right atrial and right ventricular (RV), left atrial stimulation was reached via the CS. In the early years, this approach was associated with considerable morbidity (Khan et al., 2009). After the beginning of the CRT era, several inventions were made to achive a more comfortable, feasable and safe procedure. All the other CRT techniques originate from this procedure to overcome the different limitations of the combined epicardial and endocardial lead implantations. The need of genearal anaesthesia, transeosophageal echocardiography controll during the operation, epicardial fat and fixating the epicardial lead on a moving target are disadvantages. The surgical trauma and the recoverey time is appreciably greater than the transvenous LV lead implantation. The most dangerous problem of the surgically implanted epicardial leads, usually used as a rescue technique, is the possibility of chronic increase of threshold, even the loss of permanent CRT. The different surgical epicardial lead implantation reports confirmed excellent long-term results on the basis of the 3 and 6-7 month follow up, but during the 1-5 year follow-up epicardial leads might have a significantly higher failure rate, than the CS leads (Lau, 2009). The benefit of this approach is the direct visual control of the latest contracting segment during the implantation, there is no limitation of the coronary venous anatomy for lead placement and the smaller incidence rate of lead dislodgment and phrenic nerve stimulation. Less flouroscopy and avoidance of intravenous contrast are also advantages over the transvenous approach. There are several currently used surgical approaches to implant the LV pacing leads: the full left thoracotomy with the widest accessibility of the free lateral LV wall, the minimal invasive limited left lateral thoracotomy with smaller postoperative pain and recovery time, the video-assisted thoracoscopy and the robotically assisted left ventricular epicardial lead implantation technique. After development and continous improvement of the transvenous LV implantation to the CS, the open chest access for the surgical epicardial lead placement has become a second line approach. Nevertheless at planned coronary artery bypass graft surgery, valve repair or replacement, epicardial surgical approach might still remain the first choice. The surgical implantation may be preferred in patients with congential heart disease, where the venous anatomy can interfere the transvenous approach.

5.1 Minimal thoracotomy

This epicardial LV lead implantation procedure is performed in an operating room, under general anaesthesia, single-lung ventilation and beating heart. Transeosophageal echocardiography (TEE) control is needed throughout the procedure. A 3 to 5 cm incision is made over the 4th or 5th intercostal space anterior to the midaxillary line. The lung is pushed back with a wet towel and the pericardium is opened anterior to the phrenic nerve. After mapping the left ventricle for optimal pacing site one or two epicardial unipolar or bipolar leads are attached to the target area with implantation tools (Mair et al., 2005). After testing the leads the capped terminal pins are tunneled submuscular to the provisional pocket and the pacemaker is then connected. A chest tube is required postoperativly and can be discontinuated within 48 hours. A recent investigation (Patwala, 2009) described this technique safe and acceptable option, but declaired to remain a second line procedure.

5.2 Video-assisted thoracoscopy (VATS) and epicardial lead implatation

This minimal invasive approach is a routine endoscopic procedure in thoracic surgery. It uses two or three incisions for the ports within the 4th or 5th intercostal space along the aterior and midaxillary line. General anaesthesia and single lung ventilation enables the deflatation of the left lung. The camera and the manipulating instruments are inserted through the different ports. Under visual control the pericardium is opened laterally to the phrenic nerve, the obtus marginalis as landmarks help to identify the desired site and an epicardial lead is screwed into the lateral wall of the LV. After TEE control and pacing threshold test the proximal end of the lead is passed through the medial incision and is tunneled subcutaneously to the pocket. The average operation time was reported 55±16 minutes (Gabor et al., 2005). The procedure is well tolerated, it has minimal postoperative recovery and a very good cosmetic results.

5.3 Robotically assisted left ventricular epicardial lead implantation

This is an emerging second line, effective technique performed with endoscopic assistace (DeRose et al., 2003). The daVinci Robotic Surgical System (Intuitive Surgical Inc., Sunnyvale, California) is composed of a surgeon control console and a surgical arm, that positions and directs the micro-instruments. The instrument is inserted into the chest cavity through two 8 mm ports and the endoscope is inserted through a third 10 mm port in the seventh intercostal space in the posterior axillary line. The surgeon controls the instruments away from the operating field and views the site through a magnified, real three dimensional eyepiece. Computer interfacing allows the scaled motion, eliminates tremor and provides incredibly accurate surgical precision. This technique also needs genearal anaesthesia, single lung intubation and TEE. The left and right arms are placed in the 5th and 9th intercostal space. The pericardium is opened posterior to the phrenic nerve and the region of the obtus marginals is identified to find the latest activating area with a temporary pacing electrode. Two leads are implanted, the second one is for back-up purpose. Both leads are tunneled to the axillar region and the active lead chosen by the best threshold result is connected to the pacemaker. The second lead is capped in case of need of future use. The chest tube for evacuating the air is removed and extubation is performed before leaving the operation room. After short surgical recovery time, the patients are usually discharged at the first postoperative day. Follow-up results of 42 patients comfirmes the operation time on the plateau of the learning curve at 45±13 minutes, while the 3 and 6 month clinical response was 81% and 70%. Three patients experienced loss of lead capture at 1, 9, and 14 months where the second lead had to be activated (Joshi et al., 2005). This procedure comfirmed to be safe and effective allowing minimal invasive rescue therapy after failed transvenous CS lead implantation. Despite of all the benefits of this technique, the greatest disadvantage is the limited accessability and experience with robotic systems. Nowadays only few centres are able to perform the robotic technique with enough experience.

6. Transapical endocardial lead implantation

This new technique combines the minimal invasive surgical approach and the advantage of endocardial pacing. The transapical endocardial approach was invented for the patients with extensive epicardial adhesions, which disabled the epicardial lead implantation (Kassai et al., 2008). Under general anaesthesia, selective bronchial intubation, after transthoracic echocardiographic location of the LV apex, an infraclavicular pocket and a small left thoracotomy is performed. The apex of the left ventricle is punctured and with a Seldinger technique an active fixating lead is inserted into the cavitiy of the left ventrical (Fig. 19. A, B). The bleeding is controlled with purse-string sutures. The guidance of the lead is achieved with a J shaped guide wire under flouroscopy (Fig. 19. C).

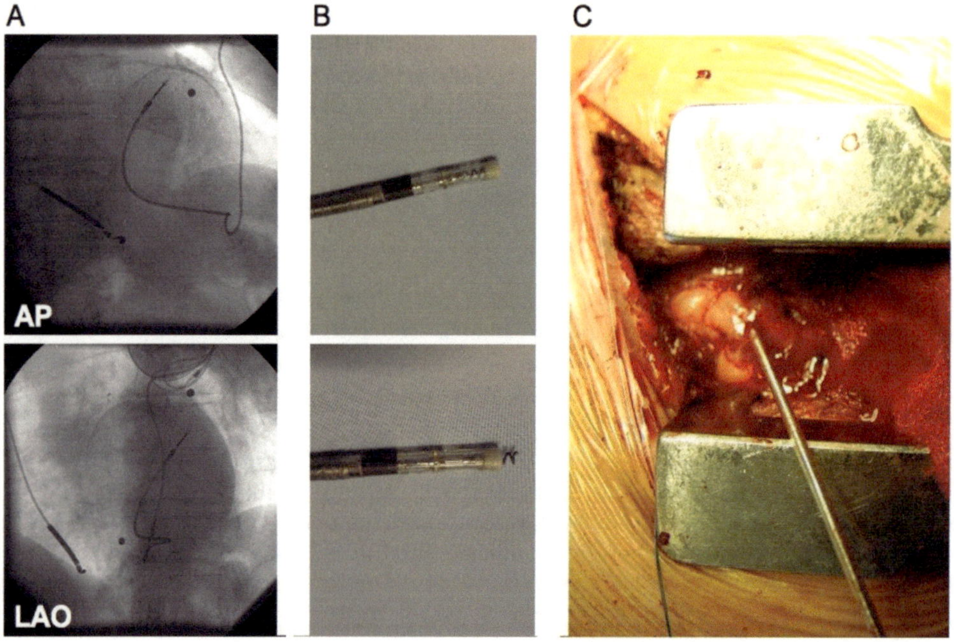

Fig. 19. A. AP and LAO projection of the LV lead, B. Tip of the active fixation lead, C. Intraoperative picture of the apex of the heart with the endocardial lead. (with permission from Kassai)

This allows wide range of manipulation of the lead in the LV cavitiy to find the latest activating, optimal segment. The transapical endocardial lead implantation does not involve the mitral valve, therefore the risk of mitral valve endocarditis is reduced. The lead is conducted into a subcutaneous tunnel up to the pocket of the previously implanted device. Oral anticoagulation is essential, the recommended INR level is identical to other mechanical prothesis.

The advantage of the this technique is the best accessibility of the endocardial segments without the limitations of the anatomy of the tributaries of CS or the surgical difficulties to reach the most delayed segment of the lateral wall. Phrenic nerve stimulation has not been observed. Though this technique is minimal invasive, the need for general anaesthesia and cardiac surgent is fundamental. The risk of oral anticoagulation and thromboemolic complication is thought to be identical to other mechanical valve prothesis or the transseptal endocardial CRT system. The limited experiences (Kassai et al., 2009) restrict this technique as a last resort where other CRT implantation techniques fail.

7. Conclusion

Event though various techniuqes are described to facilitate the LV lead delivery and positioning, the increasing number of CRT continues to pose numbers of challenging cases. The first line approach remains the transvenous epicardial technique with the interventional supplements and with the limitation of the coronary venous anatomy. Alternative approaches remain for the second line options. Incrased experience can help the implanter to choose the best second approach. Surgical access is commonly used, while transseptal and transapical endocardial lead implantations are in the learning curve phase. Stenting of the electrode using a coronary stent might be an effective method to prevent dislocation or phrenic nerve stimulation for selected patients. The possibility of the need of lead extraction should be considered during the selection of the approach. Further research and exprience is needed for the safety and long term efficacy of the alternative techniques.

8. References

Alonso, C. (2009) In the field of cardiac resynchronization therapy is left ventricular pacing via the coronary sinus a mature technique. *Europace.* Vol. 11., No. 5. (May 2009) 544-545. Epub 2009 Mar 18. Print ISSN: 1099-5129, Online ISSN: 1532-2092

Borleffs CJ, van Bommel RJ, Molhoek SG, de Leeuw JG, Schalij MJ, van Erven L. (2009). Requirement for coronary sinus lead interventions and effectiveness of endovascular replacement during long-term follow-up after implantation of a resynchronization device. *Europace.* Vol. 11., No. 5., (May 2008) 607-611. Print ISSN: 1099-5129, Online ISSN: 1532-2092

Cazeau, S., Ritter, P., Bakdach, S., Lazarus, A., Limousin, M., Hernao, L., Mundler, O., Daubert, JC., Mugica, J. (1994) Four chamber pacing in dilated cardiomyopathy. *Pacing Clinical Electrophysiology.* Vol. 11. Pt 2. (Nov 1994) 1974-9. Print ISSN: 0147-8389, Online ISSN: 1540-8159

DeRose, J.J. Jr.; Ashton, R.C. Jr.; Belsley, S.; Swistel, D.G.; Vloka, M.; Ehlert, F.; Shaw, R.; Sackner-Bernstein, J.; Hillel, Z.; Steinberg, J.S. (2003) Robotically assisted left ventricular epicardial lead implantation for biventricular pacing. *Journal of the American College of Cardiology.* Vol. 41., No. 8., (Apr 2003) 1414-1419. ISSN: 0735-1097

Foley, P.W.; Leyva, F.; Frenneaux, M.P. (2009) What is treatment success in cardiac resynchronisation therapy? *Europace* Vol.11., Suppl. 5., (Nov 2009) 58-65. Print ISSN: 1099-5129, Online ISSN: 1532-2092

Gabor, S.; Prenner, G.; Wasler, A.; Schweiger, M.; Tscheliessnigg, K.H.; Smolle-Jüttner, F.M.; (2005) A simplified technique for implantation of left ventricular epicardial leads for biventricular re-synchronization using video-assisted thoracoscopy (VATS). *European Journal of Cardio-thoracic Surgery.* Vol. 28., Iss. 6. (Dec 2005) 797-800. ISSN: 1010-7940

Garrigue, S.; Jaïs, P.; Espil, G.; Labeque, J.N.; Hocini, M.; Shah, D.C.; Haïssaguerre, M.; Clementy J. (2001) Comparison of chronic biventricular pacing between epicardial and endocardial left ventricular stimulation using Doppler tissue imaging in patients with heart failure *American Journal of Cardiology* Vol. 88., Iss.8 (Oct 2001) 858-862. Print ISSN: 0002-9149

Joshi, S.; Steinberg, J.S.; Ashton, R.C. Jr.; Balaram, S.; Fischer, A.; DeRose, J.J. Jr. (2005) Follow-up of robotically assisted left ventricular epicardial leads for cardiac resynchronization therapy. *Journal of the American College of Cardiology.* Vol. 46., No. 12., Vol. 46. No. 12 (Dec 2005) 2358-2359. ISSN: 0735-1097

Kassai I.; Foldesi C.; Szekely A.; Szili-Torok T. (2008). New method for cardiac resynchronization therapy: transapical endocardial lead implantation for left ventrical free wall pacing. *Europace.* Vol.10., No. 7., (Jul 2008) 882-3. Epub 2008 Apr. 17. Print ISSN: 1099-5129, Online ISSN: 1532-2092

Kassai I., Mihalcz A., Foldesi C., Kardos A., Szili-Torok T. (2009) A Novel Approach for Endocardial Resynchronization Therapy: Initial Experience with Transapical Implantation of the Left Ventricular Lead. *Heart Surg Forum.* Vol. 12., No.3., (Jun 2009.) 137-140. ISSN:1522-6662

Khan, F.Z.; Virdee, M.S; Fynn, S.P.; Dutka, D.P. (2009). Left ventricular lead placement in cardiac resyncrnisation therapy: where and how? *Europace.* Vol. 11., No. 5., (May 2009) 554-561. Print ISSN: 1099-5129, Online ISSN 1532-2092

Lau, W.E. (2009) Achieving permanent left ventricular pacing – options and choice. *Pacing Clinical Electrophysiology.* Vol. 32. Iss. 11. (Nov 2009) 1466-1477. Print ISSN: 0147-8389 Online ISSN: 1540-8159

Mair, H.; Sachweh, J.; Meuris, B.; Noller, G.; Schmockel, M.; Schuetz, A.; Reichart, B.; Daebritz, S.; Surgical epicardial left ventricular lead versus coronary sinus lead placement in biventricular pacing. *European Journal of Cardiothoracic Surgery.* Vol.: 27. Iss.2. (Feb 2005) 235-242. ISSN: 1010-7940

Pasquié J.L.; Massin, F.; Macia, J.C.; Gervasoni, R.; Bortone, A.; Cayla, G; Grolleau, R.; Leclercq F. (2007) Long-Term Follow-Up of Biventricular Pacing Using a Totally Endocardial Approach in Patients with End-Stage Cardiac Failure. *Pacing Clinical Electrophysiology* Vol. 30. Suppl. 1. (Jan 2007) S31-33. Print ISSN: 0147-8389 Online ISSN: 1540-8159

Patwala, A.; Woods, P.; Clements, R.; Albouaini, K.; Rao, A.; Goldspink, D.; Tan, L.-B.; Oo, A.; Wright, D. (2009) A prospective longitudinal evaluation of the benefits of epicardial lead placement for cardiac resynchronization therapy. *Europace.* Vol.: 11. Iss.: 10. (2009) 1323-1329. Print ISSN: 1099-5129

Szilagyi Sz.; Merkely B.; Roka A.; Zima E.; Fulop G.; Kutyifa V.; Szucs G.; Becker D.; Apor A.; Geller L. (2007). Stabilization of the coronary sinus electrode position with coronary stent implantation to prevent and treat dislocation. *J.Cardiovasc Electrophysiology.* Vol.18., No.3., (Mar 2007) 303-7. ISSN: 1540-8167

Szilagyi Sz.; Merkely B.; Zima E.; Kutyifa V.; Szucs G.; Fulop G.; Molnar L.; Szabolcs Z.; Geller L. (2008). Minimal invasive coronary sinus lead reposition technique for the treatment of phrenic nerve stimulation. *Europace.* Vol. 10., No. 10., (Oct 2008) 1157-60. Epub 2008 Aug 14. Online ISSN 1532-2092, Print ISSN: 1099-5129

Van Gelder BM, Scheffer MG, Meijer A, Bracke FA. (2007) Transseptal endocardial left ventricular pacing: An alternative technique for coronary sinus lead placement in cardiac resynchronization therapy. *Heart Rhythm.* Vol. 4. No. 4.,(2007) 454–460. ISSN: 1547-5271

4

The Alternative Atrial Pacing Sites

Jacek Gajek, Przemysław Skoczyński and Agnieszka Sławuta
Department of Cardiology, Wroclaw Medical University, Wrocław, Poland

1. Introduction

A permanent pacemaker implantation changes the electrophysiological and hemodynamic conditions in the heart. The electric system of the pacemaker meets the two main functions of the device, i.e. the stimulation - pacing and sensing of own cardiac rhythm. The possibility of an atrial stimulation sending the electric impulses for the whole heart is the most physiologic pacing mode. The pacing site is no longer determined by the technical and anatomical limitation since the introduction of active fixation leads enables the lead positioning and fixation in almost each place within the heart muscle. Different electrophysiological properties of various parts of the atria influence the pacing and sensing in different ways. The physiologic conduction of an electrical wave front from the sinus node to the atria and then to the atrio-ventricular node and the ventricles favours the optimal hemodynamic function of various parts of the heart muscle, changing additionally with regard to the basic rhythm and metabolic demands during a physical activity.

The physiologic electrical activation of the atria originates within the sinoatrial node, located in front of and medially from the superior vena cava ostium to the right atrium, then spreads ahead and down across the right atrium and to the left atrium throughout the conducive tissue band called Bachmann's bundle. This leads to a rush and efficient activation of the left atrium resulting in single P wave in electrocardiogram, not separating the both atria conduction. The interatrial conduction takes place also within the posterior part of fossa ovalis and coronary sinus. This kind of activation leads to the proper mechanical sequence of contraction covering firstly the free right atrial wall, then interatrial septum and subsequently posterior, anterior and lateral left atrial walls at the same time. The physiologic delay of left atrial contraction in relation to the right atrium amounts to 22+/-11 ms (1-3). The Bachmann's bundle is the fastest way to carry the activation from the right to the left atrium and its dysfunction or a complete block is connected with an unfavourable sequence of electrical and hemodynamic changes. This results in an impaired electrical and mechanical function of the left atrium leading usually to atrial fibrillation. Other causes and diseases such as arterial hypertension, inflammatory process and fibrosis take part in a deterioration of an atrial muscle function favouring the arrhythmia (4, 5).

2. The functions of atrial pacemaker

The ideal atrial stimulation should provide an optimal interplay among the three functions of the device: the pacing of the heart, mechanic or hemodynamic atrial function and antiarrhythmic influences on the atrial muscle. The different locations of the atrial electrode influence these functions in different ways depending on atrial pacing and sensing as well as atrioventricular conduction.

3. The electrical properties of pacemaker-atria unit

The implantation of atrial electrode changes the electrophysiological conditions within the atria. Many studies have shown that the altered electrophysiology could be potentially harmful or beneficial with regard to the hemodynamic and arrhythmogenic properties. The stimulation of coronary sinus was the subject of several studies. Betts et al. assessed the right atrium activation during coronary sinus pacing in experimental conditions in porcine model. They concluded that the site of the earliest activation of the right atrium depends on the part of coronary sinus where the electrode is located, but the main part of the right atrial muscle was activated via posterior wall rather than from the coronary sinus ostium (6). The total atrial activation time was studied by Roithinger et al. (7) in 28 patients without a structural heart disease. The study was performed after catheter ablation of supreventricular arrhythmias. The authors showed that the shortest total activation time could be achieved during Bachmann's bundle pacing in comparison to other stimulation sites such as distal coronary sinus, its ostium as well as high and low right lateral atrium. The influence of different right atrial pacing site on intracardiac signal-averaged electrocardiogram was studied by Kutarski et al. (8) in 24 patients undergoing biatrial pacing system implantation. The authors concluded that right atrial appendage pacing prolongs the duration of atrial potential recorded in external and internal leads. Coronary sinus stimulation is not inferior as compared to sinus rhythm and biatrial pacing carries potential benefits with regard to late potential elimination and arrhythmia protection.

4. The hemodynamic properties of the paced atria in relation to different pacing sites.

Patients with indications to atrial or atrioventricular pacing are not a homogenous group. Both dysfunctions: the impulse generation disturbances or conductive tissue disease as the indications for pacing in general as the patient's co-morbidities as well make the choice of appropriate atrial pacing site difficult. It is even more difficult to prove one of them being superior over the other ones. The important factor influencing the results of the studies and the clinical outcome in a particular patient are the interatrial conduction disturbances resulting in an electrical and hemodynamic deterioration and a subsequent atrial fibrillation. The results of small studies suggest that the interatrial conduction disorders affect approximately 30% of patients with the sick sinus syndrome and up to 12% of patients with atrioventricular conduction disorders (9). The most special group of patients are those subjected to the cardiac resynchronisation, in whom the proper depolarization sequence of atria and ventricles is particularly important and subtle differences in an interatrial and interventricular conduction delay may determine the effectiveness of the whole procedure. As far as the interventricular delay can be the subject of device programming, the differences in the interatrial conduction during pacing and sensing with regard to a different atrial lead position are of a particular interest. The choice of an atrial lead implantation site influences the electrical and mechanical properties of both atria. The time of an electrical activation of both atria and subsequent hemodynamic depends on the location of its origin, so the distance to reach the whole atrial muscle and the conductive properties of the muscle. The artificial pacing resulting in the stimulation of working myocardium leads a priori to the slower conduction of a depolarization wave. The extent of this slowing depends on the muscle properties, the conductive tissue status as well as on the distance of the pacing site to the conductive structures. The dimensions of the atria and the degree of their remodelling - fibrosis or myocytes loss - also play an important role. The duration of both atria activation influences their hemodynamic function. Interatrial and intraatrial conduction disturbances result in a loss of an atrial contraction synchrony, being in particular expressed in the left atrium. The deleterious effects of the interatrial conduction slowing and a non-physiological conduction affect the mechanical and electrical left atrial function. The mechanical results of an improper contraction sequence of the left atrium structures influence its systolic function. The inappropriate time relation of the left atrium and the left ventricle systolic and diastolic function leads to the pressure overload of the left atrium and its remodelling and enlargement (10). The locally activated renin-angiotensin-aldosterone system contributes to the mechanical and electrical remodelling as much as the coexistence of arterial hypertension and myocardial ischemia in some patients. A longer time of the left atrial activation could lead to its contraction during a partial mitral valve closure. Such circumstances contribute to an even more pronounced pressure overload and could be easily detected by the echocardiographic assessment of a mitral diastolic flow, showing sharp A wave cut by ventricular systole. The presence of electrical remodelling resulting from the described pathophysiologic processes ends in conduction and refractoriness dispersion both being substrates for re-entrant arrhythmias maintenance (11, 12). The systolic dysfunction of the left atrium originates in asynchronous contraction of its structures, as the improper timing of its systole with regard to ventricular diastole diminishes the contribution to the left ventricle endsystolic filling. This is particularly important in patients with diastolic dysfunction of the left ventricle, being the other independent factor of an atrium enlargement. All the influences could lead to atrial fibrillation and a complete loss of an active hemodynamic atrial function. Therefore the optimization of atrial pacing site is of a special importance in sicker patients with an initial inter- and intraatrial conduction disturbances, a poorer mechanical function and a greater risk of its further deterioration.

As already mentioned above the population of patients undergoing the permanent pacemaker implantation shows atrial conduction abnormalities as well as the chronotropic dysfunction or atrioventricular block being the primary cause of device implantation. Non-optimal atrial electrode placement in patients with such pre-existing disorders results in its increase and the progression of pathophysiologic process. The prolongation of the interatrial conduction during pacing can be observed in the surface electrocardiogram as the prolonged and deformed P wave. There are many small studies regarding the different atrial pacing sites and the duration of P wave. It was shown that the stimulation of the right atrial appendage results in the longest activation of both atria in comparison to the Bachmann's bundle (13) and interatrial septum pacing site (7, 14-16). The stimulation of septum is considered in many papers to be the best pacing place with regard to the both atria activation time (17-19), which seems to be concordant with a theoretical model. In some papers this kind of atrial stimulation site was also combined with the prevention of paroxysmal atrial fibrillation (20, 21). On the other hand the right atrium appendage pacing provides a better hemodynamic response - better left ventricle filling and a higher cardiac output in comparison to the right atrium free wall stimulation. This last location seems to be the worst pacing site (22). The shortening of the depolarization of both atria and the subsequent shortening of P wave duration related to the optimization of pacing site does not always carry the measurable benefits - both hemodynamic and antiarrhythmic ones. In a number of small studies it was shown that the benefit of such a stimulation was observed only in patients with initially larger interatrial conduction disturbances and/or paroxysmal atrial fibrillation because of the fact that none of the atrial pacing settings will be better than the own physiological conduction in the sinus rhythm and the non-disturbed conductive system (13, 23). In one randomized trial of Hermida et al. the benefits of low septum pacing were shown only in the group of patients with paroxysm of atrial fibrillation during three months before pacemaker implantation (24). A significant shortening of left atrium depolarization requires programming of shorter atrioventricular delays which in turn does not allow to avoid the ventricular stimulation. Moreover the non-physiological spreading of the activation wave front from the mitral annulus because of the proximity of coronary sinus can also be responsible for the limited benefits of this kind of pacing (25, 26). The advantageous hemodynamic response from interatrial septum pacing was observed in the study of Miyazaki et al. (27). They showed that the shortening of atrial depolarization by such pacing mode also shortens the difference in both atria contraction assessed as the time difference between the peak of A wave in mitral and tricuspid diastolic flow. In a 24-month-long follow-up period the mitral diastolic flow improved and the left atrium dimensions decreased. But the patients included in this study already had the documented history of paroxysmal atrial fibrillation and interatrial conduction delay (27). In the study of Di Pede et al. assessing the usefulness of interatrial pacing in patients with cardiac resynchronization there was no superiority in comparison to the right atrium appendage pacing but the patients did not have significant interatrial conduction delay. In patients treated with cardiac resynchronization therapy the increased atrioventricular conduction time results in a greater percentage of a ventricular stimulation which in turn paradoxically could contribute to the better hemodynamic result (28).

In most of the mentioned studies the results of different atrial pacing locations were assessed in acute settings or with a relatively short observation period. It can be assumed that the beneficial effects could only be seen in a longer time or the patients with less pronounced interatrial conduction abnormalities will benefit from such pacing mode later because of the progressive nature of the sick sinus syndrome and paroxysmal atrial fibrillation. On the other hand the development of the deleterious results of non-optimal atrial electrode location resulting in atrial systolic dysfunction can occur in a time period much longer than the follow-up of most studies.

Another factor influencing the described results in patients with resynchronization could be the difference between pacing and sensing of sinus rhythm. In this subgroup of patients the usually observed tachycardia leads mostly to the atrial sensing ventricular pacing mode of a pacemaker action. In this case and normal or nearly normal interatrial conduction the specific location of atrial electrode does not matter at all.

The solution of an increased atrial conduction time and non-physiologic activation pattern could be the biatrial pacing. However the beneficial effects of this kind of atrial pacing were shown only in patients with initially pronounced interatrial conduction disturbances (29-31, 32). The various electrode configuration studied always included the one implanted in the coronary sinus ostium and the other located in the right atrium appendage or Bachmann's bundle. Similarly as in the interatrial septum stimulation it was shown that biatrial stimulation results in shortening of both atria depolarization and shorter P wave duration in surface electrocardiogram. Matsumoto el al. observed a significant improvement of atrial systole synergy using the strain doppler imaging technique to assess the local myocardium movements (33). In the largest study published Dąbrowska-Kugacka et al. assessed the impact of different pacing configuration - single and biatrial - on the electromechanical sequence. They proved that the most beneficial single right atrium pacing location in patients with interatrial conduction disturbances is the Bachmann's bundle region of atrial roof, carrying similar results as biatrial pacing. The right atrium appendage location was related to the latest left atrium walls activation and contraction, whereas the stimulation of coronary sinus admittedly led admittedly to the earliest left atrium activation but resulted also in the significant dyssynchrony within the right atrium (34). These surprising results are difficult to comment because the mechanical function of the right atrium has not been extensively studied. It seems quite probable that the function of low pressure system of right heart does not really benefit or worsen from any kind of optimization of right atrium pacing. In the paper mentioned, in comparison to the work of Wang et al. (1) there was no dyssynchrony within the right atrium observed during the right atrium appendage stimulation. This could be in part the result of different assessment techniques of both studies. Wang et al. used the M-mode view and Dąbrowska-Kugacka et al. studied the atrial synchrony using the tissue doppler imaging. The results of the latter study showed explicitly that the biatrial pacing of both coronary ostium – right atrium appendage and coronary ostium – Bachmann's bundle led to the most physiological effect. Moreover, Stockburger et al. showed that biatrial pacing (coronary ostium – right atrium appendage) contributes to the better left atrium systolic function assessed by the transesophageal echocardiography. Unfortunately they also observed more disturbed diastolic mitral flow. The E wave velocity diminished in comparison to the sinus rhythm, what could be in part the result of the higher pacing frequency (35). The better systolic function of the left atrium appendage can be responsible for lower thrombosis and embolisation rate. Prakash et al. showed that the biatrial stimulation within the right atrium results in a faster activation and a better hemodynamic function of the left atrium, as well as higher A wave velocity in mitral diastolic flow spectrum which could lead to better left ventricle filling and higher cardiac output (36). The observation of Takagi et al. confirmed that biatrial pacing in combination with higher pacing rates promote the sinus rhythm maintenance after direct current cardioversion, prevent atrial fibrillation paroxysms and shorten the atrial stunning period (37).

5. The antiarrhythmic properties of atrial pacing

The atrial stimulation in patients with the sick sinus syndrome eliminates bradycardia as a clinical problem per se and on the other hand prevents bradycardia related dispersion of refractoriness and premature atrial beats eliminating the substrate and triggers for atrial fibrillation. The standard location of an atrial electrode in the right atrium appendage does not fit the physiologic electrical activation direction which occurs normally from the sinus node, so from the rear roof towards the front and lateral wall, to the interventricular septum and left atrium. This is the cause for the lengthening of both atria activation observed as broadening of P wave in the surface electrocardiogram. The optimal positioning of atrial lead or leads can take into account the results of studies examining the electrocardiographic predictors of atrial fibrillation.

The atrial activation parameters were studied by Bennet (14) using an invasive electrophysiological study with single and 2 points stimulation within the right atrium. The studied positions included right atrium appendage, coronary sinus ostium, interatrial septum and simultaneously: right atrium appendage and coronary sinus ostium. The studied parameters were the duration of both atria activation, the atrioventricular conduction time and the synchronous activation of both atria. The total activation of both atria took much longer during right atrium appendage stimulation in comparison to septum, coronary sinus ostium and biatrial stimulation. The right atrium appendage pacing resulted also in a slightly longer atrioventricular conduction. The conclusions from this study taking into account the similar results of septal, coronary sinus and biatrial stimulation strongly suggest the benefits from interatrial septum pacing, keeping in mind the relative simplicity of the implantation procedure in comparison to the cannulation of coronary sinus. These results are also against the biatrial stimulation because of the use of two electrodes and without carrying additional benefits from this pacing mode. The placement of an atrial electrode within the coronary sinus ostium can have another potential disadvantage because of the difficulties or the impossibility to place there another electrode for left ventricle stimulation in order to achieve ventricular resynchronization. The upgrading of pre-existing pacing device in patients suffering from heart failure in such conditions could be particularly difficult or demanding the placement of left ventricle epicardial electrode surgically. In the light of this study and the technical implication the best location of single lead atrial pacing seems to be interventricular septum.

The simplest method of an electrical activity assessment within the atria is the measurement of the duration of P wave in surface electrocardiogram. There is a certain evidence that the prolongation of P wave duration indicates the intra- and interatrial conduction disturbances and is related to more frequent and longer paroxysmal atrial fibrillation occurrence in comparison to patients without this finding. The conduction abnormalities are most probably not uniform, location dependent leading to the differences in P wave duration in different ECG leads. The marker of these differences is the so called P wave dispersion being beside the P wave duration the well established predictor of atrial fibrillation in selected groups of patients. The sole prolongation of the P wave duration was related with a greater risk of paroxysmal atrial fibrillation, a risk of postoperative atrial fibrillation (38-40), and the P wave duration of more than 120 ms with typical inferior leads morphology (notched (+/+) or biphasic (+/-)) is a marker of interatrial conduction block and an increased risk of any atrial tacharrhythmia (38, 41, 42). In the study of Kristensen et al. (43) the described parameters were assessed during the sinus rhythm and 70 bpm and 100 bpm atrial stimulation with the electrode placed on the interatrial septum and the high right atrium. The P wave duration during high right atrium pacing was significantly longer as compared to septal location. During pacing with the higher rate 100 bpm the P wave duration was significantly longer than during pacing 70 bpm in both electrode locations. The main result of the study was that neither P wave duration nor P wave dispersion were the predictors of atrial fibrillation paroxysm in patients with the sick sinus syndrome. De Sisti et al. (44) assessed the influence of the P wave duration on atrial fibrillation burden after a permanent pacemaker implantation. The study group consisted of 140 patients with the sick sinus syndrome with pacing indications and the medical history of at least 2 episodes of atrial fibrillation within the preceding 1 year. The results showed that the prolonged duration of P wave is an independent marker of a risk of atrial fibrillation after implantation. The P wave assessment included not only the duration but also the morphology of P wave. The background for this study were the investigations of Bayes de Luna et al. (38) indicating that the presence of broadened and biphasic P wave is the marker of advanced interatrial conduction disturbances in 4% of the studied population whereas the additional presence of notched P wave in inferior leads considered as less pronounced conduction disorders increased the percentage of patients with interatrial conduction disturbances to 16. In the study of De Sisti et al. the presence of abnormal P wave (notched or biphasic) was a strong predictor of chronic atrial fibrillation after the pacemaker implantation. In a statistical analysis only the left atrial dimensions positively correlated with the P wave duration but in multiregresion Cox hazard ratio neither left atrium dimensions nor the other clinical parameters studied increased an atrial fibrillation risk. The P wave duration was also assessed in the study of Endoh et al. (45). The study was carried out in 57 patients undergoing the pacemaker implantation and aimed to assess the P wave duration in the sinus rhythm and stimulation with the right atrium appendage electrode. The patients were divided into two groups according to the presence of episodes of atrial fibrillation in the medical history (group I and II) and without such events (group III). The group III - without atrial fibrillation - was further divided into patients with the paced P wave duration of less (IIIa) and more (IIIb) than 130 ms. The duration of the P wave during the sinus rhythm in group III was longer than in group I and II, but the paced P wave in group IIIa was similar than in groups I and II. The results indicated the prognostic value of the prolonged P wave duration for atrial fibrillation episodes. Stabile et al. showed the protective value against atrial fibrillation recurrences of single lead atrial pacing in patients with a right atrium conduction delay and an increased dispersion of refractoriness (46).

The duration of the P wave during various site atrial pacing was also assessed in the study of Hung-Fat Tse et al. (47). The electrode was placed in right atrium appendage, high interatrial septum, coronary sinus ostium and distal coronary sinus. In comparison to the duration of the P wave during the sinus rhythm the duration was significantly prolonged during right atrium appendage as well as distal coronary sinus and showed no significant difference during septal, coronary sinus ostium, biatrial: simultaneous right atrium appendage and coronary sinus ostium stimulation. Moreover, the P wave duration was significantly shorter during the stimulation of the septum and both biatrial sites: right atrium appendage and coronary sinus ostium and right atrium appendage and distal coronary sinus in comparison to the right atrium appendage pacing. The results indicate that the septal location or biatrial pacing may reduce or slow down the development of the atrial substrate for fibrillation through the reduction of both atria activation time or make it slower. The results of the studies indicate that the interatrial septum pacing may exert some antiarrhythmic action on the atria, even without any antiarrhythmic pacing algorithms. De Voogt et al. (48) extensively studied the stability of pacing and sensing parameters in relation to the location of atrial electrode - right atrium appendage versus low interatrial septum. Six weeks after the implantation procedure and then after 3 and 6 months the pacing threshold did not differ between the studied groups. After 3 and 6 months the higher voltage of the P wave in the low interatrial septum reached the statistical significance. After 6 weeks the electrodes inserted in the right atrium appendage showed a higher resistance but the difference was no longer statistically significant after 6 months of follow-up. The voltage of the far field R wave during ventricular pacing was higher in right atrium appendage location after 6 weeks but after 3 and 6 months was higher in low interatrial septum site. The far field R wave signals of more than 0,5 mV were observed in both groups/electrode locations (right atrium appendage 88% and low interatrial septum 93%). Even if the far field R wave voltage significantly differed between the groups it had no clinical significance. The interval between the ventricular stimulus and the far field R wave sensing on the atrial electrode was slightly longer in the right atrium appendage location as compared to the septal location and was probably caused by the depolarization vector direction. Nevertheless the voltage of far field R wave exceeding 0,5 mV in most patients in both studied groups did not allow to set the atrial sensing below 0,5 mV, which seems to be necessary for the confirmation of atrial fibrillation. The results indicate that the long-term pacing of the interatrial septum is a feasible, safe and beneficial alternative of the atrial electrode location. The assessment of the influence of septal pacing was also the purpose of the study of Hakacova et al. (49). Group 1 (n=22) received atrial pacing using a single-active fixation lead in the atrial septum above the bundle of His near the foramen ovale and group 2 (n=22) received 'standard' right atrium pacing - a single - active fixation lead was placed in the high right atrium. Devices were programmed in a standardized manner. There were 43 patients who completed 6 months of the follow-up and 22 patients who completed 12 months of the follow-up. The important limitation of the study was a relatively small number of patients in both groups. The atrial fibrillation burden was assessed by the number of mode-switch events of the devices and the arrhythmia duration. In the group of right atrium appendage electrode location there was a greater number of mode-switch episodes and a longer total arrhythmia duration in comparison to the group 1 but the difference was pronounced but not statistically significant only after the 12-month-long follow-up. The small number of 12 months observations could be responsible for that finding but the study rather support the concept of an interatrial septum stimulation in patients with atrial fibrillation as the preventive measure.

The location of great expectations regarding the antiarrhythmic influences of atrial pacing is the Bachmann's bundle – the group of muscle fascicles originating from crista terminalis in the proximity of the sinus node and aiming toward the left atrium in the atrial roof above the interatrial septum. The bundle divides into the fascicles going to the anterior and posterior left atrial wall. Some of the fascicles penetrate the left atrium appendage and other ones dissolve among pulmonary veins ostia. The Bachmann's bundle makes the way for impulses to travel between the right and the left atrium. The histological structure of the Bachmann's bundle fascicles resembles more the Purkinje fascicle than the working muscle cells resulting in a faster interatrial conduction and thus shortening the P wave duration (50). The stimulation of the Bachmann's bundle shortens both atria electrical activation, shortens the P wave, improves the symmetry of the left atrial activation, shortens also the sinus node recovery time (18). The long-term electrophysiological properties (sensing, pacing threshold, resistance) of the Bachmann's bundle region in terms of permanent pacing are comparable with that of right atrium appendage. In the study of Bailin et al. (13) the group of 57 patients with the atrial electrode located in the right atrium appendage was compared to the 63 patients with Bachmann's bundle pacing. The paced P wave duration was significantly shorter during the Bachmann's bundle stimulation as compared to the sinus rhythm whereas the right atrium appendage pacing showed a longer P wave. Patients with Bachmann's bundle pacing had longer atrial fibrillation free survival in comparison to the other electrode location. The time of the implantation procedure did not differ significantly between the two approaches indicating the feasibility and safety of the Bachmann's bundle region implantation. There were also no differences with regard to pacing thresholds, sensing parameters and impedance between the studied group during the procedure and after 6 weeks, 6 and 12 months. Nigro et al. (51) studied the stability of sensing and pacing parameters of atrial electrodes implanted in the Bachmann's bundle and right atrium appendage in a group of patients with type I myotonic dystrophy. The point of interest was raised because of sensing and pacing problems in patients with Steinert disease after right atrium appendage electrode insertion. The same authors already confirmed in another study better sensing and pacing parameters in the region of high interatrial septum and/or the Bachmann's bundle in comparison to the right atrium appendage during the implantation procedure (52). The subsequent study in patients with type I myotonic dystrophy was a prospective one. The initial amplitude of sinus P wave was the same in both groups but after the 12- and 24-month-long follow-up the values increased significantly in the Bachmann's bundle stimulation. The pacing threshold was similar during the implantation and it rose significantly during the follow-up in patients with right atrium appendage electrode location. There were no differences of other parameters such as electrodes impedance, the presence of far field R wave and the frequency of electrodes dislodgement.

In the PASTA study (53) the analysis was performed to assess the influence of alternative pacing sites on the events of atrial fibrillation in patients with the sick sinus syndrome. The study was carried out in 142 patients with atrial electrode located in: right atrium free wall, right atrium appendage, coronary sinus ostium and biatrial pacing in right atrium appendage and coronary sinus ostium. Thus the model included the standard pacing sites and the alternative ones. There was no difference in the burden of atrial fibrillation with regard to different sites of atrial pacing. The prevalence of the ventricular stimulation was about 60% and slightly less but not significant with the right free wall electrode location. The percentage of ventricular pacing was relatively high with recommended parameters of atrioventricular delay of 30 ms more than a spontaneous conduction but as the values were similar in all groups there are no reasons to assume that this could influence the obtained results. The coronary sinus and biatrial location was combined with more dislodgements and a significantly longer implantation procedure time.

Taking into accounts the results of the studies of Saksena et al. (54, 55), Prakash et al. (36), Delfaut et al. (56) and Bailin et al. (57) the alternative atrial pacing sites could be of a possible interest in the secondary prevention of atrial fibrillation and could be beneficial in comparison to standard atrial electrode location. However, the concept of antiarrhythmic properties of interatrial septum or biatrial stimulation has many limitations, some of them mentioned already before. The main limitations in the interpretation of the obtained results are the small number of studied subjects and non-homogenous groups of patients. In the study of Delfaut et al. (56) the patients with symptomatic recurrent atrial fibrillation were included whereas the study of Bailin et al. (57) included patients with paroxysmal atrial fibrillation. In the second study the results showed that the Bachmann's bundle pacing resulted in slowing the progression of paroxysmal atrial fibrillation in its permanent form without pharmacotherapy. In the studies of Delfaut et al. and Saksena et al. (54, 55, 56) the pacing prolonged the time to first atrial fibrillation recurrence in the patients treated with class I and III antiarrhythmic drugs.

In their studies de Voogt et al. (58) and Padeletti et al. (23, 59) have obtained different results in comparison to those previously mentioned. The studied hypothesis was the impact of different atrial pacing sites on the secondary prevention of atrial fibrillation. There were no differences between the stimulation of low interatrial septum and right atrium appendage with respect of arrhythmia recurrences in patients with indications to atrial pacing and paroxysmal atrial fibrillation. The main difference between the discussed studies is a huge difference between the incidence of permanent atrial fibrillation development in PASTA study (53) (3-6%) and Bailin et al. study (57), where in the right atrium appendage group it was as high as 50% and in the Bachmann's bundle group it amounted to 25% during the follow-up. It is possible that the lack of influence of alternative pacing sites on atrial fibrillation depends mainly on this low incidence of arrhythmia recurrence and maintenance. The low incidence of atrial fibrillation paroxysm could indicate that these groups were initially free of arrhythmia, because other studies suggest the strong correlation of previous episodes of the arrhythmia and subsequent episodes following the pacemaker implantation (60, 61). Such a correlation was confirmed in the already mentioned study of Endoh et al. (45). The authors of PASTA study concluded that the small incidence of atrial fibrillation and the lack of differences among various atrial electrode locations could be caused by the beneficial effect of the atrial stimulation per se what could not be confirmed in other sick sinus syndrome patients requiring pacing without the pacemaker implantation. It seems probable that the verification of the concept will need a much more numerous study group in those low atrial fibrillation risk patients.

6. References

[1] Wang K, Xiao HB, Fujimoto S, Gibson DG. Atrial electromechanical sequence in normal subjects and patients with DDD pacemakers. Br Heart J 1995;74:403-7.
[2] Rein AJ, O'Donnel CP, Colan SD, Marx GR. Tissue velocity Doppler assessment of atrial and ventricular electromechanical coupling and atrioventricular time intervals in normal subjects. Am J Cardiol 2003;92:1347-50.
[3] Zhang Q, Kum LC, Lee PW, Lam YY, Wu EB, Lin H, Yip GW, et al. Effect of age and heart rate on atrial mechanical function assessed by Doppler tissue imaging in healthy individuals. J Am Soc Echocardiogr 2006:19;422-8.
[4] Papageorgiou P, Monahan K, Boyle NG, Seifert MJ, Beswick P, Zebede J, Epstein LM, Josephson ME. Site-dependant intra-atrial conduction delay: relationship to initiation of atrial fibrillation. Circulation 1996;94:384-9.
[5] O'Donnell D BJ, Furniss SS. Interatrial transseptal electrical conduction: comparison of patients with atrial fibrillation and normal controls. J Cardiobvasc Electrophysiol 2002;13:1111-7.
[6] Betts TR, Ho SY, Sanchez-Quintana D, Roberts PR, Anderson RH, Morgan JM. Characteristics of right atrial activation during coronary sinus pacing. J Cardiovasc Electrophysiol. 2002; 13: 794-800.
[7] Roithinger FX, Abou-Harb M, Pachinger O, Hintringer F. The effect of the atrial pacing site on the total atrial activation time. Pacing Clin Electrophysiol 2001;24:316.
[8] Kutarski A, Głowniak A, Szczęśniak D, Ruciński P. Effects of different atrial pacing modes evaluated by intracardiac signal-averaged ECG. Cardiol J 2008; 15: 129-142.
[9] Ausubel K, Klementowicz P, Furman S. Interatrial conduction during cardiac pacing. Pacing Clin Electrophysiol 1986;9:1026-31.
[10] Satoh T, Zipes DP. Unequal atrial stretch id dogs increases dispersion of refractoriness conductive to developing atrial fibrillation. J Cardiovasc Electrophysiol 1996;9:833-42.
[11] Misier AR, Opthof T, van Hemel NM, Defauw JJ, de Bakker JM, Janse MJ, van Capelle FJ. Increase dispersion of refractoriness in patients with idiopathic paroxysmal atrial fibrillation. J Am Coll Cardiol 1992;19:1531-5.

[12] Wijffels MC, Kirchhof CJ, Dorland R, Allessie MA. Atrial fibrillation begets atrial fibrillation: a study in awake chronically instrumented goats. Circulation 1995;92:1954-68.
[13] Bailin SJ, Adler S, Giudici M. Prevention of chronic atrial fibrillation by pacing in the region of Bachmann's bundle: results of a multicenter randomized trial. J Cardiobvasc Electrophysiol 2001;12:912-7.
[14] Bennett DH. Comparision of the acute effects of pacing the atrial septum, right atrial appendage, coronary sinus os, and the latter two sites simultaneously on the duration of atrial activation. Heart 2000;84:193-6.
[15] De Voogt WG, van Mechelen R, Scheffer M, van Miltenburg van Zijl AJM, Elhendy AA. Electrocardiographic characteristics in low atrial septum pacing. Journal of Electrocardiology 2005;38:166-70.
[16] Skoczyński P, Sławuta A, Gajek J, Mysiak A. Influence of different atrial lead positions on interatrial and atrioventricular conduction and percentage of ventricular stimulation in population with SSS treated by atrioventricular pacing. Eur Heart J 2010; 31 (Abstract Supplement): 263
[17] Spencer WH, Zhu DW, Markowitz T, Badruddin SM, Zoghbi WA. Atrial septal pacing: A method for pacing both atria simultaneously. Pacing Clin Electrophysiol 1997;20:2739-45.
[18] Katsivas A, Manolis AG, Lazaris E, Vassilopoulos C, Louvros N. Atrial septal pacing to synchronize atrial depolarization in patients with delayed interatrial conduction. Pacing Clin Electrophysiol 1998; 21: 2220-5.
[19] Roithinger FX, Abou-Harb M, Pachinger O, Hintringer F. The effect of the atrial pacing site on the total atrial activation time. Pacing Clin Electrophysiol 2001;24:316-22.
[20] Padeletti L, Porciani MC, Michelucci A, Colella A, Ticci P, Vena S, Costoli A et al. Interatrial septum pacing: a new approach to prevent recurrent atrial fibrillation. J Intrrv Card Electrophysiol 1999;3:35-43.
[21] Manolis AG, Katsivas AG, Vassilopoulos C, Koutsogeorgis D, Louvros NE. Prevention of atrial fibrillation by inter-atrial septum pacing guided by electrophysiological testing, in patients with delayed interatrial conduction. Europace 2002;4:165-74.
[22] Van Campen CM, de Cock CC, Kamp O, Visser CA. Differences in pacing from the atrial appendage and the lateral atrial free wall on left ventricular filling and haemodynamics during DDD pacing. Europace 2001;3:52-5.
[23] Padeletti L, Pieragnoli P, Ciapetti C, Colella A, Musilli N, Porciani MC, Ricci R, Pignalberi C et al. Randomized crossover comparison of right atrial appendage pacing versus interatrial septum pacing for prevention of paroxysmal atrial fibrillation In patients with sinus bradycardia. Am Heart J 2001;142:1047-55.
[24] Hermida JS, Kubala M, Lescure FX, Delonca J, Clerc J, Otmani A, Jarry G, Rey JL. Atrial septal pacing to prevent atrial fibrillation in patients with sinus node dysfunction: Results of a randomized controlled study. Am Heart J 2004;148(2):312-17.
[25] Kindermann M, Schwaab B, Berg M, Frohling G. The influence of right atrial septal pacing on the interatrial contraction sequence. Pacing Clin Electrophysiol 2000;23:1752.
[26] Hermida JS, Carpentier C, Kubala M, Otmani A, Delonca J, Jarry G, Rey JL. Atrial septal versus atrial appendage pacing: feasibility and effects on atrial conduction,

interatrial synchronization, and atrioventricular sequence. Pacing Clin Electrophysiol 2003;26:26.
[27] Miyazaki H, Noma K, Date T, Kobayashi A, Koga M, Kuno M, Takeda S, Iwano K, Seki S, Inada K, Matsuo S, Miyanaga S, Abe K, Yamane T, Sugimoto K, Mochizuki S. Atrial septal pacing to resynchronize atrial contraction and improve atrial transport function. J Cardiol 2005;45:239-46.
[28] Di Pede F, Gasparini G, De Piccoli B, Yu Y, Cuesta F, Raviele A. Hemodynamic effects of atrial septal pacing in cardiac resynchronization therapy patients. J Cardiovasc Electrophysiol 2005;16(12):1273-78.
[29] Fragakis N, Shakespeare CF, Lloyd G, Simon R, Bostock J, Holt P, Gill JS. Reversion and maintenance of sinus rhythm in patients with permanent atrial fibrillation by internal cardioversion followed by biatrial pacing. Pacing Clin Electrophysiol 2002;25:278-286.
[30] Enjoji Y, Sugi K, Noro M, et al. Evaluation of bi-atrial pacing and single site pacing for prevention of atrial fibrillation. Circ J 2002;66:70-74.
[31] Gilligan DM, Fuller IA, Clemo HF, Shepard RK, Dan D, Wood MA, Ellenbogen KA. The acute effects of biatrial pacing on atrial depolarization and repolarization. Pacing Clin Electrophysiol 2000;23:1113-1120.
[32] Lewicka-Nowak E, Kutarski A, Dąbrowska-Kugacka A, Ruciński P, Zagożdżon P, Raczak G. A novel method of multisite atrial pacing, incorporating Bachmann's bundle area and coronary sinus ostium, for electrical atrial resynchronization in patients with recurrent atrial fibrillation. Europace 2007;8:805-11.
[33] Matsumoto K, Ishikawa T, Simita S, Matsushita K, Inuoue N, Kobayashi T, Uchino K, Kimura K, Umemura S. Assessment of atrial regional wall motion using strain Doppler imaging during biatrial pacing in the bradycardia-tachycardia syndrome. PACE 2006;29:220-225.
[34] Dąbrowska-Kugacka A, Lewicka-Nowak E, Ruciński P, Zagożdżon P, Raczak G, Kutarski A. Atrial electromechanical sequence and contraction synchrony Turing single- and multisite atrial pacing In patients with brady-tachycardia syndrome. PACE 2009;22:591-603.
[35] Stockburger M, Bartels R, Gerhardt L, Butter C. Dual-site right atrial pacing increases left atrial appendage flow in patients with sick sinus syndrome and paroxysmal atrial fibrillation. PACE 2007;30:20-27.
[36] Prakash A, Saksena S, Ziegler PD, Lokhandwala T, Hettrick DA, Delfault P, Nanda NC, Wyse DG. Dual site right atrial pacing can improve the impact of standard dual chamber pacing on atrial and ventricular mechanical function in patients with symptomatic atrial fibrillation: further observations from the dual site atrial pacing for prevention of atrial fibrillation trial. J Interv Card Electrophysiol 2005;12:177-87.
[37] Takagi M, Doi A, Shirai N, Hirata K, Takemoto Y, Takeuchi K, Yoshikawa J. Acute improvement of atrial mechanical stunning after electrical cardioversion of persistent atrial fibrillation: comparison between biatrial and single atrial pacing. Heart 2005;91:58-63.
[38] Bayes de Luna A, Cladellas M, Oter R. Interatrial conduction block and retrograde activation of the left atrium and paroxysmal supraventricular tachyarrhythmia. Eur Heart J 1988; 9: 1112–1118.

[39] Buxton A, Josephson M. The role of P-wave duration as a predictor of post-operative atrial arrhythmias. Chest 1981; 80: 68–73.
[40] Frost L, Lund B, Pilegaard H, Christiansen EH. Re-evaluation of the role of Pwave duration and morphology as predictors of atrial fibrillation and flutter after coronary artery bypass surgery. Eur Heart J 1996;17: 1065–1071
[41] Watson RM, Josephson ME. Atrial flutter. 1. Electrophysiologic substrate and mode of initiation and termination. Am J Cardiol 1980; 45: 732–736.
[42] Cohen J, Scherf B. Complete interatrial block (atrial dissociation). Am Heart J 1965; 70: 24–34.
[43] Kristensen L, Nielsen JC, Mortensen PT, Christensen PD, Vesterlund T, Pedersen AK, Andersen HR. Sinus and paced P wave duration and dispertion as predictors of atrial fibrillation after pacemaker implantation inpatients with isolated sick sinus syndrome. Pace 2004; 27: 606-614.
[44] De Sisti A, Leclercq JF, Stiubei M, Fiorello P, Halimi F, Attuel P.: P Wave diuration and morphology predict atrial fibrillation recurrence in patients with sinus node dysfunction and atrial-based pacemaker. PACE 2002;25: 1546-1554.
[45] Endoh Y, Nakamura A, Suzuki T, Mizuno M, Takara A, Ota Y, Kasanuki H. Clinical significance of prolonged P wave width after right atrial appendage pacing In sick sinus syndrome. Circ J 2003; 67: 485-489.
[46] Stabile G, Senatore G, De Simone A, Turco P, Coltorti F, Nocerino P, Vitale DF, Chiariello M. Determinants of efficacy of atrial pacing in preventing atrial fibrillation recurrences. J Cardiovasc Electrophysiol 1999; 10: 2-9.
[47] Tse HF, Hettrick DA, Mehra R, Lau CP. Improved atrial mechanical efficiency during alternate- and multiple-site atrial pacing compared with conventional right atrial appendage pacing: implications for selective site pacing to prevent atrial fibrillation. J Am Coll Cardiol. 2006; 47: 209-12.
[48] de Voogt WG, van Mechelen R, van den Bos A, Scheffer M, van Hemmel NM, Levine PA. Electrical characteristics of low atrial septum pacing compared with right atrial appendage pacing. Europace 2005; 7: 60-66.
[49] Hakacova N, Velimirovic D, Margitfalvi P, Hatala R, Buckingham TA. Septal atrial pacing for the prevention of atrial fibrillation. Europace 2007; 9: 1124–1128.
[50] Savitt MA, Rankin JS., Use of Bachmann's Bundle for bipolar atrial pacing. Ann Thorac Surg 1993; 56:183-184.
[51] Nigro G, Russo V, Politano L, Cioppa N, Manfredi D, Chianese R, de Chiara A, Rago A, Arena G, Palladino A, Calabro R. Right atrial appendage versus Bachmann's Bundle stimulation: A two-year comparative study of electrical parameters in myotonic dystrophy type-1 patients. PACE 2009; 32: 1191-1196.
[52] Nigro G, Russo V, Vergara P, D'Andrea A, Di Gregorio G, Politano L, Nigro G, Calabrò R. Optimal site for atrial lead implantation in myotonic dystrophy patients: The role of Bachmanns Bundle. Pacing Clin Elektrophysiol 2008; 31: 1463-1466.
[53] Spitzer S, Wacker P, Gazarek S, Malinowski K, Schibgilla V. Primary prevention of atrial fibrillation: Does the atrial lead position influence the incidence of atrial arrhythmias In patients with sinus node dysfunction? Results from PASTA study. PACE 2009; 32: 1553-1561.
[54] Saksena S, Prakash A, Ziegler P, Hummel JD, Friedman P, Plumb VJ, Wyse DG, Johnson E, Fitts S, Mehra R; DAPPAF Investigators. Improved suppression of recurrent

atrail fibrillation with dual-site right atrial pacing and antiarrhythmic drug therapy. J Am Coll Cardiol 2002; 40:1140-1150.
[55] Saksena S. The role of multisite atrial pacing in rhythm control in AF: Insights from subanalises of the dual-site atrial pacing for prevention of atrial fibrillation study. Pacing Clin Electrophysiol 2003; 26: 1565.
[56] Delfaut P, Saksena S, Prakash A, Krol RB. Long-term outcome of patients with drug refractory atrial flutter and fibrillation after single- and dual-site right atrial pacing for arrhythmia prevention. JACC 1998;32: 1900-1908.
[57] Bailin S. Is Bachmann's bundle the only site for single-site pacing to prevent atrial fibrillation? Results of multicenter randomized trial. Card Electrophysiol Rev 2003;7: 325-328.
[58] de Voogt W, van Hemel N, de Vusser P, Mairesse GH, van Mechelen R, Koistinien J, Van Den Bos A, et al. No evidence of automatic atrial overdrive pacing on reduction of paroxysmal atrial fibrillation. Europace 2007; 798-804.
[59] Padeletti L, Pürerfellner H, Adler SW, Waller TJ, Harvey M, Horvitz L, Holbrook R, Kempen K, Mugglin A, Hettrick DA; Worldwide ASPECT Investigators. Combined efficacy of atrial septal lead placement and atrial pacing algorithms for prevention of paroxysmal atrial tachyarrhythmia. J Cardiovasc Electrophysiol 2003;14: 1189-1195.
[60] Andersen HR, Nielsen JC, Thomsen PE, Thuesen L, Mortensen PT, Vesterlund T, Pedersen AK. Long-term follow-up of patients from a randomized trial of atrial versus ventricular pacing for sick-sinus syndrome. Lancet 1997;350: 1210-1216.
[61] D'Allonnes GR, Pavin D, Leclercq C, Ecke JE, Jauvert G, Mabo P, Daubert JC. Long-term effects of biatrial synchronous pacing to prevent drug refractory atrial tachyarrhythmia: A nine-year experience. J Cardiovasc Electrophysiol 2000;11:1081-1091.

5

Left Ventricular Endocardial Pacing Techniques as an Alternative for Ineffective Cardiac Resynchronization Therapy and the Role of Acute Hemodynamic Evaluation

Berry M. van Gelder[1], Patrick Houthuizen[1], Mike G. Scheffer[2], Lukas Dekker[1] and Frank A. Bracke[1]
[1]*Catharina hospital, Eindhoven*
[2]*Maasstad hospital, Rotterdam*
The Netherlands

1. Introduction

Cardiac resynchronization therapy (CRT) has become an important treatment for patients with heart failure and left ventricular dyssynchrony (Cazeau et al., 2001; Abraham et al., 2002; Auricchio et al., 2002; Cleland et al., 2005). For left ventricular (LV) pacing in CRT, transvenous placement of a lead into one of the posterolateral tributaries of the coronary sinus (CS) is the first choice. However, even with growing experience and improvement of available materials and tools placement of a lead into the coronary venous system may fail.

Failures can be due to inability to engage the coronary sinus, absence of suitable side branches in the posterolateral area, coronary vein stenosis, lead instability, high stimulation threshold, phrenic nerve stimulation or a combination (Auricchio et al., 2004; Bentkover et al., 2003; Gras et al., 2002).

As alternative for surgical epicardial lead implantation, in case of failed coronary sinus implant, atrial transseptal approaches with endocardial LV lead placement have been described, using a modified transseptal puncture technique from either the right jugular vein (Jaïs et al., 1998; Jaïs et al., 2000; Leclercq et al., 1999; Jaïs et al., 2006) or from the left axillary vein (Sen et al., 2004).

We modified the atrial transseptal technique for endocardial LV lead placement by using a standard transseptal puncture from the femoral vein, dilatation of the atrial septum and subsequent passage of the lead through the septum via the subclavian vein (Van Gelder et al., 2007). Shortly after, a second alternative technique was described for LV endocardial implantation, using a limited lateral thoracotomy with transapical insertion of the lead (Kassai et al., 2009). We also used this transapical technique in a number of patients in whom the trans-atrial septum implant was unsuccessful or contraindicated due to the presence of an artificial valve in mitral position.

Besides being an alternative for failed coronary sinus implants, the flexibility of lead positioning by both endocardial techniques also offers the possibility of an endocardial implant at a different LV site in patients not responding to CRT. The efficacy of the

endocardial lead position at different locations can be evaluated in an acute hemodynamic study using a sensor tipped pressure wire for invasive measurement of LVdP/dtmax, prior to permanent implantation (Van Gelder et al., 2004).
In this chapter we describe the technique and results of the transseptal and transapical implant. The technical aspects and results of the temporary LV endocardial pacing and hemodynamic studies in patients that were nonresponders are described in detail.

2. The atrial transseptal technique

2.1 Patients and methods

In the period from January 2006 to May 2010 we attempted implantation of an endocardial LV lead in 20 patients, (10 males; mean age 68±8.6 years). All patients had standard indications for implantation of a CRT-P or CRT-D device. Clinical details are summarized in table 1.

	Sex	Age (years)	CM	NYHA	EF (%)	PQ (ms)	QRS (ms)	ACT
Pt. 1	M	54	ICM	III-IV	18	176	169	Yes
Pt. 2	F	71	DCM	III-IV	20	182	200	Yes
Pt. 3	M	58	DCM	III	23	188	142	Yes
Pt. 4	M	65	ICM	IV	28	212	168	Yes
Pt. 5	F	78	DCM	III	35	168	156	No
Pt. 6	F	68	DCM	III	45	230	118	No
Pt. 7	M	82	ICM	III	21	152	174	Yes
Pt. 8	F	80	ICM	III	25	AF	200	Yes
Pt. 9	F	62	DCM	III	30	190	170	Yes
Pt. 10	F	76	ICM	III-IV	15	143	156	Yes
Pt. 11	M	74	ICM	III-IV	18	VP	198	Yes
Pt. 12	M	70	DCM	III-IV	22	240	280	Yes
Pt. 13	V	72	DCM	III-IV	20	195	175	Yes
Pt. 14	M	74	ICM	III	23	238	198	Yes
Pt. 15	M	55	DCM	IV	13	AF	173	Yes
Pt. 16	V	55	ICM	III	25	138	140	Yes
Pt. 17	V	62	DCM	III	21	159	194	Yes
Pt. 18	M	66	ICM	III	21	VP	220	Yes
Pt. 19	M	76	ICM	III	27	VP	265	Yes
Pt. 20	V	64	ICM	III	33	129	122	Yes

ACT = anti coagulant therapy; AF = Atrial fibrillation; CM = Cardiomyopathy DCM = Dilated cardiomyopathy; EF = Ejection fraction; ICM = Ischemic cardiomyopathy; VP = Ventricular pacing

Table 1. Patient characteristics.

Of notice, 18 patients were on anticoagulant therapy before the implantation. None of the patients had echocardiographic evidence of left atrial or left ventricular thrombi. After the initial implantation attempt of the CS lead, 11 out of the 20 patients had developed one or more of the following complications. A high stimulation threshold (4 patients), phrenic nerve stimulation (4 patients), and/or one or more lead dislodgements (3 patients) during short term follow-up with no alternative CS locations. The remaining 8 patients had an unsuccessful implantation of a coronary sinus lead. In 6 of these patients, the right atrial and ventricular lead together with the CRT devices were implanted during the first procedure with the port of the LV lead sealed with an IS-1 plug. A transseptal procedure was performed on a later date.

In 2 patients the transseptal procedure was performed during primo implantation, when coronary sinus lead implantation was unsuccessful. In all patients we were convinced that either persuading in the primo procedure or a new attempt in the failures at follow-up, would not lead to a successful procedure. Under these conditions, the options of an alternative implant route, either epicardial with a lateral thoracotomy, or a transseptal endocardial approach were discussed with patient and/or relatives.

2.2 Implantation technique

The pacemaker or ICD pocket was made or reopened under local anesthesia. In primo implants right ventricular and right atrial lead were implanted first. Subsequently the subclavian vein was punctured and a 10 F sheath (Safe Sheath) was inserted, allowing obtaining access to the right atrium with an Attain Deflectable 6226 or 6227 DEF Catheter Delivery System (Medtronic Inc. Minneapolis, MN, USA). In 18 out of 20 patients implants were performed from the left pectoral area, in 2 patients from the right.

In 19 patients a standard transseptal puncture employing a Adult Transseptal (Medtronic Inc. Minneapolis, MN, USA) or a Preface 8F 307803M (Biosense Webster, Inc. Diamond Bar CA 91765, USA) sheath was performed from the right femoral vein. After transseptal puncture patients were anticoagulated with an intravenous injection of 5000 international units of heparin. A 0.035" guide wire with a length of 260 cm was inserted into the left atrium and advanced into one of the pulmonary veins or the left ventricle.

At that time the dilator of the transseptal sheath was removed from the system and a 4 cm long 6mm angioplasty balloon (Cordis Corporation - Endovascular, Warren, New Jersey, USA) inserted into the left atrium. The transseptal sheath was withdrawn into the right atrium and the balloon positioned across the septal puncture site. The balloon was inflated with contrast medium and the inflation was stored on X-ray in order to identify the indentation of the balloon as a marker of the atrial septum puncture location (Fig.1-A). This picture was used as a road map during the procedure. The balloon was deflated and withdrawn into the transseptal sheath while the guide wire was kept in the left atrium.

The deflectable catheter inserted from the pectoral area was advanced in the right atrium and the tip curved in a rigid J-shape pointing in a left-cranial direction. Using fluoroscopy from a right and left anterior oblique view the tip of the deflectable catheter was positioned towards the atrial septum puncture side guided by the transseptal guide wire and the reference image of the balloon inflation. As a result, the deflectable catheter pointed towards the atrial septum from an inferior direction. In the first 2 patients different catheters and guide wire combinations were used to enter the left atrium through the deflectable catheter. A standard 6F right Judkins or internal mammary artery angiography catheter together with a 0.035" hydrophilic stiff guide wire (Terumo Europe NV, Leuven, Belgium) inserted in the deflectable catheter turned out to be the best combination to enter the left atrium and was used as the first choice in the succeeding procedures (Fig. 1-B).

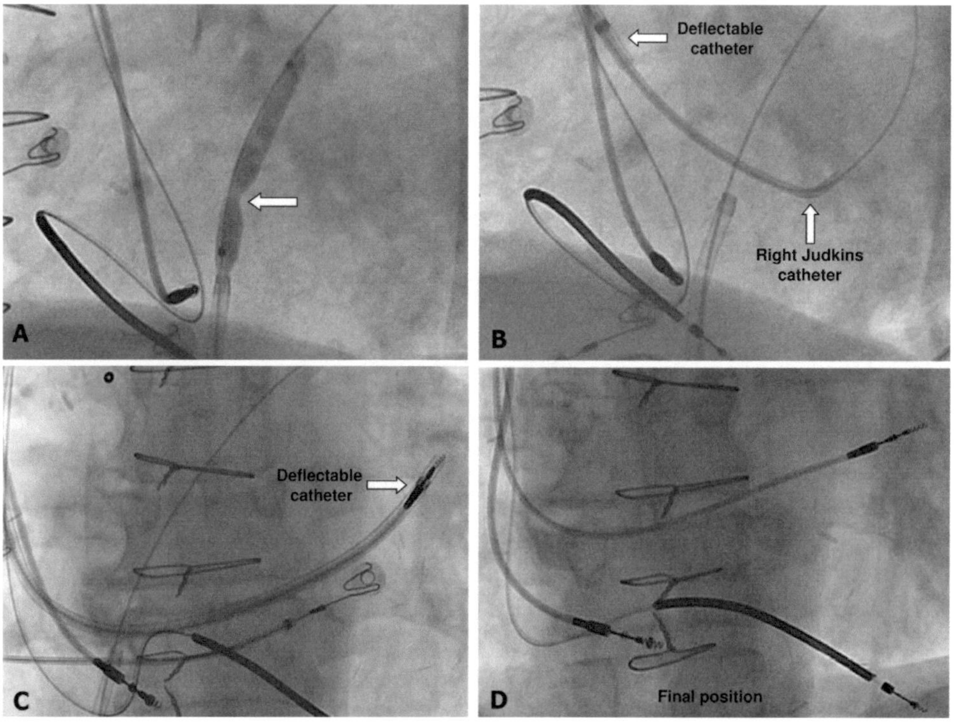

Fig. 1. Inflation of the 6 mm balloon at the level of the right atrial septum (arrow), panel A. Atrial septum crossed with a 6F right Judkins catheter and Terumo guide wire, panel B. Atrial septum crossed with deflectable catheter, panel C. Final position Medtronic 4076 screw-in lead position in left posterolateral area, panel D.

Different directions of the tip of the guide wire could be obtained by advancing and rotating the right Judkins catheter just outside the deflectable catheter. When the hydrophilic guide wire was in the left atrium an additional inflation of the balloon in the atrial septum was performed to ensure adequate access to the left atrium and subsequently the balloon again was withdrawn into the right atrium. Now the right Judkins catheter was advanced over the hydrophilic guide wire into the left atrium. After passing the atrial septum, the tip of the right Judkins catheter was turned in an inferior position, allowing advancement of the guide wire and the right Judkins catheter into the left ventricle. Hereafter the deflectable sheath was advanced through the atrial septum and positioned in the left ventricle at the posterolateral area (Fig. 1-C).

Occasionally, after entrance of the guide wire into the left atrium, additional dilatation of the septum with the balloon advanced from superior through the deflectable sheath was necessary to create the right direction of the slit in the septum to allow passage of the sheath. After removal of the right Judkins catheter, a standard bipolar screw-in lead Medtronic 4076-65 cm (Medtronic Inc. Minneapolis, MN, USA) was subsequently implanted through the deflectable sheath in the posterolateral area (Fig.1-D).

After testing for pacing and sensing thresholds and excluding phrenic nerve stimulation at maximal output of the pacing system analyzer (10.0 V), the deflectable catheter was removed using a longitudinal slitter tool, which is a standard device in removing coronary sinus sheaths. The lead was sutured to the pectoral muscle and connected to the CRT device. Anticoagulant therapy was (re)instituted immediately after the procedure: dalteparine in therapeutic dose until adequate anticoagulation with an oral vitamin K antagonist (INR between 3.0 and 4.0) was obtained.
In the last patient the right Judkins was exchanged for an Attain Select catheter (Medtronic Inc, Minneapolis MN, USA), allowing insertion of a 4F Select Secure pacing lead.

2.3 Results

Successful implant of a LV endocardial lead was obtained in 19 out of the 20 patients. In the patient that failed (pt. 2) the atrial septum could not be traversed with the deflectable catheter in combination with the right Judkins catheter and hydrophilic guide wire, even after successful transseptal puncture and dilatation of the atrial septum with a 6 mm balloon. In the remaining 19 patients it was relatively easy to find the atrial perforation with the hydrophilic guide wire.

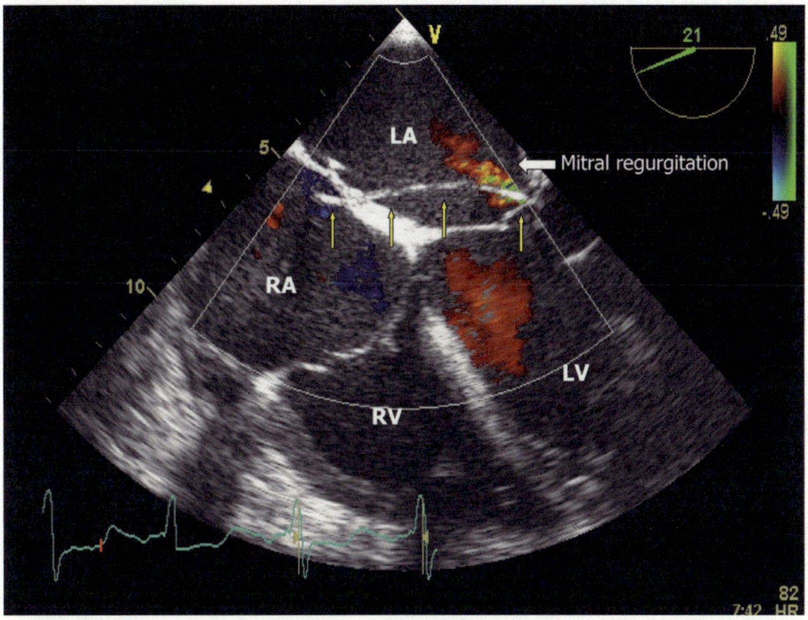

Fig. 2. Trans esophageal echocardiogram showing the position of the LV pacing lead crossing the atrial septum and mitral valve (arrows). There is a low grade mitral regurgitation at the site of the pacing lead.

After entering the left atrium with the hydrophilic guide wire it was sometimes difficult to pass the right Judkins catheter and the deflectable guiding catheter into the left atrium. When this problem was encountered, an additional inflation of the 6 mm balloon prior to advancement of the deflectable catheter facilitated this maneuver. If advancement still failed, inflation of a 6 mm balloon in the atrial septum, inserted from superior over the hydrophilic guide wire through the deflectable catheter, was sufficient to enable passage of

deflectable catheter. As indentation of the balloon was still visible at these additional inflations, it became apparent that there was significant elastic recoil around the dilatation site. After these maneuvers, the deflectable catheter could easily be passed into the LV towards the posterolateral wall in all 19 patients, followed by positioning and fixation of the lead. The mean stimulation threshold after fixation of the lead was 0.78±0.24 V, 1.2±0.5 mA at 0.5 ms pulse width, and the amplitude of the intracardiac electrogram was 14.2±9.7 mV with a slew rate of 3.1±1.0 V/s. Stimulation with 10.0 V did not result in phrenic nerve stimulation in any of the patients.
In 2 out of the first 4 patients dislodgement of the lead was observed within 24 hours after implantation. In one patient the lead could be repositioned by insertion of a stylet, in the second re-insertion of the deflectable catheter was necessary. Insufficient slack in the lead was considered as the main cause of the dislodgements. After paying attention to this phenomenon no further dislodgements were observed. Chronic stimulation threshold 2 months after implantation was 1.48±0.35V at 0.063±0.027 ms pulse width. Echocardiographic studies after implant did not show a transseptal shunt in any of the patients. In 2 patients an increase in mitral regurgitation was observed after implantation from grade I to II-III and from grade II to III. Average mitral regurgitation for the first 10 patients was grade 1.6±0.8 pre implant and 2.0±0.9 post implant (p=0.19) (Fig.2).
There were no clinical signs of thrombo-embolic events in an average follow-up period of 32.8 ± 17.5 months. All patients improved clinically with at least 1 NYHA class. Three patients died during follow-up.

2.4 Atrial septum perforation from the pectoral area

In the previous paragraph access to the left atrium was obtained by a traditional transseptal puncture followed by dilatation of the atrial septum with a 6 mm balloon.

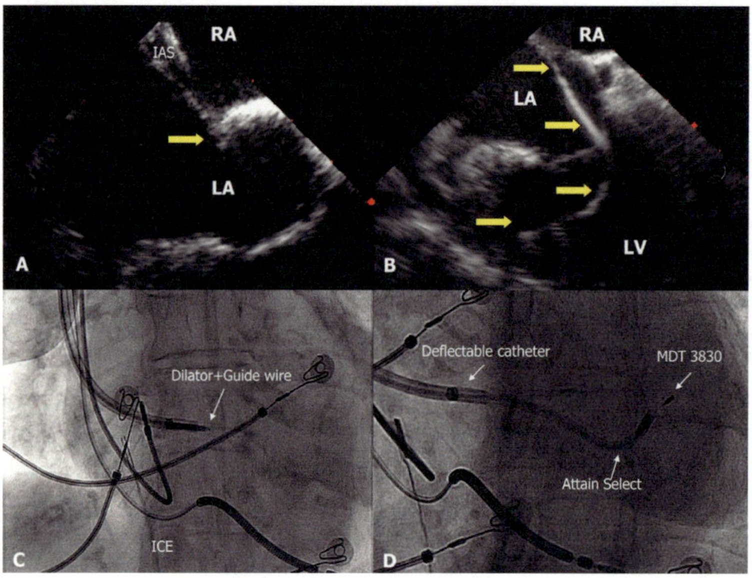

Fig. 3. Intra Cardiac Echo (ICE) demonstrating tenting position (arrow) of the deflectable catheter with dilator and guide wire against the fossa ovalis (A, C). Positioning of the Medtronic 3830 lead in the posterolateral area through the Attain Select catheter (B, D).

A more elegant approach, avoiding working in 2 separated sterile fields, would be perforation of the septum from the device implant site. There is only one case report describing atrial septum puncture from the left pectoral area using a modified Brockenbrough needle (Sen et al., 2004). We recently performed a perforation with access to the left atrium from the left pectoral area in a 64 year old female patient, NYHA class III, with an ischemic cardiomyopathy, left bundle branch block, QRS width 132 ms, ejection fraction 28%. She had a coronary sinus lead implant in the mid cardiac vein as only accessible side branch. Unfortunately she developed untreatable phrenic nerve stimulation, which necessitated a new intervention. Due to the lack of suitable coronary sinus side branches, a transseptal approach was chosen.

After positioning a deflectable catheter (Medtronic DEF 6227) , with a dilator and guide wire against the fossa ovalis using moderate pressure, tenting of the fossa ovalis was observed on intra cardiac echo (ICE), (Fig. 3). In this position 40 Watt RF energy from a electrosurgical unit ERBE ICC 200 (ERBE Elektromedizin GmbH, D-72072 Tuebingen, Germany) was applied for 2 seconds, where after the guide smoothly passed the inter atrial septum.

Advancement of the guide wire was followed by introduction of the Attain Select catheter (Medtronic Inc., Minneapolis, MN, USA) into the left atrium and subsequently into the left ventricle. After positioning the Attain Select catheter against the posterolateral wall of the left ventricle, a Medtronic SelectSecure lead was implanted in this area. After obtaining satisfactory values for pacing and sensing, the Attain Select catheter and the deflectable catheter were removed employing standard catheter slitting techniques.

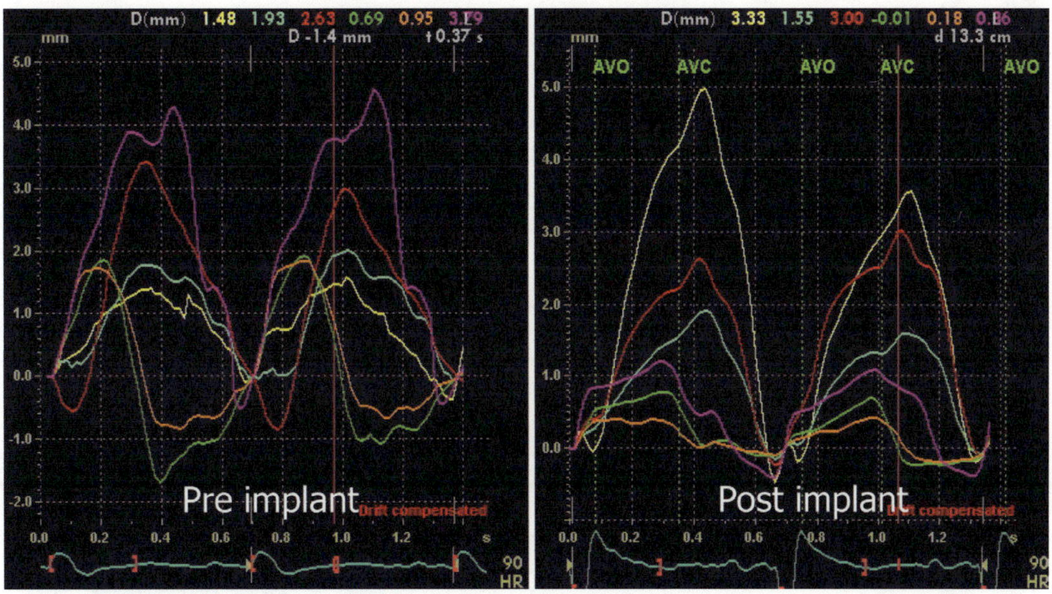

Fig. 4. Tissue tracking traces of the patient with the septal perforation from the pectoral area, showing restoration of synchrony after optimization.

Patient recovered quickly and the system was optimized in the referring hospital (Dr.MGS) using echocardiographic techniques (Fig. 4). In the follow-up the patient was responder to CRT demonstrated by improvement in clinical signs of heart failure, reduction in NYHA class and reduction of LV dimensions on echocardiography.

3. The transapical implantation technique

3.1 Introduction

In our experience with transseptal LV endocardial implants, occasionally we failed to implant the LV lead. In 2 cases where introduction of the guide wire and /or catheter into the left atrium after dilatation of the atrial septum was unsuccessful; in a third patient with failure of an epicardial LV lead and a persistent left superior vena cava and one patient with a failed CS implant and an artificial valve in the mitral position, which is a contra indication for the transseptal approach, we performed a transapical implant. In these 4 patients we used a slight modification of the technique described by Kassaï et al. (Kassaï et al., 2009) to perform a transapical approach.

3.2 Implantation technique

The transapical implant is performed under total anesthesia with a left lateral thoracotomy at the side of the left ventricular apex. When apical pulsations are not palpable the apex can be located by transthoracic echocardiography. After opening of the thorax a small pericardial incision is made over the LV apex. Next, LV apex is visualized and a purse string suture is applied around the apex. LV is punctured though the purse string suture with an 18G needle allowing introduction of a 0.035" guide wire into the LV cavity. Over this guide wire an 8.4 F Medtronic C304-59 SelectSite deflectable catheter with a dilator is introduced into the left ventricle.

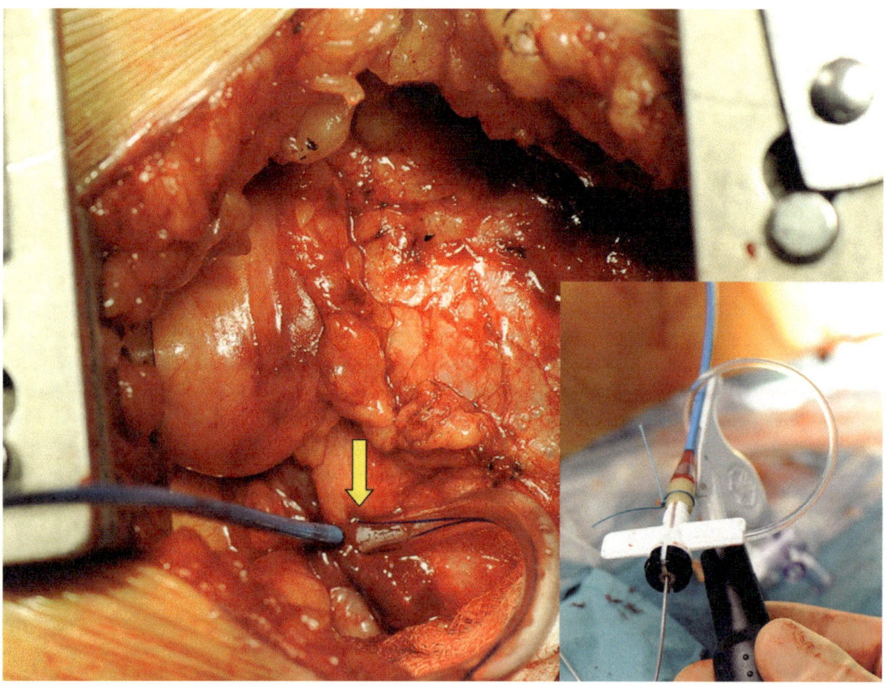

Fig. 5. Insertion place of the SelectSite deflectable lead after lateral thoracotomy. Catheter is inserted through a previous placed purse string suture around the apex (arrow). Inset shows the control mechanism of the deflectable catheter in detail. Distal curve of the deflectable catheter can be controlled by rotation of the black handle.

The external handle at the proximal end enables the operator to curve the distal end of the catheter and together with torqability of the catheter all endocardial positions can be reached. After positioning the deflectable catheter against the selected site of the LV wall, a Medtronic SelectSecure 3830-74 was screwed to the endocardium.

After obtaining satisfactory values for pacing and sensing, the deflectable catheter was removed employing standard catheter slitting techniques. Of note, the intracardiac EGM of the LV lead should display an injury pattern already before screwing, which increases after screwing and is maintained during removal of the deflectable catheter. During removal of the deflectable catheter care should be taken to preserve enough slack of the lead inside the LV cavity to prevent early dislocation.

Bleeding from the left ventricle insertion side can be controlled by the purse string suture around the puncture hole. In case of continuous bleeding an extra purse string suture with pledge material may be used to gain hemostasis.

After closure of pericardium and ribs, the lead is also fixed to muscular structures around the ribs, employing the standard fixation sleeve, leaving some extra length between both fixation points. From this place the lead is tunneled to a subcutaneous or muscular pocket located in the left pectoral region in all patients. The postoperative anticoagulant regimen was identical to the protocol for transseptal implants.

The postoperative hospitalization for these four patients was 5.8±1.0 days, which is significantly longer than after a transseptal procedure. One patient needed a re-thoracotomy at day 2 postoperative due bleeding at the site of the thoracotomy. There were no hemodynamic complications during follow up. Radiographic control revealed a stable position of the LV endocardial lead at 2 months follow-up. One example is displayed in figure 6.

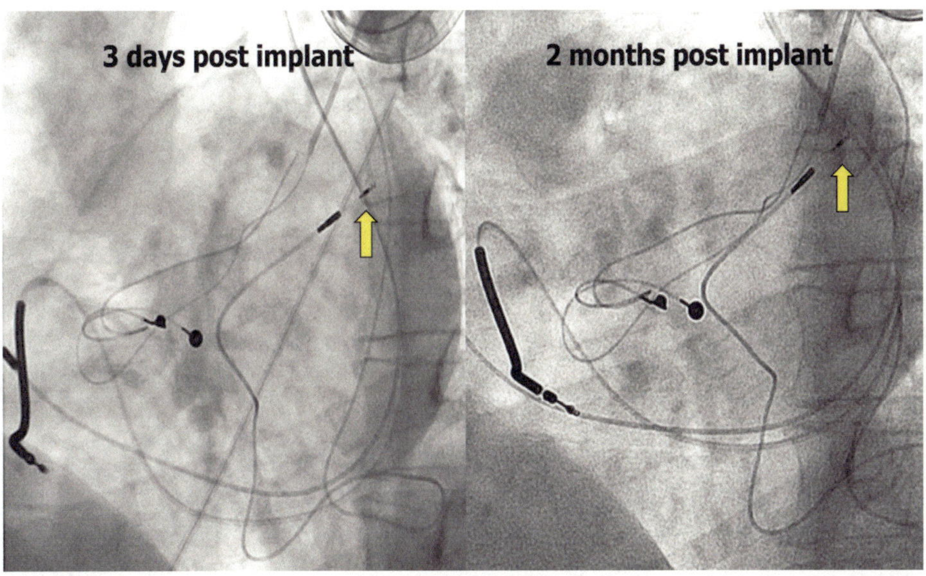

Fig. 6. Left anterior oblique view of one of the patients with a transapical implantation. The left panel shows the lead position of the SelectSecure lead in the posterolateral area (arrow) 3 days after implant (left panel) and 2 months after implant in the right panel. Comparison shows the stability of the lead inside the LV cavity and at both fixation points.

3.3 Discussion and conclusion LV endocardial implantation

LV endocardial pacing can be considered as an alternative for failed coronary sinus implants, which still has a failure rate at implant of 8.4% (Leon et al., 2005). The combined failure rate at implant and short term follow-up is estimated between 10 and 15%. Although the current standard alternative for failed transvenous coronary sinus implants is a surgical epicardial approach, LV endocardial lead placement is an alternative in selected patients, either by transseptal or transapical technique.

The transseptal technique, first described by Jaïs et al., was later modified by Leclerq et al. using a transseptal puncture from the right jugular vein (Jaïs et al. 1998; Leclercq et al., 1999). Engagement of the fossa ovalis and the absence of classical anatomical landmarks make a superior approach challenging. Further, in case of implant through the jugular vein subcutaneous tunneling of the lead over the clavicle and sternum in left pectoral implants is necessary, which increases the risk of skin erosion and lead damage.

Our technique resembles the initial idea of Jaïs et al. but is easier to perform and has the advantage over the transseptal puncture from the jugular vein that entrance created by balloon dilatation can be used from all upper thoracic veins that are used for implantation from the right as well as the left side. Balloon dilatation of the atrial septum has been reported with a 8 mm balloon used during mitral balloon valvotomy, which did not result in a hemodynamic relevant left to right shunt at follow-up (McKay et al., 1987; Cequier et al., 1988; Palacios et al. 1989) and would therefore be unlikely with the smaller 6 mm balloon.

The risk of thrombo-embolic complications from left ventricular endocardial lead placement is a major concern for application of this technique. Not intended and unnoticed left ventricular endocardial lead placement is a potential source for thromboembolism that might result in neurological complications in patients not receiving anticoagulant therapy (Sharifi et al., 1995; Van Gelder et al., 2000). Anticoagulant therapy with a recommended target INR between 2.5 and 3.5 is mandatory in these patients, although the risk of thrombo-embolic complications seems to diminish 3 years after implantation, suggesting complete endotheliazation after this period (Sharifi et al., 1995). Long term follow-up showed no thrombo-embolic complications as long as anticoagulant therapy was maintained (Pasquié et al., 2007). In our series ninety percent (18 out of 20 patients) had already an indication for anticoagulant therapy before the decision for CRT, as is common in this patient population. During the follow-up of 32.8±17.5 months in this study no thrombo-embolic complications with permanent damage have been noticed so far.

Mitral valve dysfunction due to the presence of the endocardial lead passing the mitral valve was only observed in 2 of the first 10 patients, in whom conventional 7F screw-in leads were used. Application of a very soft and flexible 4F lead (Medtronic SelectSecure 3830) gave a further reduction of mechanical effects on mitral valve function.

The generally accepted alternative for failed coronary sinus pacing is surgical epicardial placement of the LV lead through a limited lateral thoracotomy or a thoracoscopic approach. However, thoracotomy can be contraindicated due to previous cardiac surgery or poor general condition. Further, complications of surgery can be anticipated as well. Joshi et al. reported post operative complications after a robotically assisted left ventricular lead placement in 7 out of 42 patients (Joshi et al., 2005). Koos et al. reported the comparison of coronary venous lead placement versus a limited lateral thoracotomy, which was in favor of the transvenous lead placement with respect to post implant hospitalization, increase in functional capacity and mortality at 1 year follow-up (Koos et al., 2004).

Apart from 2 dislodgement of the left ventricular lead in our early experience with transseptal lead placement, there were no procedure related complications in this cohort. Our preliminary results therefore suggest the feasibility and safety of LV transseptal endocardial lead implantation. A main advantage is the possibility in case of a failed coronary sinus lead positioning to implant the left ventricular lead during the same procedure from the already created sub pectoral entry site, either from the right or left pectoral area.

Considerations regarding anticoagulant regimen and freedom of selecting any pacing site inside the LV of the transseptal approach can also be applied to the transapical approach. There are 2 main differences between both techniques. First, the transapical approach has the advantage that the LV lead is not crossing the mitral valve with the potential to cause dysfunction, which was, however, almost completely eliminated by using very flexible 4F leads.

The risk of mitral valve endocarditis as mentioned by Kassaï et al., due to close and permanent contact between lead and the mitral valve, is not supported by the long-term follow-up of LV endocardial leads as reported by Pasquié et al. (Kassaï et al., 2008; Kassaï et al., 2009; Pasquié et al., 2007). It will be clear that in the presence of an artificial mitral valve the transseptal approach is contra indicated. In our limited experience the transapical approach has a 100% success rate and a predictable operation time of approximately 1.5 hour. A second difference is that the impact on hospitalization and morbidity is higher for the transapical approach due to the lateral thoracotomy. The average postoperative hospitalization was 5.8±1.0 days versus 1 day for transseptal approaches.

It can be concluded that both technique are safe and feasible as an alternative for failed CS implants. The preference of the operator determines the choice of the technique; whereas both methods have there specific advantages and disadvantages which may play a role in the final choice.

4. Acute hemodynamic testing and ineffective CRT

4.1 Introduction

Left ventricular endocardial pacing is initially considered for patients with failed coronary sinus implants or preliminary lead failure during follow-up. However, nonresponders in CRT can be related to patient selection, LV lead placement, presence of scar tissue, or inadequate optimization of the atrio-ventricular (AV) and/or interventricular (V-V) interval (Yu et al., 2005).

The application of LV endocardial pacing either by transseptal or transapical approach offered the operator the freedom of selection the optimal pacing site. A second argument for LV endocardial pacing is the superior hemodynamic effect as compared to epicardial pacing. (Garrigue et al., 2001; van Deursen et al., 2008).

After our initial experience with transseptal LV endocardial lead implantations for failed implants or early lead failure, the following questions were raised:

1. Is there a role for LV endocardial pacing in nonresponders?
2. Can the hemodynamic effect of resynchronization be improved by endocardial pacing and/or an optimal lead position?
3. Can the hemodynamic effect be predicted prior to implantation from a temporary hemodynamic pacing study?
4. Can all pacing modalities be performed in a temporary set up?

The use of LVdP/dtmax for selecting the optimal pacing site and evaluation of the optimal setting of AV and V-V interval has been shown in the past (Butter C et al. 2001; Soliman et al. 2009; van Gelder et al., 2007b). The results of the measurements, which are not depending on the operator's interpretation, are immediately available during the study. This implies that the method is extremely suitable during decision making at implantation to determine the hemodynamic effect of a left ventricular pacing site. The rapid hemodynamic stabilization after changing pacing parameters also enables the operator to perform a high number of measurements in a relative short period of time, which makes the method less sensitive to changing baseline conditions as demonstrated in the majority of our studies (Fig. 7).

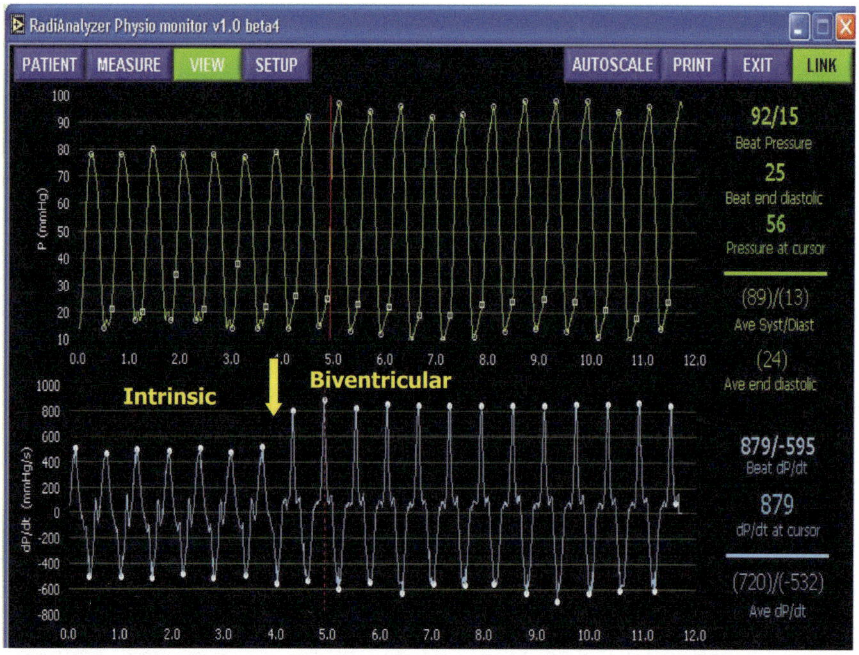

Fig. 7. Recording of LV pressure (upper tracing) and LVdP/dt (lower tracing) showing the transition for intrinsic to biventricular pacing. The example shows the rapid hemodynamic stabilization after extreme hemodynamic changes.

The procedure is minimal invasive and requires only 2 hours immobilization for the patient, which makes it also suitable for use in an out-patient setting. Supported by this knowledge we started hemodynamic evaluation of nonresponders with a temporary pacing study at multiple endocardial LV locations.

4.2 Patients and methods

Twelve patients, all males, age 75.4±7.4 years, 1 dilated and 11 ischemic cardiomyopathy, NYHA class III-IV; ejection fraction 20.1±6.2% underwent a temporary hemodynamic pacing study. Eight patients were nonresponders, 3 were failed CS implants and 1 was evaluated as a candidate for CRT. The latter patient had a dual chamber ICD and progressive heart failure associated with right bundle branch block (RBBB). There were 2 more patients with a RBBB, 5 with a LBBB and 4 with RV pacing as baseline rhythm.

In all patients the hemodynamic effect of LV endocardial pacing was evaluated from the posterolateral (PL) basal, the PL mid, the apical and mid septal LV segment, employing LVdP/dtmax measured with a 0.014" RADI pressure wire and a temporary pacing wire positioned retrograde or transseptal into the LV. The set-up for the temporary study is schematically shown in the following figure. (Fig. 8)

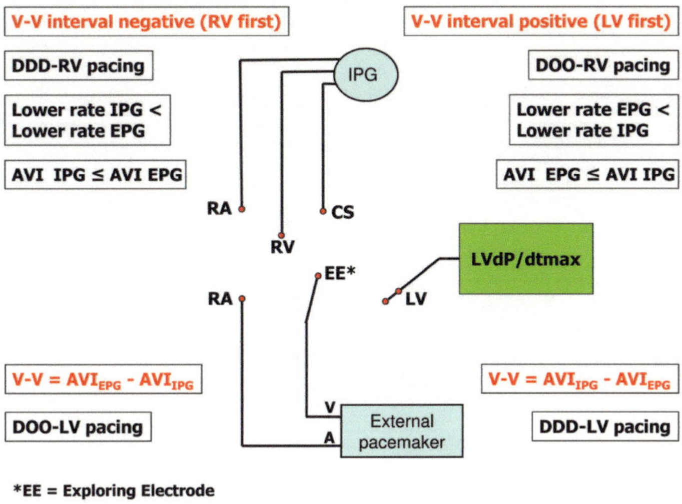

Fig. 8. Schematic presentation of the temporary hemodynamic pacing study.

The exploring electrode is used for temporary LV pacing either AV sequentially, or combined with the implanted system in a biventricular mode with the option of using a V-V interval.

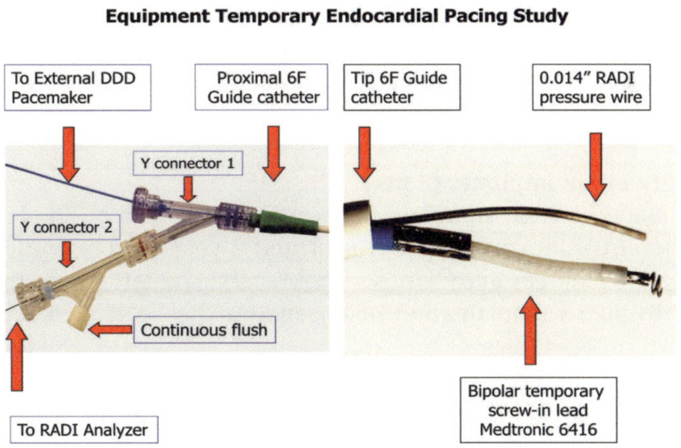

Fig. 9. Set up of the 6F guide catheter with RADI pressure wire and temporary bipolar screw-in lead both inserted through the guide catheter.

For hemodynamic evaluation of a selected pacing site the AV (for LV pacing) and AV and V-V (for BiV pacing) were optimized. A temporary atrial electrode has to be inserted to synchronize the external and implanted system. In the transseptal set-up a 6F guide catheter, multipurpose or internal mammary catheter, are inserted through the 8F transseptal sheath. For femoral or radial approach the same guide catheter can be used employing a 6F sheath at the arterial entrance site, as shown in figure 9.

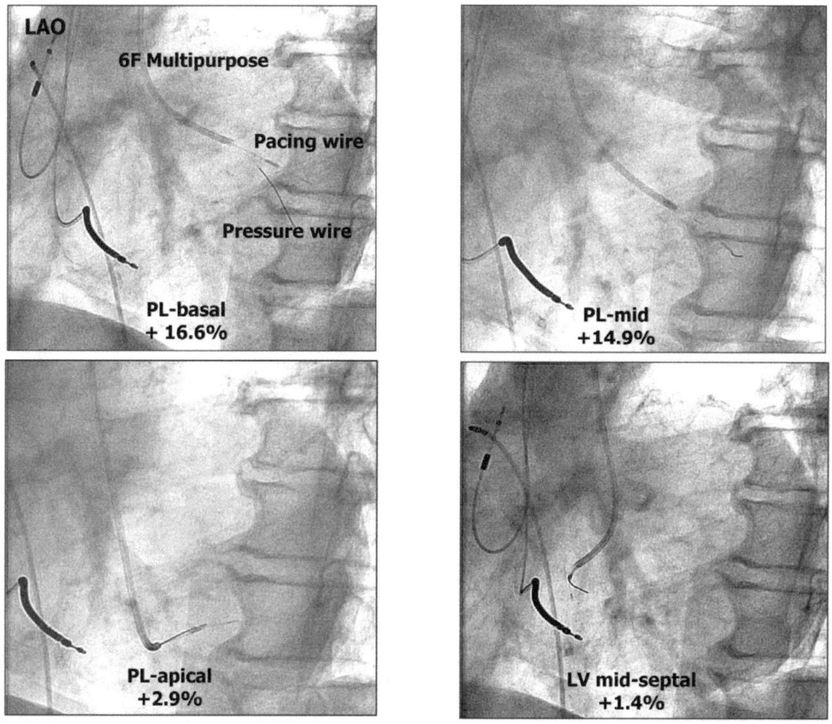

Fig. 10. Example of radiographic pictures in a left anterior oblique position of the 4 locations that were hemodynamically tested during the temporary pacing study. The percentage increase in LVdP/dt compared to baseline is mentioned for every position.

4.3 Results

4.4 Failed coronary sinus implants (2 pts)

Two patients developed a high stimulation threshold, approaching the level of exit block. Both had a successful CS implant respectively 1 and 2 years before with placement of the lead in the only accessible coronary sinus side branch. The latter was the reason for the temporary study to justify implantation of an endocardial lead as a replacement of the failing CS lead.

In the first patient, a 76 year old male with ICM, who was pacemaker dependent LVdP/dtmax decreased to 321 mmHg/s when programmed to RV pacing, thus imitating complete failure of the LV lead. Biventricular pacing from PL-basal, PL-mid, LV apex, LV septum resulted in a LVdPdtmax of respectively 994, 933, 741, and 813 mmHg/s, whereas the CS lead, which was in a PL basal position resulted in 967 mmHg/s. Patient underwent a successful transseptal implant of an endocardial LV lead in the PL-basal area.

The second patient with an extreme high LV threshold, had a 17% increase in LVdP/dt with the CS lead, which was positioned in a PL basal position. Temporary pacing from other endocardial positions did not improve this increase. CS pacing could be maintained at maximum LV output setting. A LV endocardial lead will be implanted at generator change to avoid premature battery depletion of the new device.

4.5 Nonresponders (10 pts)

In 2 patients 74 and 79 years old, both with ICM, and an ECG with right bundle branch block (RBBB), QRS duration 170 and 175 ms did not respond to CRT with leads positioned in the CS. The hemodynamic pacing study revealed no improvement in LVdP/dtmax with the implanted system. LV pacing from the 4 endocardial positions could not increase LVdP/dt above the intrinsic baseline value in both patients.

In one patient with a dual chamber ICD and increasing heart failure, but with a RBBB, implantation of a CRT system was considered. Prior to implant a temporary pacing study was performed to evaluate the hemodynamic effect of CRT. LV endocardial pacing showed an increase in LVdP/dtmax when pacing from the PL basal area of 17%. CS angiography showed a suitable side branch in the target area and a successful implant was performed in the preselected location.

Four patients, 1 with DCM and 3 with ICM, with LBBB in 3 patients and RV pacing in 1 patient, were all nonresponders. The mean ejection fraction prior to implant was 17.5±6.5%. Hemodynamic pacing study revealed an increase of LVdP/dtmax at the optimal endocardial location of 25.2±4.8%. In 3 patients the optimal location was PL-basal, and PL-mid in 1 patient. The patients with the lowest ejection fraction of 13 and 12% underwent a successful transseptal and transapical implant respectively. One of these patients with DCM, turned out to be superresponder with a reduction of NYHA class IV to II, an increase in ejection fraction from 13 to 45% and a decrease in the end-diastolic and systolic diameter to 61 and 47 mm, respectively, with only minor mitral regurgitation (Bracke et al. 2010).

In one nonresponder (LBBB, QRS duration 206 ms), who was not optimized but programmed to a standard setting with a V-V interval of 40 ms (LV pre-activation), LVdP/dtmax was 1017 mmHg/s. During hemodynamic testing LVdP/dtmax with RV pacing was 1113 mmHg/s, whereas CS pacing resulted in a LVdP/dtmax of 870 mmHg/s. All endocardial positions except LV apex had a lower LVdP/dtmax than with RV pacing. LV apex had the same LVdP/dt as RV pacing, which was not surprising, because of the similarity in anatomical positions of bot pacing modalities. Changing the V-V timing to -40 ms (RV pre-activation), and selecting the proximal CS electrode increased LVdP/dtmax for biventricular pacing to 1193 mmHg/s (+17.3%). Patient clinically improved after optimization with 1 NYHA class.

In one patient who showed increasing heart failure after initial response to CRT, was referred to our institution for hemodynamic evaluation. Hemodynamics at the current setting showed a LVdP/dtmax value of 720 mmHg/s. After optimization of the AV and V-V interval and selecting the proximal CS electrode of the dual unipolar lead instead of the distal electrode LVdP/dtmax could be increased with 11.5%, which resulted in a significant clinical improvement with loss of weight and reduction of diuretics.

The last patient, male 87 years, NYHA class III, ejection fraction 25%, LBBB with QRS duration of 154 ms presented as a clinical nonresponder. Baseline LVdP/dt was 827 mmHg/s and increased with 45% by optimized biventricular pacing employing the implanted CS lead. In the best endocardial position (PL-basal) a gain of 51% could be obtained. Although left ventricular remodeling with reduction of end-diastolic and systolic diameter was significant, patient did subjectivally not improve. Presumably, patient's symptoms were most probably associated with increasing age depending physical limitations instead of failing CRT.

4.6 Hemodynamic effect related to pacing site

The effect of LV pacing as related to the investigated pacing sites, posterolateral-basal (PL-bas), posterolateral-mid (PL-mid), LV apical (LV-apic) and LV midseptal (LV-sept) position is illustrated in fig. 11.

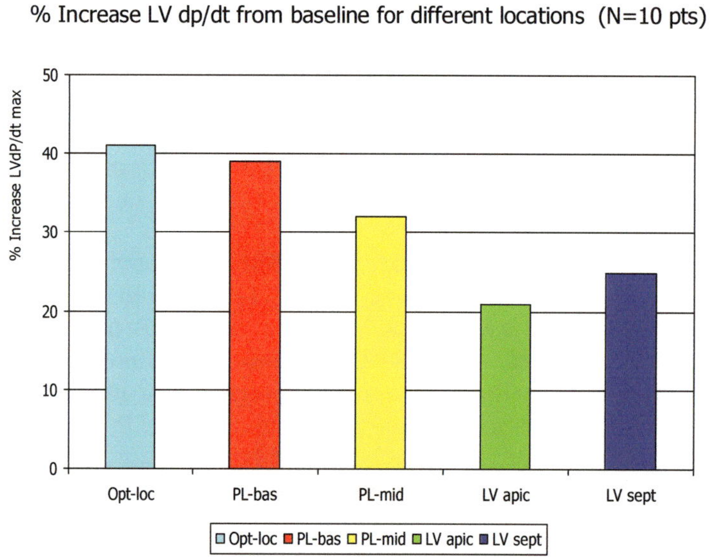

Fig. 11. Graphic display of percentage increase of LVdP/dt at 4 endocardial LV locations. The average of the optimal location (Opt-loc) is displayed in the left bar.

The posterolateral basal position is on average the best position, demonstrated by the maximum increase in LVdP/dt in 7 out of the 10 patients. In 1 patient the posterolateral-mid position gave the best result. In 2 patients LV pacing from the LV apex had the highest LVdP/dt. Of note, one patient with the highest value of LVdP/dt with LV apex pacing was one of the patients with a RBBB. The second patient was the patient in whom all LV endocardial locations resulted in a lower LVdP/dt than RV apex pacing, but LV apex was the best of 4 locations, which is reasonable because LV apex pacing has the best similarity with RV apex pacing.

In the all nonresponders where the effect of LV epicardial pacing from the CS was compared to the effect at the endocardial counterpart, we could not find a significant difference between epicardial and endocardial stimulation in this small series of patients. Epicardial stimulation from the CS position resulted in an increase in LVdP/dt of +7.1%±2.5%, whereas from the endocardial counterpart an increase of 6.7%±4.1% was measured, an observation which is in contrast with other studies (Garrigue et al., 2001; Van Deursen at al., 2007; Van Deursen et al., 2008).

In all nonresponders the increase in LVdP/dt by CS pacing was below 10%. In 4 nonresponders a low response could be anticipated because of lead positions in the antero-lateral vein (2 pts) and mid cardiac vein (2 pts).

5. Discussion

LV endocardial pacing is an alternative for failed coronary sinus implants as illustrated in the first section of this chapter. The choice for application of endocardial LV pacing in case of failed CS implant is based on a risk analysis in which factors like age, physical condition, degree of heart failure and the presence of anticoagulant therapy play a role.

Remains the question, should hemodynamic testing for the evaluation of the effect of LV pacing in patients with failed CS implants be performed prior to the LV endocardial implant?

The answers that we get from the temporary hemodynamic studies are twofold. First, it is a quantification of the improvement that can be obtained with LV endocardial pacing, expressed as the increase in LVdP/dtmax. Second, the pacing site where this optimal effect is obtained is determined and is used as the target area for the permanent implant.

The latter justifies hemodynamic testing in failed implants with proper patient selection, or short term failure in patients that are responding to CRT during this short follow-up, in whom a transseptal implant is considered.

In patients not responding to CRT due to a suboptimal position of the CS lead, implant of an endocardial LV lead can be considered. Hemodynamic evaluation in a temporary setting seems to be mandatory prior to the implant procedure, in order to determine the effect on contractility at the optimal endocardial site and the location of this site. This temporary study prevents implants of a LV endocardial lead in patients in whom, based on the outcome of the temporary study, with an increase in LVdP/dtmax of less than 10% no clinical improvement can be anticipated. On the other hand, patients that show an increase in LVdP/dt over 15% from an endocardial location are suitable candidates for an endocardial implant and the optimal site in the temporary study determines the target area for the permanent implant.

Implantation of an additional CS lead, thus creating triple site ventricular stimulation in nonresponders is suggested by Leclercq et al., who demonstrated improvement in cardiac volumes by echocardiographic techniques in this configuration over biventricular stimulation (Leclercq et al., 2008). Although the effect and technique of triple ventricular stimulation needs further investigation (Auricchio & Prinzen, 2008), the technique is not feasible in the patient category with failed CS implants or short term failure of a single CS lead.

From our experience it became obvious that in patients with LBBB the postero-lateral basal area is the optimal site with a significant lower hemodynamic response from different locations like the septal and apical segment. From this experience it is difficult to understand that in larger studies (MADIT CRT), with no specific focus on this item, is concluded that the location of LV stimulation has no effect on clinical outcome.

In spite of the small number of patients and a non-homogeneous patient population according to their electrocardiographic presentation, it is clear that in nonresponders an increase in LVdP/dt of less than 10% is objectivated. If pacing from a different LV location with a rise in LVdP/dt over 15% is initialized these patients became responders to CRT.

After measurement of the hemodynamic effect on LVdP/dt in a nonresponder at the programmed pacing parameters, optimization of AV and V-V interval should be performed to exclude a suboptimal setting of AV and V-V interval as a contributor to non response. If the patient also has a CS dual unipolar lead, the effect of selecting a different stimulation electrode should also be evaluated. In 2 of our patients improvement in LVdP/dtmax as well as clinical status could be obtained by optimization of AV, V-V interval and selection of the CS pacing electrode. One can speculate that development of quadripolar CS leads with programmable pacing configurations may contribute to a further optimization of CRT.

6. Conclusion

LV endocardial pacing from a transseptal or transapical approach can be considered after failed CS implant or non responsiveness to CRT. The tentative benefit of a LV endocardial implant can be hemodynamical evaluated by measurement of LVdP/dt in a temporary set up. The endocardial postero-lateral area proved to be significant better than apical and mid-septal locations in patients with LBBB. In this small series the superior effect of endocardial pacing compared to the epicardial counterpart could not be objectivated from the hemodynamic evaluation.

7. References

Abraham WT, Fisher WG, Smith AL, Delurgio DB, Leon AR, Loh E, Kocovic DZ, Packer M, Clavell AL, Hayes DL, Ellestad M, Messenger J, for the MIRACLE Study Group. Cardiac resynchronization in chronic heart failure. *N. Engl. J. Med.* 2002;346:1845-1853.

Auricchio A, Ding J, Spinelli JC, Kramer AP, Salo RW, Hoersch W, KenKnight BH, Klein HU, for PATH-CHF Study Group. Cardiac resynchronization therapy restores optimal atrioventricular mechanical timing in heart failure patients with ventricular conduction delay. *J. Am. Coll. Cardiol.* 2002;39:1163–1169.

Auricchio A, Abraham WT. Cardiac resynchronization therapy: current state of the art. Cost versus benefit. *Circulation* 2004;109:300–307.

Aurichio A, Prinzen FW. Cardiac Resynchronization Therapy: The more pacing sites, the better the outcome ? *J. Am. Coll. Cardiol.* 2008;51;1463-1465.

Bentkover JD, Stewart EJ, Ignaszewski A, Lepage S, Liu P, Cooper J. New technologies and potential cost savings related to morbidity and mortality reduction in Class III / IV heart failure patients in Canada. *Int. J. Cardiol.* 2003;88:33-41.

Bracke FA, Houthuizen P, Rahel BM, and van Gelder BM. Left ventricular endocardial pacing improves the clinical efficacy in a non-responder to cardiac resynchronization therapy: role of acute haemodynamic testing. *Europace* 2010; doi:10.1093/europace/euq043.

Butter C, Auricchio A, Stellbrink C, Fleck E, Ding J, Yu Y, Huvelle E., Spinelli J. Effect of resynchronization therapy stimulation site on the systolic function of heart failure patients. Circulation 2001;104:3026-3029.

Cazeau S, Leclercq C, Lavergne T, Walker S, Varma C, Linde C, Garrigue S, Kappenberger L, Haywood G, Santini M, Bailleul C, Daubert JC, for the Multisite Stimulation in Cardiomyopathies (MUSTIC) Study Investigators. Effects of multisite biventricular pacing in patients with heart failure and intraventricular conduction delay. *N. Eng. J. Med.* 2001;344: 873-880.

Cequier A, Bonan R, Dyrda I, Crépeau J, Dethy M, Petitclerc R, Waters D. Atrial shunting after percutaneous mitral valvuloplasty. Circulation 1988;78: II-488 (Abstract).

Cleland JGF, Daubert JC, Erdmann E, Freemantle N, Gras D, Kappenberger L, Tavazzi L, for the cardiac resynchronization on morbidity and mortality in heart failure (CARE-HF) study investigators. *N. Eng. J. Med.* 2005;352(15):1539-1549.

Garrigue S, Jaïs P, Espil G, Labeque J-N, Hocini M, Shah DC, Haïssaguerre M, Cleménty J. Comparison of chronic biventricular pacing between epicardial and endocardial left ventricular stimulation using Doppler tissue imaging in patients with heart failure. *Am. J. Cardiol.* 2001; 88: 858-862.

Gras D, Leclercq C, Tang AS, Bucknall C, Luttikhuis HO, Kirstein-Pedersen A. Cardiac Resynchronization Therapy in advanced heart failure; the multicenter InSync clinical study. *Eur. J. Heart Fail.* 2002;4:311–320.

Jaïs P, Douard H, Shah DC, Barold S, Barat J-L, Clémenty J. Endocardial biventricular pacing. *Pacing Clin. Electrophysiol.* 1998;21:2128-2131.

Jaïs P, Takabashi A, Garrigue S, Yamane T, Hocini M, Shah DC, Barold SS, Deisenhofer I, Haïssaguerre, Clémenty J. Mid-term follow-up of endocardial biventricular pacing. *Pacing Clin. Electrophysiol.* 2000;23:1744-1747.

Jaïs P, Sacher F, Laborderie J, Reuter S, Bordachar P, Hsu L-F, Sanders P, Hocini M, O'Neill MD, Johnsson A, Takahasi, Y, Haissaguerre M, Clementy J. Tailored endocardial left ventricular pacing is superior to coronary sinus in heart failure patients needing cardiac resynchronization. *Heart Rhythm* 2006;3:S247.(abstract).

Joshi S, Steinberg JS, Ashton RC, Balaram S, Fischer A, and DeRose JJ. Follow-up of robotically assisted left ventricular epicardial leads for cardiac resynchronization therapy. *J. Am. Coll. Cardiol.* 2005;46:2358-2359.

Kassaï I, Szili-Torok . Concerns about the long-term outcome of transseptal cardiac resynchronization therapy: what have we learned from surgical experience. Europace 2008;10:121-122.

Kassaï I, Foldesi C, Szekely A,, Szili-Torok T. Alternative method for cardiac resynchronization therapy. Transapical lead implantation. *Ann. Thoracic. Surg.* 2009;87(2):650-652.

Koos R, Sinha A-M, Markus K, Breithardt O-A, Mischke K, Zarse M, Scmid M, Autschbach R, Hanrath P and Stellbrink C. Comparison of left ventricular lead placement via the coronary venous approach versus lateral thoracotomy in patients receiving cardiac resynchronization therapy. *Am. J. Cardiol.* 2004;94:59-63.

Leclercq C, Gadler F, Kranig W, Ellery S, Gras D, Lazarus A, Clementy J, Boulogne E, Daubert J-C for the TRIP-HF (Triple Resynchronization in Paced Heart Failure patients). A randomized comparison of triple-site versus dual site ventricular stimulation in patients with congestive heart failure. *J. Am. Coll. Cardiol.* 2008;51:1455-1462.

Leclercq F, Hager FX, Macia JC, Mariottini CJ, Pasquié JL, Grolleau R. Left ventricular lead insertion using a modified transseptal catheterization technique: a totally endocardial approach for permanent biventricular pacing in end-stage heart failure. *Pacing Clin. Electrophysiol.* 1999;22:1570-1575.

Leon AR, Abraham WT, Curtis AB, Daubert JP, Fisher WG, Gurley J, Hayes DL, Lieberman R, Petersen-Stejskal S, Wheelan K. Safety of transvenous cardiac resynchronization system implantation in patients with chronic heart hailure: combined results of over 2000 patients from a multicenter study program. *J. Am. Coll. Cardiol.* 2005;46:2348-2356.

McKay RG, Lock JE, Safian RD, Come PC, Diver DJ, Baim DS, Berman AD, Warren SE, Mandell VE, Royal HD, Grossman W. Balloon dilatation of mitral stenosis in adult patients: Postmortem and percutaneous mitral valvuloplasty studies. *J. Am. Coll. Cardiol.* 1987;9:723-731.

Palacios IF, Block PC, Wilkins GT, Weyman AE. Follow-up of patients undergoing percutaneous mitral balloon valvotomy. Analysis of factors determining restenosis. Circulation 1989;79:573-579.

Pasquié JL, Massin F, Macia J, Gervasoni R, Bortone A, Cayla G, Grolleau R, and Leclercq F, Grolleau R. Long-term follow-up of biventricular pacing using a totally endocardial approach in patients with end-stage cardiac failure. *Pacing Clin. Electrophysiol.* 2007; 30:S31–S33.

Sen JI, Cesario DA, Swerdlow CD, and Shivkumar K. Left ventricular endocardial lead placement using a modified transseptal technique. *J Cardiovasc Electrophysiol* 2004; 15:234–236.

Sharifi M, Sorkin R, Sharifi V, et al. Inadvertent malposition of a transvenous-inserted pacing lead in the left ventricular chamber. *Am. J. Cardiol.* 1995;76:92-105.

Soliman MH, van GelderBM, Bracke FA, AAJ van Zundert, van Straten AHM. Acute hemodynamic effects of cardiac resynchronization therapy in patients with poor left ventricular function during cardiac surgery. *J. Card. Surg.* 2009;24:585-590.

Van Deursen C, Van Hunnik A, Kuiper M, Prinzen FW. Endocardial left ventricular pacing improves cardiac resynchronization therapy in canine LBBB hearts (abstr). *Circulation* 2007;116 Suppl II:2515.

Van Deursen C, van Geldrop I, van Hunik A, Auricchio A, Echt D, Prinzen FW. Improved myocardial repolarization, and left ventricular systolic and diastolic function during endocardial cardiac resynchronization therapy. *Heart Rhythm* 2008;5:S188 (Abstract).

Van Gelder B, Bracke F, Oto A, Yildirir A, Haas PC, Seger JJ, Stainback RF and Meijer A. Diagnosis and management of inadvertently placed pacing and ICD leads in the left ventricle: A multicenter experience and review of the literature. *Pacing Clin. Electrophysiol.* 2000;23:877 – 883.

Van Gelder BM, Bracke FA, Meijer A, Lakerveld LJM, and Pijls NHJ.Effect of Optimizing the VV interval on Left Ventricular Contractility in Cardiac Resynchronization Therapy. *Am. J. Cardiol.* 2004;93:1500-1503.

Van Gelder BM, Scheffer MG, Meijer A, Bracke FA. Transseptal endocardial left ventricular pacing: An alternative technique for coronary sinus lead placement in cardiac resynchronization therapy. *Heart Rhythm* 2007; 4:454-460.

Van Gelder BM, Bracke FA, van der Voort PH, Meijer A. Optimal sensed AV interval determined by the paced QRS complex. *Pacing and Clin Electrophysiol* 2007;30:476-481.b.

Yu C-M, Wing-Hong Fung J, Zhang Q, and Sanderson JE. Understanding nonresponders of cardiac resynchronization-Current and future perspectives. *J Cardiovasc. Electrophysiol.* 2005;16:1117-1124.

6

Pacing Therapy in Infants and Children with Congenital and Acquired Complete Atrioventricular Block: Optimal Pacing Strategies, Management, and Follow-up.

Floris E.A. Udink ten Cate and Narayanswami Sreeram
Department of Paediatric Cardiology, Heart Center Cologne, University Hospital of Cologne, Cologne, Germany

1. Introduction

Bradycardia due to high-degree atrioventricular (AV) block remains the main indication for permanent cardiac pacing in childhood. Although there are major differences in the etiology of AV block in children and adults, the same pacing systems and leads are used in both age groups. The first pacemaker was implanted in a child in the late 1960s (Martin et al., 1966). Nowadays, implantation of a permanent pacing system is a straightforward and safe procedure with excellent pacemaker performance during follow-up, even in infants and small children (Welisch et al., 2010).

Applying permanent pacing therapy in the young can be challenging. Many paediatric issues, such as patient size, body growth, coexistence of congenital heart disease, presence of residual intracardiac shunts and life style, have to be considered. Selecting the best pacing system for a child requires a firm understanding of modern pacing design, pacing indications, advantages and drawbacks of epicardial and endocardial lead pacing, and possible complications. The aim of this chapter is to give a dedicated overview of the practical implications of pacing in children with complete AV block.

2. Etiology of atrioventricular block in childhood

Before we describe the techniques and management of pacing in children, an overview of the most important causes of complete AV block in children is given. Having a complete understanding of the etiology and prognosis of complete AV block in childhood should improve best pacing practice in the paediatric age group. A summary of the causes of complete AV block in childhood is presented in Table 1.

2.1 Postoperative complete atrioventricular block

Complete AV block is an important complication of surgical correction of congenital heart disease (Gross et al., 2006). Due to advances in surgical techniques and improved anatomic knowledge of the course of the conduction system in various congenital heart diseases, the incidence of postoperative complete AV block has decreased significantly during the last decades (Gross et al., 2006). Although complete AV block was found in more than 10% of children in the 1960s, a study from the early 1970s reported that this incidence had fallen to around 2% (Fryda et al., 1970). In the current era, 1 - 3% of all children undergoing surgery for congenital heart disease develop complete AV block. Importantly, it has been shown that surgical complete AV block is associated with significant morbidity and decreased survival. (Gross et al., 2006; Driscoll et al., 1979). Therefore, all children should receive a pacemaker device when complete AV block does not resolve in the early postoperative course (Gross et al, 2006).

Surgical acquired AV block	VSD, AVSD, TOF LVOT obstruction, ccTGA discordant AV connections
Isolated congenital complete AV block	maternal anti-SSA/Ro - SSB/La antibodies, NLE abnormal development of AV conduction
AV block associated with structural cardiac abnormalities	ccTGA heterotaxy, left atrial isomerism
	single ventricle physiology, Fontan palliation D-TGA after Mustard or Senning operation
Infectious disease	bacterial viral EBV, varicella, Coxsackie B Rheumatic fever Chagas' disease Lyme disease HIV
Neuromuscular disease	Myotonic dystrophy Emery-Dreifuss muscular dystrophy Duchenne muscular dystrophy
Metabolic disease	Carnitine deficieny Kearns-Sayre syndrome
Syndromes	Holt-Oram syndrome 18p-syndrome
Others	long-QT syndrome post-Ablation hypertrophic cardiomyopathy percutaneous VSD closure myocarditis connective tissue disease sarcoidosis amyloidosis cardiac tumors

AVSD = atrioventricular septal defect, AV = atrioventricular, ccTGA = congenitally corrected transposition of the great arteries, D-TGA = dextro-transposition of the great arteries, EBV = Ebstein-Barr virus, HIV = human immunodeficiency virus, LVOT = left ventricular outflow tract, NLE = neonatal lupus erythematosus, TOF = tetralogy of Fallot, VSD = ventricular septal defect.

Table 1. Causes of complete atrioventricular block in neonates, infants and children.

The greatest risk for complete AV block is associated with corrective surgical procedures for ventricular septal defects (VSD), usually as part of more complex congenital heart disease, atrioventricular septal defects (AVSD), left ventricular outflow tract obstruction, L transposition of the great arteries, tetralogy of Fallot (TOF), and discordant atrioventricular connections (Batra et al., 2003; Gross et al., 2006). Most children who require pacing for surgically induced AV block are less than 1 year old.

Of importance, several studies report spontaneous resolution of complete AV block in the early postoperative period, most often occurring between 7 and 14 days. Complete AV block may resolve spontaneously in 43 - 92% of children (Gross et al, 2006). Factors associated with a spontaneous recovery of AV nodal function are currently not known. Hence, late recovery of complete AV block has also been reported in approximately 10% of cases (Batra et al., 2003). Recovery of AV conduction was identified within the first 30-day postoperative interval in most children. Recurrence of high-degree AV block or complete AV block is not observed in these children, although different studies have shown inconsistent findings (Batra et al., 2003; Gross et al., 2006). On the contrary, late onset complete AV block (> 30 days postoperatively) has been described after cardiac surgery for congenital heart disease (Goldman et al., 1985.; Liberman et al., 2008). Complete AV block was identified at a mean of 4.7 years after surgery in one study (Goldman et al., 1985), occurring as late as 16 years after cardiac surgery (Liberman et al., 2008). Close monitoring of AV conduction seems mandatory in all patients after surgery for congenital heart disease.

2.2 Congenital complete AV block

Congenital complete AV block (CCAVB) is a rare cardiac conduction disorder with an estimated incidence of 1 in 11.000 to 22.000 live births (Michaelson & Engle, 1972). In 25% of cases, coexisting congenital heart disease can be identified. Congenital heart diseases in which AV conduction is particularly at risk include heterotaxy syndrome with left atrial isomerism, atrioventricular septal defect with common atrioventricular junction, and congenitally corrected transposition of the great arteries (ccTGA) (Anderson et al., 1974; Stephenson & Kaltman, 2006). Complete AV block in these patients may be present at birth, or may develop later in life. When complete AV block is not present at birth, close monitoring of the cardiac conduction system is mandatory in these patients (Stephenson & Kaltman, 2006 & Graham et al, 2000). Notwithstanding, most patients with CCAVB have structurally normal hearts, and CCAVB in these cases is therefore referred to as 'isolated' CCAVB. Although abnormal embryological development of the cardiac conducting system have been identified as a cause of isolated CCAVB (Anderson et al., 1977; Lev et al., 1971), most patients have autoimmune, anti-SSA/Ro - SSB/La-antibody-induced CCAVB (Buyon & Winchester, 1990; McCue et al., 1977).

Since an association between maternal connective tissue disease and anti-SSA/Ro - SSB/La antibodies was suggested in the late 1970s (McCue et al., 1977), efforts in clinical and experimental studies have resulted in a broad understanding of the pathogenesis and clinical outcome of autoimmune-associated CCAVB (Boutjdir et al., 1998; Buyon & Clancy, 2005; Jaeggi et al., 2010). Maternal anti-SSA/Ro - SSB/La autoantibodies enter the fetal circulation between 16 and 24 weeks gestation (Buyon et al., 1995), and may induce injury to the developing cardiac conducting system and myocardial tissue in a subset of fetuses. Autoimmune CCAVB develops in 1 - 2% of these antibody-positive pregnancies. Of importance, the estimated recurrence risk of women who had a previous child with CCAVB is 16 - 25% (Buyon et al., 2009). Although 30 - 50% of these women have clinically manifest

connective tissue diseases, such as systemic lupus erythematosus or Sjögren's syndrome, the majority of antibody-positive women who gave birth to an infant with CCAVB, are asymptomatic (Julkunen & Eronen, 2001).
Anti-SSA/Ro - SSB/La antibody-induced CCAVB is associated with substantial morbidity and mortality during gestation and infancy, with more than 60% of infants requiring permanent pacemaker therapy in their first year of life (Buyon et al., 1998; Breur et al., 2002). The most common indication for pacemaker placement in the neonatal period is congestive heart failure (Buyon et al., 1998). The natural history of isolated CCAVB was addressed in a prospective multicenter study, involving 102 children and adults (Michaelsson et al., 1995; Michaelsson et al., 1997). All children were asymptomatic during their 15 years of life. Of concern, 10 patients without a pacemaker died, of which 6 CCAVB related deaths occurred without preceding symptoms. The mortality rate was significantly lower in paced compared to non-paced patients. Therefore, the authors concluded that the prognosis of isolated CCAVB may be improved when patients are paced earlier in life (Michaelsson et al., 1997). A recent study supported the concept of earlier 'prophylactic' pacing in children with isolated CCAVB (Balmer et al., 2002). At present, more than 94% of children with CCAVB are paced before they reach the age of 15 years (Villain et al., 2006).
Another important prognostic issue in children with autoimmune-associated CCAVB is the development of dilated cardiomyopathy (Moak et al., 2001; Udink ten Cate et al., 2001). We and others have demonstrated that as many as 6 - 11 % of paced children with autoimmune-associated CCAVB develop dilated cardiomyopathy during a follow-up period of 10 ± 7 years (Moak et al., 2001; Udink ten Cate et al., 2001; Kim et al., 2007). Risk factors may include presence of anti-SSA/Ro - SSB/La antibodies, increased heart size at initial evaluation and the absence of pacemaker-associated normalization of left ventricular size during follow-up (Udink ten Cate et al., 2001). Although pacemaker-induced ventricular dysfunction has been offered as an etiologic factor in the pathogenesis of dilated cardiomyopathy in these patients (Janousek et al., 2004), some children with anti-SSA/Ro - SSB/La antibody-induced CCAVB develop dilated cardiomyopathy before being paced (Nield et al., 2002; Villain et al., 2006). These data suggest that children with anti-SSA/Ro - SSB/La antibody-induced CCAVB may have preexisting myocardial damage, which increases their risk of pacemakerinduced dilated cardiomyopathy. Close monitoring of their ventricular function during follow-up is mandatory.
The prognosis of non-autoimmune CCAVB seems to be different compared to autoimmune-associated CCAVB (Cruz et al., 2004; Villain et al., 2006). Patients are commonly diagnosed later in life, the AV block is often progressive, and these children have a good prognosis after pacemaker implantation (Villain et al, 2006).
Moreover, connective tissue disease is not found in these mothers, and the recurrence risk in future pregnancies is low. Pacemaker-induced heart failure does not seem to occur during medium follow-up (Cruz et al., 2004). For these reasons, a new definition of congenital complete AV block was recently proposed: 'an AV block is defined as congenital if it is diagnosed in utero, at birth or within the neonatal period' (Brucato et al., 2003).

3. Pacing indications and patient selection

Specific recommendations for pacemaker implantation have been published in several guidelines by the American College of Cardiology, the American Heart Association, and the Heart Rhythm Society, with an update in 2008 (Epstein et al., 2008). The European Society of

Cardiology, and the European Heart Rhythm Association have also recently published a guideline for permanent pacing and cardiac resynchronization therapy (Vardas et al., 2007). Pacing recommendations for children are also a part of these published guidelines, and have been very useful in daily practice. It should be remembered however, that the level of evidence for these recommendations is low. Most recommendations for children requiring permanent pacing are not based on prospective clinical studies, but rather rely on expert opinion.
The main indications for pacing in children are (1) symptomatic sinus node dysfunction, (2) bradycardia-tachycardia syndrome, (3) congenital, surgical or acquired complete AV block, and (4) advanced second-degree AV block. Because this chapter is dedicated to AV block in children, pacing recommendations for this specific conduction disorder are summarized in Table 2.

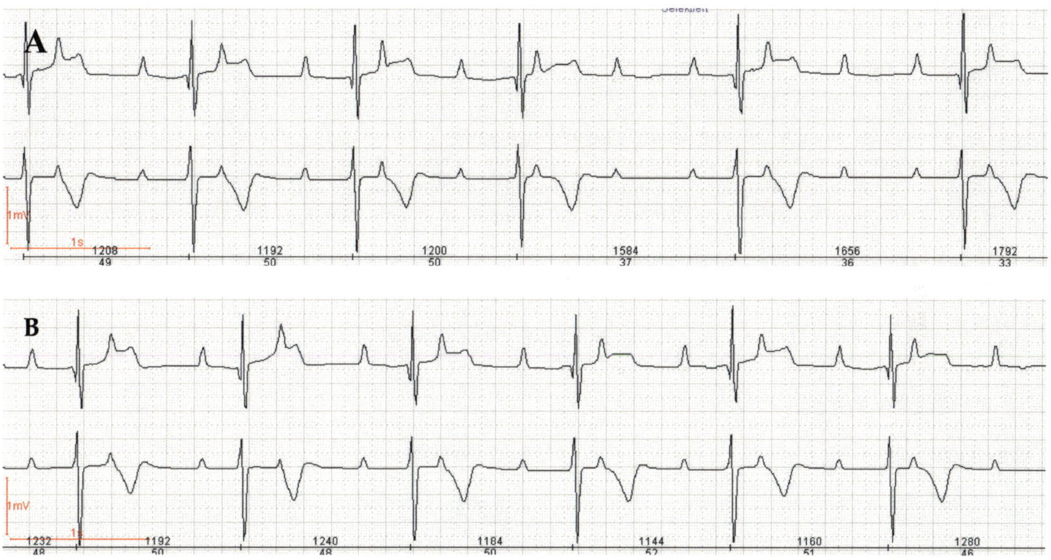

Fig. 1. Rhythm strip showing complete atrioventricular block (**A**) and second-degree atrioventricular block in a 2-year-old boy with bradycardia-related symptoms (**B**). The child underwent permanent pacemaker implantation (single chamber) using the transvenous approach. A lumenless 4.1-F endocardial lead inserted.

Surgical second-degree or complete AV block persisting beyond 7 days postoperatively, not expecting to resolve spontaneously, is considered to be a Class I indication for permanent pacemaker implantation (Vardas et al., 2007; Epstein et al., 2008). There are two important reasons for not delaying pacemaker implantation in these patients, although there is reasonable evidence that AV conduction may recover in the first 30 postoperative days (Batra et al., 2003). The prognosis of surgically induced complete AV block is poor (Gross et al, 2006, Simon et al., 1982). The second consideration is that there have been enormous improvements in pacing systems and battery longevity. A pacemaker can now be safely implanted in most small infants.
Advanced second-degree or complete CAVB with symptomatic bradycardia (Figure 1), ventricular dysfunction, or low cardiac output, is also considered to be a Class I indication for pacemaker insertion. One has to keep in mind that symptoms of bradycardia can be subtle in children, (Balmer & Bauersfeld, 2003). Therefore, many investigators have tried to

predict the need for future pacemaker therapy in isolated CCAVB, using diagnostic tests, such as serial ECG recordings and ambulatory Holter monitoring (Esscher & Michaellson, 1983; Dewey et al., 1987; Breur et al, 2006). Interpretation of these parameters remains difficult.

Class I, permanent pacemaker implantation is indicated for:

1. Advanced 2nd or 3rd AV block with symptomatic bradycardia, ventricular dysfunction, or low cardiac out put.
2. Postoperative advanced 2nd or 3rd degree AV block that is not expected to resolve or persists > 7 days after cardiac surgery.
3. Congenital complete AV block with a wide QRS escape rhythm, complex ventricular ectopy, or ventricular dysfunction.
4. Congenital complete AV block in the infant with aventricular rate less than 55 betas per minute (bps) or with congenital heart disease and a ventricular rate les s than 70 bps.

Class IIa, permanent pacemaker implantation is reasonable for:

1. Congenital complete AV block beyond the first yearof life with an average heart rate less than 50 bp m, abrupt pauses in ventricular arte that are 2 or 3 times the basic cycle length, or associated with sym ptoms due to chronotropic incompetence.
2. Congenital heart disease and impaired hemodynamics due to sinus bradycardia or loss of AV synchrony.
3. Unexplained syncope in the patient with prior congenital heart surgery complicated by transient complete heart block with residual fascicular block after careful eveluation to exclude other causes of syncope.
4. Long QT syndrome with 2:1 or complete AV block.

Class IIb, permanent pacemaker implantation may be considered for:

1. Transient postoperative third-degree AV block thatreverts to sinus rhythm with residual bifascicularblock.
2. Congenital complete AV block in asymptomatic childen or adolescents with an acceptable rate, narrow QRS complex, and normal ventricular function.
3. Neuromuscular diseases with any degree of AV block (including first-degree AV block) due to risk of unpredictable progression of AV conduction disease.

Class III, permanent pacemaker implantation is not indicated for:

1. Transient postoperative third-degree AV block withreturn of normal AV conduction within 7 days.
2. Asymptomatic postoperative bifascicular block with and without first-degree AV block.
3. Asymptomatic type I (Wenckebach) second-degree AV b lock

---

* Adapted from Epstein AE, DiMarco JP, Ellenbogen KA, et al. ACC/AHA/HRS 2008 guidelines for device-based therapy of cardic rhythm abnormalities: executive summary. Heart Rhythm 2008;5:e1-62; and Vardas PE, Auricchio A, Blanc JJ, et al. Guidelines for cardiac pacing and cardiac resynchronization therapy: the task force for cardiac pacing and cardiac resynchronization therapy of the European Society of Cardiology. Developed in collaboration with the European Heart Rhythm Association. Eur Heart J 2007;28:2256-2295.

Table 2. Indications for permanent pacemaker implantation in children and adolescents with high-degree or complete AV block with or without congenital heart disease*.

Several studies have shown that monitoring of heart size and cardiomegaly in children with isolated CCAVB is of use in daily practice in deciding if a child requires a pacemaker (Beaufort-Krol et al., 2007; Breur et al., 2002; Sholler & Walsh, 1989). We favour implantation of a pacemaker in a child with isolated CCAVB in whom the heart size progresses during follow-up, even when the heart rate criteria for pacemaker implantation are not met.

4. Selecting a pacing system: single or dual chamber device?

The aim of permanent pacing therapy in patients with complete AV block is to restore heart rhythm and rate, relieve the patient from bradycardia-related symptoms, provide haemodynamic stability, and thereby improve patient well-being and clinical outcome. These objectives can only be met when the best of 'two pacing worlds' are combined: a single or dual chamber device with an epicardial or transvenous pacing lead. Selecting a pulse generator and pacing lead for a child who needs life-long pacing for complete AV block depends on several important factors. It should be remembered that the risks of pacemaker placement are related to the size of the patient, making patient size an important consideration in selecting an appropriate pacing system. Issues regarding the selection of a single or dual chamber are addressed in this part of the chapter. Considerations related to epicardial or endocardial lead system selection are subsequently discussed.

4.1 Modern pulse generators: size and location of pacemaker pocket

Many of the shortcomings of pacing in children have been overcome in the last two decades. Pulse generators have become smaller and battery longevity has increased. Also the programmability of many pulse generators has seen major advances.

Due to these advances, pacemaker therapy can be applied safely to small infants and even preterm infants weighing less than 2000 g (Ohmi et al., 1992; Kammeraad et al 2004,; Inoue et al., 2005). Although most of these infants will receive a single chamber device (VVI mode) with an epicardial pacing lead because of their small size, single lead endocardial pacing systems also have been successfully implanted with an abdominally located pacemaker pocket (Hoorntje et al., 2000).

The abdominal pocket is the preferred pulse generator location in neonates, infants and small children receiving an epicardial pacing system. Subpectoral and prepectoral subcutaneous pockets are used in children and adolescents for placement of their transvenous pacing system. In general, the subpectoral pocket is preferred in young active children in whom a pulse generator implanted in a prepectoral subcutaneous pocket is more prone to trauma. Moreover, the risk of deep pocket infections seem to be less when the pulse generator in inserted under the pectoralis major muscle (Gillette et al., 1991; Cohen et al., 2002).

4.2 Programming a pacing device: heart rate limits and rate-responsive pacing

Most modern pulse generators have a large flexibility in programming. Several pacemaker options are available which may help achieving better pacemaker performance, longevity, and optimize patient needs in daily life.

Upper and lower heart rate settings are important in children. Physiologically, the average heart rates in children differ from the adult heart rate requirements. An upper heart rate limit of 180 beats per minute is required in most small children. The selected pulse generator should be capable of providing high upper rate limits. Another important topic is the programmed minimal heart rate. Particularly in neonates and small infants, programming the heart rates in the normal physiological range may induce ventricular dysfunction (Chen et al., 2008). After programming a pacemaker in a specific heart rate range, these settings should be re-evaluated at every pacemaker follow-up visit. Pacemaker programming must be tailored to the individual paediatric patient.

Another important function is the rate-responsive pacing mode. The advantage of rate-responsive pacing lies in the presumed augmentation of cardiac output with exercise. Ideally, rate-responsive or rate-adaptive sensors in pacemakers sense changes in activity level and adapt heart rate to the new level of activity. An adequate chronotropic response to exercise has been demonstrated in adult patients with a VVIR pacing mode (Oldroyd et al., 1991). Another study in adults showed that DDDR pacing resulted in a slight improvement in cardiopulmonary performance compared to VVIR pacing, probably due to a better atrial contribution to cardiac output on exercise in DDDR paced patients (Vogt et al, 1988). Although, a normal increase in heart rate during exercise is more important than AV synchrony, the addition of AV synchrony does provide an additional benefit, supporting the use of DDDR pacing mode in adults (Benditt et al., 1987).

As with many topics in paediatric cardiology, results from large adult studies are often extrapolated to paediatric patients. However, limited data regarding rate-responsive pacing exist in children. One study showed that minute ventilation sensors, used for sensing the chronotropic response, closely matched intrinsic sinus node function during exercise in healthy children, supporting the appropriateness of rate-responsive pacing in children requiring permanent pacing therapy (Cabrera et al., 2002). Ventricular rate-responsive pacing is feasible, effective and safe in children with complete atrioventricular block (Ragonese, et al., 1994). Therefore, most pacemakers in children with complete AV block are programmed to a rate-responsive mode.

4.3 Battery longevity and autocapture-controlled pacing

In general, battery longevity is good with modern pacemakers. A pacemaker battery may last for 5 - 10 years in most paediatric patients (Udink ten Cate et al., 2002; Welisch et al., 2010). Battery survival is influenced by many factors, of which pacing mode, programmed heart rate, pacing lead performance, and percentage of cumulative stimulation are the most important (Maginot et al., 2000.; Batra & Balaji, 2006). The higher heart rate requirements of infants and children compared with adults result in less battery durability. Moreover, epicardial pacing systems, which are frequently implanted in infants and small children, have higher acute and chronic pacing thresholds, further limiting battery longevity (Khairy et al., 2006).

An important tool in reducing energy drain and extending battery life in infants and children is the use of automatic algorithms for pacing threshold measurement, such as AutoCapture and Ventricular Capture Management (Bauersfeld et al, 1999; Cohen et al., 2004; Silvetti et al, 2007a). These algorithms measure atrial and/or ventricular pacing thresholds throughout the day. The system responds to increases and decreases of pacing thresholds and subsequently regulates battery output. These pacing algorithms can be used in both epicardial and transvenous lead systems. A recent study demonstrated that autocapture pacing in children with epicardial lead systems extended the calculated battery life up to 15% (Tomaske et al, 2007). Automatic pacing threshold determination might be an important technological tool to prolong battery longevity and increase pacemaker safety. Patients with high or fluctuating pacing thresholds benefit the most. However, not all pacemakers are equipped with this function.

4.4. Single and dual chamber pacemakers

The positive haemodynamic effects of AV synchronous pacing have been well described in adults. A properly timed atrial contraction, resulting in AV synchrony, augments ventricular filling and cardiac output through the Frank-Starling relationship, improves venous return, and assists AV closure (Buckingham et al., 1992). The value of AV synchrony was already recognized in the early 1970s in patients with AV block following cardiac surgery and acute myocardial infarcts (Chamberlain et al., 1970; Hartzler et al., 1977).

While evidence exists that DDD pacing might be superior to VVI pacing in adults, no similar data are available in children, in whom a single chamber device offers the advantage of lower cost, ease of implantation and extended battery longevity. With AV asynchronous pacing, the atria may contract against closed AV valves, causing atrial distension with subsequent increases in pulmonary wedge pressure and jugular venous pressure (Horenstein et al., 2004). This might provoke signs and symptoms of fullness, dyspnea, headache, fatigue, syncope and exercise intolerance, the so-called pacemaker syndrome (Furman, 1994).

Pacemaker syndrome however, is exceedingly uncommon in young children. The development of symptoms attributable to the pacemaker syndrome in children with single chamber devices is a time related event (Horenstein et al., 2003; Horenstein et al., 2004). Although more than 50% of children with single chamber devices may develop pacemaker syndrome, those children who became symptomatic had been paced for a median of 11 years. These data were confirmed in another study (Horenstein et al., 2003). Based on these findings, single chamber pacing device is preferably implanted as the initial pacing mode in young children, particularly in those with a structurally normal heart, isolated complete AV block and normal ventricular function. Early establishment of AV synchrony in this patient population offers no added benefit.

Some data exists on VDD pacing in children, a pacing mode which combines the advantages of AV synchrony and the smaller size of single chamber pacing systems (Rosenthal et al., 1997a; Seiden et al., 1997). In this pacing mode, a single implanted transvenous lead is used for AV synchronous pacing, with the extra proximally located electrode being used for atrial sensing. The acute results of this pacing mode are similar to others used in the conventionally used pacing modes (Rosenthal et al., 1997a; Seiden et al., 1997). There are two major practical difficulties in applying VDD pacing mode in children: (1) with growth, atrial sensing is lost in many patients due to loss of contact between the atrial sensing electrode and the myocardium, and (2) only large diameter adult leads are available. Therefore, most centers have abandoned this pacing technique in children.

4.5 Specific considerations in selecting single or dual chamber device

4.5.1 Ventricular dysfunction

An important consideration in selecting a pacing system is the presence of ventricular dysfunction. The ventricular dysfunction may worsen when a child receives a single chamber device. Therefore, a dual chamber system should be selected in patients with ventricular dysfunction with or without congenital heart disease.

4.5.2 Single ventricle morphology and Fontan palliation

Specific considerations are required for permanent pacing systems in patients after the Fontan procedure. Currently, the Fontan operation is the surgical approach of choice for children with single ventricle physiology (Barber et al., 2005). Sinus node dysfunction and complete AV block are common indications for permanent pacing in patients after Fontan palliation. Studies have estimated that approximately 10% of these patients need pacemaker insertion during follow-up (Barber et al., 2005; Cohen et al., 2001a). Due to the limitations in venous access to the heart after the Fontan procedure, most patients receive an epicardial pacing system (Cohen et al., 2001a). Although various pacing modes have been described in these patients (Warfield et al., 1999), a recent haemodynamic study performed in the early postoperative period showed clearly that AV synchrony is vital in patients with Fontan physiology (Barber et al., 2005). Whether novel pacing techniques, such as multisite pacing to improve ventricular synchrony, have advantages over dual chamber pacing in these patients warrants further study.

5. Selecting a pacing system: epicardial or endocardial pacing leads?

Both transvenous and epicardial pacemaker leads are being used in paediatric patients with good early and long-term results. Because published guidelines on pacing indications in children and adults do not address selection of the type of pacing lead, choosing a transvenous or epicardial pacing lead depends on several considerations. An overview is presented on lead selection, the relative advantages of transvenous and epicardial pacing systems, complications and lead longevity.

5.1 Anatomic considerations

A unique aspect of pacing practice in children is that many patients have associated congenital heart disease. Coexisting anatomic vascular abnormalities in both surgically corrected and uncorrected congenital heart disease can influence the choice of the pacing lead system. Venous abnormalities associated with limited or difficult access to the heart include persistent left superior vena cava, various systemic venous abnormalities, single ventricle physiology after a modified Fontan procedure and presence of superior vena cava vein stenosis or obstruction in patients after Mustard or Senning operations for transposition of the great arteries. An epicardial lead system may be preferable in some of these patients.

However, several options for alternative vascular access have been proposed in various types of corrected congenital heart disease (Gillette et al., 1986; Rosenthal et al., 1995; Adwani et al., 1997; Emmel et al., 2007). Pacing following the Fontan procedure for single ventricular physiology is usually accomplished using an epicardial lead system. Some authors have implanted endocardial pacing leads in the coronary sinus or using the transhepatic pathway in patients with a Fontan circulation (Rosenthal et al., 1995; Adwani et al., 1997). However, these techniques can be used only in a limited subset of patients with single ventricular physiology.

Another example of transvenous lead implantation in a difficult venous anatomic setting is in patients with D-transposition of the great arteries palliated with a Mustard or Senning operation. Although progressive loss of sinus rhythm and sinus node dysfunction has been well documented in a significant proportion of patients following the Mustard or Senning operation, AV conduction abnormalities, higher-degree AV block and surgical complete AV block have also been noted at follow-up (Hayes & Gersony, 1986; Vetter et al., 1987). Superior vena cava obstruction appears postoperatively in 5 - 22% of patients with a Mustard or Senning type repair (Turley et al., 1988; Khairy et al., 2004). Because an obstruction in the venous pathway used for transvenous lead implantation can be present without signs and symptoms, detailed venography, computerized tomographic scans or magnetic resonance imaging investigations are warranted in patients selected for an transvenous pacing system. When a venous stenosis or obstruction is encountered, implantation of a vascular stent may relief the stenosis, and allows implantation of a transvenous pacing system (Emmel et al., 2007). The intermediate term results of the 'stent-and-pace' procedure are good.

5.2 Intracardiac right-to-left shunting: a contraindication for transvenous pacing?

Thrombus formation and paradoxical embolization may adversely affect patients with transvenous pacing systems. Although risk factors and data on the prevalence of thrombus formation on endocardial leads in children are lacking, several studies support the concept of paradoxical embolization (Silka & Rice, 1991; Johnson & Galindez, 1998; Barakat et al., 2000). A recent study identified the risk of systemic thromboemboli associated with transvenous pacing systems in adult patients with intracardiac shunts (Khairy et al., 2006). This study showed that patients with transvenous pacing systems and intracardiac shunts have a greater than two-fold increased risk of systemic thromboemboli. Of concern was that there was no apparent protective value of chronic aspirin or warfarin therapy in these patients. Independent risk factors for paradoxical systemic embolic events were older age, atrial fibrillation or flutter, and ongoing phlebotomy. A limitation of the study was that standardised methods for assessing right-to-left shunting were not uniformly adopted in all participating centers.

The authors of this study suggested that efforts to eliminate right-to-left shunting should be pursued before transvenous pacing is applied, and if this may not be feasible, the epicardial pacing approach should be considered (Khairy et al., 2006).

5.3 Endocardial or epicardial pacing system?

The introduction of modern steroid-eluting bipolar leads has resulted in improved lead performance and survival of both epicardial and endocardial leads (Goldman-Cutler et al., 1997; Johns et al, 1992; Udink ten Cate et al, 2002). The addition of steroid elution limits the inflammatory response at the electrode-tissue interface, resulting in better acute and chronic stimulation thresholds and improved battery longevity (Mond & Stokes, 1992). Both pacing lead systems offer effective pacing options in infants and children. Moreover, implantation of a transvenous or epicardial pacing system are safe and feasible procedures in most children. Although, the epicardial approach remains essential in children with congenital heart disease in whom venous access is not available, a transvenous lead system is most commonly advocated in children of adequate size (Fortescue et al., 2004; Kammeraad et al., 2004).

An endocardial pacing system is preferably implanted in children weighing more than 15 kg (Fortescue et al., 2004; Alexander 2004), although implantation at a smaller patient size has been reported (Kammeraad et al., 2004; Sachweh et al., 2000). Several patient and lead related features should be weighed before an optimal decision regarding an epicardial or endocardial lead system can be made.

Advantages of the epicardial approach include the avoidance of vascular injury and risk of venous occlusion, absence of lead problems associated with somatic growth, and no risk of endocarditis (Cohen et al., 2001b; Fortescue et al., 2004). Moreover, a dual chamber device can be implanted more easily in small children with or without congenital heart disease using the epicardial approach. Transvenous pacing systems offer the advantages of avoidance of a surgical procedure (thoracotomy or sternotomy), excellent lead survival, and lower acute and chronic pacing thresholds, and thereby increased battery longevity (Kammeraad et al., 2004; Udink ten Cate et al., 2002).

Major concerns regarding epicardial and endocardial lead systems include lead survival in epicardial leads, and risk of venous thrombosis and long-term vascular integrity after endocardial lead placement (Cohen et al., 2001; Kammeraad et al., 2004). Although modern steroid-eluting epicardial leads offer acceptable acute and chronic performance, they are prone to exit-block or non-capture due to high thresholds at the lead tip (Alexander, 2004). Several possible reasons for epicardial lead failure have been suggested, such as recurrent minor traumas imposed on the leads due to the active lifestyle of children (Figure 2), and presence of scarred epicardium after surgery for congenital heart disease (Silvetti et al., 2007b). Current lead survival is 90% at 2 years after implantation, and 74% at 5 years for epicardial leads. A recent study showed a 5-year lead survival of 90% for endocardial leads (Fortescue et al., 2004). However, when a reanalysis was made of all leads placed in children who were less than 1 year of age at implant, the estimated 2-year and 5-year endocardial lead survivals were 90% and 78%, respectively.

Endocardial lead systems carry a significant risk of venous thrombosis in infants and small children. The concern of venous patency in children who need life-long pacing has been an argument for a more conservative approach of selecting a lead system, preferring the epicardial approach (Bracke et al, 2003; Bar-Cohen et al., 2006).

Complete venous obstruction has been documented in 11 - 21% of children at medium-term follow-up (Bar-Cohen et al., 2006; Figa et al. 1997, Kammeraad et al., 2004). Partial venous obstruction may be seen in another 12% of children receiving an endocardial pacing system

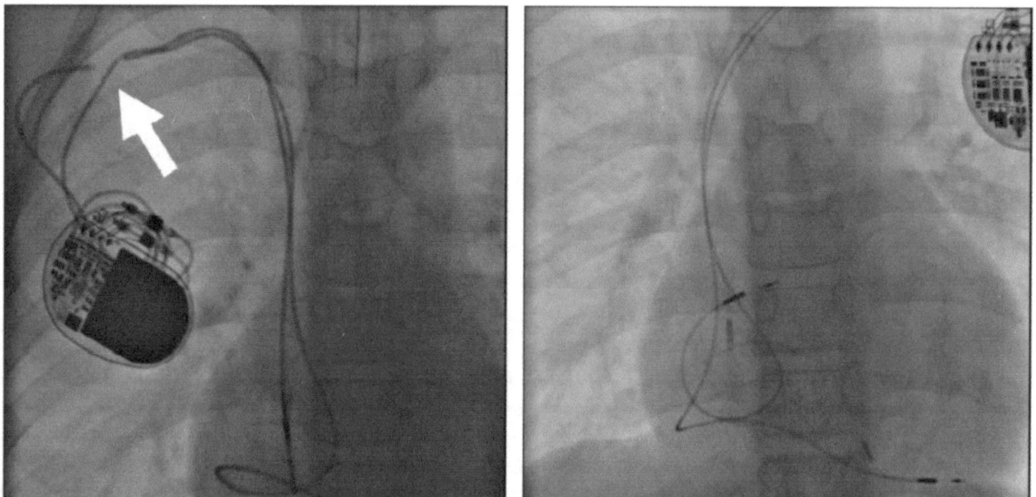

Fig. 2. In the example above, a 12 year old active boy presented with acute failure of the atrial lead 5 years following upgrade from single chamber to dual chamber pacing. The original ventricular lead had been partially abandoned in the heart. The atrial lead clearly shows a fracture, probably related to lead compression stress between the clavicle and the first rib. Four weeks later, the ventricular electrode had also failed, and he presented with a junctional escape rhythm at a rate of 35 to 40 beats per minute. The leads were entirely removed using a combined subclavian and femoral venous approach, and a new DDD system was implanted via the left subclavian vein, using 2 thin lumenless leads.

at young age. The location of thrombosis varied throughout the venous anatomy, with most venous obstruction occurring in the left innominate vein (Bar-Cohen et al., 2006). However, not all studies found venous obstruction in children after endocardial pacing (Gillette et al., 1988).

Venous thrombosis is most often asymptomatic (Bar-Cohen et al., 2006; Kammeraad et al., 2004). Nevertheless, it may cause superior vena cava syndrome in some patients. An important corollary, particularly in young patients requiring future lifelong pacing, is that every effort must be made to remove and replace nonfunctional leads in the vascular system. This often means the use of a variety of extraction systems, and occasionally transcatheter recanalization of stenosed or occluded vessels.

Risk factors for venous thrombosis are not yet known. A recent study showed that patient age, body size, and lead characteristics at implant did not clearly predict venous occlusion (Bar-Cohen et al., 2006). However, an earlier study concluded that if the lead size indexed to body surface area was more than 6.6 mm2/m2, venous thrombosis could be predicted with a sensitivity of 90% and specificity of 84% (Figa et al, 1997). The recent development of a lumenless 4.1 F endocardial lead is a promising new lead design, which may decrease the risk for venous occlusion in children (Chakrabarti et al., 2009).

In summary, many arguments exist for and against the use of epicardial or endocardial pacing systems in different subgroups of paediatric patients. In general, most neonates and small infants weighing < 10 kg receive initially an epicardial pacing system. At subsequent generator replacement, and depending on the child's size, an endocardial pacing system may be implanted.

5.4 Patient size and somatic growth issues in children

Transvenous pacing implantation in children requires special attention to their amazing somatic growth potential. It has been estimated that approximately 190 mm of additional right ventricular pacing lead in infants and 100 mm in 10-year-old children is needed to enable growth to adulthood (Gheissari, et al., 1991). Moreover, an 80-mm right atrial lead loop will allow 6 to 12 years of growth in infants and older children (Sanjeev & Karpawich, 2006).

To enable safe future growth in children with reliable transvenous single or dual chamber pacing, an additional amount of lead can be advanced into the heart during pacemaker implantation. Several options for creating such a redundant lead loop have been described (Rosenthal et al., 1997b; Gasparini, et al., 2000). A redundant lead loop may be placed in the right atrium or in the inferior vena cava. An example of a redundant lead loop in the inferior vena cava is shown in Figure 3.

If necessary, additional lead can be advanced during an elective pulse generator replacement. When transvenous pacing is applied in neonates or small infants, the length of the redundant lead loop is insufficient for most of these patients to grow into adulthood. Elective lead advancement is often needed. Lead advancement during the first 2 years after pacemaker implantation was necessary in 4/36 (11%) infants weighing < 10 kg who received transvenous leads (Kammeraad et al., 2004). In one of these, lead advancement failed and the lead was replaced.

5.5 Active or passive lead fixation

A stable position of the lead tip is pivotal to provide excellent acute and chronic thresholds and lead performance. The development of passive and active fixation mechanisms has

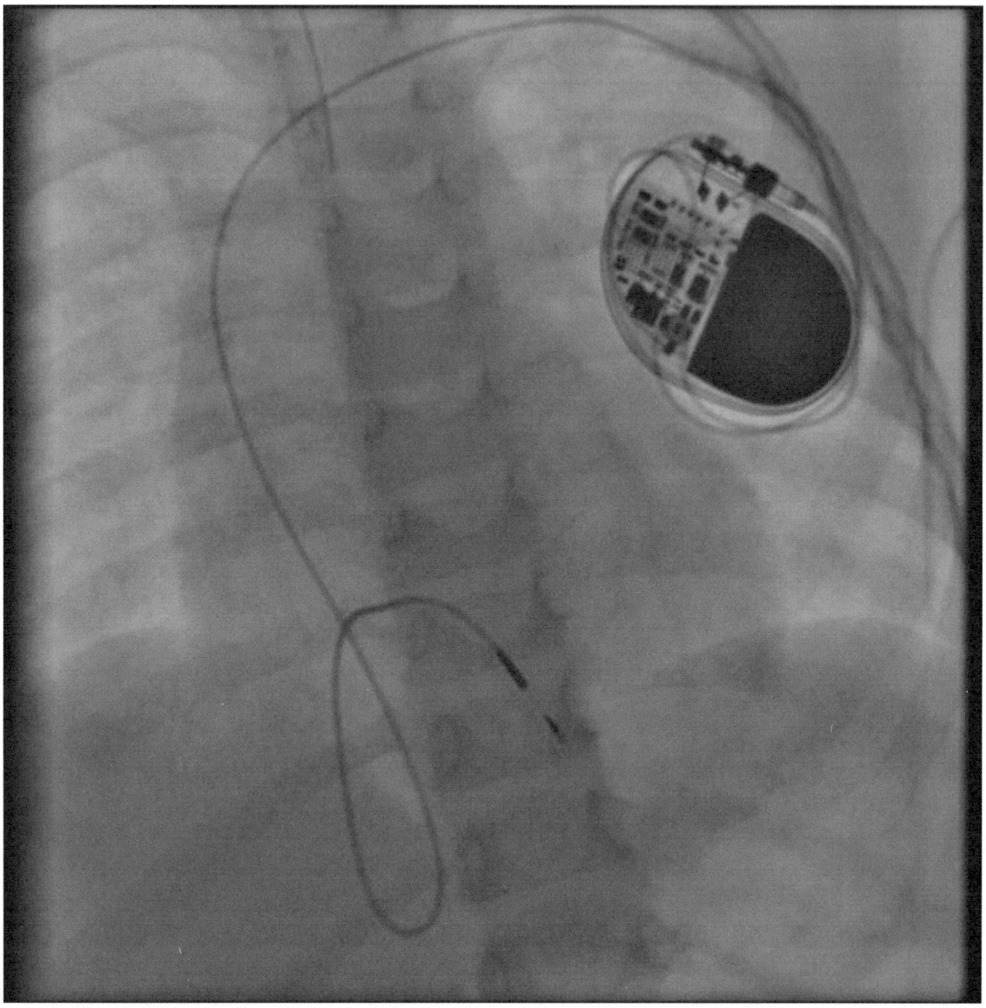

Fig. 3. Posteroanterior chest X ray of a child with congenital complete atrioventricular block who received a single chamber transvenous pacing system after developing bradycardia-related symptoms. The child's weight was 12 kg. A redundant lead loop for future somatic growth was placed in the inferior vena cava.

resulted in a tremendous reduction of the need for lead repositioning during follow-up (Furman et al., 1979). Passive fixation leads can be used for lead placement in the right ventricular apex. These leads can be easily positioned within the trabeculae of the right ventricle. The chronic pacing thresholds of passive fixation leads tend to be slightly better than those of active fixation leads (Hidden-Lucet et al., 2000). A disadvantage of passive fixation leads is that future lead extraction and replacement are more difficult, and this is an important issue in children (Hidden-Lucet et al., 2000).

Active fixation leads, usually equipped with a screw-in helix mechanism can be fixed more easily at almost any position in the atrium and ventricle, making this lead type ideal for selective site pacing (Chakrabarti et al., 2009). Active fixation may also prevent lead displacement when a redundant atrial loop is used, which is again of particular relevance to young children (Rosenthal & Bostock, 1997). In specific anatomic situations, such as transvenous pacing after the Mustard or Senning procedure, where the leads have to be securely positioned at unusual anatomic sites, active fixation is preferable.

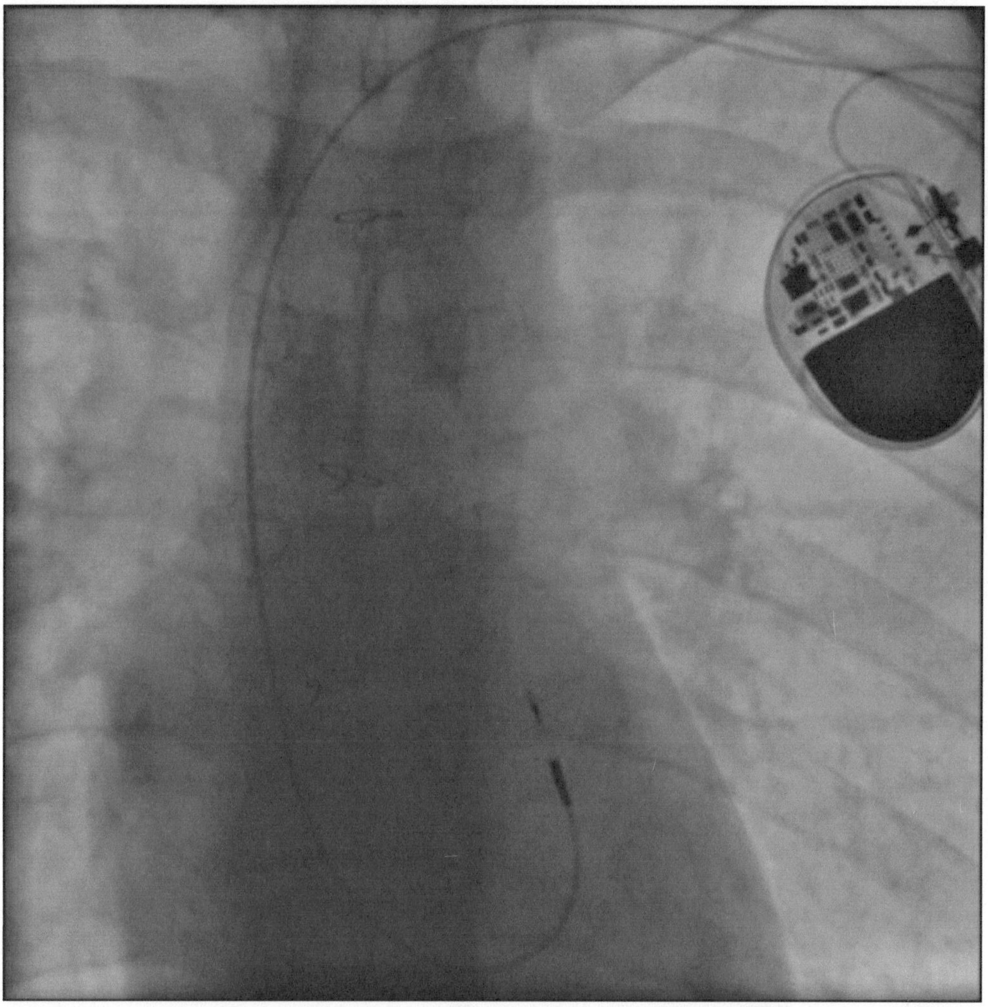

Fig. 4. The chest x ray shows an active fixation lead implanted in the roof of the native left atrium in a young patient who had undergone a Mustard operation for palliation of transposition of the great arteries.

5.6 Unipolar and bipolar leads

Epicardial and endocardial leads are available in unipolar or bipolar electrical configurations (Breivik et al., 1982; Breivik, et al., 1983; Mond, 1991). In general, the external diameter of a unipolar lead is usually smaller, because each coil is separated using insulating material. Although unipolar epicardial leads are still being used in paediatric pacing practice, most modern endocardial leads have a bipolar electrical configuration (Udink ten Cate et al., 2002).

The advantages of the unipolar lead configuration are lower pacing impedance, smaller size, and better lead survival and probably pacemaker longevity. With recent advances in lead design, the differences in pacing longevity between unipolar and bipolar lead systems have become marginal (Breivik et al., 1983; Mond, 1991). In addition, the lead diameter of bipolar leads has significantly decreased. Pectoral muscle stimulation, which may occur in unipolar pacing systems, is not often encountered in bipolar pacing systems. Bipolar leads are also less likely to detect far-field signals and electromagnetic interference (Mond, 1991).

6. Pacing and lead complications in children: implications for follow-up

6.1 Lead fractures, dislodgements, non-capture and insulation breaks

Possible mechanisms of epicardial and endocardial lead failure include lead fracture, dislodgement, high thresholds and insulation break. A recent retrospective study of 1007 implanted epicardial and endocardial leads in children with and without congenital heart disease requiring permanent pacing therapy found that lead fracture and exit-block were common complications seen with epicardial leads, whereas insulation breaks and lead dislodgements occurred more frequently in transvenous pacing systems (Fortescue et al., 2004). In this study, 15% of the leads failed during follow-up, affecting 23% of the patients. Of these patients, 28% experienced multiple lead failures. The most common lead failure types were lead fracture and insulation break. The rates of lead failure are in accordance with those noticed in several other studies, reporting lead failure rates ranging between 2 - 28% of implanted leads (Sachweh et al., 2000; Cohen et al., 2001b; Udink ten Cate et al., 2002; Bakhtiary et al., 2007; Welisch et al., 2010). Lead longevity of epicardial pacing systems were lower in most studies (Sachweh et al., 2000; Udink ten Cate et al., 2002; Fortescue et al., 2004; Welisch et al., 2010).

Risk factors for lead failures in children may include younger age at implant and presence of congenital heart disease (Fortesue et al., 2004). Epicardial pacing leads are associated with a higher risk of lead failure. An explanation for these findings is that children undergo rapid linear growth and are more physically active than adults, thereby placing additional stress on the pacing lead system and increasing the risk for lead failure.

Interestingly, it has been observed that only a minority of children (8%) report symptoms of pacing lead failure (Fortescue et al., 2004). Symptoms included skeletal muscle stimulation, palpitations, dizziness, or syncope. The remainder of patients were found to have pacemaker lead failure during regular pacemaker interrogation, routine chest radiography, or intraoperative lead examination. Routine and regular pacemaker follows up and interrogation are of upmost importance for optimal patient care.

6.2 Pacemaker pocket infections and endocarditis

Although pacemaker infections are uncommon in the paediatric population, deep pocket infection and pacemaker endocarditis are serious and life-threatening complications. When pacemaker-related infections occur, removal of the infected pulse generator and pacing leads are often required for infection control (Klug et al., 1997). Infections may be divided into superficial cellulitis, pocket infection, and endocarditis (defined as positive blood cultures). Pacemaker-related infections may develop in children before hospital discharge, or during early follow-up. Early pacemaker infections probably result from wound contamination during implantation (Cohen et al., 2002). In one paediatric retrospective study, the incidence of pacemaker-related infection was 7.8% for the whole cohort. The incidences of superficial cellulitis, deep pocket infection and pacing lead infection were 4.9%, 2.3%, and 0.5%, respectively (Cohen et al., 2002). The authors concluded that the incidence of deep pocket infections was similar to those seen in adult studies (Kiviniemi et al., 1999; Klug et al., 1997), while more superficial infections occurred in their paediatric cohort. Moreover, Down syndrome was identified as an independent risk factor for pacemaker related infections. Patients with Down syndrome were 4 times as likely to develop an infection. The more severe pacemaker-related infections are most often seen following revision of a pulse generator with or without pacemaker lead exchange (Cohen et al., 2002; Fortescue et al., 2004).

Most superficial infections can be managed with (intravenous) antibiotic therapy alone. Appropriate management of deep pocket infections and pacemaker lead infection, or endocarditis, involves complete removal of the entire pacemaker system and long-term intravenous antibiotic therapy. With aggressive and appropriate therapy, mortality rates in children with pacemaker infection are minor. A subpectoral pocket may be preferable for transvenous pacing systems in children, because infection seems to be less likely (Gillette et al., 1991; Cohen et al, 2002).

6.3 Postpericardiotomy syndrome after pacemaker implantation

Postpericardiotomy syndrome (PSS) is a well known complication after cardiac surgery. It has been observed in 10 - 50% of patients following open heart procedures (Miller et al., 1988). PPS may also occur after pacemaker implantation (Polin et al., 2006). PPS occurs in 2 - 6% of children following initial pacemaker implantation of both epicardial and transvenous lead systems (Udink ten Cate et al., 2002; Zeltser et al., 2004). Acute PPS may also develop after a subsequent lead revision in a small subset of children (Zeltser et al., 2004). Patients typically present with respiratory distress, chest pain, fever, and lethargy. Cardiovascular compromise was often seen. Most PPS episodes occurred within 14 days after pacemaker placement (Zeltser et al, 2004). In some instances, PPS may have a late onset (Spindler et al., 2001).

PPS can be successfully managed with medical therapy that includes both anti-inflammatory agents (NSAIDs) and diuretics. Pericardiocentesis is an option when cardiovascular compromise is present. The clinical outcome of PPS in children after permanent pacemaker implantation is excellent.

6.4 Pacing induced ventricular remodelling and dysfunction

The right ventricular (RV) apex has been the conventional site for endocardial ventricular pacing in children and adults (Karpawich, 2004). Recent studies have demonstrated that pacing from the RV apex may induce left ventricular dyssynchrony (Thambo et al., 2004; Tops et al., 2007; Cheng et al., 2009). It has long been recognized that ventricular dyssynchrony caused by a variety of cardiovascular diseases, including heart failure, ventricular preexcitation, and left bundle branch block mediate ventricular remodelling and subsequently myocardial dysfunction (Prinzen et al., 1995; Kass, 2008; Udink ten Cate et al., 2010a; Udink ten Cate et al., 2010b). Evidence is now emerging that pacing-induced ventricular dyssynchrony disturbs myocardial regional workload and wall stress, which may result in wall motion abnormalities, myocardial perfusion defects, changes in coronary blood flow, increased left ventricular cavity volume, and asymmetrical changes in left ventricular wall thickness (Karpawich, 2004; Kass, 2008; Cheng et al., 2009). Moreover, interstitial and cellular histopathological alterations have been demonstrated in the hearts of animals and patients after long-term right ventricular apical pacing (Karpawich et al., 1999; Cheng et al., 2009).

The concept of pacemaker-induced heart failure is particularly important when permanent pacing is applied to young children, who often need life-long pacing. Dilated cardiomyopathy may develop in 6 – 11% of paced children with autoimmune CCAVB during follow-up (Moak et al., 2001; Udink ten Cate et al., 2001; Kim et al., 2007). In addition, heart failure associated with prolonged pacemaker therapy was found in 46% of adolescents with repaired congenital heart disease (Nothroff et al., 2006). Although other risk factors may play an additional role in the pathogenesis of cardiomyopathy in these patients, pacing-induced LV dyssynchrony is an important but under-recognised contributor.

6.4.1 Strategies to minimize ventricular pacing

Identification of risk factors for pacing-induced cardiomyopathy, unravelling its pathogenesis, and developing pacing strategies to avoid the adverse effects of right ventricular apical and lateral wall pacing are crucial. The detrimental effects of pacing on right ventricular function are in part related to the cumulative percentage of ventricular pacing (Sweeney et al., 2005). An infant in whom the right ventricle is paced for 100% of the time is at a higher risk for developing ventricular dysfunction compared to an infant who is only paced for 50% of the time. This has prompted the search for novel pacing strategies that reduce unnecessary ventricular pacing, and thereby reducing the cumulative percentage of ventricular pacing (Kaltman et al., 2008; Sweeney et al., 2004).

Managed ventricular pacing (MVP) and AAISafeR modes are new pacing algorithms designed for reducing cumulative percentage of ventricular pacing, with established benefits in the adult population (Mansour et al., 2006; van Mechelen & Schoonderwoerd, 2006). This pacing strategy requires the implantation of a dual chamber device, programmed in DDD or DDDR mode. Patients who have sinus node disease, second-degree AV block, or high-degree AV block with intermittent complete AV block are thought to benefit most of this pacing algorithm (Kaltman et al., 2008).

MVP is an atrial based pacing mode (AAI or AAIR). It primarily paces the atrium and monitors the ventricle for loss of AV conduction. When no ventricular beats are sensed between two consecutive atrial sensed or paced beats, MVP automatically mode switches to DDD or DDDR backup pacing (Kaltman et al., 2008; Mansour et al., 2006). Adverse effects have been described in the adult population, including tachyarrhythmias, ventricular fibrillation and failure of mode switch to ventricular backup pacing (Mansour et al., 2006; van Mechelen & Schoonderwoerd, 2006). The experience with MVP in children is limited. There is one retrospective study evaluating the safety and effectiveness of MVP in reducing unnecessary ventricular pacing in a large group of children with various diseases, including congenital and acquired AV block (Kaltman et al., 2008). Congenital heart disease was present in 64% of the children in the study group. MVP was effective in reducing the cumulative percentage of ventricular pacing, and only 1 MVP-related adverse effect was reported. Frequent nonconducted atrial depolarizations were noted in a patient with intermittent AV block. No proarrhythmic effect of MVP was noted in this study. Although there are no large randomized prospective trials in paediatric patients, MVP seems to be a promising pacing strategy for a subgroup of children of AV block.

6.4.2 Should right ventricular apical pacing be avoided in children at all cost?

The important question which has arisen following recent reports of pacing-induced cardiomyopathy is: should permanent pacing from the RV apex (for transvenous systems) or RV anterior free wall (for epicardial systems) be abandoned in children with complete AV block? This is not an easy question to answer. First, a large proportion of children are at risk of developing ventricular dysfunction due to pacing, not all of them develop heart failure. Several studies have been undertaken to assess the incidence of ventricular dysfunction in paced children with CCAVB, and to identify potential risk factors (Udink ten Cate et al., 2001; Moak et al., 2006; Beaufort-Krol et al., 2007; Kim et al., 2007; Vatasescu et al., 2007; Gebauer et al., 2009). Most studies found an incidence of dilated cardiomyopathy and LV dilation in 6.0 to 13.4% of children after long-term pacing. Risk factors for development of dilated cardiomyopathy and LV dilation with ventricular dysfunction may include presence of anti-SSA/Ro - SSB/La antibodies, increased heart size at initial evaluation and the absence of pacemaker-associated normalization of left ventricular size during follow-up, prolonged QRS duration, and transvenous pacing location (RV apex and RV free wall worse compared to RV septum). The interpretation of these results is troublesome, because most studies involved small groups of patients. Interestingly, recent studies have demonstrated physiologically benefits of alternative site pacing, including RV septal, outflow tract, or Hisbundle pacing (Karpawich, 2004). The degree of pacing-induced LV dyssynchrony is lower with these pacing strategies. However, large clinical paediatric studies are needed to determine if selective RV pacing sites are superior to pacing the RV apex, which is still most frequently used in clinical practice.

6.4.3 Echocardiographic follow-up of children with permanent pacemaker therapy

Serial echocardiographic investigations are important in the management of children with permanent pacemaker therapy. Although shorthening fraction, left heart size and ejection fraction can be easily measured, these conventional echocardiographic parameters are not sensitive enough to identify paced children at risk for development of dilated cardiomyopathy at an early stage in the disease process. However, this should be the ultimate goal for selection of children who may benefit from upgrading their pacing system to DDD pacing, biventricular pacing or selective site pacing. Tissue Doppler echocardiography and speckle tracking imaging may be used for measuring LV dyssynchrony, regional and global ventricular function (Figure 5). When LV dyssynchrony, regional and global myocardial function deteriorates, we might be able to identify patients who are at the highest risk for development of dilated cardiomyopathy. Although more research work needs to be done, these new techniques may guide crucial improvements in the management of children with permanent pacing devices.

7. Conclusions

Pacing in children with congenital or acquired AV block is a safe and feasible therapy. Selecting an appropriate pacemaker system for a child with complete AV block remains challenging. Several patient-related and pacemaker-related issues should be considered, including patient size, cardiac anatomy, pacing indication, pulse generator capabilities and pacing lead characteristics.

A single chamber pacemaker is the preferably initial pacing mode in young children with complete AV block and normal ventricular function. Early establishment of AV synchrony in the young patient with a structurally normal heart and normal ventricular function is not thought to be beneficial. Conversely, single chamber devices should not be implanted in children following the Fontan operation or with ventricular dysfunction.

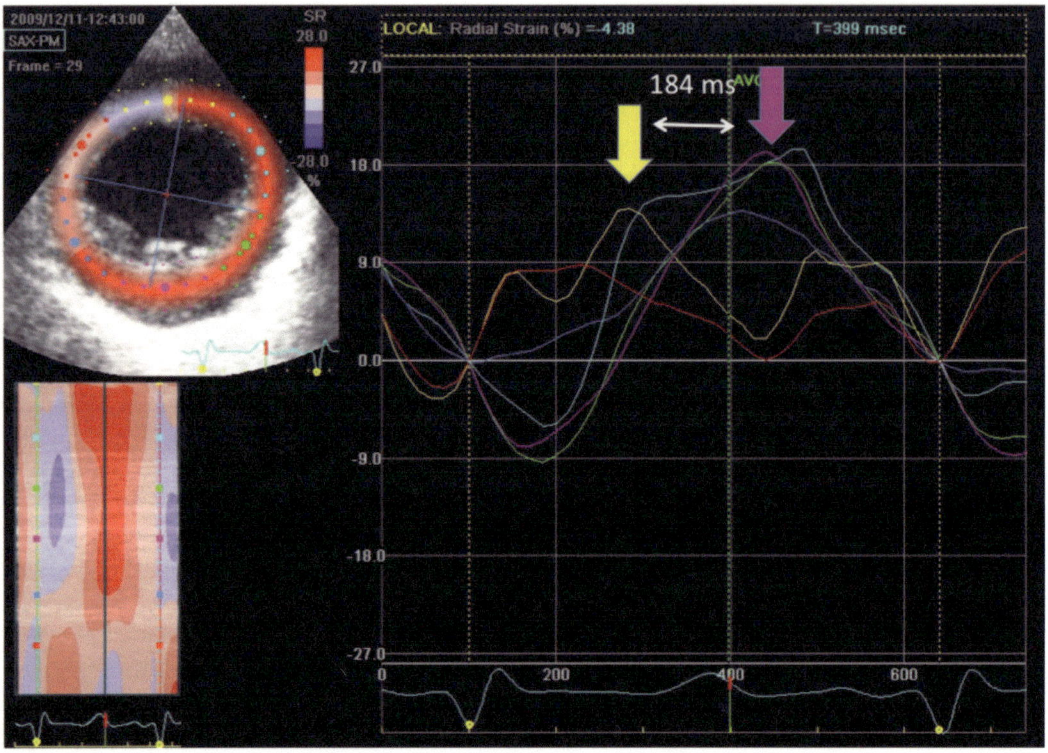

Fig. 5. This image shows a parasternal short-axis view at the mid-ventricular level of a child with permanent right ventricular pacing for congenital complete AV block. The ventricular walls are divided into six myocardial segments (farb-coded). During one cardiac cycle, the time to systolic peak radial strain can be measured. The time delay between the septal and posterior wall (yellow and purple arrows, respectively), a parameter of LV dyssynchrony is estimated. There is significant LV dyssynchrony in this patient (184 ms, normally the time delay is < 130 ms). In addition, there is an inhomogeneous pattern of radial strain, with severely reduced peak radial strain values for all myocardial segments. (Radial peak strain values are presented as positive values).

Excluding children weighing less than 15 kg, transvenous pacing systems may be safely implanted in children with structurally normal hearts. Active fixation endocardial leads are preferred in most children. Epicardial pacing is preferred in neonates and small infants, or when coexisting congenital heart disease exists with difficult venous access of the heart. Pacemaker-induced ventricular dysfunction and adverse remodelling are of concern in children who need life-long pacing. Definitive risk factors are to be determined. The concept of pacemaker-induced heart failure will have important implications in the way we treat and manage children with permanent pacemakers, with selective site pacing being likely to play a more important role.

8. References

Adwani, SS.; Sreeram, N. & DeGiovanni, JV. (1997). Percutaneous transhepatic dual chamber pacing in children with Fontan circulation. *Heart*, 77:574-575.

Alexander, ME. (2004). Transvenous pacing in infants: a faith based initiative? *Pacing Clin Electrophysiol,* 27:1463-1465.

Anderson, RH.; Becker, AE.; Arnold, R. & Wilkinson, JL. (1974). The conducting tissues in congenitally corrected transposition. *Circulation,* 50:911-923.

Anderson, RH.; Weninck, ACG.; Losekoot, TG. & Becker, AE. (1977). Congenitally complete heart block: developmental aspects. *Circulation,* 56:90-101.

Bar-Cohen, Y.; Berul, CI.; Alexander, ME.; et al. (2006). Age, size, and lead factors alone do not predict venous obstruction in children and young adults with transvenous lead systems. *J Cardiovasc Electrophysiol,* 17:754-759.

Bakhtiary, F.; Dzemali, O.; Bastanier, CK.; Moritz, A. & Kleine, P. (2007) Medium-term follow-up and modes of failure following epicardial pacemaker implantation in young children. *Europace,* 9:94-97.

Balmer, C.; Fasnacht, M.; Rahn, M.; Molinari, L. & Bauersfeld, U. (2002). Long-term follow-up of children with congenital complete atrioventricular block and impact of pacemaker therapy. *Europace,* 4:345-349.

Balmer, C. & Bauersfeld U. (2003). Do all children with congenital complete atrioventricular block require permanent pacing? *Indian Pacing Electrophysiol J,* 3:178-183.

Barakat, K.; Robinson, NM. & Spurrell, RA. (2000). Transvenous pacing lead-induced thrombosis: a series of cases with a review of the literature. *Cardiology,* 93:142-148.

Barber, BJ.; Batra, AS.; Burch, GH.; et al. (2005). Acute hemodynamic effects of pacing in patients with Fontan physiology: a prospective study. *J Am Coll Cardiol,* 46:1937-1942.

Batra, AS.; Wells, WJ.; Hinoki, KW.; Stanton, RA. & Silka, MJ. (2003). Late recovery of atrioventricular conduction after pacemaker implantation for complete heart block associated with surgery for congenital heart disease. *J Thorac Cardiovasc Surg,* 125:1291-1293.

Batra, AS. & Balaji, S. (2006). Pacing in adults with congenital heart disease. *Expert Rev Cardiovasc Ther,* 4:663-670.

Bauersfeld, U.; Nowak, B.; Molinari, L.; et al. (1999). Low energy epicardial pacing in children: the benefit of autocapture. *Ann Thorac Surg,* 68:1380-1383.

Beaufort-Krol, G.; Schasfoort-Van Leeuwen, MJM.; Stienstra, Y. & Bink-Boelkens MThE. (2007). Longitudinal echocardiographic follow-up in children with congenital complete atrioventricular block. *Pacing Clin Electrophysiol,* 30:1339-1343.

Benditt, DG.; Milstein, S.; Buetikofer.; et al. (1987). Sensor-triggered, rate-variable cardiac pacing. *Ann Intern Med,* 107:714-724.

Boutjdir, M.; Chen, L.; Zhang, ZH.; Tseng, CE.; El-Sherif, N. & Buyon, JP. (1998). Serum and immunoglobulin G from the mother of a child with congenital heart block induce conduction abnormalities and inhibit L-type calcium channels in a rat heart model. *Pediatr Res,* 44:11-19.

Bracke, F.; Meijer, A. & van Gelder, B. (2003). Venous occlusion of the access vein in patients referred for lead extraction: influence of patient and lead characteristics. *Pacing Clin Electrophysiol,* 26:1649-1652.

Breivik, K.; Engedal, H. & Ohm, OJ. (1982). Electrophysiological properties of a new permanent endocardial lead for uni- and bipolar pacing. *Pacing Clin Electrophysiol,* 5:268-274.

Breivik, K.; Ohm, OJ. & Engedal, H. (1983). Long-term comparison of unipolar and bipolar pacing and sensing, using a new multiprogrammable pacemaker system. *Pacing Clin Electrophysiol,* 6:592-600.

Breur, JM.; Udink ten Cate, FE.; Kapusta, L.; et al. (2002). Pacemaker therapy in isolated congenital atrioventricular block. *Pacing Clin Electrophysiol,* 25:1685-1691.

Breur, JM.; Udink ten Cate, FE.; Kapusta, L.; et al. (2006). Potential additional indicators for pacemaker requirement in isolated congenital atrioventricular block. *Pediatr Cardiol,* 27:564-568.

Brucato, A.; Jonzon, A.; Friedman, D.; et al. (2003). Proposal for a new definition of congenital complete atrioventricular block. *Lupus,* 12:427-435.

Buckingham, TA.; Janosik, DL. & Pearson, AC. (1992). Pacemaker hemodynamics: clinical implications. *Prog Cardiovasc Dis,* 34:347-366.

Buyon, JP. & Winchester, R. (1990). Congenital complete heart block: a human model of passively acquired autoimmune injury. *Arthritis Rheum,* 33:609-614.

Buyon, JP.; Waltuck, J.; Kleinman, C. & Copel, J. (1995). In utero identification and therapy of congenital heart block. *Lupus,* 4:116-21.

Buyon, JP.; Hiebert, R.; Copel, J.; et al. (1998). Autoimmune-associated congenital heart block: demographics, mortality, morbidity, and recurrence rates obtained from a national neonatal lupus registry. *J Am Coll Cardiol,* 31:1658-1666.

Buyon, JP. & Clancy, RM. (2005). Autoantibody-associated congenital heart block: TGFbeta and the road to scar. *Autoimmun Rev,* 4:1-7.

Cabrera, ME.; Portzline, G.; Aach, S.; Condie, C.; Dorostkar, P. & Mianulli, M. (2002). Can current minute ventilation rate adaptive pacemakers provide appropriate chronotropic response in pediatric patients? *Pacing Clin Electrophysiol,* 25:907-914.

Chakrabarti, S.; Morgan, GJ.; Kenny, D.; et al. (2009). Initial experience of pacing with a lumenless lead system in patients with congenital heart disease. *Pacing Clin Electrophysiol, 32:*1428-1433.

Chamberlain, DA.; Leinbach, RC.; Vassaux, CE.; et al. (1970). Sequential atrioventricular pacing in heart block complicating acute myocardial infarction. *N Engl J Med,* 282:577-582.

Chen, CA.; Chang, CI.; Wang JK.; et al. (2008) Restoration of cardiac function by setting the ventricular pacing at a lower range in an infant with congenital complete atrioventricular block and dilated cardiomyopathy. *Int J Cardiol,* 131:e38-e40.

Cheng, A.; Helm, RH. & Abraham, TP. (2009). Pathophysiological mechanisms underlying ventricular dyssynchrony. *Europace,* 11:v10-v14.

Cohen, MI.; Vetter, VL.; Wernovsky, G.; et al. (2001a). Epicardial pacemaker implantation and follow-up in patients with a single ventricle after the Fontan operation. *J Thorac Cardiovasc Surg,* 121:804-811.

Cohen, MI.; Bush, DM.; Vetter, VL.; et al. (2001b). Permanent epicardial pacing in pediatric patients: seventeen years of experience and 1200 outpatient visits. *Circulation,* 103:2585-2590.

Cohen, MI.; Bush, DM.; Gaynor, JW.; Vetter, VL.; Tanel, RE. & Rhodes, LA. (2002). Pediatric pacemaker infections: Twenty years of experience. *J Thorac Cardiovasc Surg,* 124:821-827.

Cohen, MI.; Buck, K.; Tanel, RE.; et al. (2004). Capture management efficacy in children and young adults with endocardial and unipolar epicardial systems. *Europace,* 6:248-255.

Cruz, RB.; Viana, VS.; Nishioka, SA.; Martinelli, FM. & Bonfa, E. (2004). Is isolated congenital heart block associated to neonatal lupus requiring pacemaker a distinct cardiac syndrome? *Pacing Clin Electrophysiol,* 27:615-620.

Dewey, RC.; Capeless, MA. & Levy, AM. (1987). Use of ambulatory electrocardiographic monitoring to identify high risk patients with congenital complete heart block. *N Eng J Med,* 316:835-839.

Driscoll, DJ.; Gilette, PC.; Hallman, GL.; Cooley, DA. & McNamara, DG. (1979). Management of surgical complete atrioventricular block in children. *Am J Cardiol,* 43:1175-1180.

Emmel, M.; Sreeram, N.; Brockmeier, K. & Bennink, B. (2007). Superior vena cava stenting and transvenous pacemaker implantation (stent and pace) after the Mustard operation. *Clin Res Cardiol,* 96:17-22.

Epstein, AE.; DiMarco, JP.; Ellenbogen, KA.; et al. (2008). ACC/AHA/HRS 2008 guidelines for devicebased therapy of cardiac rhythm abnormalities. *Heart Rhythm,* 5:e1-e62.

Esscher, E. & Michaelsson, M. (1983). QT interval in congenital complete heart block. *Pediatr Cardiol,* 4:121-124.

Figa, FH.; McCrindle, BW.; Bigras, JL.; Hamilton, RM. & Gow, RM. (1997). Risk factors for venous obstruction in children with transvenous pacing leads. *Pacing Clin Electrophysiol,* 20:1902-1909.

Fortescue, E.; Berul, CI.; Cecchin, F.; et al. (2004). Patient procedural and hardware factors associated with pacemaker lead failures in pediatrics and congenital heart disease. *Heart Rhythm,* 1:150-159.

Fryda, R. & Kaplan, S. (1970). Postoperative heart block in children. *Am J Cardiol* 25:96.

Furman, S.; Pannizzo, F. & Campo, I. (1979). Comparison of active and passive adhering leads for endocardial pacing. *Pacing Clin Electrophysiol,* 2:417-427.

Furman, S. (1994). Pacemaker syndrome. *Pacing Clin Electrophysiol,* 17:1-5.

Gasparini, M.; Mantica, M.; Galimberti, P.; Coltorti, F.; Ceriotti, C. & Priori, S. (2000). Inferior vena cava loop of the implantable cardioverter defibrillator endocardial lead: A possible solution to the growth problem in pediatric implantation. *Pacing Clin Electrophysiol,* 23:2108-2112.

Gebauer, RA.; Tomek, V.; Salameh, A.; et al. (2009). Predictors of left ventricular remodelling and failure in right ventricular pacing in the young. *Eur Heart J,* 30:1097-1104.

Gheissari, A.; Hordof, AJ. & Spotnitz, HM. (1991). Transvenous pacemakers in children: relation of lead length to anticipated growth. *Ann Thorac Surg,* 52:118-121.

Gillette, PC.; Wampler, DG.; Shannon, C. & Ott, D. (1986). Use of cardiac pacing after the Mustard operation for transposition of the great arteries. *J Am Coll Cardiol,* 7:138-141.

Gillette, PC.; Zeigler, V.; Bradham, GB. & Kinsella, P. (1988). Pediatric transvenous pacing: a concern for venous thrombosis? *Pacing Clin Electrophysiol,* 11:1935-1939.

Gillette, PC.; Edgerton, J.; Kratz, J. & Zeigler, V. (1991). The subpectoral pocket: the preferred implant site for pediatric pacemakers. *Pacing Clin Electrophysiol,* 14:1089-1092.

Goldman, BS.; Williams, WG.; Hill, T.; et al. (1985). Permanent cardiac pacing after open heart surgery: congenital heart disease. *Pacing Clin Electrophysiol,* 8:732-739.

Goldman-Cutler, N.; Karpawich, PP.; Cavitt, D.; et al. (1997). Steroid-eluting epicardial pacing electrodes: six year experience of pacing thresholds in a growing pediatric population. *Pacing Clin Electrophysiol*, 20:2943-2948.

Graham, TP Jr.; Bernhard, YD.; Mellen, BG.; et al. (2000). Long-term outcome in congenitally corrected transposition of the great arteries: a multi-institutional study. *J Am Coll Cardiol*, 36:255-261.

Gross, GJ.; Chiu, CC.; Hamilton, RM.; Kirsh, JA. & Stephenson, EA. (2006). Natural history of postoperative heart block in congenital heart disease: implications for pacing intervention. *Heart Rhythm*, 3:601-604.

Hartzler, GO.; Maloney, JD.; Curtis, JJ.; et al. (1977). Hemodynamic benefits of atrioventricular sequential pacing after cardiac surgery. *Am J Cardiol*, 40:232-236.

Hayes, CJ. & Gersony, WM. (1986). Arrhythmias after the Mustard operation for transposition of the great arteries: A long-term study. *J Am Coll Cardiol*, 7:133-137.

Hidden-Lucet, F.; Halimi, F.; Gallais, Y.; Petitot, JC.; Fontaine, G. & Frank, R. (2000). Low chronic pacing thresholds of steroid-eluting active fixation ventricular pacemaker leads: a useful alternative to passive fixation leads. *Pacing Clin Electrophysiol*, 23:1798-1800.

Hoorntje, T.; Kammeraad, J.; Bennink, G. & Sreeram, N. (2000). Transvenous permanent pacemaker implantation in neonates. *Int J Cardiol*, 75:103-104.

Horenstein, MS. & Karpawich, PP. (2004). Pacemaker syndrome in the young: Do children need dual chamber pacing as the initial pacing mode? *Pacing Clin Electrophysiol*, 27:600-605.

Horenstein, MS.; Karpawich, PP. & Tantengco, MVT. (2003). Single versus dual chamber pacing in the young: noninvasive comparative eveluation of cardiac function. *Pacing Clin Electrophysiol*, 26:1208-1211.

Inoue, S.; Mizobuchi, M.; Yoshimura, N.; Yamaguchi, M. & Nakao, H. (2005). Succesful perinatal management of a very low birthweight infant with congenital complete atrioventricular block. *Am J Perinat*, 22:387-390.

Jaeggi, E.; Laskin, C.; Hamilton, R.; Kingdom, J. & Silverman, E. (2010). The importance of the level of maternal anti-Ro/SSA antibodies as a prognostic marker of the development of cardiac neonatal lupus erythematosus a prospective study of 186 antibody-exposed fetuses and infants. *J Am Coll Cardiol*, 55:2778-2784.

Janousek, J.; Tomek, V.; Chaloupecky, V. & Gebauer, RA. (2004). Dilated cardiomyopathy associated with dual-chamber pacing in infants: improvement through either left ventricular cardiac resynchronization or programming the pacemaker off allowing intrinsic normal conduction. *J Cardiovasc Electrophysiol*, 15:470-474.

Johns, JA.; Fish, FA.; Burger, JD.; et al. (1992). Steroid-eluting epicardial pacing leads in pediatric patients: encouraging early results. *J Am Coll Cardiol*, 20:395-401.

Johnson, C. & Galindez, L. (1998). Multiple systemic emboli complicating the course of a patient with an atrial septal defect, an atrial septal aneurysm and an endocardial right atrial pacemaker lead. *P R Health Sci J*, 17:281-284.

Julkunen, H. & Eronen, M. (2001). Long-term outcome of mothers of children with isolated heart block in Finland. *Arthritis Rheum*, 44:647-652.

Kaltman, J.; Ro, P.; Zimmerman, F.; et al. (2008). Managed ventricular pacing in pediatric patients and patients with congenital heart disease. *Am J Cardiol*, 102:875-878.

Kammeraad, J.; Rosenthal, E.; Bostock, J.; et al. (2004). Endocardial pacemaker implantation in infants weighing < 10 kg. *Pacing Clin Electrophysiol,* 27:1466-1474.

Karpawich, PP. (2004). Chronic right ventricular pacing and cardiac performance: the pediatric perspective. *Pacing Clin Electrophysiol,* 27:844-849.

Karpawich, PP.; Rabah, R. & Haas, JE. (1999). Altered cardiac histology following apical right ventricular pacing in patients with congenital atrioventricular block. *Pacing Clin Electrophysiol,* 22:1372-1377.

Kass, DA. (2008). An epidemic of dyssynchrony. But what does it mean? *J Am Coll Cardiol,* 51:12-17.

Khairy, P.; Landzberg, MJ.; Lambert, J. & O'Donnell, CP. (2004). Long-term outcomes after the atrial switch for surgical correction of transposition: a meta-analysis comparing the Mustard and Senning procedures. *Cardiol Young,* 14:284-292.

Khairy, P.; Landzberg, MJ.; Gatzoulis, M.; et al. (2006). Transvenous pacing leads and systemic thromboemboli in patients with intracardiac shunts: a multicenter study. *Circulation,* 113:2391-2397.

Kim, JJ.; Friedman, RA.; Eidem, BW.; et al. (2007). Ventricular function and long-term pacing in children with congenital complete atrioventricular block. *J Cardiovasc Electrophysiol,* 18:373-377.

Kiviniemi, MS.; Pirnes, MA.; Eranen, HJK.; Kettunen, RVJ. & Hartikainen, JEK. (1999). Complications related to permanent pacemaker therapy. *Pacing Clin Electrophysiol,* 22:711-720.

Klug, D.; Lacroix, D.; Savoye, C.; et al. (1997). Systemic infection related to endocarditis on pacemaker leads: Clinical presentation and management. *Circulation,* 95:2098-2107.

Lev, M.; Silverman, J.; Fitzmaurice, FM.; Paul, MH.; Cassells, DE. & Miller, RA. (1971). Lack of connection between the atria and the more peripheral conduction system in congenital atrioventricular block. *Am J Cardiol,* 27:481-490.

Llanos, C.; Izmirly, PM.; Katholi, M.; et al. (2009). Recurrence rates of cardiac manifestations associated with neonatal lupus and maternal/fetal risk factors. *Arthritis Rheum,* 60:3091-3097.

Liberman, L.; Pass, RH.; Hordof, AJ. & Spotnitz, HM. (2008). Late onset of heart block after open heart surgery for congenital heart disease. *Pediatr Cardiol,* 29:56-59.

Maginot, KR.; Mathewson, JW.; Bichell, DP. & Perry, JC. (2000). Applications of pacing strategies in neonates and infants. *Progr Pediatr Cardiol,* 11:65-75.

Mansour, F.; Talajic, M.; Thibault, B. & Khairy, P. (2006). Pacemaker troubleshooting: when MVP is not the most valuable parameter. *Heart Rhythm,* 5:612-614.

Martin, MV.; Lime, AB.; Almeida, CS; et al. (1966). Implantation of Chardack-Greatbatch adjustable rate and current pacemaker in a 4 month old infant. *Pediatrics,* 37:323-328.

McCue, CM.; Mantakas, ME.; Tingelstad, JB. & Ruddy, S. (1977). Congenital heart block in newborns of mothers with connective tissue disease. *Circulation,* 56:82-90.

van Mechelen, R. & Schoonderwoerd, R. (2006). Risk of managed ventricular pacing in a pacing with heart block. *Heart Rhythm,* 11:1384-1385.

Michaelsson, M. & Engle, MA. (1972). Congenital complete heart block: an international study of the natural history. *Cardiovasc Clin,* 4:86-101.

Michaelsson, M.; Jonzon, A. & Riesenfeld, T. (1995). Isolated congenital complete atrioventricular block in adult life: a prospective study. *Circulation,* 92:442-449.

Michaelsson, M.; Riesenfeld, A. & Jonzon, A. (1997). Natural history of congenital complete atrioventricular block. *Pacing Clin Electrophysiol,* 20:2098-2101.

Miller, GL.; Horneffer, PJ.; Gardner, TJ.; Rykiel, MF. & Pearson, TA. (1988). The epidemiology of the postpericardiotomy syndrome: a common complication of cardiac surgery. *Am Heart J,* 116:1323-1329.

Moak, JP.; Barron, KS.; Hougen, TJ.; et al. (2001). Congenital heart block: development of late-onsetcardiomyopathy, a previously underappreciated sequela. *J Am Coll Cardiol,* 37:238-242.

Moak, JP.; Hasbani, K.; Ramwell, C.; et al. (2006). Dilated cardiomyopathy following right ventricular pacing for AV block in young patients: resolution after upgrading to biventricular pacing systems. *J Cardiovasc Electrophysiol,* 17:1068-1071.

Mond, HG. (1991). Unipolar versus bipolar pacing – poles apart. *Pacing Clin Electrophysiol,* 14:1411-1424.

Mond, HG. & Stokes KB. (1992). The electrode-tissue interface: the revolutionary role of steroid elution. *Pacing Clin Electrophysiol,* 15:95-107.

Nield, LE.; Silverman, ED.; Taylor, GP.; et al. (2002). Maternal anti-Ro and anti-La antibodyassociated endocardial fibroelastosis. *Circulation,* 105:843-848.

Nothroff, J.; Norozi, K.; Alpers, V.; et al. (2006). Pacemaker implantation as a risk factor for heart failure in young adults with congenital heart disease. *Pacing Clin Electrophysiol,* 29:386-392.

Ohmi, M.; Tofukuji, M.; Sato, K.; et al. (1992). Permanent pacemaker implantation in premature infants less than 2,000 grams of body weight. *Ann Thorac Surg,* 54:1223-1225.

Oldroyd, KG.; Rae, AP.; Carter, R.; Wingate, C. & Cobbe, SM. (1991). Double blind cross over comparison of the effects of dual chamber pacing (DDD) and ventricular rate adaptive (VVIR) pacing on neuroendocrine variables, exercise performance and symptoms in complete heart block. *Br Heart J,* 65:188-193.

Polin, GM.; Zado, E.; Nayak, H.; et al. (2006). Proper management of pericardial tamponade as a late complication of implantable cardiac device placement. *Am J Cardiol,* 98:223-225.

Prinzen, FW.; Cheriex, EM.; Delhaas, T.; et al. (1995). Asymmetric thickness of the left ventricular wall resulting from asynchronous electrical activation. A study in patients with left bundle branch block in dogs with ventricular pacing. *Am Heart J,* 130:1045-1053.

Ragonese, P.; Guccione, P.; Drago, F.; Turchetta, A.; Calzolari, A. & Formigari, R. (1994). Efficacy and safety of ventricular rate responsive pacing in children with complete atrioventricular block. *Pacing Clin Electrophysiol,* 17:603-610.

Rosenthal, E.; Qureshi, SA. & Crick, JC. (1995). Successful long-term ventricular pacing via the coronary sinus after the Fontan operation. *Pacing Clin Electrophysiol,* 18:2103-2105.

Rosenthal, E.; Bostock, J.; Qureshi, SA.; Baker, EJ. & Tynan, M. (1997a). Single pass VDD pacing in children and adolescents. *Pacing Clin Electrophysiol,* 20:1975-1982.

Rosenthal, E. & Bostock, J. (1997b). Use of an atrial loop to extend the duration of endocardial pacing in a neonate. *Pacing Clin Electrophysiol,* 20:2489-2491.

Sachweh, JS.; Vazquez-Jiminez, JF.; Schondube, FA.; et al. (2000). Twenty years experience with pediatric pacing: epicardial and transvenous stimulation. *Eur J Cardiothorac Surg,* 17:455-461.

Sanjeev, S. & Karpawich P. (2006). Superior vena cava and innominate vein dimensions in growing children: An aid for interventional devices and transvenous leads. *Pediatr Cardiol,* 27:414-419.

Seiden, HS.; Camunas, JL.; Fishburger, SB.; et al. (1997). Use of single lead VDD pacing in children. *Pacing Clin Electrophysiol,* 20:1967-1974.

Simon, A.; Dick, M 2nd.; Stern, A.; Behrendt, D. & Sloan, H. (1982). Ventricular pacing in children. *Pacing Clin Electrophysiol,* 5:836-844.

Silka, MJ. & Rice, MJ. (1991). Paradoxic embolism due to altered hemodynamic sequencing following transvenous pacing. *Pacing Clin Electrophysiol,* 14:499-503.

Silvetti, MS.; De Santis, A.; Grovale, N.; Grutter, G.; Baccarini, A. & Drago, F. (2007a). Ventricular pacing threshold variations in the young. *Pacing Clin Electrophysiol,* 30:175-181.

Silvetti, MS.; Drago, F.; De Santis, A.; et al. (2007b). Single-centre experience on endocardial and epicardial pacemaker system function in neonates and infants. *Europace,* 9:426-431.

Sholler, GF. & Walsh EP. (1989). Congenital complete heart block in patients without anatomic cardiac defects. *Am Heart J,* 118:1193-1198.

Spindler, M.; Burrows, G.; Kowallik, P.; Ertl, G. & Voelker, W. (2001). Postpericardiotomy syndrome and cardiac tamponade as a late complication after pacemaker implantation. *Pacing Clin Electrophysiol,* 24:1433-1444.

Stephenson, EA. & Kaltman, JR. (2006). Current state of the art for use of pacemakers and defibrillators in patients with congenital cardiac malformations. *Cardiol Young,* 16:151-156.

Sweeney, MO.; Shea, J.; Fox, V.; et al. (2004). Randomized pilot study of a new atrial-based minimal ventricular pacing mode in dual-chamber implantable-cardioverter-defibrillators. *Heart Rhythm,* 1:160-167.

Sweeney, MO.; Ellenbogen, KA.; Casavant, D.; et al. (2005). Multicenter, prospective, randomized safety and efficacy study of a new atrial-based managed ventricular pacing mode (MVP) in dual chamber ICDs. *J Cardiovasc Electrophysiol,* 16:811-817.

Thambo, JB.; Bordachar, P.; Garrigue, S.; et al. (2004). Detrimental ventricular remodelling in patients with congenital complete heart block and chronic right ventricular apical pacing. *Circulation,* 110:3766- 3772.

Tomaske, M.; Harpes, P.; Pretre, E.; Dodge-Khatami, A. & Bauersfeld, U. (2007). Long-term experience with AutoCapture-controlled epicardial pacing in children. *Europace,* 9:645-650.

Tops, LF.; Schalij, MJ.; Holman, ER.; van Erven, L.; van der Wall, EE. & Bax, JJ. (2006). Right ventricular pacing can induce ventricular dyssynchrony in patients with atrial fibrillation after atrioventricular node ablation. *J Am Coll Cardiol,* 48:1642-1648.

Turley, K.; Hanley, FL.; Verrier, ED.; et al. (1988). The Mustard procedure in infants (less than 100 days of age). Ten year follow-up. *J Thorac Cardiovasc Surg,* 96:849-853.

Vardas, PE.; Auricchio, A.; Blanc, JJ.; et al. (2007). Guidelines for cardiac pacing and cardiac resynchronization therapy: the task force for cardiac pacing and cardiac resynchronization therapy of the European Society of Cardiology. Developed in collaboration with the European Heart Rhythm Association. *Eur Heart J*, 28:2256-2295.

Vatasescu, R.; Shalganov, T.; Paprika, D.; et al. (2007). Evolution of left ventricular function in paediatric patients with permanent right ventricular pacing for isolated congenital heart block: a medium term follow-up. *Europace*, 9:228-232.

Vetter, VL.; Tanner, CS. & Horowitz, LN. (1987). Electrophysiologic consequences of the Mustard repair of D-transposition of the great arteries. *J Am Coll Cardiol*, 10:1265-1273.

Villain, E.; Coastedoat-Chalumeau, N.; Marijon, E.; et al. (2006). Presentation and prognosis of complete atrioventricular block in childhood, according to maternal antibody status. *J Am Coll Cardiol*, 48:1682-1687.

Vogt, P.; Goy, JJ.; Kuhn, M.; Leuenberger, P. & Kappenberger, L. (1988). Single versus double chamber rate responsive cardiac pacing: comparison by cardiopulmonary noninvasive exercise testing. *Pacing Clin Electrophysiol*, 11:1896-1901.

Warfield, DA.; Hayes, DL.; Hyberger, LK.; Warnes, CA. & Danielson, GK. (1999). Permanent pacing in patients with univentricular heart. *Pacing Clin Electrophysiol*, 22:1193-1201.

Welisch, E.; Cherlet, E.; Crespo-Martiney, E. & Hansky, B. (2010). A single institution experience with pacemaker implantation in a pediatric population over 25 years. *Pacing Clin Electrophysiol*, 33:1112-1118.

Udink ten Cate, FE.; Breur, JM.; Cohen, MI.; et al. (2001). Dilated cardiomyopathy in isolated congenital complete atrioventricular block: early and long-term risk in children. *J Am Coll Cardiol*, 37:1129-1134.

Udink ten Cate, FE.; Breur, JM.; Boramanand, N.; et al. (2002). Endocardial and epicardial steroid lead pacing in the neonatal and paediatric age group. *Heart*, 88:392-396.

Udink ten Cate, FE.; Kruessell MA. ; Wagner, K. ; et al. (2010a). Dilated cardiomyopathy in children with ventricular preexcitation : the location of the accessory pathway is predictive of this association. *J Electrocardiol*, 43:146-154.

Udink ten Cate, FE.; Wiesner, N. ; Trieschmann, U. ; Khalil, M. & Sreeram, N. (2010b). Dyssynchronous ventricular activation in asymptomatic Wolff_parkinson-White: a risk factor for development of dilated cardiomyopathy. *Indian Pacing Electrophysiol J*, 10:248-256.

Zeltser, I.; Rhodes, LA.; Tanel, RE.; et al. (2004). Postpericardiotomy syndrome after permanent pacemaker implantation in children and young adults. *Ann Thorac Surg*, 78:1684-1687.

Advantages of Right-Sided Implantation of Permanent Cardiac Pacemakers Performed by a Surgeon

Davor Horvat
General Hospital in Karlovac,
Croatia

1. Introduction

A pacemaker is a medical device which uses electrical impulses, delivered by electrodes contacting the heart muscles, to regulate the beating of the heart. The primary purpose of a pacemaker is to maintain an adequate heart rate, either because the heart's native pacemaker is not fast enough, or there is a block in the heart's electrical conduction system (Fig. 1,2a,2b,3) (McWilliam, JA. 2007., Gregoratos, G. 2005).

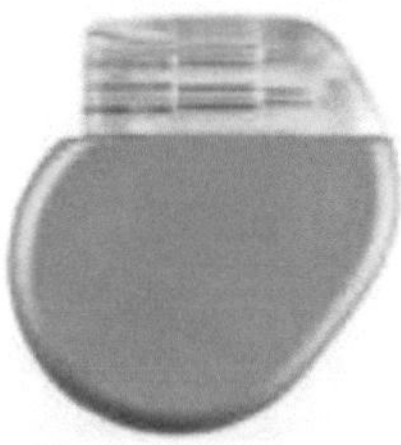

Fig. 1. A puls generator of a pacemaker

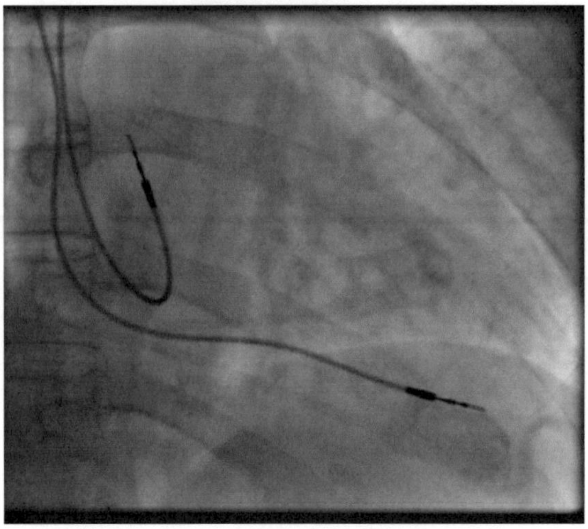

Fig. 2a. A leads of a pacemaker

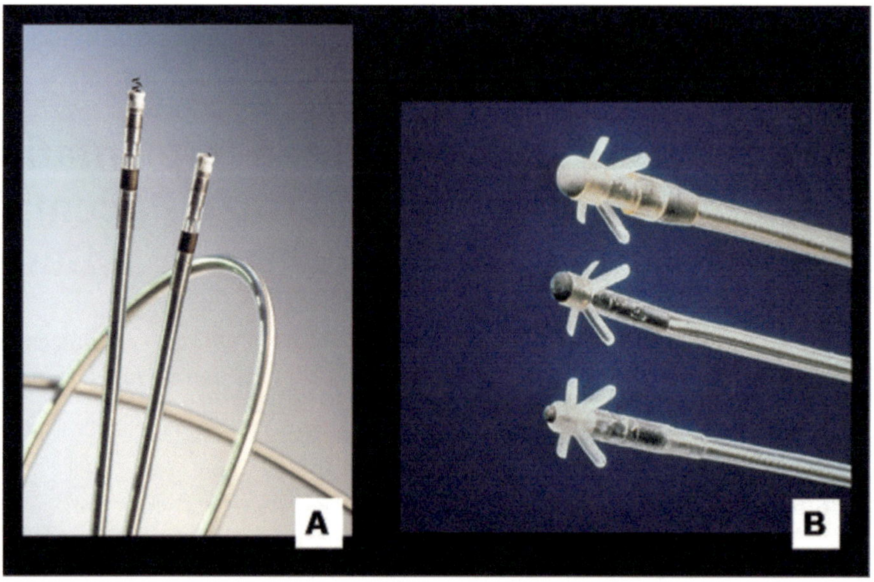

Fig. 2b. A leads of a pacemaker

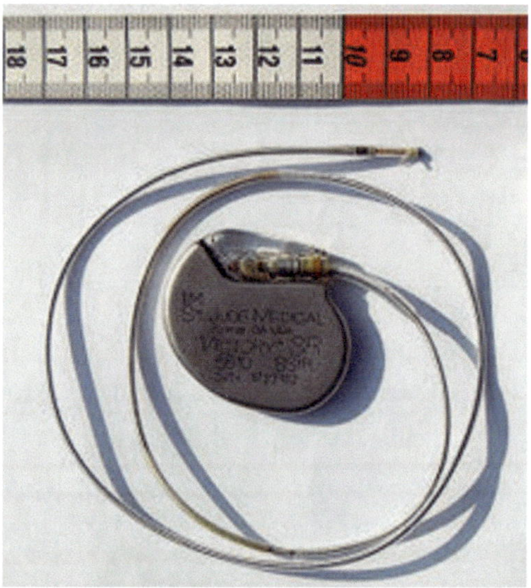

Fig. 3. A puls generator of a pacemaker with electrode

The first use of transvenous pacing in conjunction with an implanted pacemaker was by Parsonnet in the USA (Parsonnet, V. 1978, a Parsonnet, V.; Zucker, IR. & Asa, MM. 1962, b Parsonnet, V; Zucker, IR. & Asa, MM.1962)., Lagergren in Sweden (Lagergren, H. 1978., Lagergren H, & Johansson, L.1963) and Jean-Jaques Welti in France (Welti, JJ. 2009) in 1962-63. The transvenous procedure involved incision of a vein into which was inserted the catheter electrode lead under fluoroscopic guidance, until it was lodged within the trabeculae of the right ventricle. This method was to become the method of choice by the mid-1960s (McWilliam, JA. 2007).). Permanent pacing with an implantable pacemaker involves transvenous placement of one or more pacing electrodes within a chamber, or chambers, of the heart. The procedure is performed by incision of a suitable vein into which the electrode lead is inserted and passed along the vein, through the valve of the heart, until positioned in the chamber. The procedure is facilitated by fluoroscopy which enables the physician or cardiologist to view the passage of the electrode lead. After satisfactory lodgement of the electrode is confirmed the opposite end of the electrode lead is connected to the pacemaker generator. There are three basic types of permanent pacemakers, classified according to the number of chambers involved and their basic operating mechanism. In single-chamber pacemaker type, only one pacing lead is placed into a chamber of the heart, either the atrium or the ventricle. In dual-chamber pacemaker type, wires are placed in two chambers of the heart. One lead paces the atrium and one paces the ventricle. This type more closely resembles the natural pacing of the heart by assisting the heart in coordinating the function between the atria and ventricles ("Heart Rhythm Society", 2004). A pacemaker is typically inserted into the patient through a simple surgery using either local anesthetic or a general anesthetic. The patient may be given a drug for relaxation before the surgery as well. An antibiotic is typically administered to prevent infection (de Oliveira, JC et al. 2009). In most cases the pacemaker is inserted in the left shoulder area where an incision is made below the collar bone creating a small pocket where the pacemaker is actually housed in the patient's body. The lead or leads (the number of leads varies depending on the type of pacemaker) are fed into the heart through a large vein using a fluoroscope to monitor the progress of lead insertion. A temporary drain may be installed and removed the following day. The actual surgery may take about an hour (McWilliam, JA. 2007).

2. Important

2.1 What is the problem?

The aim of this paper is to point out the advantages of right-sided implantation of cardiac pacemakers, to stress the advantages of the cooperation with a surgeon while preparing the pacemaker's layer as well as to critically judge the frequency of developed complications in such a treatment. The second problem is to show the better place for the generator's implantation.

2.2 What has been done by other researchers and where you can contribute?

In today's practice implantation of the generator of cardiac pacemakers beneath the right clavicle by means of surgical preparation of the layer is not so often used as a method of implantation of cardiac pacemakers.

The reason for this is greater practicality of the left-sided implantation due to a simpler anatomic position of the subclavian vein as well as easier organisation of work in case only a cardiologist performs an operation without the help of a surgeon.

2.3 What have you done and which method or tools were used ?

However, in case of right-sided implantation of a cardiac pacemaker, the position of an electrode is in the form of the letter «S», which means that the electrode bends in two contralateral curves which is in contrast to left-sided implantation where the electrode has only one curve on its path from the generator to the peak of the heart. It is these two curves of the electrode that cause its better stability and a fewer number of post-operative dislocations.

An example of such a way of implantation of an electrode of a cardiac pacemaker is presented in Figure 4. This Figure also shows right-sided implantation of an atrium electrode where each of these two arrows indicates one of the two curves of the electrode. The same principle can also be applied to the ventricular electrode and as a result of these two curves of the electrode better stability of the electrodes is achieved (Fig. 5).

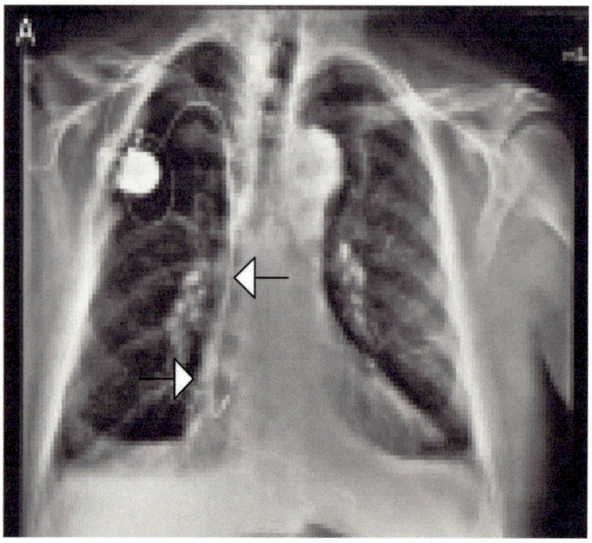

Fig. 4. Right-sided implantation of an atrial electrode

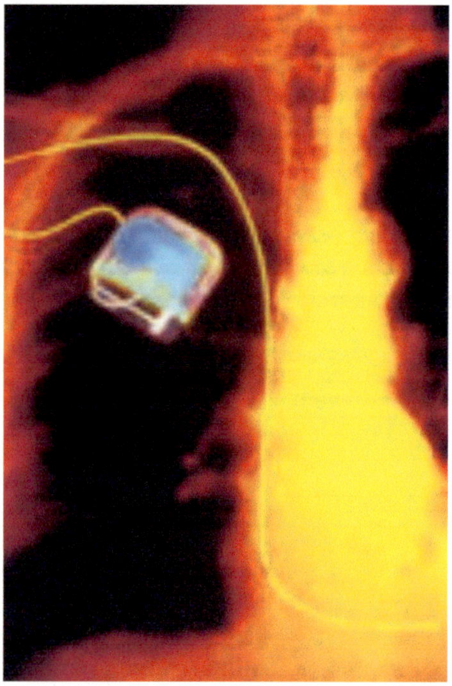

Fig. 5. Right-sided implantation of a ventricular electrode

In contrast to this, Figure 6 shows left-sided way of implantation of a ventricular electrode where only one bigger curve of the electrode is visible. However, such one curve of the electrode cannot give satisfactory stability of the electrode of a cardiac pacemaker (Fig. 7a,7b). Finally, due to greater instability of the electrode, this causes greater possibility of dislocations (8). Moreover, additional efforts for displacing the electrode are needed in such a case. This requires some extra time, new expenses, and partly, it affects the self-conficence of the operator.

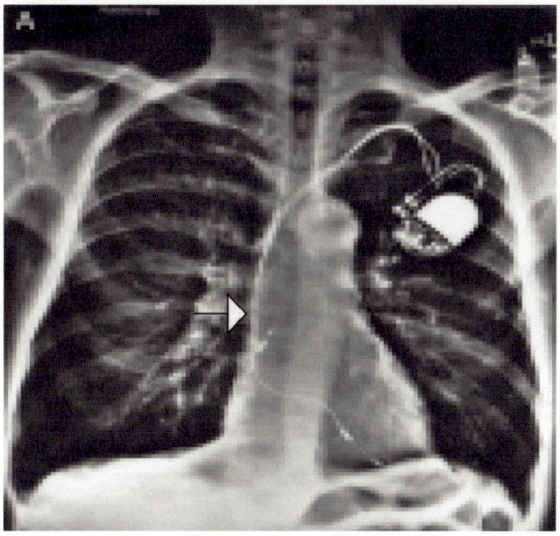

Fig. 6. Left-sided implantation of a ventricular electrode

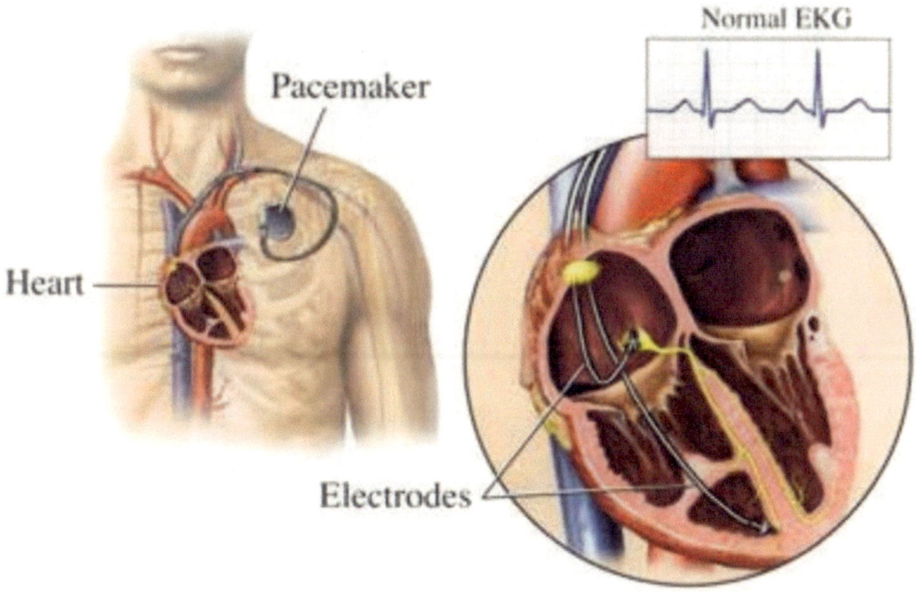

Fig. 7a. The scheme of left-sided electrodes implantation

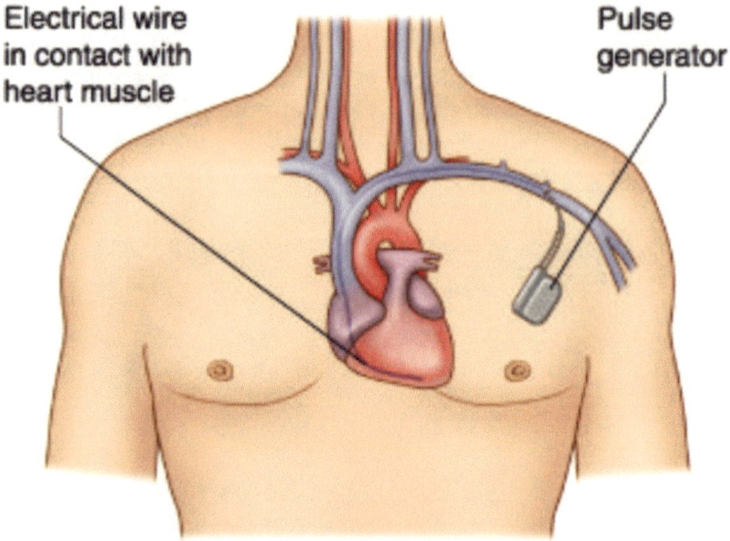

Fig. 7b. The scheme of left-sided electrodes implantation

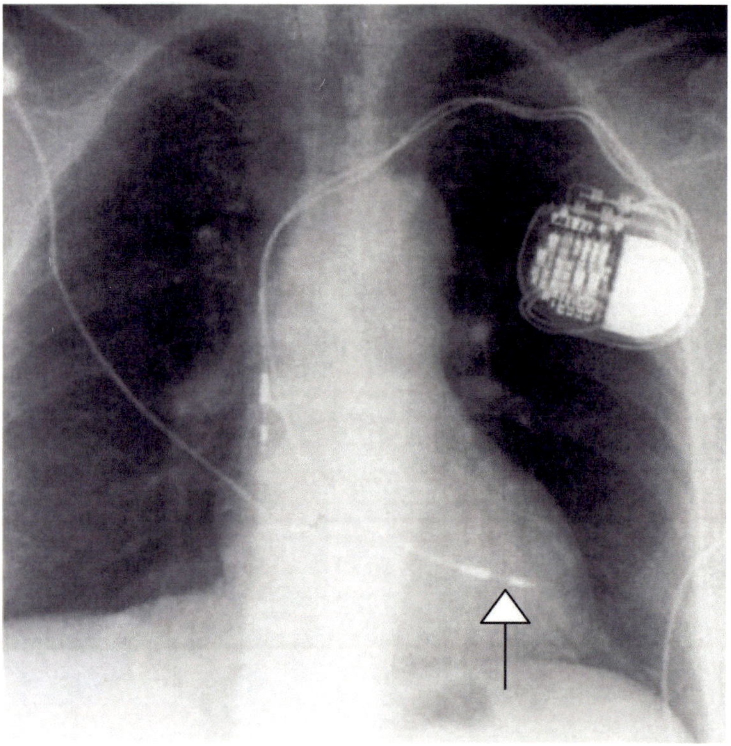

Fig. 8. Chest radiograph obtained after pacemaker implantation shows that ventricular lead is displaced superiorly in left ventrlcle

Also, the surgeon's help while implanting a cardiac pacemaker beneath the clavicle makes it possible for the generator's layer to be formed between the big and the small pectoral muscle. In such a way a better aesthetic impression for the patient is achieved because the place of implantation cannot be practically seen from the outside at all. Furthermore, frequency of decubitus of the skin is reduced due to prolapse of the generator in thin patients as well as frequency of the puncture of the subclavian vein is reduced, too. Namely, the vena cephalica is shown by a surgical approach through which placing of the electrode into the subclavian vein is made possible. In this way the possibility of complications such as haematomae and iatrogenic pneumothorax (Fig. 9) is reduced because the access through the vena cephalica is considerably less traumatic than a direct access through the subclavian vein.

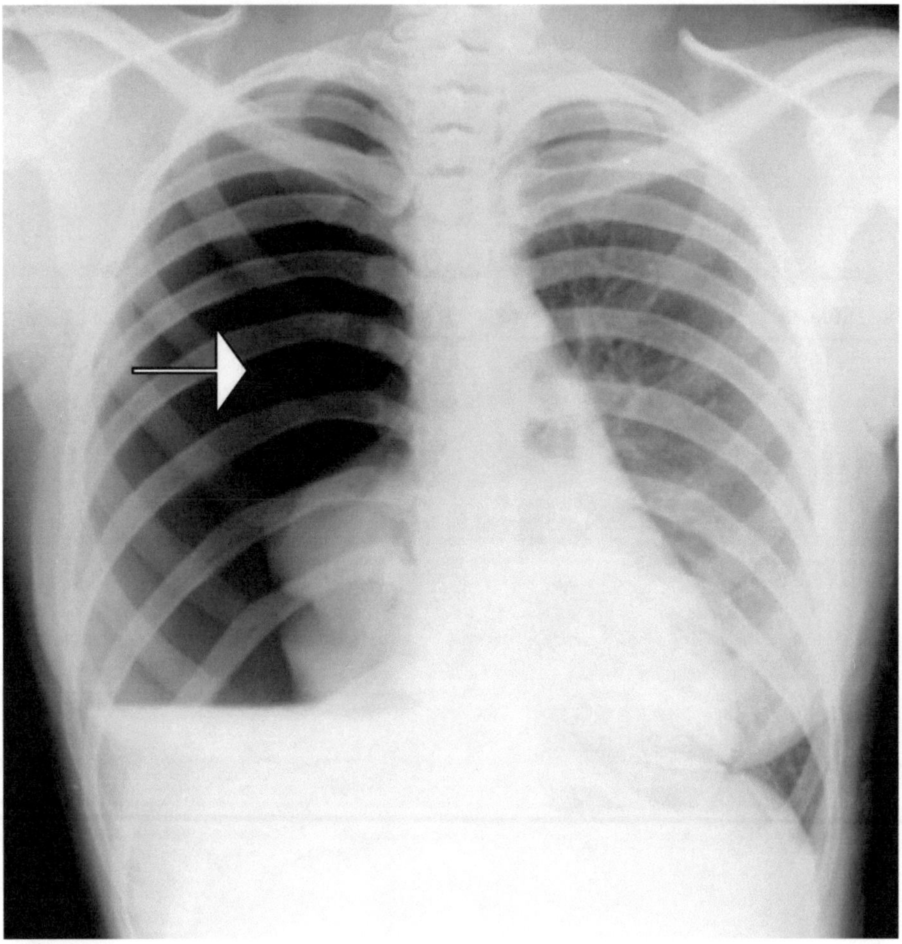

Fig. 9. Iatrogenic pneumothorax

Such an example of «deep» implantation of the generator of a cardiac pacemaker is presented in Figures 10a,10b,10c. Namely, a formed layer of the generator of a cardiac pacemaker beneath the pectoral muscle means that above the very generator one can see a muscle which additonally stabilizes it.

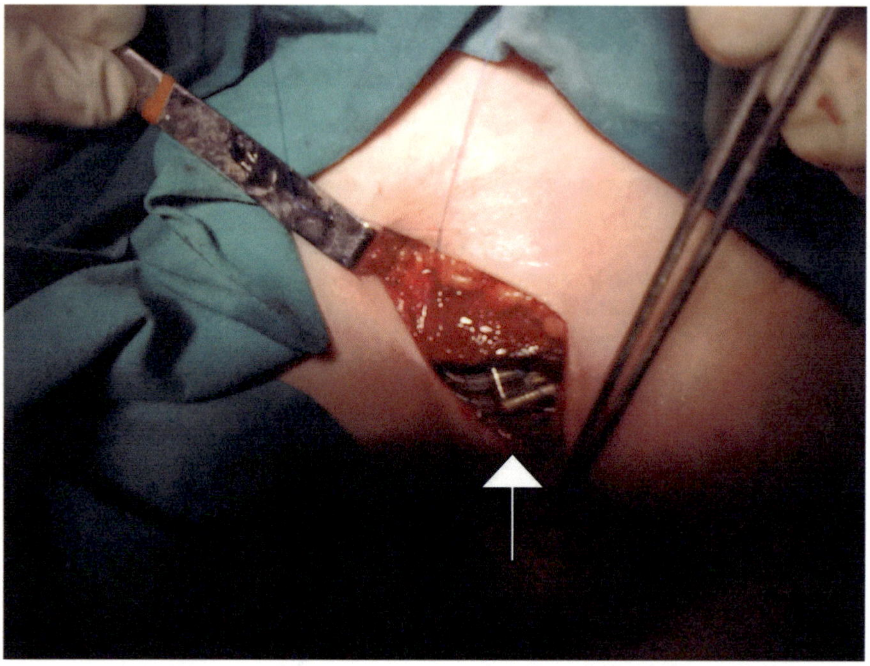

Fig. 10a. Implantation of the pulse generator of a cardiac pacemaker beneath a pectoral muscle

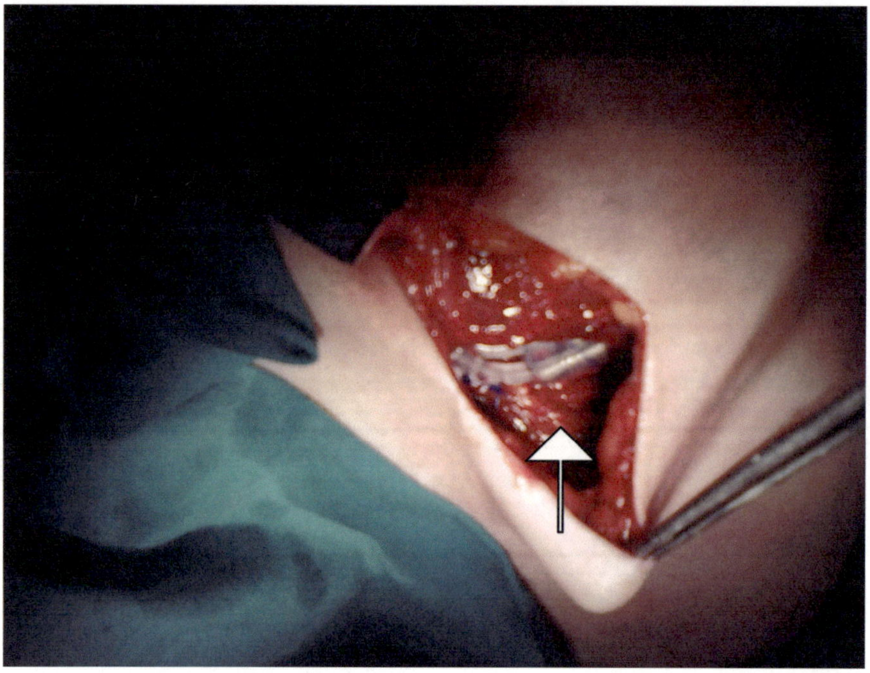

Fig. 10b. Implantation of the pulse generator of a cardiac pacemaker beneath a pectoral muscle

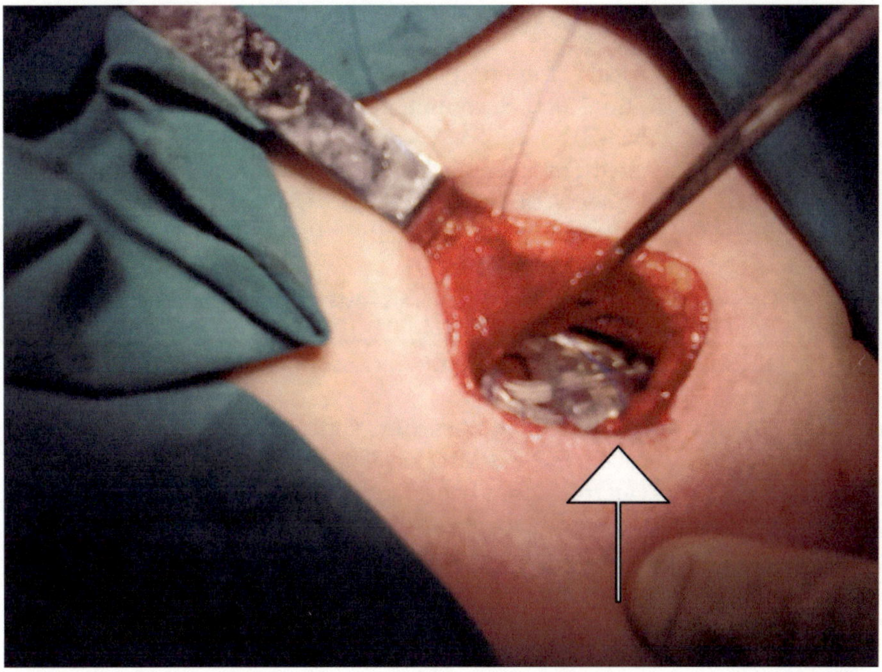

Fig. 10c. Implantation of the pulse generator of a cardiac pacemaker beneath a pectoral muscle

2.4 What are my results?

In order to support this thesis from a practical point of view, a research involving 281 patients with right-sided primoimplantation of permanent cardiac pacemakers by a surgeon was carried out. The correction of dislocated electrode in the course of the first year was determined in 11 patients (3.9%). The puncture of subclavian vein due to inadequate vena cephalica was determined in 62 patients (22.1%). However, the care of the local haematomae was determined in 4 patients (1.4%) and local infections in 2 patients (0.7%). The need for an access to the other side was determined in 6 patients (2.1%). However, only 3 patients polled (1.1%) had, during a follow-up, a subjective feeling of discomfort at the place of implantation of a cardiac pacemaker.

One should especially point out that frequency of dislocation of an electrode, puncture of the vena subclaviae, changes of the side of implantation and looking after local surgical complications such as infections, haematomae and decubitus were better in our hospital than in other centres (Ellenbogen et al., 2002, Harcombe et al., 1998, Aggarwal et al., 1995).

2.5 What is new and good, what is not good?

To sum up, frequency of complications during right-sided implantation of cardiac pacemakers performed by a surgeon is satisfactory low and patients are highly satisfied. Also, the frequency of decubitus of the skin, prolapse of generator, frequency of the puncture of the subclavian vein, complications such as haematomae and iatrogenic pneumothorax are reduced. This method is complicate because a cardiologist works with a surgeon, but the positive effects are bigger.

3. References

McWilliam, JA. (2007). "Electrical stimulation of the heart in man". *Br Med J*, Vol.,1., 348-50.

Gregoratos, G. (2005). Indications and Recommendations for Pacemaker Therapy. *Am Fam Physician*, Vol.,71.,1563-70.

Parsonnet, V. (1978). "Permanent Transvenous Pacing in 1962". *PACE*, Vol.,1., 285.

a Parsonnet, V.; Zucker, IR. & Asa, MM. (1962). "Preliminary Investigation of the Development of a Permanent Implantable Pacemaker Using an Intracardiac Dipolar Electrode". *Clin Res*, Vol.,10., 391.

b Parsonnet, V; Zucker, IR. & Asa, MM. (1962). "An intracardiac bipolar electrode for interim treatment of complete heart block". *Am J Cardiol*, Vol.,10., 261-5.

Lagergren, H. (1978). "How it happened: my recollection of early pacing". *Pacing Clin Electrophysiol*, Vol.,1(1).,140-3.

Lagergren H, & Johansson, L. (1963). "Intracardiac stimulation for complete heart block". *Acta Chir Scand*, Vol.,125., 562-6. PMID 13928055.

Welti, JJ. Biography, (2009). Heart Rhythm Foundation.
http://www.wikidoc.org/index.php/Artificial_pacemaker#_ref-11
"Pacemakers, Patient and Public Information Center. Heart Rhythm Society". 2004.
http://www.hrspatients.org/patients/treatments/pacemakers.asp.

de Oliveira, JC et al. (2009). "Efficacy of antibiotic prophylaxis prior to the implantation of pacemakers and cardioverter-defibrillators: Results of a large, prospective, randomized, double-blinded, placebo - controlled trial". *Circ Arrhythmia Electrophysiol*, Vol., 2.(1), 29-34.

Ellenbogen, KA et al. (2002). Delayed Complications Following Pacemaker Implantation. *Pacing Clin Electrophysiol*, Vol., 25.(8), 1155-8.

Harcombe, A et al. (1998). Late complications following permanent pacemaker implantation or elective unit replacement. *Heart*, Vol., 80.(3), 240-4.

Aggarwal, RK et al. (1995). Early complications of permanent pacemaker implantation: no difference between dual and single chamber systems. *Br Heart J*, Vol., 73.(6), 571-5.

Part 2

Remote Monitoring

8

Telemonitoring of the Pacemaker

Umashankar Lakshmanadoss MD[1],
Abrar Shah MD[2] and James P Daubert MD[3]
[1]*Johns Hopkins Medical Institutions, Baltimore, MD,*
[2]*University of Rochester Medical Center, Rochester, NY,*
[3]*Duke University Medical Center, Durham, NC,*
USA

1. Introduction

With increasing knowledge about the cardiovascular diseases and with more advanced technology, indications for implantation of pacemakers are expanding. By the end of 2007, about 560,000 pacemakers were implanted in North America and 680,000 in Europe. With the increasing prevalence of pacemakers, management and follow up of these complex patients is becoming an ongoing issue. Close monitoring and interrogation of their pacemakers remains a main part of the complete evaluation of these patients. It is estimated that in North America and in Europe, there are 3.2 million pacemaker encounters per year. Due to huge number of patients, following all the patients in the outpatient clinic/hospital on the regular basis may not be feasible. Hence, it has been suggested that telemonitoring system could provide a practical substitute to the time-consuming and expensive in-office visits.In this chapter, we will be describing the current technologies and also provide an update on this rapidly evolving topics, by incorporating the latest data and on-going trials.

Telemonitoring is defined as the use of audiovisual and other information technologies to monitor patient status at a distance; it can be used in monitoring the cardiac and respiratory status of patients. In 1905, Einthoven transmitted Electro Cardio Gram (EKG) from a hospital to his home using a telephone line. In 1920s, Winters transmitted the heart sounds using a radio link. Later on in the 1960s, with increasing technological advances, the United States navy used the telemonitoring system to transmit their soldiers' physiologic data from the ships to their shore hospital at Florida, USA (Institute of Medicine). In the past few decades, telemonitoring attained a robust development. Recent Heart Rhythm Society / European Heart Rhythm Association expert consensus on monitoring the cardiac devices (Wilkoff et al., 2008) recommended that patients with pacemakers/defibrillators should be monitored at regular intervals based on the time elapsed after the device implantation. (Table 1)

Telemonitoring may be subdivided into:

1. Remote follow- up:

Device data will be transferred from the patient to the physician's office or to the central data processing center in a *predetermined scheduled time* using the wand / transmitter.

2. Remote monitoring:

In addition to the transmission of the data from the device on a *daily basis, unscheduled transmission of the predefined alerts* (e.g. battery depletion, improper sensing / capture), will also happen. The data from the device will be transmitted and the physician will be notified, according to the predefined settings by the physician (e.g. information given to the physician/health care provider through SMS, emails, contacting the office through phone).

Minimum frequency of monitoring of pacemakers either in person or remotely		
	Remote monitor	In person follow - up
Within 3 days of Implantation	-	X
2-12 weeks post implantation	-	X
Every 3-12 months after implantation	X	X
Every 1-3 months at signs of battery depletion	X	X
Annually until depletion of battery	-	X

Table 1. Timeline for follow up of the Pacemakers
X – Recommended; - Not recommended

3. Bidirectional telemetry:
In addition to the remote monitoring of the pacemakers, *remote interrogation and remote programming* of the pacemakers can be done with newer revolutionary technologies.

2. Importance of monitoring the pacemaker:

Monitoring of pacemakers is necessary for both patient- and device-related factors. Wilkoff et al. (2008) described the various important reasons and goals of monitoring pacemakers. By closely monitoring the pacemakers, the clinician would achieve the goals outlined below. (Table 2)

Patient Centered Factors
Optimize the patient's quality of life
Identify the patients at risk (based on the alerts) and appropriate follow up
Identify any abnormal brady / tachy arrhythmias
Identify non device related problems and appropriate referrals
Patient safety
Peace of mind for the patient

Device Related Factors
Optimize the pacemaker function to meet patients' need
Identify and correct abnormal device function
Identify the end of life of the battery, monitor lead dysfunction
Monitor the various alerts by the device and triage accordingly
Maintain a database for future research purpose.

Table 2. Factors effecting pacemaker placement

3. Description of the telemonitoring technology:

Implanted pacemakers are pre-equipped with a micro-antenna, which communicates with a small external device, commonly known as transmitter. A receiver or "*wand*," is attached by a wire to the programmer and positioned on the body's surface over the pacemaker implantation site to receive the telemetry signal from the pacemaker. The wand will be *talking* to the device as radiofrequency signals {either the Industrial, Scientific and Medical (ISM) band from 902–928 MHz or a subsection of the Medical Implant and Communications (MICS) band from 402–405 MHz}. The distance for radiofrequency signal communication has increased from several cm to several meters and some devices can even communicate without a wand. The transmitters are able to interrogate programmed parameters and diagnostic data stored in the device memory with active participation of patient (via a wand), or automatically (wandless), at preset time intervals. The data downloaded from the device by the transmitter is then uploaded as an encrypted data, to a secured clinical database either by a standard analog phone line or through wireless GSM (Global System for Mobile) connection. The programmer is a computer with specific software and associated hardware modifications that provide highly reliable exchange of the encrypted information and precise communication with the cardiac device. The transmission of these data may be initiated by patient (as a scheduled transmission or event triggered (symptom / alert by device).

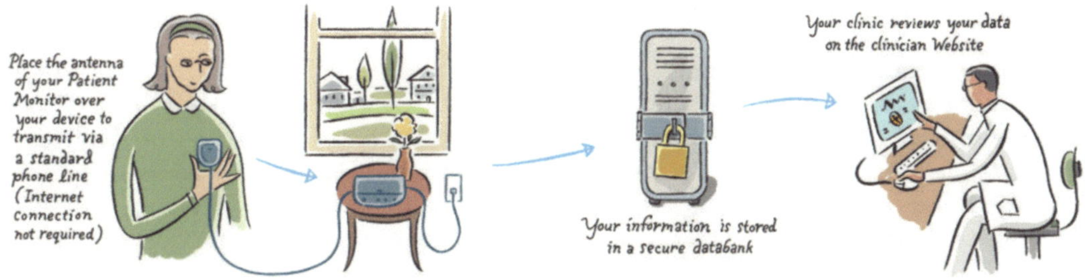

Fig. 1. Telemonitoring technology.

The data will be processed in central processing center, which is usually maintained by the device manufacturers. The data will be uploaded in a secure website and a health care provider can login and look into the events (Figure 1). In addition to the uploading of the data to website, depending on clinical urgency, the concerned health care provider will be notified via email, SMS, fax or telephone call as predefined by the physicians. Moreover, some manufacturers follows a traffic light like system, in which the alerts will be sent to the clinician in varying colors like red, yellow and green, depending on the magnitude of the problem. Otherwise, after initiating manual transmission, patient also can call the physician, who can login to the password protected secure website and look into the events.

Typically, the following informations are transmitted to database: heart rate, battery status, lead integrity, pacing lead impedance, episodes of arrhythmias, delivered antitachycardia pacing, percent pacing, histogram, real-time and magnet Electrograms (EGM), stored EGMs

and arrhythmia summary with mode switch duration. These data will help the clinician to diagnose any active problems. In addition, monitoring of the silent events like asymptomatic atrial fibrillation is *very important* as these arrhythmias are proven to be an independent risk factor for increased mortality in patients with heart failure. In addition to these data, patient can also enter his blood pressure measurements, body weights and other symptoms related to heart failure (in patients with Cardiac Resynchronization Therapy {CRT}). Based on these data, physicians would be able to make changes in the management of the patient's condition.
Programmers can also communicate the interrogated data to a remote printer for a hard copy presentation or be transferred to a database or Electronic Medical Record (EMR). To connect to the database or to EMR, the data are saved and then transferred via disc, CD ROM, USB drive, directly by a network cable, Bluetooth or Wi-Fi communication to an internet or intranet network connection. The ISM and MICS radiofrequency communication is used only for connecting the pacemaker to the programmer or remote telemetry device and not for connecting the programmer to printers, saved files, the database, EMR or registries.

4. Types of remote transmission:

4.1 Patient initiated remote transmission:

In this mode of transmission, the initiation of data transfer from the pacemaker is done by the patient himself / herself. This may be a regular, scheduled transmission or an unscheduled transmission, triggered either by the patient symptoms (like shortness of breath, lightheadedness, syncope, palpitations) or in response to an alert given by the pacemaker (usually an audible sound or vibration).

4.2 Device initiated remote transmission:

In this mode of transmission, initiation of data transfer from the pacemaker is done by the pacemaker itself. Data will be transferred on a regular scheduled basis, at fixed time intervals (often at night, when the patient is lying in bed). Usually, the patient need not place the wand over the pacemaker. The pacemaker itself will "talk" to the home monitor/ communicator and initiate transfer. If there is any change in patient's physiologic data or any new alerts by the pacemakers, there will be an unscheduled initiation of the data transfer from the pacemaker, even without the knowledge of patient.

4.3 Transtelephonic monitoring without interrogation:

This is one of the older techniques. This technology is solely limited to pacemaker follow-up. In this method of transmission, patient must initiate data transmission through a telephone. Each transmission usually includes an initial rhythm strip and then a rhythm strip demonstrating magnet rate of pacing system. Telephone transmissions provide only a brief snapshot of cardiac rhythm and thus intermittent problems may not be detected. It still has some value in monitoring the pacemakers approaching end of life and in need of elective replacement of the battery.

5. Types of various tele monitors by 4 major companies:

The following four types of remote monitors are produced by the various pacemaker manufacturers:

5.1 Biotronik

In 2001, Biotronik introduced wireless remote monitoring of cardiac devices. Biotronik Home Monitoring uses three simple colours to quickly and automatically convey a wealth of vital information to physicians who need on-the-spot patient data anywhere, any time. When activated, Home Monitoring ® (Biotronik & Co. KG, Berlin, Germany) transmits data systematically on a daily basis, at a fixed time of day (usually in the night times), via a special cell phone-like instrument (CardioMessenger®, Biotronik Figure 2)) kept within 2 m from the implanted device. The transmission utilizes state-of-the-art encrypted SMS technology to transfer worldwide data to a dedicated center.

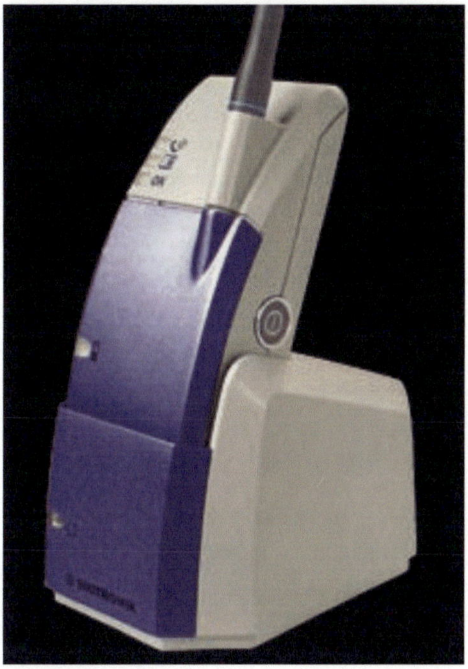

Fig. 2. CardioMessenger® from Biotronik

Event notifications are assigned by the physician with a red or yellow colour-code to ensure that only serious or important patient status changes are alerted to the physician. The "red-dot" principle serves as a simple navigator that lets physicians quickly assess the patient's status at a glance while allowing them to focus only on those cases with clinically relevant events. In addition to color-coded messages on the internet, the physician receives a notification via email, fax, or text message in case of serious changes in the patient's status.

Red indicates a severe deviation from a defined threshold with high priority.

Yellow indicates an important deviation from a defined threshold with priority.

White indicates the absence of any severe or important change.

When a clinically relevant status change occurs, Biotronik Home Monitoring® generates an event alert via email, SMS, or fax to the physician while simultaneously displaying the severity of the patients' status on the secure Biotronik Home Monitoring® website. It also offers information that might allow the detection of adverse events on average of 2 and 5 months earlier than feasible by standard care in patients followed quarterly and biannually, respectively (Ellery et al., 2006). The majority of the alerts are disease-related, prompted by atrial fibrillation, ventricular arrhythmias, and ICD or CRT therapy, in particular.

5.2 CareLink®

CareLink® is produced by Medtronic, Minneapolis, MN, USA. The monitor produced by CareLink® is very small, about a pound in weight and easy to carry in a brief case. On the scheduled day, patients have to simply connect their monitor to a regular phone line, push the start button, and hold the antenna over heart device. The monitor sends the device information and turns itself off when the transmission is done. Data will be transferred to the secure central data collecting system; from there, the information will be passed on to the health care personnel as guided by the urgency of the information.

If patients have a Medtronic heart device with Conexus Automatic Monitoring, the device data may be sent automatically, usually while the patient is sleeping. These transmissions are scheduled by the clinical team. On the scheduled night, the device "wakes up" and communicates with the monitor. The monitor silently sends the device data, without assistance from the patient.

Heart devices with automatic monitoring are able to send a CareAlert® notification to the database, when certain conditions are met, such as low battery or an irregular heartbeat. This information will be appropriately transmitted to medical team (Figure 3).

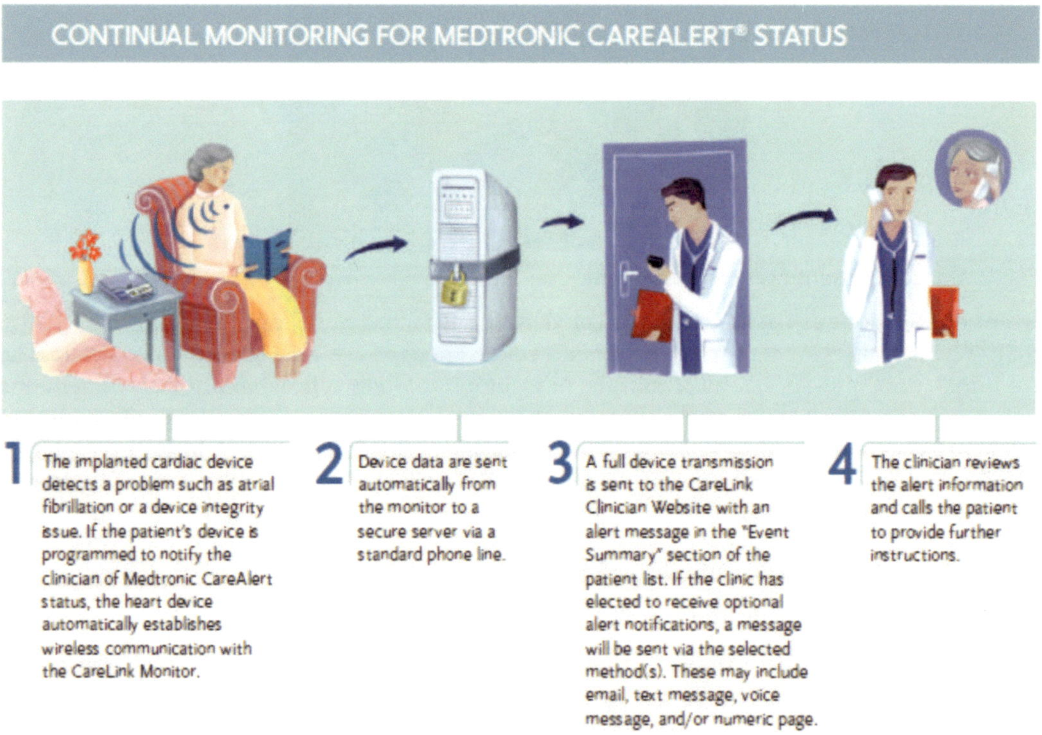

Fig. 3. CareAlert®

5.3 Latitude

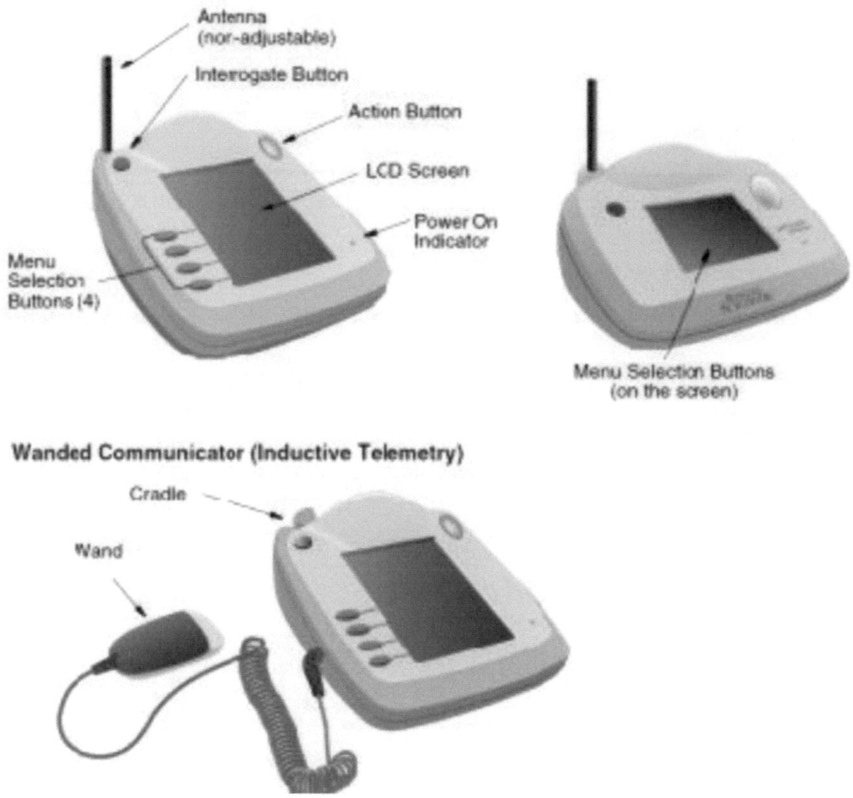

Fig. 4. Latitude Home Monitoring System

Latitude system uses a wireless (e.g. radio frequency or Bluetooth®) feature that offers daily and/or weekly status checks with physician notification. This feature can be activated for patients who have a device that uses ZIP Wandless Telemetry, and/or for patients who use the weight scale from the Latitude Heart Failure Management system.

There are two levels of alert conditions: red alerts and yellow alerts. The alerts are designed to provide the physician advance notification of a potential health or device problem. Conditions that could potentially leave the patient without available device therapy result in declaration of a red alert (Table 3). Notification of red alerts is not configurable, as the device-following physician will always be notified if a red alert is detected on the Latitude secure server. By default, notification is sent by telephone, but there are several notification options for red alerts as described in "Red Alert Notification Preferences."

Daily Measurement Red Alerts
• High or low shock lead impedance
• High or low right ventricular pacing lead impedance
Red Alerts Indicating Potential Loss of Therapy
• Device battery has reached end of life (EOL)
• Remote monitoring disabled due to limited battery capacity
• High or low shock lead impedance detected when attempting to deliver a shock
• High voltage detected on shock lead during charge
• Ventricular tachycardia mode change due to magnet
• Ventricular tachycardia mode set to value other than monitor + therapy
• Possible malfunction
• Device parameter error

Table 3. Red alert notifications occur for the above conditions, depending on device model

Device battery has reached Elective Replacement Indicator (ERI)
Explant indicator reached
Voltage was too low for projected remaining capacity
Ventricular pacing leads
• Low right ventricular intrinsic amplitude
• High right ventricular intrinsic amplitude
• Low left ventricular intrinsic amplitude
• High left ventricular intrinsic amplitude
• Low left ventricular pacing lead impedance
• High left ventricular pacing lead impedance
Atrial pacing leads
• Low atrial intrinsic amplitude
• High atrial intrinsic amplitude
• Low atrial pacing lead impedance
• High atrial pacing lead impedance
Arrhythmias
• Shock therapy delivered to convert arrhythmia (ventricular)
• Accelerated arrhythmia episode (ventricular)
• Atrial arrhythmia burden within a 24-hour period
Patient triggered event stored
Pacing
• Cardiac resynchronization therapy pacing percentage
• Right ventricular pacing percentage
An average daily weight change of 2 pounds or more over multiple days
Change of 5 pounds or more any time within a week

Table 4. Yellow alert notifications occur for the above conditions, depending on device model and on the physicians' preference

Notification of yellow alerts is optional by the physicians. Notification for yellow alerts is provided through the Latitude website and, optionally by other methods such as fax. A physician may choose to receive some, all, or none of the yellow alerts. Yellow alert notifications can be configured for the above conditions, depending on device model (Table 4).

5.4 Merlin@Home®:

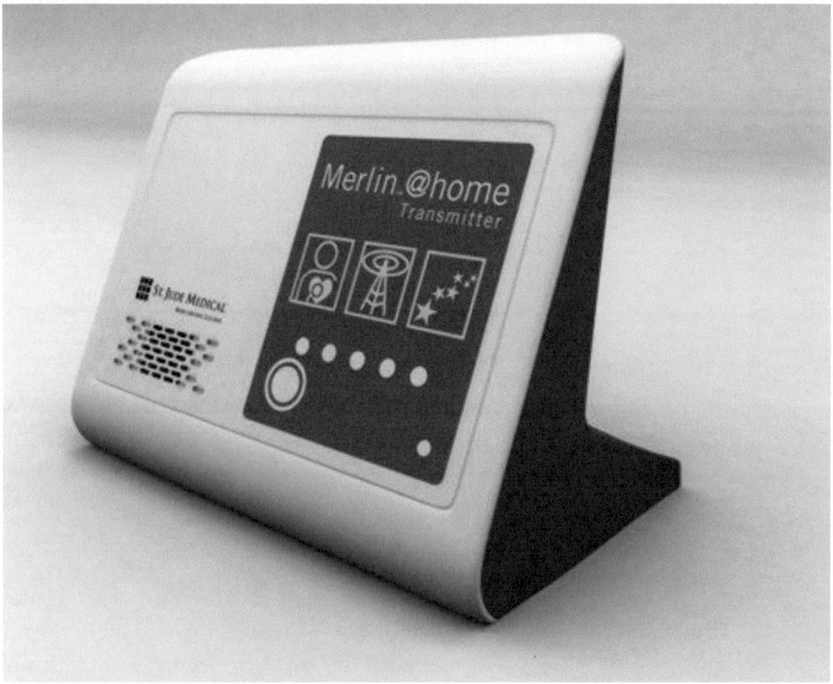

Fig. 5. Merlin@ home Transmitter®

In 2008, St Jude got FDA approval for Merlin@ home transmitter® (Figure 5), a radio frequency wireless technology that remotely monitors patients' implanted cardiac devices. The Merlin@ home transmitter's ®wireless technology gives patients the additional comfort of having devices automatically checked. Since the transmitter initiates scheduled follow-up and uses radio frequency wireless telemetry to download data from device, entire follow-up procedure is conducted without any direct patient involvement. The only requirement is that each patient remains within range of the transmitter while it reads his or her device. Patients also may initiate data transmissions as instructed by their physicians. Data downloaded by the Merlin@home transmitter® is sent to Merlin.net, a secure, internet-based data management system, where it is stored for review by the patient's physician. The data can also be linked in to the Electronic Health Record / Electronic Medical Record directly and can be stored there for future references.

Table comparing the 4 types of available remote monitors:

Major differences among the available systems include degree of patient involvement in data transmission, transmission modality, transmission scheduling, and patient alerts as detailed in Table 5.

	Biotronik	Medtronic	Boston Scientific	St Jude
System Name	Home Monitoring™	CareLink™	Latitude™	Merlin.net™
System Activation	Automatic	Automatic / Manual	Automatic/ Manual	Automatic / Manual
Approved in	America and Europe	America and Europe	America and Europe	America and Europe
Device to Programmer	Wireless	Wand / Wireless	Wand / Wireless	Wand / Wireless
Programmer to Server	4 - band GSM network (Cellular network)	Analogue phone line	Analogue phone line	Analogue phone line
Patient involvement	No	Yes	Yes	No
Patient device characteristics	Portable	Stationary	Stationary	Stationary
Frequency of transmissions	Daily FU; Alert events	Scheduled FU; Alert events	Scheduled FU; Alert events	Scheduled FU; Alert events
Remote follow up	Yes	Yes	Yes	Yes
Remote Monitor	Yes	Yes	Yes	Yes
Data storage	Website long term	Website long term	Website long term	Website long term
Data presentation	Processed as graphs and tables	Standard as in Programmer	Standard as in Programmer	Standard as in Programmer
Real - time /stored EGM (duration)	45 seconds	10 seconds	10 seconds	30 seconds
Transmission time	<0.5 minute	<3 minutes	5 minutes	< 3 minutes
Feedback to the patient via transmitter	LED indicating the status	LED indicating the status	Automatic text and audio messages	LED indicating the status
Special Features	Wireless PMs	Configurable red and yellow alerts	Configurable red and yellow alerts	Automated phone calls to patients

Table 5. Comparison of the four different available remote monitors

6. Benefits of telemonitor

According to the Heart Rhythm Society Task Force on Device Performance Policies and Guidelines (Wilkoff et al., 2008), the primary goal of these remote, automated, wireless, or internet- based cardiac rhythm device monitoring systems is to identify the abnormal device behavior in a more timely fashion, automatically and accurately determining the status of certain implanted device functions, thereby decreasing the reliance on reporting by the patients and physicians. However, in addition to the primary goal of earlier diagnosis, it does have other various advantages as described below.

6.1 Reduction in clinic visits

In a study by Brugada (2006), 271 patients with a Biotronik ICD and Home monitoring systems were routinely followed every three months over the course of a year. Retrospective analysis of the Biotronik Home Monitoring data showed that as many as half of the regular scheduled visits may have been skipped, without impairing patient safety. In addition to reducing the scheduled clinic visits, remote follow-up may avoid unscheduled visits following an ICD shock. After a shock / alert, the patient may perform manual transmission of the data to the physician for determining the appropriateness of the shock, and it may be then decided whether the patient should be seen for device reprogramming or modification of drug therapy.

6.2 Early diagnosis of worsening clinical scenarios:

Implantable cardiac devices can play a key role in the early detection and treatment of atrial fibrillation (AF) / atrial tachyarrhythmia (AT), which is an important marker of cardiac mortality. The possibility of early detection of AT/AF remains poor when relying on patient symptoms alone. Furthermore, reliance on patient symptoms alone may result in inappropriate medical therapy such as early discontinuation of anticoagulation. Intermittent monitoring via long-term event recorders or Holter monitors can be inadequate in documenting paroxysmal atrial tachyarrhythmias. Given the morbidity and mortality associated with AT/AF and the fact that AT/AF is often asymptomatic, early treatment and close monitoring may be helpful in reducing the risk of stroke and in monitoring treatment efficacy.

These devices can accurately detect and continuously monitor for atrial tachyarrhythmias. The devices also have extensive reporting capabilities and can provide an objective picture of the cumulative length of time that a patient experiences atrial tachyarrhythmias.Hoppe et al. (2006) did a retrospective analysis of the Cardiac Resynchronization in Heart Failure (CARE-HF) study involving 409 patients with CRT devices. They found that AF was documented without the aid of the device in 16.1% of the patients, while the device-based diagnostics detected AT/AF in an incremental 22% (93/409) of the patients during a mean follow-up of 29.4 months. In a study of patients with AT/AF who also had an AT500R pacemaker (Medtronic, Inc., Minneapolis, MN) or a GEMR III ICD (Medtronic, Inc., Minneapolis, MN), Purerfellner et al. (2004) found that the devices had AT/AF episode detection accuracy of 95.3% and 95.7%, respectively, and an AT/AF burden sensitivity of 95.3%.

High ventricular rates in a patient with atrial arrhythmias are indicative of poor rate control. Poor rate control in itself can lead to the development of HF and can exacerbate existing HF. Additionally, poor rate control has been linked to earlier time to first hospitalization, HF exacerbation, and inappropriate ICD shocks, as noted by Hoppe et al (2006). In people with CRT devices, a fast ventricular response to AF can lead to a loss of biventricular pacing as the device mode switches to asynchronous pacing. Given that patients with HF can derive benefits from even small changes in hemodynamic status, the amount of biventricular pacing should be as close to 100% as possible in order to maximize patient benefit from the therapy.

Therefore, early identification of poor ventricular rate control allows for more rapid clinical interventions including changes in drug regimen or other treatment modalities (e.g., ablation) to optimize rate control with the goal of reducing hospitalizations and unnecessary shocks as well as helping to maximize the delivery of biventricular pacing in people with a CRT device.

6.3 Improved patient satisfaction

Most patients readily accept remote monitoring, and feel secured by the use of this technology to improve their healthcare. Studies have shown a high patient satisfaction rate, ease of use, and compliance with the use of remote monitoring systems (Joseph et al 2004). Patients feel reassured being consistently in contact with hospital. In an Italian multi center trial by Marzegalli et al (2008), with the CareLink® system,9 9% of patients rated the monitor setup as very or somewhat easy since their first transmission. About 98% of the patients found the antenna very easy or somewhat easy to position since the first transmission, and the time required for the procedure rated as brief or very brief in all after a short practice. Personal knowledge of the nurse who actually calls the patient in case of problems tremendously increases patient assurance and compliance.

6.4 Cost saving

The economic aspects have not been evaluated extensively. A study from France examined the potential cost savings for long-term care of ICD recipients assisted by Home Monitoring (www.theheart.org). A multicenter database for this study included 502 patients from six university hospitals. Costs of conventional ICD follow-up examinations were compared with the expected costs of follow-up coupled with telemonitoring. Assuming that telemonitoring may obviate up to 2 visits per year, the expected decrease in costs for follow-up visits was estimated at $2,149 per patient during the 5 years of expected service life of the device. Transportation expenses were the main component of the overall costs, and the savings due to telemonitoring were particularly significant when the distance between the patient home and the medical facility is longer. However, these results must be viewed with caution as this is looking only at expected, not actual costs and there is no robust data available at this time.

6.5 Time saving

As all the data gathered during a normal in-office device interrogation can be sent remotely to the device clinic for evaluation, the patients and accompanying persons save time by using the remote monitoring network. In a study conducted by Raatikainen et al. (2008), the average time saved was about 3 hours per patient per visit and it was directly related to the travelling distance to the device clinic. Also, the physicians on average save 20 minutes and other office staff saved 45 minutes for each visit, delivering the same care through the remote network.

7. Drawbacks:

7.1 Non compliance

Some elderly people have difficulty when using transmission systems for which manual transmission is requested and need assistance from their relatives. A minority of patients do not accept remote monitoring. Reasons for that include concern about privacy, fear of technology, and concern about the risk of losing human contact with the nurses and physicians. Some patients showed lower compliance post implantation, perhaps by forgetting to send transmissions or by switching off the transmitter. These are usually patients who did not accept their disease and device implantation. For them, psychological support and counseling are recommended.

7.2 Patient safety due to technical problems:

Transmission failures due to technical issues are rare. Infrequent transmission failures (2%) were observed due to mobile phone network defects or patients' absence from home.Technical problems related to the mobile phone, e.g., battery depletion or a deactivated monitor were rarely reported. In a study of 93 patients, Wallbrück et al. (2002) assessed the feasibility of an automatic long-distance monitoring system for pacemaker patients, and the clinical relevance of transmitted data. Automatic daily transmission (mostly during the night) and patient triggered transmission were enabled. The number of received and sent messages was compared. To check data integrity, the transmitted data were compared with those collected by the pacemaker programmer. Three patients (3.2%) were excluded due to insufficient mobile net coverage at their living site. The authors showed that 89.7% of the messages automatically generated by the implanted devices and 64.8% of patient-triggered messages were received at the Home Monitoring Service Center. Various reasons could explain message failure: patient away from home at the time of transmission, monitor was switched off, device not correctly loaded, device too far away from the patient bed, or GSM network coverage unreliable. The interruption in the sequence of messages ranged from 1 to more than 4 days. In another study, Toselli et al. (2004) reported the data obtained from 894 scheduled reports, of which 876 (98%) were successful. When the investigators compared the Home Monitoring data with those retrieved during conventional ICD interrogation at the time of in-clinic follow-ups, they did not observe any difference.

7.3 Patient confidentiality

Data confidentiality is an issue of particular importance for the device company and for the physician. Since the data are now transmitted via internet in the vast majority of cases, the system is secured at each step of transmission - from the patient to the home monitoring service centre and from there to the physician. As with any advanced transmission technology, hacking is a potential issue. Hackers could transmit the same radio signals - causing a defibrillator to shock or shut down, or divulge a patient's medical information - without needing a programmer. It is widely believed that the risk of unauthorized access to an ICD is unlikely, given the considerable technical expertise required. (Wireless ICD programming vulnerable to hackers, report claims. http://www.theheart.org/ article/847781.do).

7.4 Patient-physician relationship

Joseph et al (2004) have shown a high patient satisfaction rate, ease of use, and compliance with the use of remote monitor. However, some patients may find difficulty in using the technology and they may feel that they lost the human contact with a health care provider. Proper explanation and psychological support to them holds the key.

7.5 Legal issues

As with any technology, patients should be informed about the advantages and disadvantages. Home Monitoring was developed to allow earlier detection of technical or arrhythmic events, but it does not protect the patient against such events nor does it allow any remote intervention by a physician. In case of an event, in addition to the use of the monitor, the patient must activate the Emergency Medical Services (EMS) as appropriate. Home monitoring devices are not a replacement for EMS. A written informed consent form should be used to ensure that the patient has been properly informed about the system and that the patient agreed to use of it.

8. Reimbursement:

In the USA, on June 9, 2006, Centers for Medicare & Medicaid Services (CMS) published a transmittal stating that physicians should use (and carriers should pay for) existing Current Procedural Terminology codes 93731, 93734, 93741 and 93743 (the in-office pacemaker and ICD interrogation codes) for remote monitoring of cardiac devices. Reimbursement rates vary from state to state, and in some instances are the same as an in-office visit without device programming. In Germany, the procedural reimbursement for remote monitoring is nearly the same as that offered for standard follow-up visits. Furthermore, there is currently no limit to the number of remote interrogations by physicians, who can either monitor the patient status at regular intervals (e.g., every 3 months), or in response to selected special events, or both. United Kingdom offers no reimbursement for remote monitoring. In France, the fees are fixed, and clinics and hospitals are reimbursed according to levels of activities. In Italy, the Italian Association on Arrhythmias and Cardiac Pacing is working with the National Public Health Service to develop reimbursement codes for remote monitoring.

9. Ongoing trials in telemonitoring of the Cardiac devices

Remote monitoring may be particularly useful in patients with cardiac resynchronization therapy, as they are most likely to have transmissions of medically related events. As detailed in table 6, a number of different randomized trials are currently underway to assess the utility of telemonitoring of pacemakers and defibrillators specifically looking for signs of volume overload, heart failure, shocks etc

Study Title	Condition	Device	Status
CareLink® Evaluation	Heart Failure	Medtronic CareLink®	Not yet recruiting
Clinical Evaluation Of Remote Monitoring With Direct Alerts To Reduce Time From Event To Clinical Decision	ICD / CRT	Merlin.NET®	Recruiting
A Randomized Trial of Remote Monitoring of Implantable Cardioverter Defibrillators Versus Quarterly Device Interrogations in Clinic	VT / VF	CareLink®monitoring system	Active, not recruiting
Telemedical Interventional Monitoring in Heart Failure	Heart Failure		Active, not recruiting

European Health Economic Trial on Home Monitoring in ICD Therapy (EuroEco)	VT / VF	Home Monitoring provided by Biotronik ICD devices	Recruiting
MOnitoring REsynchronization deviCes and cARdiac patiEnts (MORE CARE)	Heart Failure	Medtronic CareLink®	Recruiting
Benefits of Implantable Cardioverter Defibrillator Follow-up Using Remote Monitoring	VT / VF / Heart Failure	Home Monitor ®	Active, not recruiting
Home-Monitoring in Implantable Cardioverter Defibrillator (ICD) Patients	VT / VF	Home-monitoring provided by LUMAX ICD device and CardioMessenger II®	Recruiting
Effects of Remote Patient Monitoring on Heart Failure Management	Heart Failure	Heart failure remote patient monitoring system	Recruiting
Remote Follow-up of Patients Receiving Implantable Cardioverter Defibrillator for Prophylactic Therapy	VT / VF	ICD	Completed
TRIAGE-CRT Telemonitoring in Patients With CHF and Indication of CRT-D	Heart Failure/ CRT	Kronos™ LV-T, Lumax™ HF-T	Completed
Follow-up of Patients With Implantable Cardioverter Defibrillators by Home Monitoring (ANVITE)	VT / VF / Heart Failure	ICD / CRT / Home Monitor™	Recruiting
RAPID-RF: Remote Active Monitoring in Patients With Heart Failure	Heart Failure / Atrial Fibrillation	ICD / CRT	Completed
Supporting Care and Independence at Home	Heart Failure	Chronic heart failure monitoring system / Device: Lifestyle monitoring system	Recruiting
Home Monitoring in Cardiac Resynchronisation Therapy	Heart Failure	ICD / CRT	Completed
Psychosomatic Effects of Implantable Cardioverter Defibrillator With Home Monitoring Function (QUANTUM)	Arrhythmia/ Quality of Life	BIOTRONIK Lexos-T™ ICD with home monitoring/ Device: Lumos-T® ICD with home monitoring	Recruiting
Evolution of Management Strategies of Heart Failure Patients With Implantable Defibrillators	Heart Failure / SCD / ICD	Medtronic CareLink® system	Recruiting

Comparison Between Remote Patient Management and Standard Care in CRT-D and ICD-patients to Assess the Impact on Hospital Length of Stay Because of Heart Failure	Heart Failure / VT / VF	CareAlert® / ICD / CRT	Recruiting
Evaluation of the " Tele-follow-up " for the Follow-up of Implantable Defibrillators	Tele- follow-up of CHF	ICD / Telemedicine	Active, not recruiting
Actions elicited by In-hospital Follow-up of Cardiac Devices	In-hospital follow-up of cardiac device	ICD / Pacemaker	Recruiting

Table 6. Data from www.clinicaltrials.gov; accessed on July 22nd 2010

ICD: Implantable Cardioverter Defibrillator
VT: Ventricular Tachycardia
VF: Ventricular Fibrillation
SCD: Sudden Cardiac Death
CRT: Cardiac Resynchronization therapy

10. Remote programming

Bidirectional telemetry uses encoded and encrypted radiofrequency signals which allows transmission of information from the pacemaker to the programmer and from the programmer to the pacemaker. In this way, the clinician can "talk" to the pacemaker, interrogate and get the necessary data from it and if needed, he/she can reprogram the device by sending signals to the pacemaker to optimize pacemaker function. Despite sound technology to program the pacemakers remotely, it is not yet implemented due to concerns over patient safety and privacy. This concern is related to the limited ability to respond to potential changes in the patient's condition as a result of the altered device parameters. As greater experience with remote monitoring is gained and as a secure support system for remote management of patients is developed, this technology will likely be implemented. Moreover, patient safety is a concern as, if some one may hack in to the secure system and change the settings / deactivate the devices. There have been no reports to date of hacking of implantable devices.

11. Future directions

In the future, the use of telemonitoring might dramatically reduce hospitalization rates of patient after pacemaker or ICD implantation. As mentioned in the table 6, there are many ongoing trials researching the benefit of earlier detection of a patient's deterioration in clinical status (mainly heart failure) with the aid of Home monitoring. Clinical data such as trends in patients' daily activity, in the mean heart rate and in the occurrence of arrhythmia, along with technical parameters will be correlated with major cardiovascular events - death and hospitalization.

12. Conclusions

Rapidly evolving technological advances in wireless communication allow for the development of miniaturized devices and new techniques in telemonitoring. The safety of telemonitoring has been demonstrated in various trials. The clinical use of tele monitoring is very promising based on the ongoing trials. This novel feature seems to be very important and might impact costs and therapeutic decisions. The relationship between patients and their physicians who perform pacemaker and ICD follow-up with telemonitoring should be more clearly defined so that patient - physician relationship is maintained. Remote programming of the pacemakers is a possibility in future. However patient safety due to hacking is a real concern.

13. References

Brugada, P. (2006). What evidence do we have to replace in-hospital implantable cardioverter defibrillator follow-up? *Clin Res Cardiol* Vol 95, III3–9.

Ellery S, Pakrashi T, Paul V, Sack S. Predicting mortality and rehospitalization in heart failure patients with home monitoring--the Home CARE pilot study. Clin Res Cardiol. 2006;95 Suppl 3:III29-35.

Hoppe, UC, et al. (2006). Effect of cardiac resynchronization on the incidence of atrial fibrillation in patients with severe heart failure. *Circulation*. Vol 114, No 1,18-25.

Joseph, G. K., Wilkoff, B. L., Dresing, T., Burkhardt, J., & Khaykin, Y. (2004). Remote interrogation and monitoring of implantable cardioverter defibrillators. Journal of Interventional Cardiac Electrophysiology: An International Journal of Arrhythmias and Pacing, 11(2), 161-166.

Institute of Medicine (U.S.). Committee on Evaluating Clinical Applications of Telemedicine and Field,MJ. *Telemedicine: a guide to assessing telecommunications in health care.* Washington, D.C.: National AcademyPress. 1996: xiv, 271.

Love CJ. (2007). Pacemaker troubleshooting and follow-up. In: *Clinical Cardiac Pacing, Defibrillation, and Resynchronization Therapy. Third edition,* Ellenbogen, KA; Kay, GN; Lau, C-P; Wilkiff, BL (Ed.). Chapter 24, Saunders Elsevier, Philadelphia.

Marzegalli, M et al. (2008). Remote monitoring of CRT-ICD: The multicenter Italian CareLink evaluation— ease of use, acceptance, and organizational implications. *Pacing Clin Electrophysiol,*Vol 31,1259 –1264

Purerfellner, H et al. (2004). Accuracy of atrial tachyarrhythmia detection in implantable devices with arrhythmia therapies. *Pacing Clin Electrophysiol.*,Vol 27, No 7,983-992

Raatikainen, M.J.P. et al. (2008). Remote monitoring of implantable

Cardioverter defibrillator patients: a safe, time-saving, and cost-effective means for follow-up. *Europace,* Vol 10, 1145–1151

Toselli T, Regoli F, Pratola C et al. (2004). Implantable cardioverter-defibrillator and Home Monitoring technology. *Ital Heart J,* Vol 5, SSuppl. 1,30S–31S

Wallbrück K, Stellbrink C, Santini M et al. (2002). The value of permanent follow- up of implantable pacemakers–first results of a European trial. *Biomed Tech,* Vol 47, Suppl 1, Pt 2,:950–953

Guler NF, Ubeyli ED. Theory and applications ofbiotelemetry. *J Med Syst* 2002;26:159–17

Wilkoff, B. L., A. Auricchio, J. Brugada, M. Cowie, K. A. Ellenbogen, A. M. Gillis, D. L. Hayes, et al. 2008. HRS/EHRA expert consensus on the monitoring of cardiovascular implantable electronic devices (CIEDs): Description of techniques, indications, personnel, frequency and ethical considerations. Heart Rhythm: The Official Journal of the Heart Rhythm Society 5 (6) (Jun): 907-25.

Wireless ICD programming vulnerable to hackers, report claims. http://www.theheart.org/article/847781.do.

9

Remote Monitoring in Patients with Pacemakers and Implantable Cardioverter-Defibrillators: New Perspectives for Complex Therapeutic Management

Axel Müller[1], Thomas M. Helms[2], Hans-Jürgen Wildau[3], Jörg Otto Schwab[4] and Christian Zugck[5]

[1]Klinik für Innere Medizin I der Klinikum Chemnitz gGmbH Bürgerstr. 2, D-09113 Chemnitz,

[2]Deutsche Stiftung für chronisch Kranke, Alexanderstraße 26, D-90762 Fürth,

[3]BIOTRONIK SE Co,Woermannkehre 1, D-12359 Berlin,

[4]Universitätsklinikum Bonn, Medizinische Klinik und Poliklinik II, Sigmund-Freud-Str. 25, D-53105 Bonn,

[5]Universitätsklinikum Heidelberg, Innere Medizin III (Kardiologie, Angiologie und Pulmologie), Im Neuenheimer Feld 410, D-69120 Heidelberg, Germany

1. Introduction

For more than 50 years, antibradycardia pacemakers have been implanted. Technological developments have led to an improvement, extension of diagnostic and treatment options (such as holter function for detecting arrhythmias and biosensors), and to an increasingly more automated device management (control of sensing and stimulus thresholds). Furthermore, it was possible to extend the runtime of the pacemaker assembly.

In 1980, the first implantable cardioverter-defibrillator (ICD) has been implanted in a human being with the objective of secondary prevention of sudden cardiac death. Meanwhile, advances in technology have led to a size reduction of the device assembly and to the possibility of transvenous implantations. Due to the MADIT II-study, published in 2002, the ICD-implantation indications have broadened to include patients with coronary artery disease in the primary prevention of sudden cardiac death (A.J. Moss et al., 2002).

Since the 1990´s, biventricular pacemakers and ICDs enabled with Cardiac Resynchronization Therapy (CRT) are being implanted in patients with reduced left ventricular ejection fraction, prolonged QRS-complex, and advanced heart failure.

These patients undergoing CRT perceived improvement in heart failure symptoms (M.R. Bristow et al, 2004). Clinically asymptomatic patients with reduced left ventricular pump function and prolonged QRS-complexes are now also being considered candidates for implantation of biventricular pacemakers and ICDs to prevent cardiac decompensations (C. Linde et al., 2008; A. J. Moss et al. 2009).

In recent years, national and international associations have drawn up guidelines for implantation of antibradycardia, ICD, and CRT devices (biventricular pacemakers and

ICDs) (A.E. Epstein et al., 2008). Recently, implantation rates for antibradycardia pacemakers, ICD and CRT devices have constantly increased.
In the USA, the expansion of indications for ICD and CRT implantations to include *primary prevention* of sudden cardiac death led to an amplification of ICD and CRT implantations.
Device therapy is increasingly used even in elderly multimorbid patients. While the number of pacemaker aggregate replacements remained constant in 1992-2006, the number of ICD aggregate replacements decreased during this period, due to runtime extension of ICD aggregates (C. Zhan et al., 2007, S.M. Kurtz et al, 2010).
However, despite technical improvements in implantation and devices complications are to be expected. Alter et al. studied 440 ICD patients with a median follow-up of 46 (+/- 36) months and found a complication rate of 31%. This primarily involved peripoerative complications (10%), inadequate shock outputs (12%), ICD-lead related complications (12%) and complications caused by the aggregate (6%) (P. Alter et al., 2005).
Pacemaker and ICD annual reports submitted to the FDA revealed high annual malfunction replacement rates for pacemakers (1.4 - 9.0 replacements per 1000 implants) and for ICD´s (7.9 – 38.6 replacements per 1000 implants). The annual pacemaker malfunction replacement rate per 1000 implants decreased significantly during the study period 1990-2002. In contrast, the ICD malfunction replacement rate per 1000 implants increased markedly during the same period. In recent years, the problems surrounding the sprint fidelis lead showed the risk of lead and aggregate failures (M. Maytin et al., 2010). Defects of ICD-leads may even occur after implantation. Data presented by Kleemann and his colleagues who reported on survival of transvenous defibrillation leads during long-term follow-up revealed that the annual failure rate increased progressively with time after implantation and reached 20% in 10-year-old leads (T. Kleemann et al., 2007)

- increasing rates of implantation (especially for ICD- and CRT-systems)
- growing number of patients with implanted pacemakers, ICD-, and CRT-systems (follow-up appointments, aggregate replacement)
- growing number of elderly patients with comorbid conditions
- new diagnostic options (arrythmia management, biosensor technology)
- trend towards automated aftercare (e.g. automatic stimulus treshold determination)
- risk of device-related malfunctions (e.g. lead defects)
- fast transitions to new models in complex ICD- and CRT-systems

Table 1. Trends and problems in device therapy

The current developments and risks in device therapy (table 1) prescribe requirements to be met in terms of patient safety, follow-up appointments, and an increasingly complex management of ICD- and CRT-patients.
A device-based remote-monitoring represent an important contribution to meet these requirements and fulfill the needs.

2. Principle and development of technology

Remote monitoring overcomes the spatial separation between patient and physician. In the meantime, device-based remote monitoring has become a classical field for telemedical applications in cardiology, in addition to diagnostics of cardiac arrhythmia and telemonitoring of chronic heart failure (CHF)-patients.

Already in the mid of the 1970s, first examinations of transtelephonic monitoring of patients with antibradycardia pacemakers were carried out. At first, ECGs were recorded and transmitted via telephone to a receiving centre. A transmission of pacemaker function was, however, not possible (C. H. Klingenmaier et al., 1973). Medtronic "CareLink 2090" and St. Jude Medical "Housecall" were the first systems to allow remote monitoring. The CareLink-System enabled the computer in the monitoring centre to connect via telephone to the device. Thus, remote monitoring bridged the spatial distance between two different observers and thus a consultation without any active intervention in programming became possible.

St. Jude Medical developed the "Housecall"-System to transmit data from the ICD and the CRT-D to the physician. The system allows the patient to gather and transmit information to the practitioner about the ICD using the Housecall Plus Transmitter. The information provided by the IEGM and the online intracardiac ECG allows realtime ICD-surveillance for the first time. Either the patient or the physician can initiate the call to transmit via the small transmitter up-to-the-second information about how the patient's heart and ICD are working. The system enables the physician to monitor device performance. A determination of stimulus thresholds and a programming of the ICD settings, however, were not possible yet.

In the 1990s, BIOTRONIK started the development of the "Home Monitoring"-technology. First pacemakers were implanted in 2000. Today, hundreds of thousands of BIOTRONIK Home Monitoring systems have been implanted. The Home Monitoring System is the only remote monitoring system in which the transmission of data to the CardioMessenger requires no action by either the patient or the practitioner. The CardioMessenger transmits the data to BIOTRONIK's Service Center via a cell phone. The Service Center analyzes the data and forwards it to the patient's physician either by sms, email or fax. The Home Monitoring concept has been modified slightly and extended, and nowadays it represents the technological basic principle for telemonitoring for patients with electrical implants. All telemonitoring systems consist of the following components: Implanted device, patient monitor, the provider´s data server, data presentation for the physician (figure 1).

In the meantime, almost all manufacturers (BIOTRONIK, Medtronic, St. Jude Medical, Boston Scientific) have developed their own concepts for remote monitoring of pacemakers, ICD´s and CRT-systems, which in spite of their uniform structure vary in their technical realization and features (table 2).

Data can be transmitted from the implant to the patient monitor in various ways. This includes, for instance, transmissions that can be initiated automatically without any user interaction (Home Monitoring, BIOTRONIK) or by radio frequency (RF) wireless telemetry that is used to download data from the device (Merlin.net, St. Jude Medical; LATITUDE, Boston Scientific). In contrast, data can be transmitted manually by the patient (CareLink, Medtronic). Figure 2 shows patient monitors both for automated and manual data transmission.

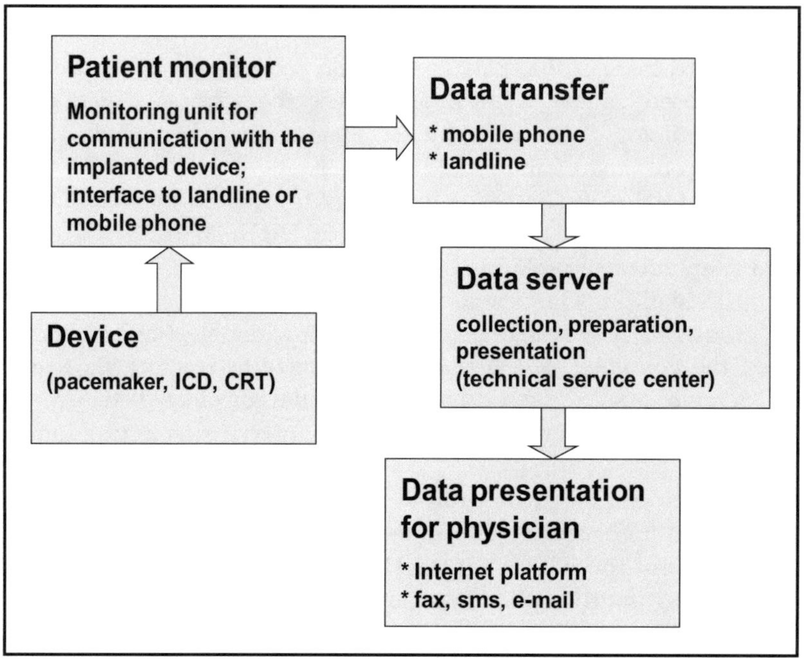

Fig. 1. Individual components of a device-based remote monitoring for patients with pacemakers, ICD´s and CRT-systems

System (manufacturer)	Implants	Patient monitor (data transfer from the implanted device)	Transfer to data server	Data presentation to the physician	Integration into the EHR	Specifics
Home Monitoring (BIOTRONIK)	PM, ICD, CRT	Cardio-Messenger (automatic)	GSM, GPRS	Internet, alerts via sms, e-mail, fax	Possible	IEGM-online-transmission, Heart-Failure-monitor
CareLink (Medtronic)	PM, ICD, CRT (backward compatible)	CareLink-monitor (manual and automatic)	Telephone line	Internet, alerts via sms	Possible	OptiLink-system (intrathoracic impedance measurement), IEGM, Cardiac Compass
Merlin.net(St. Jude Medical)	Specific ICDs, CRTs	Merlin@home (manual and automatic)	GSM, telephone line	Internet, alerts via sms, e-mail, fax	Possible	Holistic data-management-system, line-transmission
LATITUDE (Boston Scientific)	Specific ICDs, CRTs	LATITUDE-Communicator (manual and automatic)	Telephone line	Internet	Possible	Integration of external sensors (weight scale, blood pressure monitor)

Table 2. Overview of different systems for remote monitoring of pacemakers (PM), ICD´s and CRT-systems

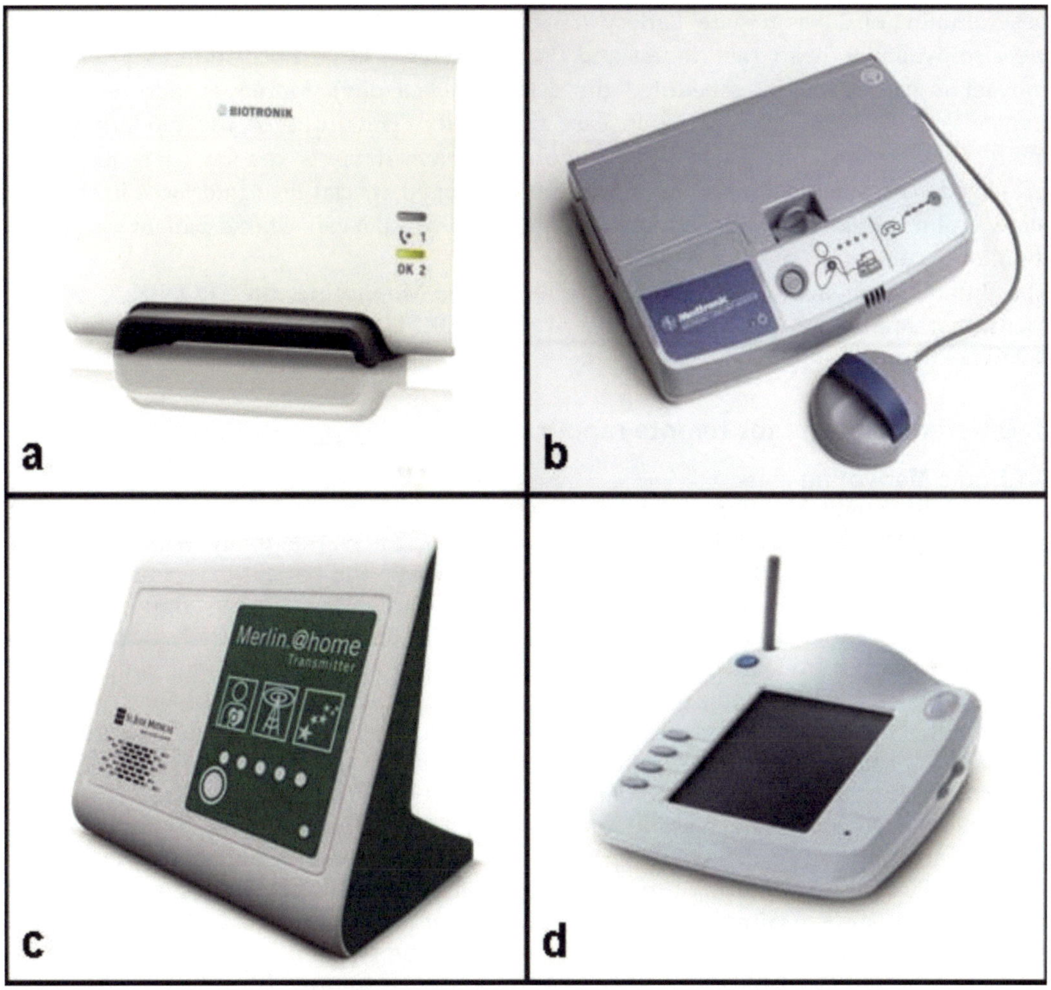

Fig. 2. Various patient monitors for remote monitoring of implants (a: CardioMessenger, BIOTRONIK; b: CareLink-Monitor, Medtronic; c: Merlin@home, St. Jude Medical; d: LATITUDE Communicator, Boston Scientific)

The patient monitor is the interface between the implant and the data servers. The data transmission from the patient monitor to the manufacturer´s data servers can be carried out via landline or mobile phone. Individual providers use both ways. The advantages of data transfer via mobile phone are the independence of location and the absence of a fixed telephone line.

In future, however, the mobile phone technology is certainly going to be the dominant model. The provider´s data servers collect the data and present it to the physician. There is no active processing of the medical data. In addition, all transmitted data are saved in the servers according to the requirements with data security.

The treating physician can receive the data via fax, sms or internet. In the meantime, all vendors have developed password protected internet platforms. This permits an access to patient data from any computer. Apart from data concerning system integrity (actual

programming of the aggregate, battery status, thresholds, impedances etc.) diagnostic data are also available (heart rate at rest and during exercise, atrial fibrillation etc.). The data transfer is carried out at scheduled times (e.g. once a day). Moreover, additional data transmissions can be carried out in case of ICD-Rx. Thus, due to the modern remote monitoring systems offered by the vendors complete datasets can be transmitted and presented. The manufacturers have therefore developed special user interfaces in order to allow an immediate data review. Furthermore, the physician can ask the patient via patient monitor to contact the physician by phone.
The different systems for remote monitoring (Home Monitoring, BIOTRONIK; CareLink, Medtronic; Merlin.net, St. Jude Medical; LATITUDE, Boston Scientific) are described in detail below.

3. Different systems for remote monitoring

3.1 Home Monitoring

BIOTRONIK Home Monitoring System is the first wireless, mobile remote monitoring system for patients with implantable cardiac devices on the market today. All devices have an integrated antenna in the header, enabling an automatic and patient-independent remote and wireless telemetry to a transmitter device (CardioMessenger®, figure 2). Data transmission is initiated at times predetermined by the physician, normally during night-time. Data transfer from the implant to the CardioMessenger® is provided via ULP-AMI (ultra low-power active medical implants) operating in the 402-405 MHz Band, which is worldwide standardized; its terms of use are laid down in relevant standards. In Europe, the standard ETSI EN 301 839-1 V1.2.1 (2007-07) is applied. The data are transmitted from the patient monitor via a mobile phone network to the BIOTRONIK Service Center. There, the data are put into an easily accessible form and can then be viewed by the physician online via the internet on a password protected website (Home Monitoring Platform®). BIOTRONIK Home Monitoring uses an intuitive, color-coded, web-based system (red and yellow) physicians and clinic staff, which allows for automatic patient classification aimed at significantly simplifying clinic workflow. In addition, the types of events which trigger an alert can be customized for each patient. The physician is informed by e-mail, sms, fax or phone messages whenever critical data or pre-defined, individual events are available for consultation. In addition to exporting data in CSV files, files can be exported using the Portable Document Format (PDF) standard. Data transfer is fully automated and requires no manual support by the patient. Furthermore, the system provides the opportunity to configure individual filter settings for data transfer according to individual patient needs and the desired level of safety. As an additional feature, IEGM Online HD®, a high-definition intracardiac ECG, can also be transmitted for patients with implanted ICD and CRT-devices (figure 3).
In addition, mathematical modeling enables the integration of different parameters (e.g. heart rate, right ventricular impedance, intrathoracic impedance measurement) into a complex monitoring concept (Heart Failure Monitor®). This unique system allows the attending physician to monitor each patient with dual-chamber pacemaker or CRT devices very closely and to react in time to prevent potential cardiovascular events at an early stage. Home Monitoring has, however, the disadvantage that only aggregates using an antenna integrated in the device can be monitored; external sensors (blood pressure monitor, weight scale etc.) cannot be integrated into the system.

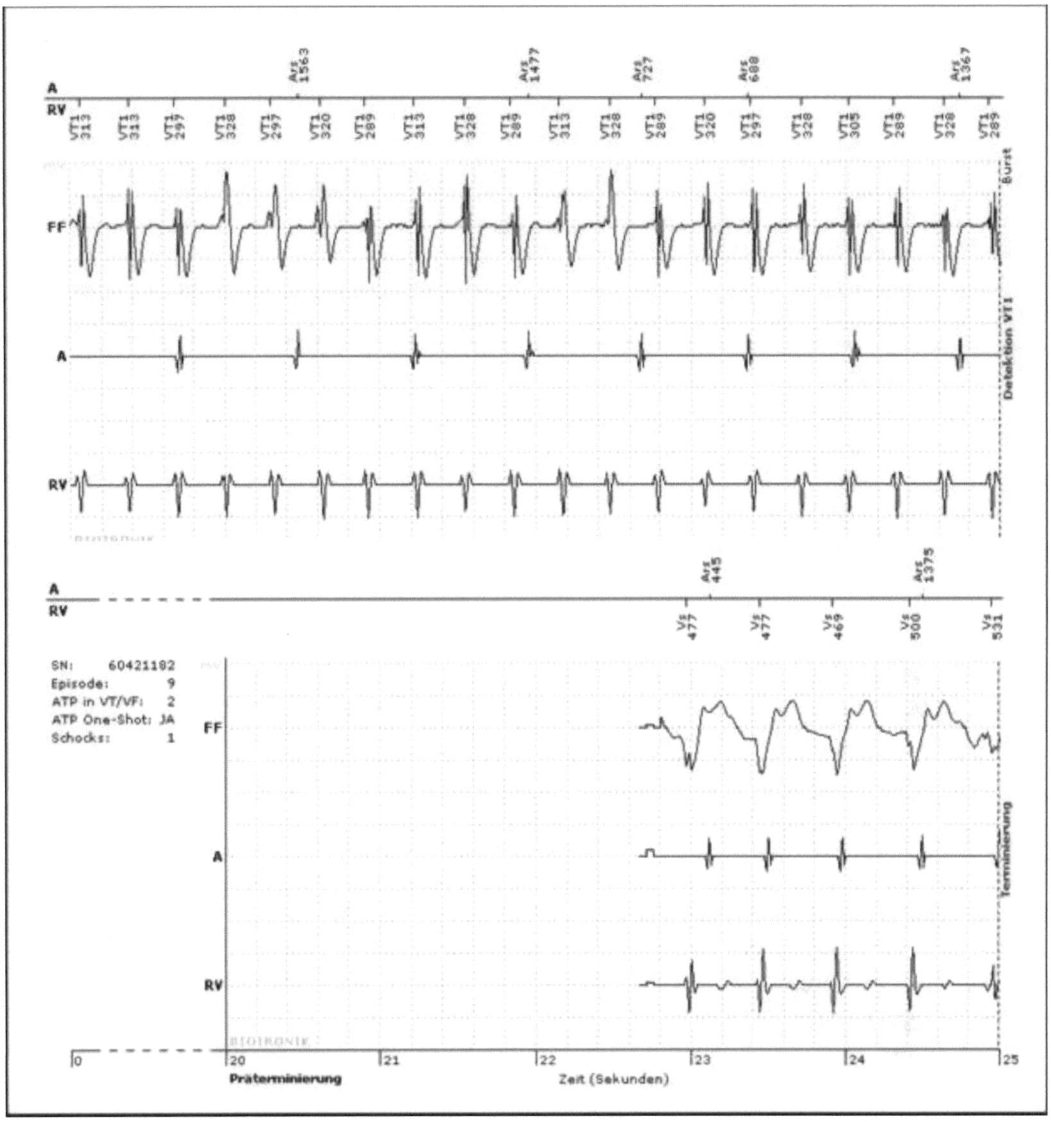

Fig. 3. Intracardiac ECG (IEGM), transmitted via Home Monitoring: detection of a sustained ventricular tachycardia (above) - Termination after shock (below)

3.2 CareLink

Medtronic CareLink has evolved from the Remote-View-System. The patient can collect data by holding an antenna over his implanted device. The system is backward compatible, so that patients with older devices can also be monitored. The data are captured by the antenna, downloaded by the monitor (CareLink-Monitor®) and transferred to the Medtronic CareLink Network (figure 2). Through this network, patient data are transmitted from their implantable device using a portable monitor that has to be connected to a standard telephone line. The patient's physician can view the data on a secure internet website (figure 4).

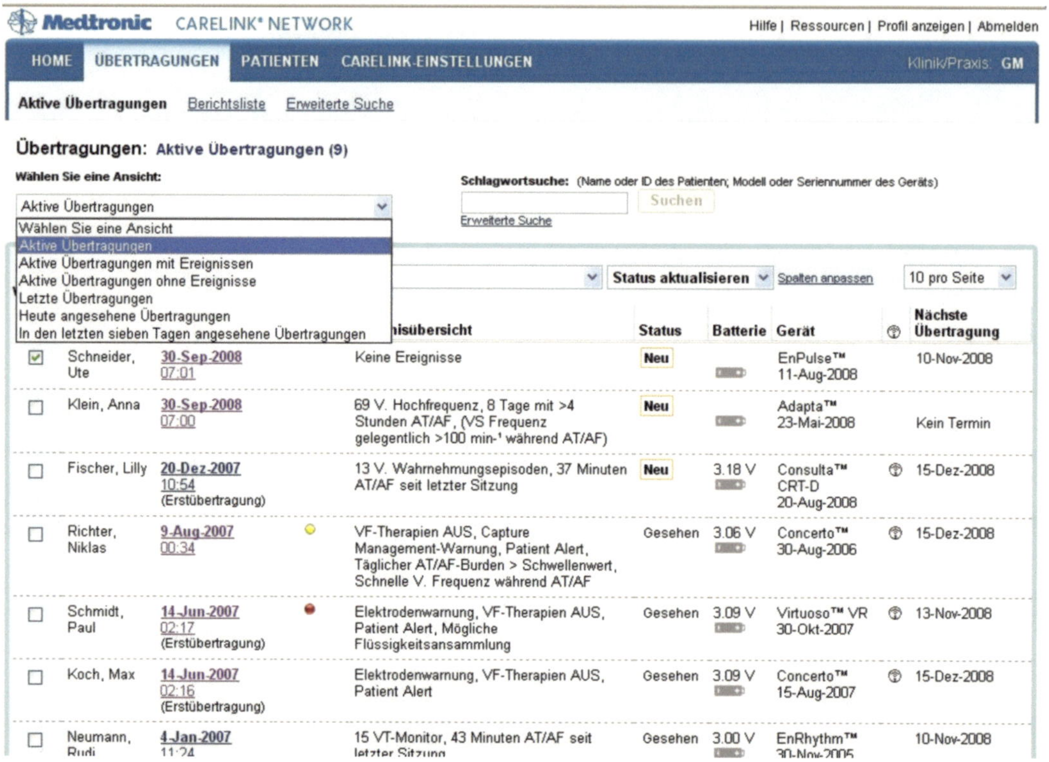

Fig. 4. Password-protected internet platform of the CareLink-system (source: Medtronic)

The network also allows Medtronic CareAlert® notifications to be transmitted when any of the programmable alert conditions from a patient's implanted device has occurred. The data transfer performs via standard telephone line. The system can be used for remote monitoring of implantable event recorders (Medtronic Reveal®). CareLink allows to transmit information on system and diagnostic data (Cardiac Compass®) and IEGM´s (event-triggered and on demand).

Another option for remote monitoring is OptiLink®, which incorporates CareLink and OptiVol®. The latter was developed to monitor patients with implanted CRT-D devices and to detect possible cardiac decompensations at early stage. The system measures the drop of intrathoracic impedance upon intrapulmonary fluid accumulation. Data are reliably transmitted via Medtronic's exclusive Conexus Wireless Telemetry®. This provides the physican with helpful tools to prevent cardiac decompensation. This may also lead to prevent hospitalizations for acute decompensated heart failure.

3.3 Merlin.net

St. Jude Medical Merlin.net is the successor to the Housecall Plus®-Remote Patient Monitoring. The monitor Merlin@home® is the core of the system (figure 2). Data are transmitted daily wirelessly (via RF) to the Merlin@home® Transmitter and from there via telephone to the internet-based Merlin.net server. Merlin@home supports all RF telemetry equipment (ICD, CRT-Ds).

The system also allows physicians to compile a more complete patient record, by easily transferring cardiac device data into electronic health records (EHRs), figure 5. Data transfer is compatible with IHE HL7 and IEEE 11073.

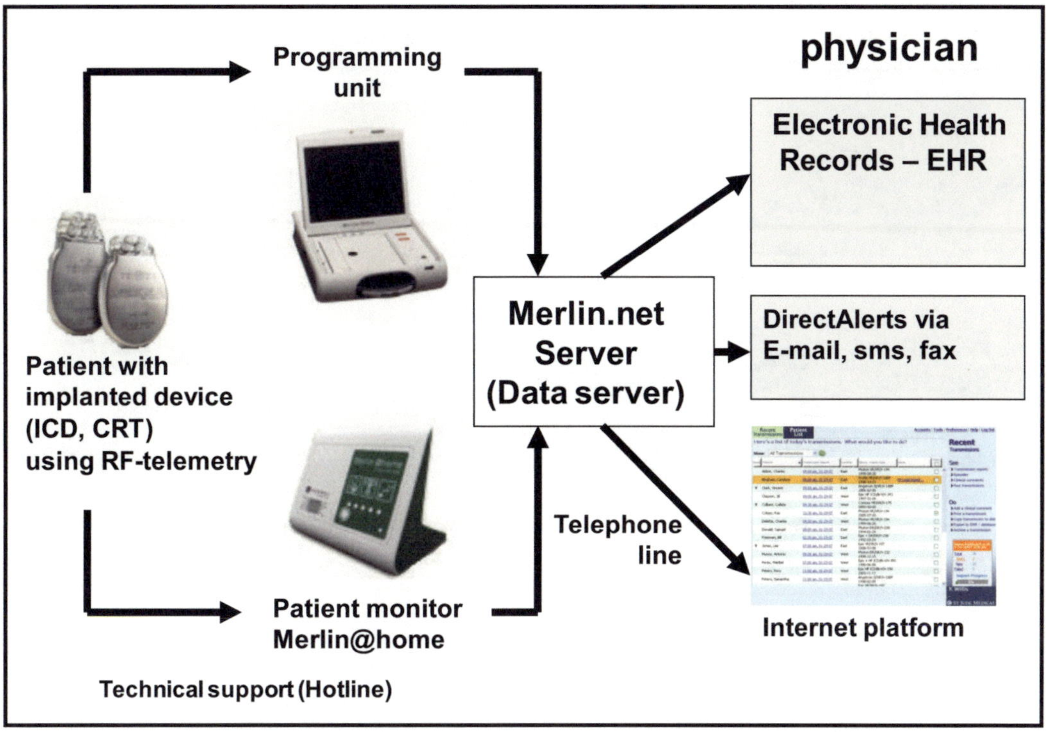

Fig. 5. Complex remote monitoring with St. Jude Medical Merlin.net - Integration of telemedical and direct aftercare (modified according to St. Jude Medical)

Data gathered during outpatient aftercare can also be integrated into the system. Additionally, St. Jude Medical provides help service that both patients and physicians may call with any technical questions or problems they may be experiencing. Merlin.net features include DirectCall® message, which provides pre-recorded messages that clinics can program to call patients to remind them of upcoming scheduled follow-ups, inform them if they have missed a follow-up, confirm that their transmitted data has been reviewed or ask them to call their physician's office or the hospital for more information. The DirectAlerts® Notification feature can be used to alert a physician to changes in the device or the patient's disease state.

3.4 LATITUDE

The Boston Scientific LATITUDE Patient Management system is being used mainly in the USA. It integrates remote monitoring of ICD- and CRT-systems (Remote Follow-up), telemonitoring, and heart failure management. Patients may initiate data transmission. LATITUDE Communicator® serves as the patient monitor (figure 2). The LATITUDE Communicator® uses RF to send and receive signals from the implanted device and a bluetooth communication system to communicate with an optional weight scale and blood

pressure monitor. The information is then transmitted via the phone line to a secure server. An Internet-based system provides easy access to diagnostic information from a patient's device and puts the physician in control of remote data collection. Design of the internet platform largely corresponds to that of the device.
The internet platform provides several care providers secure access to patient data (figure 6).

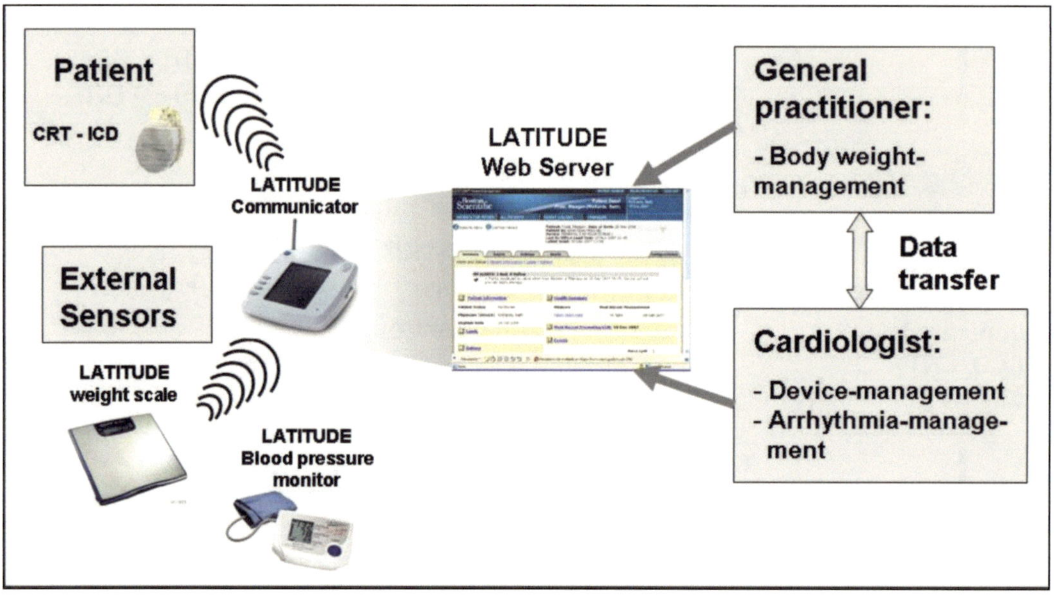

Fig. 6. LATITUDE-system (Boston Scientific) – Integration of external sensors (weight scale and blood pressure monitor) into the device-based remote monitoring (modified according to Boston Scientific)

The advantage of the LATITUDE -system is the possibility to integrate external devices (weight scale and blood pressure monitor), which reflects a fundamental part in monitoring patients with CHF.

4. Remote monitoring in clinical practice

Since the 1990s, device-based Remote Monitoring is being used in clinical practice. Now almost all pacemaker and ICD manufacturers have developed and improved internet-based solutions. Due to evidence-based medicine scientific studies are being required to prove efficacy or effectiveness and efficiency of remote monitoring.
Especially aspects concerning data security, advantages over conventional aftercare and cost efficiency have to be taken into consideration.
Clinical studies on remote monitoring of patients with pacemakers, ICDs, and CRT-systems investigated technical feasibility and safety of data transfer, first. In these breaking studies focusing on patients with implanted pacemakers, stability and safety of transtelephonic data transmission could be proved. In a study of 93 patients, Wallbrück et al. assessed the feasibility of an automatic long-distance monitoring system (Home Monitoring®, BIOTRONIK) for pacemaker patients, and the clinical relevance of transmitted data. Three patients (3.2%) were excluded due to insufficient mobile net coverage at their living site. For

the other patients, 5311 of 5911 messages were successfully registered. Interrupts in the sequence of messages occurred 331 times. Two hundred ten of these (63%) lasted just 1 day, 14 interrupts (4%) lasted 5 or more days. This rate could be reduced by providing information to the patients (K. Wallbrück et al., 2002). In a prospective study, 59 ICD-patients were followed remotely using the CareLink-system; patient acceptance of the system was high; satisfaction by the medical staff with data quality was also very favourable (M. H. Schoenfeld et al., 2004). The PREFER-study showed that the strategic use of remote pacemaker interrogation follow-up (CareLink, Medtronic) detects actionable events that are potentially important more quickly and more frequently than transtelephonic rhythm strip recordings (G.H. Crossley et al., 2009).

Stability of data transfer can be optimized in various ways:

The patient monitor can indicate disturbed data transmission through the flashing of its associated visual indicator. Another option is to use systems that remind patients to initiate data transmission (Merlin@net, St. Jude Medical). The Home Monitoring system enables the physician to define automatic and individually configurable notification if data transfer is missing. A service-hotline for patients can increase data transmission rate.

The application of unified bandwidths allows secured data transfer. However, reprogramming of the implant via remote monitoring is not possible due to law restrictions.

Device-based remote monitoring of patients with implanted antibradycardia pacemakers, ICDs and CRT-systems includes the four following aspects (figure 7):

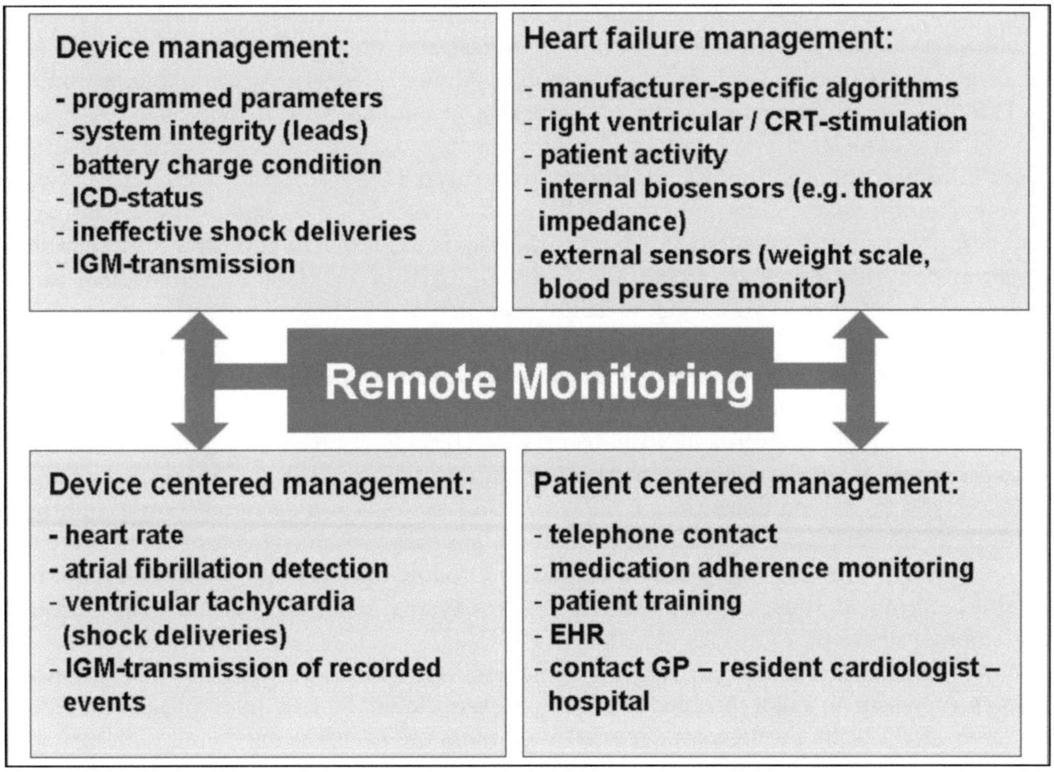

Fig. 7. Four relevant aspects of device-based remote monitoring in patients with implanted antibradycardia pacemakers, ICD, and CRT- systems

Device-management is an important tool used to monitor system integrity and to provide security of implants.
Important parameters (battery charge condition, atrial and ventricular signals, ICD-status etc.) are transferred.
Today, the complete actual device programming is transferred and visualized. This data primarily ensures patient security by enabling a complex device monitoring. In various cases, remote monitoring has been shown to confer clinical benefits.
BIOTRONIK Home Monitoring enables physicians to detect severe lead problems (e.g. lead fracture, lead micro dislocations, Twiddler-syndrome) early and to react quickly (N. J. Varma, 2008; M. L. Loricchio et al., 2008; M. F. Scholten et al., 2004). Intracardiac ECG serves as an important tool used to detect device malfunctions. Patient safety may be increased due to remote monitoring. This particularly concerns patients with highly complex devices (ICDs and CRT-systems). Nevertheless, the overall prevalence of technical problems was rather low. Nielsen et al. monitored a total of 260 patients with Home Monitoring ICDs. Technical events for single and double chamber ICDs occured only in 0.8% of patients and included invalid shock coil impedance, invalid ventricular lead impedance and special implant status (J. C. Nielsen et al., 2008). The retrospective study by Lazarus, which reported on the results of 11,624 patients implanted with a pacemaker, an ICD or a CRT-system using the BIOTRONIK Home Monitoring, revealed similar findings. Most transmitted events had medical reasons (e.g. cardiac arrhythmia) (A. Lazarus, 2007).
Arrhythmia management is an important partial aspect of device-based Remote Monitoring. It allows to detect mean patient heart rate at rest and at a workload performance and occurrences of atrial and ventricular arrhythmias. Ahmadi-Kashani et al. could show in their INTRINSIC RV study that an elevated heart rate in patients with a dual-chamber ICD is significantly associated with greater risk of achieving the primary end point of death or heart failure hospitalization. Of patients with a mean HR < 75 bpm, 5.8% died or were hospitalized for heart failure, whereas 20.9% with a mean HR > 90 bpm achieved the same end point, a 3.6-fold difference (M. Ahmadi-Kashani et al., 2009). In addition, early detection of atrial defibrillation is an important aspect in rhythm monitoring. Paroxysmal atrial tachycardias are often asymptomatic. In the presence of atrial fibrillation, thromboembolic events and progression of CHF may further deteriorate the patient's prognosis. During the CHAMP-study, 25 out of 120 patients with CRTs experienced paroxysmal atrial tachycardias, for an incidence rate of 21%. Paroxysmal atrial tachycardias were recorded in 29 and 17% of patients with and without previous history of atrial fibrillation, respectively (C. Leclercq et al, 2010). Remote monitoring allows early detection of atrial fibrillation in patients with implanted pacemakers, ICDs and CRT-systems and early reaction to optimize medical treatment (antiarrhythmic drug therapy, anticoagulation) (N. Varma et al., 2005; R. P. Ricci et al., 2009 a). Compared to scheduled follow-ups (usually every 3-6 months), remote control and, thus, an early detection of paroxysmal atrial tachycardias may lead to a reduction of stroke (R. P. Ricci et al., 2009 b).
Among patients, in whom an ICD is implanted, shocks, appropriate or inappropriate, always represent a major problem as they are associated with a poor prognosis. (M.O. Sweeney et al., 2010). Furthermore, mental and emotional health seems to fall with repeated ICD shocks. Progressive heart failure was the most common cause of death in patients who received a shock (J. E. Poole et al., 2008). Inappropriate shocks are often related to technical failure in device sensing (lead malfunction, T-wave-oversensing) or to cardiac arrhythmia.

These inappropriate shocks can be reduced through remote monitoring which is helpful for early detection of technical and medical events as well as by new algorithms to preven shocks (K.J. Volosin et al., 2010). In addition, intracardiac electrogram is also helpful (J.C.J. Res und Mitarbeiter, 2006; S. Spenker et al., 2009).

In recent years, heart failure management of patients with ICDs and particularly of those with CRT-systems, is attracting interest in clinical scientific studies. There are many complex reasons for that: New methods focussing on biosensors (e.g. intrathoracic impedance measurement) allow better monitoring of potential cardiac decompensations. Another reason is that patients often need residential treatment due to heart failure.

The latter increases costs and also results in a negatively effect quality of life.

Therefore, manufacturers have developed various concepts (e.g. Medtronic Cardiac Compass®, BIOTRONIK Heart Failure Monitor®). The aim of these concepts is to enable an "early warning system" to impeding episodes of worsening heart failure through integration of various components (e.g. heart rate at rest and in the recovery phase, patient´s physical activity, arrhythmia load, intrathoracic impedance). These concepts are currently under investigation in prospective studies. Despite promising approaches in intrathoracic impedance measurement (Optivol®, Medtronic), the method remains problematic due to limited sensitivity, specificity, and positive predictive value (D. Vollmann et al., 2007; D. Cantazariti et al., 2009). Other remote monitoring concepts (LATITUDE, Boston Scientific) are able to integrate external sensors (weight scale, blood pressure monitor via bluetooth). Thus, monitoring of ICD- and CRT-patients with CHF presents a complex problem. Therefore, device-based remote monitoring offers many possibilities and chances. Experiences already exist for Medtronic CareLink and for BIOTRONIK Home Monitoring. Tachyarrhythmia and cardiac decompensation events in patients with an implanted CRT could be treated efficiently due to CareLink. Patients benefited from an early therapeutic interventions (M. Sanitini et al., 2009).

In their "Home CARE" pilot study conducted in 123 patients with clinical indication for CRT Ellery et al. examined Home Monitoring in cardiac resynchronization therapy. In 70% of the rehospitalization events, the retrospective analysis of transmitted data via Home Monitoring revealed an increase in mean heart rate at rest and in mean heart rate over 24 h within 7 days preceding hospitalization. Both duration of physical activity and the rate of biventricular stimulation were reduced. Home Monitoring of these data may predict events leading to hospitalization (S. Ellery et al., 2006). Different studies concerning device-based remote monitoring of patients with CHF are currently being carried out (e.g. InContact-Studie, St. Jude Medical).

Patient-centered management forms a fourth aspect that has to be mentioned in this context. The concept for the monitoring and treatment of CHF is extended by various measures (telephone calls, drug adherence monitoring, patient training). Integration of special telemedical service centres enables comprehensive patient care with the centre taking the role of coordinator within the network consisting of GP, resident cardiologist and hospital. The aim is to implement medical treatment in accordance with the guidelines in order to improve the patients´ quality of life, to prevent hospitalizations and to improve patients´ prognosis. New information processing technologies allow the integration of collected data into an electronic health record (EHR) with password protection which can be accessed by individual physicians (GP, resident cardiologist and physicians at hospital).

The numbers of follow-up will increase with the number of pacemaker-, ICD- and CRT-implants and can thus become an additional exposure for resident cardiologists and hospitals.

Furthermore, high individual costs arise for patient transport. Remote monitoring can act as a contribution to individualization of follow-up scheduling. This is of particular importance in the way that different patient groups require different follow-up scenarios.

One retrospective study of 271 patients with ICD-indication followed for 12 months using Home Monitoring by Brugada et al. examined the utility of remote monitoring in forecasting the necessity of a previously scheduled routine in-clinic visit. 908 pairs of Home Monitoring data and follow-up data were evaluated. The largest fraction of 608 (67%) consisted of true negative forecasts, while a total of 141 (16%) of the forecasts turned out to be true positive in accordance with retrospective follow-up view. There was a 14% false negative rate. Problems would not have been detected without routine follow-up visits. This particularly effects is caused by an increase in ventricular or atrial pacing threshold, discovery of lead dislodgement, ventricular episodes, misinterpretation of atrial fibrillation. However, the incidence of false negative forecasts decreased over time. A patient management with additional sources of information (first follow-up, lead problems, hospitalization etc.) could decrease the number of misinterpretations and, therefore, the numbers of follow-ups (P. Burgada, 2006).

Despite these positive results, there are still some controversial issues concerning particularly the efficiency of device-based remote monitoring in reducing the number of follow-ups. Heidbüchel et al. estimated that remote monitoring could potentially lead to a decreased frequency of follow-up, if combined with clinical follow-up by the local general practitioner (H. Heidbüchel et al., 2008). In contrast, Al-Khatib et al., who assigned 151 patients with an ICD to remote monitoring versus quarterly interrogations in clinic, could found no significant differences in cardiac-related resource utilization at 1 year (S. M. Al-Khatib et al., 2010).

Yet, currently available remote monitoring systems can neither substitute an emergency service nor can they replace entirely direct contact. Device-based remote monitoring is recommended for patients with stable device-function who have no need of reprogramming (B.L. Wilkoff et al., 2008).

The potential cost/benefit of remote monitoring for patients with cardiac devices (ICDs, CRTs or pacemakers) is another important aspect which has to be taken into account. A study by Fauchier et al. showed that remote monitoring of ICDs diminished the costs of follow-up. Particularly, they calculated that remote monitoring reduced the overall cost of ICD follow-up when the distance between home and the device clinic was >100 km (L. Fauchier et al., 2005). A trial of remote monitoring by Raatikainen et al. from Finland demonstrated that compared with the in-office visits, remote ICD monitoring required less time from both patient and physician to complete the follow-up. Substitution of two routine in-office visits during the study by remote monitoring reduced the overall cost of routine ICD follow-up by 41% per patient (M.J. P. Raatikainen et al., 2008). Furthermore, it could be demonstrated in a study from France that remote monitoring decreases the duration of post-operative hospitalization after implantation of pacing systems or replacement of pulse generators (F. Halimi et al., 2008).

The issue of patient and physician acceptance of remote monitoring still remains. This specifically relates to the concern that direct patient-physician-communication may get lost.

An Italian study with 119 patients revealed a high level of acceptance and satisfaction after 1-year remote control (R. P. Ricci et al., 2010).

However, despite these promising data and possibilities, device-based remote monitoring of antibradycardia pacemaker patients has failed to diffuse so far. There are various reasons for that: Different remote monitoring systems are not backward compatible and, thus, not able to monitor old generation devices. Secondly, routine follow-ups of patients with implanted pacemakers do not impose additional burden on the clinical workload. Furthermore, antibradycardia pacemakers are primarily inserted in elderly patients; this might create a treshold to apply remote monitoring, despite the fact that experience had shown that the technology is manageable by elderly patients. The situation is different for patients with ICDs and CRTs; due to its various possibilities device-based remote monitoring will grow in importance and, moreover, the population consists of heart failure patients.

However, there are still barriers for wider adoption. Among physicians, significant barriers may be technical problems (e.g. missing internet access, different systems), suspected additional expenditure of time and missing refund of expenses. The other barrier is the flood of data produced by remote monitoring. In a study by Lazarus 3,004,763 transmissions were made by 11,624 recipients of pacemakers, defibrillators and combined ICD-cardiac resynchronization therapy (CRT-D) systems. On average, 47.6% of the patients were event-free (A. Lazarus, 2007). Theuns et al. who examined the impact of remote monitoring on clinical workload showed that despite the large number of data transmissions, remote monitoring imposed a minimal additional burden on the clinical workload. The median number of clinical events/patient/month was 0.023 (D.A.J. Theuns et al., 2009). In order to guarantee an efficient analysis and selection of relevant data, specially trained nurses are deployed. These pacing expert nurses consult the website and submit critical cases to physician (R. P. Ricci et al., 2008).

Last but not least, the acceptance of device-based remote monitoring in future will depend on the development of standards and clinical guidelines. Remote monitoring must prove to be of great value in optimizing patient care and increasing efficiency of the health system.

5. Conclusion and perspective

Device-based remote monitoring has been increasingly established for many years. This system enables data transfer from pacemakers, ICDs and CRTs to the physician. Despite technical differences between the providers, the remote monitoring systems consist of unified components. The patient monitor connects to the device and transfers the data via landline or mobile phone to the providers´ server. There, data are anonymously decoded, analysed, and uploaded to a secure internet platform. The patient's physicians have access to this platform through identity codes and personal passwords and can also be informed of critical events via e-mail, sms or fax.

Meanwhile, most manufacturers (BIOTRONIK, Medtronic, St. Jude Medical, Boston Scientific) have provided their own device-based remote monitoring systems, all of which are already used in clinical practice. Safety and stability of data transmission was proven in clinical trails. Modern remote monitoring systems are taking several aspects of patient monitoring into account; they have developed from pure device monitoring to complex patient management systems integrating device-, arrhythmia-, heart failure-, and patient centered-management resulting in comprehensive monitoring with the option of early interventions. Modern information processing technologies allow the integration of collected data into an electronic health record (EHR) providing, therefore, holistic aftercare services and patient monitoring. In the future, fast mobile communication technologies for data transfer and internet platforms will be the most important tools. Device-based remote monitoring will become standard in monitoring of patients being implanted with complex cardiac devices (ICDs, CRTs) which is in accordance to the current guidelines. The next step is the transition from monitoring management to therapeutic management. This would be of particular benefit for CHF patients. However, although proven to be technically manageable, the implementation of these possibilities essentially depends on the acceptance on the part of patients, physicians and health insurances. Problems such as data security, data storage, cost reimbursement of telemedical solutions should be resolved in this context. Further clinical studies are needed to prove the benefits of device-based remote monitoring such as patient safety, individual patient´s follow-up settings and cost/benefit.

6. References

Ahmadi-Kashani M, Kessler DJ, Day J, Bunch J, Stolen KQ, Brown S, Sbaity S, Olshansky B on behalf of the INTRINSIC RV Study Investigators. (2009). Heart rate predicts outcomes in an implantable cardioverter-defibrillator population. *Circulation*, 120, pp. 2040-2045

Al-Khatib SM, Piccini JP, Knight D, Stewart M, Clapp-Channing N, Sanders GD. (2010). Remote monitoring of implantable cardioverter defibrillators versus quarterly device interrogations in clinic: results from a randomized pilot clinical trial. *J Cardiovasc Electrophysiol*, 21, pp. 545-550

Alter P, Waldhans S, Plachta E, Moosdorf R, Grimm W. (2005). Complications of implantable cardioverter defibrillator therapy in 440 consecutive patients. *PACE*,28, pp. 926-932

Bristow MR, Saxon LA, Boehmer J, Krueger S, Kass DA, De Marco T, Carson P, DiCarlo L, DeMets D, White BG, DeVries DW, Feldman AM. (2004). Cardiac-resynchronization therapy with or without an implantable defibrillator in advanced chronic heart failure. *N Engl J Med*, 350, pp. 2140-2150

Brugada P. (2006). What evidence do we have to replace in-hospital implantable cardioverter defibrillator follow-up? *Clin Res Cardiol*, 95, Supplement 3, pp. III/3-III/9

Catanzariti D, Lunati M, Landolina M, Zanotto G, Lonardi G, Iacopino S, Oliva F, Perego GB, Varbaro A, Denaro A, Valsecchi S, Vergara G on behalf of the Italian Clinical Service Optivol-CRT Group. (2009). Monitoring intrathoracic impedance with an implantable defibrillator reduces hospitalizations in patients with heart failure. *PACE*, 32, pp. 363-370

Crossley GH, Chen J, Choucair W, Cohen TJ, Gohn DC, Johnson WB, Kennedy EE, Mongeon LR, Serwer GA, Qiao H, Wilkoff BL for the PREFER Study Investigators. (2009). Clinical benefits of remote versus transtelephonic monitoring of implantable pacemakers. *J Am Coll Cardiol*, 54, pp. 2012-2019

Ellery S, Pakrashi T, Paul V, Sack S on behalf of the Home CARE Phase 0 Study Investigators. (2006). Predicting mortality and rehospitalization in heart failure patients with Home Monitoring - the Home CARE pilot study. *Clin Res Cardiol,* 95, Supplement 3, pp. III/29-III/35

Epstein AE, Dimarco JP, Ellenbogen KA, Estes NA 3rd, Freedman RA, Gettes LS, Gillnov AM, Gregoratos G, Hammill SC, Hayes DL, Hlatky MA, Newby LK, Page RL, Schoenfeld MH, Silka MJ, Stevenson LW, Sweeney MO; American College of Cardiology/American Heart Association Task Force on Practice; American Association of Thoracic Surgery; Society of Thoracic Surgeons. (2008). ACC/AHA/HRS 2008 Guidelines for device-based therapy of cardiac rhythm abnormalities. *J Am Coll Cardiol* , 51, pp. e1-e62

Fauchier L, Sadoul N, Kouakam C, Briand F, Chauvin M, Babuty D, Clementy J. (2005). Potential cost savings by telemedicine-assisted long-term care of implantable cardioverter defibrillators recipients. *PACE,* 28, pp. S255-S259

Halimi F, Clementy J, Attuel P, Dessenne X, Amara W, on behalf of the OEDIPE trial investigators. (2008). Optimized post-operative surveillance of permanent pacemakers by home monitoring: the OEDIPE trial. *Europace,* 10, pp. 1392-1399

Heidbüchel H, Lioen P, Foulon S, Huybrechts W, Ector J, Willems R, Ector H. (2008). Potential role of remote monitoring for scheduled and unscheduled evaluations of patients with an implantable defibrillator. *Europace,* 10, pp. 351-357

Kleemann T, Becker T, Doenges K, Vater M, Senges J, Schneider S, Saggau W, Weisse U, Seidl K. (2007). Annual rate of transvenous debrillaton lead defects in implantable cardioverter-defibrillators over a period of > 10 years. *Circulation,* 115, pp. 2474-2480

Klingenmaier CH, Moyer PR, Aunon JI, Shaffer MJ, Siegel FA, Rios JC. (1973). A method of computer-assisted pacemaker surveillance from a patient's home via telephone. *Computers and Biomedical Research,* 6, pp. 327-335

Kurtz SM, Ochoa JA, Lau E, Shkolnikov Y, Pavri BB, Frisch D, Greenspon AJ. (2010). Implantation trends and patient profiles for pacemakers and implantable cardioverter defibrillators in the United States: 1993-2006. *PACE,* 33, pp. 705-711

Lazarus A. (2007). Remote, wireless, ambulatory monitoring of implantable pacemakers, cardioverter defibrillators, and cardiac resynchronization therapy systems: analysis of a worldwide database. *PACE,* 30, pp. S2-S12

Leclercq C, Padeletti L., Cihak R, Ritter P, Milasinovic G, Gras D, Paul V, van Gelder IC, Stellbrink C, Rieger G, Corbucci G, Albers B, Daubert JC on behalf of the CHAMP Study Investigators. (2010). Incidence of paroxysmal atrial tachycardias in patients treated with cardiac resynchronization therapy and continuously monitored by device diagnostics. *Europace,* 12, pp. 71-77

Linde C, Abraham WT, Gold MR, St John Suttan M, Ghio S, Daubert C on behalf of the REVERSE Study Group. (2008). Randomized trial of cardiac resynchronization in mildly symptomatic heart failure patients and in asymptomatic patients with left ventricular dysfunction and previous heart failure symptoms. *J Am Coll Cardiol,* 52, pp. 1834-1843

Loricchio ML, Castro A, Ciolli A, Sasdelli M, Ferraiuolo G. (2008). Pacing failure due to microdislodgement of ventricular pacing lead detected by home monitoring technology. *J Cardiovasc Med,* 9, pp. 946-948

Maisel WH, Moynahan M, Zuckerman BD, Gross TP, Tovar OH, Tillman D-B, Schultz DB. (2006). Pacemaker and ICD generator malfunctions. Analysis of Food and Drug Administration Annual Reports. *JAMA,* 295, pp. 1901-1906

Maytin M, Love CJ, Fischer A, Carrillo RG, Garisto JD, Bongiorni MG, Segreti L, John RM, Michaud GF, Albert CM, Epstein LM. (2010). Multicenter experience with extraction of the Sprint Fidelis implantable cardioverter-defibrillator lead. *J Am Coll Cardiol,* 56, pp. 646-650

Moss AJ, Zareba W, Hall WJ, Klein H, Wilber DJ, Cannom DS, Daubert JP, Higgins SL, Brown MW, Andrews ML. (2002). Prophylactic implantation of a defibrillator in patients with myocardial infarction and reduced ejection fraction. *N Engl J Med,* 346, pp. 877-883

Moss AJ, Hall WJ, Cannom DS, Klein H, Brown MW, Daubert JP, Estes III M, Foster E, Greenberg H, Higgins S, Pfeffer MA, Solomon SD, Wilber D, Zareba W for the MADIT-CRT Trial Investigators. (2009). Cardiac-resynchronization therapy for the prevention of heart-failure events. *N Engl J Med,* 361, pp. 1329-1338

Nielsen JC, Kottkamp H, Zabel M, Aliot E, Kreutzer U, Bauer A, Schuchert A, Neuser H, Schumacher B, Schmidinger H, Stix G, Clementy J, Danilovic, Hindricks G. (2008). Automatic home monitoring of implantable cardioverter defibrillators. *Europace,* 10, pp. 729-735

Poole JE, Johnson GW, Hellkamp AS, Anderson J, Callans DJ, Raitt MH, Reddy RK, Marchlinski FE, Yee R, Guarnieri T, Talajic M, Wilber DJ, Fishbein DT, Packer DL, Mark DB, Lee KL, Bardy GH. (2009). Prognostic importance of defibrillator shocks in patients with heart failure. *N Engl J Med,* 359, pp. 1009-1017

Raatikainen MJ, Uusimaa P, van Ginneken MME, Janssen JPG, Linnaluoto M. (2008). Remote monitoring of implantable cardioverter defibrillator patients: a safe, time-saving, and cost-effective means for follow-up. *Europace,* 10, pp. 1145-1151

Res JCJ, Theuns DAMJ, Jordaens I. (2006). The role of remote monitoring in the reduction of inappropriate implantable cardioverter defibrillator therapies. *Clin Res Cardiol* , 95, Supplement 3, pp. III/17-III/21

Ricci RP, Morichelli L, Santini M. (2008). Home monitoring remote control of pacemaker and implantable cardioverter defibrillator patients in clinical practice: impact on medical management and health-care resource utilization. *Europace,* 10, pp. 164-170

Ricci RP, Morichelli L, Santini M. (2009) a. Remote control of implanted devices through Home Monitoring technology improves detection and clinical management of atrial fibrillation. *Europace,* 11, pp. 54-61

Ricci RP, Morichelli L, Gargaro A, Laudadio MT, Santini M. (2009) b. Home monitoring in patients with implantable cardiac devices: is there a potential reduction of stroke risk? Results from a computer model tested through Monte Carlo simulations. *J Cardiovasc Electrophysiol*, 20, pp. 1244-1251

Ricci RP, Morichelli L, Quarta L, Sassi A, Porfili a, Laudadio MT, Gargaro A, Santini M. (2010). Long-term patient acceptance of and satisfaction with implanted device remote monitoring. *Europace*, 12, pp. 674-679

Santini M, Ricci RP, Lunati M, Landolina M, Perego GB, Marzegalli M, Schirru M, Belvito C, Brambilla R, Guenzati G, Gilardi S, Valsecchi S. (2009). Remote monitoring of patients with biventricular defibrillators through the CareLink system improves clinical management of arrhythmias and heart failure episodes. *J Interv Card Electrophysiol* , 24, pp. 53-61

Schoenfeld MH, Compton SJ, Mead RH, Weiss DN, Sherfesee L, Englund J, Mongeon LR. (2004). Remote monitoring of implantable cardioverter defibrillators. a prospective analysis. *PACE*, 27, pp. 757-763

Scholten MF, Thornton S, Theuns DA, Res J, Jordaens LJ. (2004). Twiddler's syndrome detected by home monitoring device. *PACE* , 27, pp. 1151-1152

Spencker S, Coban N, Koch L, Schirdewan A, Müller D. (2009). Potential role of home monitoring to reduce inappropriate shocks in implantable cardioverter-defibrillator patients due to lead failure. *Europace*, 11, pp. 483-488

Sweeney MO, Sherfesee L, DeGroot PJ, Wathen MS, Wilkoff BL. (2010) Differences in effects of electrical therapy type for ventricular arrhythmias on mortality in implantable cardioverter-defibrillator patients.*Heart Rhythm*, 7(3), pp. 353-360

Theuns DAMJ, Rivero-Ayerza M, Knops P, Res JCJ, Jordaens LJ. (2009). Analysis of 57,148 transmissions by remote monitoring of implantable cardioverter defibrillators. *PACE*, 32, pp. S63-S65

Varma N, Stambler B, Chun S. (2005). Detection of atrial fibrillation by implanted devices with wireless data transmission capability. *PACE*, 28, pp. S133-S136

Varma NJ. (2009). Remote monitoring for advisories: automatic early detection of silent lead failure. *PACE*, 32, pp. 525-527

Vollmann D, Nägele H, Schauerte P, Wiegand U, Butter C, Zanotto G, Quesada A, Guthmann A, Hill MRS, Lamp B, for the European InSync Sentry Observational Study Investigators. (2007). Clinical utility of intrathoracic impedance monitoring to alert patients with an implanted device of deteriorating chronic heart failure. *European Heart Journal*, 28, pp. 1835-1840

Volosin KJ, Exner DV, Wathen MS, Sherfesee L, Scinicariello AP, Gillberg JM. (2010). Combining shock reduction strategies to enhance ICD therapy: a role for computer modelling.*J Cardiovasc Electrophysiol*, 22., pp. [Epub ahead of print]

Wallbrück K, Stellbrink C, Santini M, Gill J, Hartmann A, Wunderlich E. (2002). The value of permanent follow-up of implantable pacemakers - first result of an European trial. *Biomedizinische Technik*, 47, pp. 950-953

Wilkoff BL, Auricchio A, Brugada J, Cowie M, Ellenbogen KA, Gillis AM, Hayes DL, Howlett JG, Kautzner J, Love CJ, Morgan JM, Priori SG, Reynolds DW, Schoenfeld MH, Vardas PE. (2008). HRS/EHRA expert consensus on the monitoring of cardiovascular implantable electronic devices (CIEDs): description of techniques, indications, personnel, frequency and ethical considerations. *Europace,* 10, pp. 707-725

Zhan C, Baine WB, Sedrakyan A, Steiner C. (2007). Cardiac device implantation in the United States from 1997 through 2004: a population-based analysis. *J Gen Intern Med*, 23, Supplement 1, pp. 13-19

10

Remote Monitoring of Implantable Pacemaker, Cardioverter Defibrillator, and Cardiac Resynchronizer

Milton E. Guevara-Valdivia[1] and Pedro Iturralde Torres[2]
[1]*Servicio de Electrofisiología y Estimulación Cardiaca. Unidad Médica de Alta Especialidad (UMAE) del Hospital de Especialidades Dr. "Antonio Fraga Mouret". Centro Médico Nacional (CMN) La Raza, Instituto Mexicano del Seguro Social (IMSS), México, D. F.*
[2]*Departamento de Electrocardiografía y Electrofisiología. Instituto Nacional de Cardiología "Ignacio Chávez" México D.F.*
México

1. Introduction

Implantable pacemakers (P), cardioverter defibrillators (CD), cardiac resynchronization systems (CRS), closed-loop recorders, and hemodynamic monitoring implantable products offer multiple programmable options, which allow storage of large quantities of diagnostic information related to the device's function. Traditionally, these mechanisms require direct interrogation to allow seeing the scheduled parameters and stored data to identify and correct possible malfunctioning and improve rescheduling therapy. Implantation of these devices (P, CD, and CRS) has been increasing day by day, thus considerably increasing patients' handling and healthcare system work load. To reduce the time that outpatient services impose and to optimize patient care, manufacturers of these devices offer increasingly more refined remote questioning instruments. Recent technological progresses and a better administration of economical resources may probably allow widening of the use of remote monitoring in the upcoming years.

2. Remote monitoring systems

Currently, there are different monitoring devices and almost all manufacturers have introduced their own version of remote monitoring systems (Figure 1); for example, Biotronik has introduced the Biotronik Home Monitoring® system; Medtronic® has introduced the CareLink® Network; Latitude® Patient Management system has been introduced by Boston Scientific®, and St. Jude Medical's Merlin.net® Patient Care Network (PCN). All these equipments can be compared according to their main characteristics (Table I), and to be implemented, they need to be equipped with an antenna that communicates to a small external device known as transmitter that is able to question the diagnosis parameters of the data stored in most of the devices, either with patient's active participation or at pre-scheduled intervals.

Parameters	Biotronik Home Monitoring®	Medtronic Carelink® Network	Boston Scientific Latitude®	Merlin.net® Patient Care Network (PCN)
FDA's date of approval	2001	2005	2006	2007
Device name	CardioMessenger®	PatientLook SentryCheck (OptiVol)	Latitude Communicator	Merlin@home
Characteristics	Portable	Stationary	Stationary, interactive	Stationary, voice-interactive
Telemetry at home USA	MICS	MICS, antenna	Antenna and wireless	MICS
Telemetry - rest of the world	MICS	Antenna	Not available	Antenna
Wireless products	All products	DAI and DAI + ResBiv	All products	DAI and DAI + ResBiv
Reminders / Manual transmission	Automatic	No	Yes	Yes
Patient takes actions in case of event	CardioMessenger® / Recall	Audio	Audio	Vibration
Telemetry range	4-GSM band, GPRS, mobile, ***analog*** line	***Analog*** line	***Analog*** line	***Analog*** line
Interaction during transmission	No	No (wireless) Yes (Analog line)	No (wireless) Yes (Analog line)	No (wireless) Yes (Analog line)
Transmission	Daily, follow-up, event messages (automatic)	Scheduled follow-up, event message (started by the patient)	Scheduled follow-up, event message (started by the patient)	Started by the patient (manual)
Event transmission route	Fax, Internet, e-mail, text message	e-mail, text message	Fax, phone	Fax, Internet, EMR
Early detection	<24 hours (all events)	<24 hours (certain kind of events)	<24 hours (certain kind of events)	Not available
Data storage	Long term	Long term	Long term	Long term
EMR interface	HL7	HL7, EMR	HL7	HL7, EMR
Data presentation	Event- and signaling-based	Event-based	Orientation in signaling	Event-based
Real-time EGM	Event-generated	Holter and pacemaker	Holter and pacemaker	Not available
Holter transmission	>45 sec.	10 sec.	10 sec.	30 sec.

Parameters	Biotronik Home Monitoring®	Medtronic Carelink® Network	Boston Scientific Latitude®	Merlin.net® Patient Care Network (PCN)
Sensor	IC monitor	OptiVol®, Cardiac Compass	Weight, BP, symptoms, pacemaker statistics	Statistics and surface ECG
Repercussion on long-lasting battery	Low	High	High	Not available

Abbreviations: MICS = Medical implant and Communications bandwidth (402-405 MHz), GSM = Global System for Mobile Communication, GPRS = General Packet Radio Service, HL7 = Interface standard, EMR = Electronic medical records, EGM = intracavitary electrocardiogram, IC = Heart failure, DAI = Implantable automatic defibrillator, DAI + ResBiv = Implantable automatic defibrillator plus biventricular resynchronizer

Table 1. Remote monitoring systems

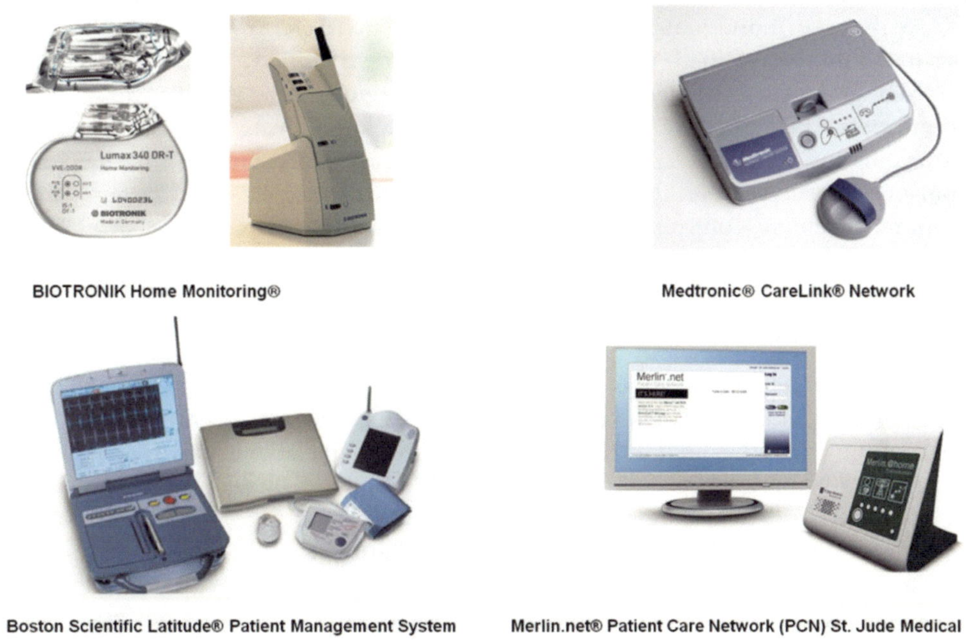

Fig. 1. The four remote monitoring systems currently in use.

Once captured, the data from that device are uploaded using a transmitter that has a standard analogical telephone line or wireless telephones, to a safe central where the data are processed. The patient receives messages or event alerts through an acoustic signal (*beep*) and/or vibrations, and in certain systems, such alerts are used to indicate that the patient should start the data manual transfer from the transmitter to a central base. During transmission, the level of participation varies depending on the manufacturers' and the patient's clinical condition, and the urgency of the processed data may trigger a rapid alert to the physician through an email, text messages, fax, or a phone call, in which a detailed report is simultaneously published in a secure website for the visualization of the physician or another authorized reviewer.

Most of the remote monitoring systems transmit patients' data through standard telephone lines, either on a weekly or fortnightly basis. Yet, we should not forget that there are other equipments, such as Biotronik Home Monitoring®, in which the transmission is based on a wireless telephone that could be carried in the belt or handbag, which is capable of capturing the stored information daily. Still, with either system, the patient's information can be continuously controlled and the variables that are included more frequently are battery status, battery impedance, electrode impedance, post-shock impedance, arrhythmia detection, therapies administered, and average heart rate. Furthermore, it is possible to record an electrogram (EGM) of the event that triggered the alert or, failing this, a change in the electrode impedance, caused by a fracture or the device elective replacement, as well as inefficiency to deliver a stimulus, onset of atrial fibrillation (AF) events, and heart failure (HF) deterioration.

Typically, transmission parameters differ among equipments; nevertheless, they are adjustable to each patient. The physician can set specific alert conditions according to the patient's base disease. Remote monitoring reports are generated and sent with different alert levels, so that the individual may answer according to their urgency. For instance, the physician could be notified within an hour (if so scheduled) in case of ventricular tachycardia or increase in ventricular extrasistolia: two events that trigger an alert of different levels. The main differences among the remote monitoring procedures relate to the data transmission frequency and reporting, the necessary level of patient participation for the transmission success, and the movement capability that they offer. No system allows the programming remote control a functionality that probably will not be available soon because of ruling issues and the legal medical rate.

3. Types of remote monitoring systems

The **Biotronik Home Monitoring®** system transmits data on a daily basis, at fixed intervals and soon after a clinically relevant event has occurred. Home Monitoring® has introduced the first equipment of this kind in 2001 and it is currently available in over 50 countries. The equipment can be programmed per event line and individual surveillance parameters. The usual events included in these devices are atrial monitoring for AF detection, HF monitoring, and high-definition intracavitary EGM (Figure 2), similar to the therapies being administered.

This system bases its functioning in three steps: The first step is the communication between the implanted generator and the patient device, named CardioMessenger (CM) (Figure 3). The generator emits a message at a medical implant-reserved frequency (402–405 MHz) to the CM, activating a radiofrequency (RF) circuit integrated to the head of the implanted equipment. On the scheduled time, the patient must be from 20 cm to 2 m far from the CM to ensure successful transmission.

The second step relates to the CM message delivery to the service central in Germany, via GSM/GPRS cellular. The CM zips and codes the information using the standard known as Digital Encryption Standard (DES), owing to which the patient can be elsewhere in the world with access to a cellular network, and the system will function normally (Figure 4).

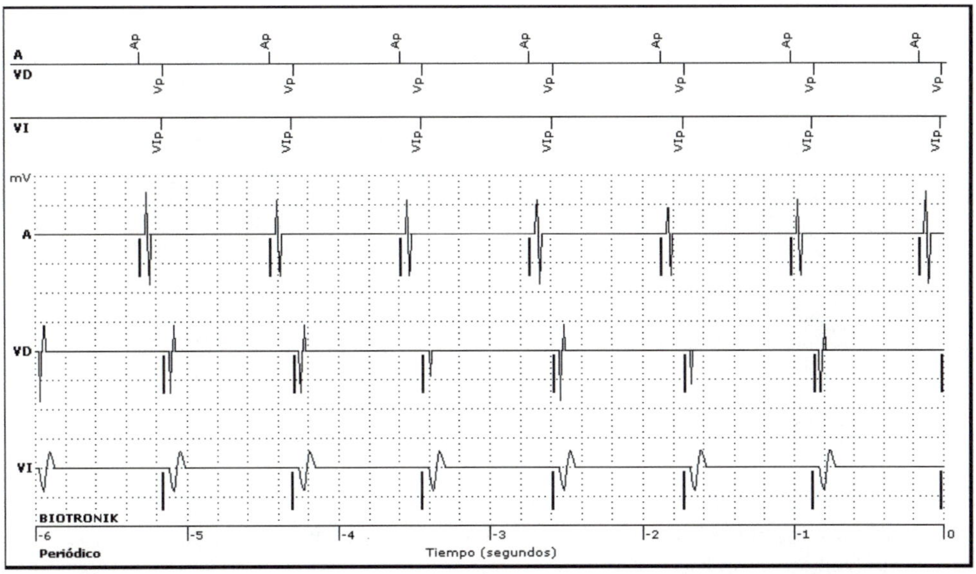

Fig. 2. An intracavitary ECG of a resynchronizer with implantable automatic defibrillator, which was sent as a device periodical report of the Biotronik Home Monitoring® system, available in the Internet. The mark channel can be observed at the top and the electrocardiograms can be found at the bottom. Abbreviations: Ap = Stimulation of the right atrium. Vp = Stimulus of the right ventricle. VIp = Stimulus of the left ventricle. A = EGM of the right atrium. VD = EGM of the right ventricle. VI = EGM of the left ventricle.

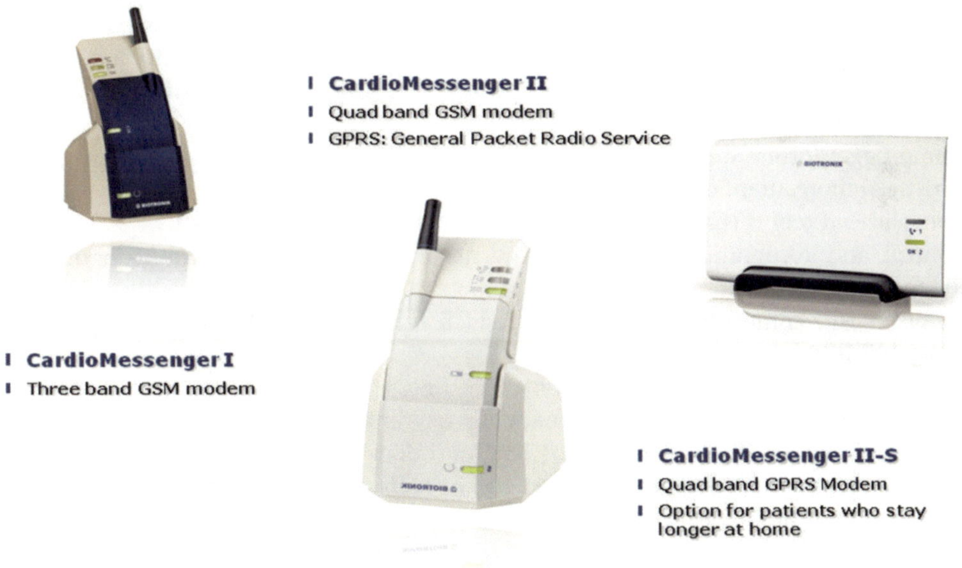

Fig. 3. Three types of CardioMessenger® of Biotronik Home Monitoring® system.

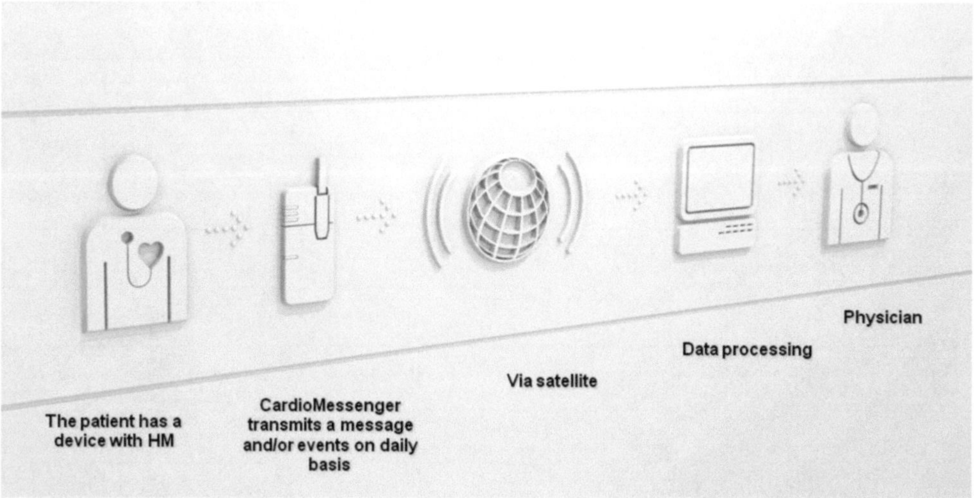

Fig. 4. Chart showing for whom the Biotronik Home Monitoring® system works. The approximate transmission time is of about 5 minutes.

This is an automatic system performing the following types of transmissions and messages:

1. Every 24 hours, at a physician-preset time, the device sends a transmission containing the data gathered along the last 24 hours and the CM issues a message to the service center.
2. When any major cardiac event or change occurs in the device's or electrodes' technical parameters, a message is immediately sent.

In the third step, the physician receives a report issued from the service center based in Germany, named CardioReport, to which he/she will have access through an internet-based secure webpage (Figure 5). He/she may also receive a text message (SMS), fax, or e-mail informing him/her that the patient must be monitored in case of an adverse event. In the internet, the physician will have access, from any computer, to whole information related to the event and/or report, and to the device and its electrodes, which will have the following characteristics:

- Home page: Intuitive platform that allows the physician to rapidly visualize patients who need more attention.
- Consolidated report (CardioReport) per patient, continuously updated.
- Control and recognition of changed events and the possibility to recognize alert changes.
- Fields to add comments and remarks, which relate to both the patient and his/her clinical history.
- Time line: history of detailed events on a time line.

The system rapidly transmits symptomatic or asymptomatic events, regardless of the patient's location, in that it is automatic, silent, and does not require his/her participation. The follow-up can be either monthly, quarterly, or half-yearly, and the physician may also access the accumulated files published in an internet-secure site for rapid review and evaluation of its evolution.

The **CareLink®Network (Medtronic®)** system is designed to perform remote monitoring of the status of the implanted device and includes a monitor and an antenna, through which the patient and/or the medical personnel may interact.

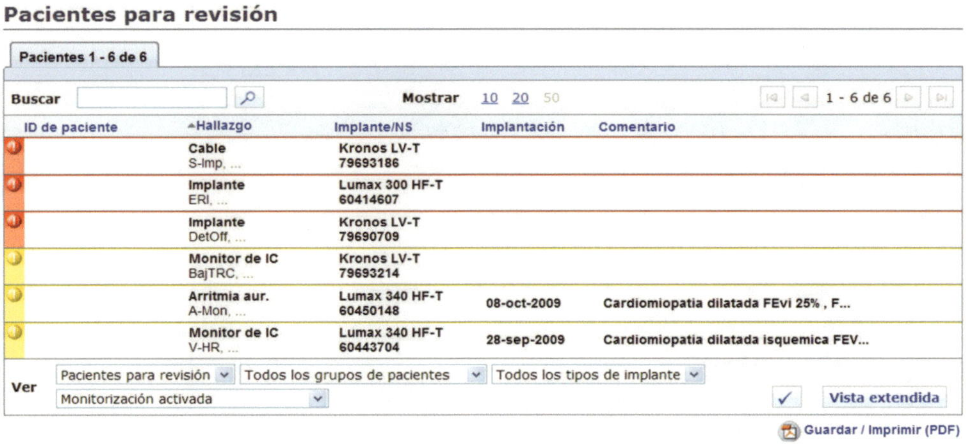

Fig. 5. Page available at the Biotronik Home Monitoring® website portal in which the patients' conditions can be observed. Red and yellow colors, characteristics of the signaling, according to the level of attention that should be addressed; in this case, yellow color indicates review and red signifies urgent review.

The monitor is small and has an antenna that connects to an analogical telephone line. The user (who may be the patient him/herself) has to press a button to switch it on and place the antenna onto the implanted device. The monitor questions and transmits the patient's technical and physiologic data stored in it and 10 seconds, in real time, of the EGM.

The monitor will automatically call a toll-free telephone number and send the information to the servers of the CareLink® system using a safe connection. To inform the patient that the transmission has successfully occurred, the monitor uses audible tones and visual indicators.

There are two types of monitors, manuals and automatics, which work in a similar way, even with some small differences. CareLink® monitors operate with a single specific implantable device, i.e. each monitor is linked to the serial number of the implanted equipment and will not work in another patient, because the server will not accept transmissions made from a CareLink® monitor associated with another device. There is a webpage where it is possible to visualize the condition of the discharged patients using a PC with Internet through a web browser (Figure 6), and only registered personnel will have access to the data of the patients followed up in that center.

The in-line format allows a detailed report, in which it counts on a Cardiac Compass® visualization system that allows visualization of up to 14 months of accumulated parameters, namely, atrial and ventricular stimulation, heart rate, atrial fibrillation events, and the response of the heart rate to the patient's activity. The CareLink®Network (Medtronic®) system includes in its follow-up those devices available in OptiVol®, a single sensor for the increase in the pulmonary fluid used for the early detection of deterioration of HF. This sensor indicates the ratio between the liquid status and the intrathoracic impedance, and the system is driven through a device-issued audible tone, which asks the patient to start a period of communication sessions in response to the events that the implanted device has detected, as well as relevant clinical changes in the system: arrhythmias, administered therapies, etc. The description customization for each patient requires the use of a programmer during the outpatient visit. Manual programming also needs to define the transmission.

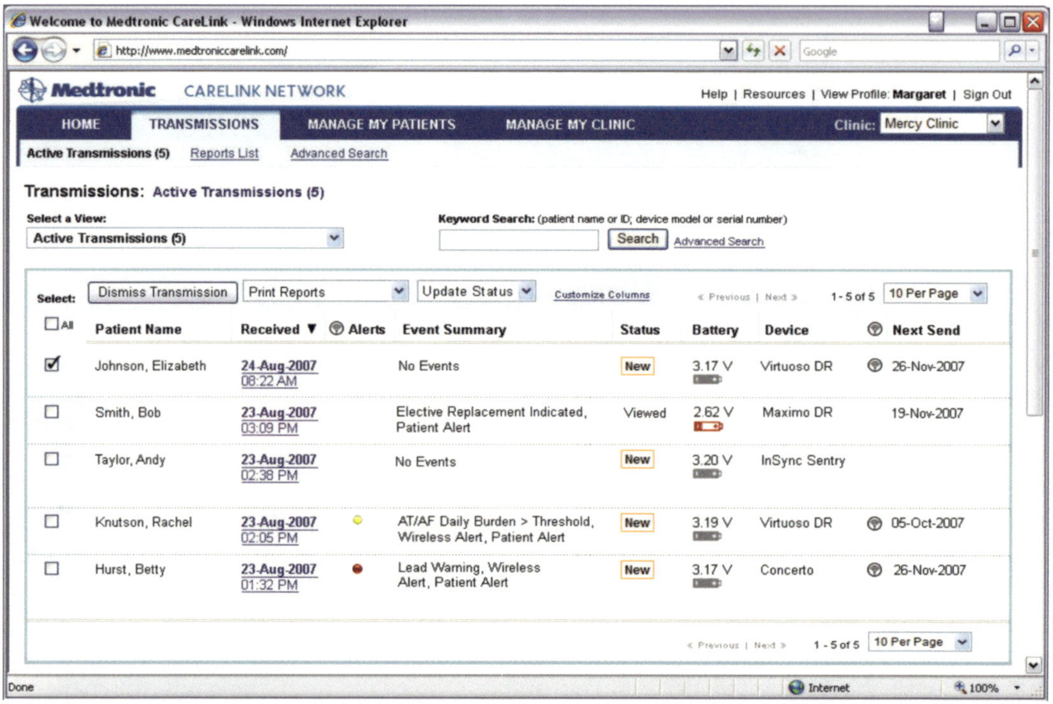

Fig. 6. Webpage of the CareLink® Network (Medtronic®) system in which a list of patients, type of alert under the signaling scheme, and type of event, battery voltage, and type of device can be observed.

Latitude® Patient Management System (Boston Scientific®) admits almost all Boston Scientific® devices, namely CD and RCS, depending on the implanted device and on the fact that it is operated through telemetry or a wireless transmitter to question the device at home, usually on a weekly basis. The transmitter also uses a ground analogical system to transmit data that can be configured to be used in several countries. A unique characteristic of this product is the possibility to wirelessly connect weight and blood pressure scales for the remote monitoring of the HF condition; also in addition, the patient may obtain an automatic weekly report of his/her condition (fatigue, ankle edema, orthopnea, etc.). Notices of events may be individually configured based on the "red" and "yellow" alerts. Furthermore, the customized data transmission system allows different physicians (general physician, cardiologist, and electrophysiologist) to improve the follow-up in HF clinics.

St. Jude Medical's Merlin.net® Patient Care Network (PCN) is an implant procedure and implantable device clinical follow-up remote transmission system that stores data for up to 7 years. The implant system is provided through InvisiLink® Wireless telemetry and the follow-up is provided through the RF Merlin@home® transmitter, which receives the DirectCall® messages; furthermore, it offers an online agenda. A useful characteristic is the possibility offered to the physician to indicate warnings and regular remainders for medical appointments in the patient's transmitter and to make automatic calls to patients with the results. The monitoring system sends daily notices known as DirectAlerts® and can export a database by integrating the Healthcare Enterprise (IHE) system. The Merlin@home® system is a small box, similar to a phone operating in the medical device band in the 402–405 MHz range. It has a start button that allows the interrogation to be started by the patient, and has status lights for both the transmitter and the transmission in one icon and connects to an analogical telephone line. On a daily basis, it checks the status of the implanted device and notification is sent to the physician through e-mail, fax, text message, phone call, or Internet (Figure 7). The device may be used in emergency rooms. In addition, there is a version that is not wireless. The system has both manual and automatic programming; pool programming is possible and it also offers DirectCall® message feature; notifications (DirectAlert®) that allow the patient's condition to be monitored may be configured either as urgent or report. It has a DirectTrend™ visualization that graphically shows the stimulation percentage trend.

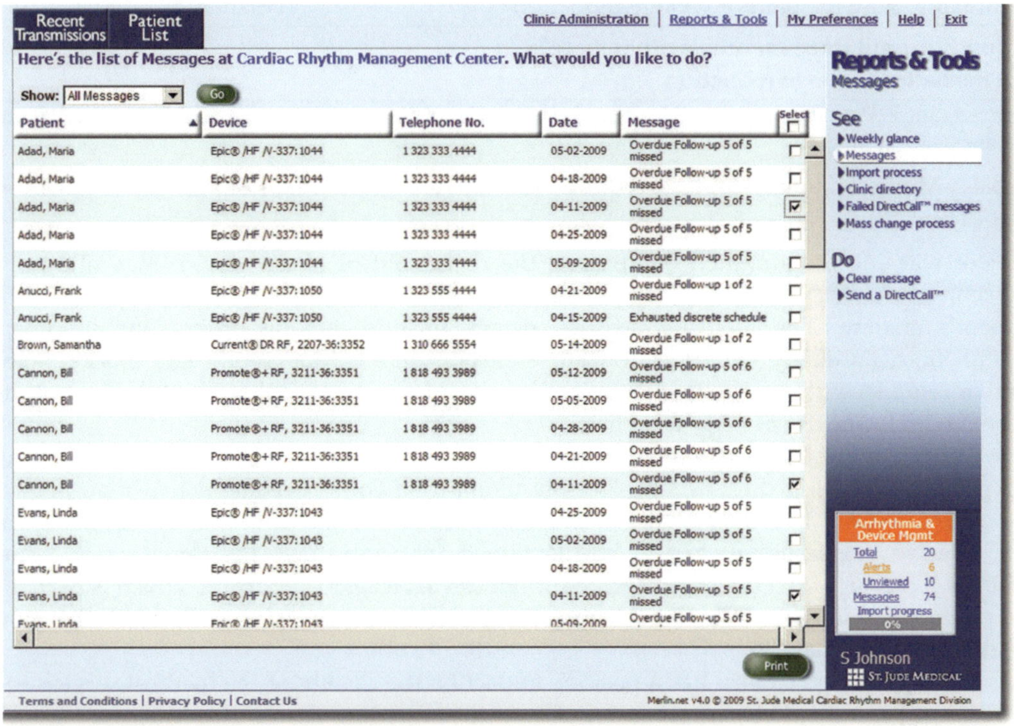

Fig. 7. Webpage of the Merlin.net® Patient Care Network (PCN) system in which the list of patients, type of devices, and other characteristics can be observed.

4. Benefits of remote monitoring

The Heart Rhythm Society (HRS) and the European Heart Rhythm Association (EHRA) have defined that the main purpose of remote monitoring is to identify the device's abnormal behavior as soon as possible to limit the sub-registration of its malfunctioning. This is how they have also established the determining factors to set the device follow-up frequency; something of utmost importance was to establish the minimum interval required to provide follow-up, either on-site or remotely (Table II).

Currently, the Biotronik Home Monitoring® seems to be the best system for the early detection of the abnormal behavior of the device. This may be particularly pertinent in the

Conditions	Type of monitoring
Within the first 72 hours after having implanted a P,CD, CRS	Personally
Two to twelve weeks after having implanted a P,CD, CRS	Personally
Three to twelve months after having implanted a P, CRS	Personally or remotely
Three to twelve months after having implanted a CRS + defibrillator and CD	Personally or remotely
Annually, until the battery voltage reduction	Personally
Monthly, until three months, with data related to the battery voltage reduction	Personally or remotely

Abbreviations: P = Pacemaker, CD = Cardioverter defibrillator, CRS = Cardiac resynchronization system

Table 2. Minimum follow-up time required for remote monitoring or onsite visit of P, CD, and CRS

case of warning-programmed equipment; the daily control of the device may allow the expecting behavior without needing to shorten the follow-up intervals, which reduces the patient's anxiety. The reported adverse events include, among others, the imminent dysfunction caused by battery worn-out, electrode defects, and inefficient shocks. Some similar remarks with other remote monitoring systems suggest a potential of similar output, even if with lower risk of early detection.

Another important target of remote monitoring is the reduction in the number of followed-up patients attending the hospital. Remote monitoring could become a tool that, maybe, could replace visits to the hospital, which may be unnecessary when remote monitoring has not detected any issues. It has to be mentioned that nowadays the remote monitoring systems have improved the data capture format as well as alert-reporting, which is partially user-defined, and simplification of their interpretation, what has enhanced the time scheduled for its analysis.

Remote monitoring can also has a positive impact on the quality of the medical service and the patient's quality of life, because:

- It allows the early detection of arrhythmias, changes in the device functioning, or changes in the patient condition during follow-up.
- It helps in providing individual programming time aimed to optimize the handling of patients having frequent arrhythmias or technical complications, cost reduction, and workloads imposed by the patients having no complications or having stable clinical conditions.
- The acceptance of patients to the state-of-the-art reliability that the implanted device operates properly, along with the advantage of reduced number of hospital visits.

Even if more exact indicators of the patient's clinical conditions have not been clearly defined, abnormal vitals, including inadequate increase in the heart rate at rest, minute ventilation, and a drop in intrathoracic impedance may be signals of HF deterioration. As adaptation to new technologies requires efforts to abandon what is already known, both hospital services and physicians are enthusiastically accepting this system.

5. Future perspectives

Remote monitoring may probably be included in the upcoming devices (P, CD, and CRS), and one can expect that new useful sensors will be made available soon. These progresses may introduce changes in the follow-up procedures and their goals, may allow the physicians to opportunely intervene to improve the clinical outcomes, and may cause reduction in medical expenses. New sensors may become necessary to prevent HF, as measure of intrathoracic impedance, intracardiac pressure, and minute ventilation. Other sensors that are potentially valuable for remote monitoring are function of the left ventricle, volume of the left ventricle and contractibility, oxygen venous saturation, muscular activity, and, finally, myocardium ischemia. The latter is related to recent publications in which one may obtain the reconstruction of a 12-derivation ECG through the implanted device (CRS, CD), obtaining a good correlation with the conventional surface ECG[7]. If we aggregate the possibility to obtain information through remote monitoring, its utility will be very helpful to discriminate myocardium ischemia, atrial and ventricle extrasistolia, and, most importantly, the possibility to distinguish between supraventricular tachycardia and ventricular tachycardia. Some of these sensors could be used in patients already implanted with P, CD, and CRS.

6. Conclusions

The remote monitoring system is a useful tool that can be used in health institutions to follow-up P, CD, and CRS, obtaining substantial benefits such as early diagnosis of arrhythmias, to adequately recommend a treatment. Reduction in the number of visits to device clinics allows the patient to freely perform his/her daily activities or travel, because he/she will be covered by continuous remote monitoring. Furthermore, there is the possibility that patients with any kind of limitation to attend the clinic, either because of any physical or transportation limitation, may find an alternative in this system. Finally, with remote monitoring, patients counting on any medical alert of *recall* could benefit from a stricter follow-up to detect possible system failures. With all these benefits, the satellite remote monitoring system offers an alternative to the on-site visit for the monitoring of the devices, though this may not replace medical visit.

7. References

Jung W, Rillig A, Birkemeyer R, Miljak T, Meyerfeldt U.(2008). Advances in remote monitoring of implantable pacemakers, cardioverter defibrillators and cardiac resynchronization therapy systems. *J Interv Card Electrophysiol,* 23:73-85.

Burri H, Senouf D., (2009). Remote monitoring and follow-up of pacemaker and implantable cardioverter defibrillator. *Europace,*11:701-709.

Nielsen JC, Kottkamp H, Zabel M, Aliot E, Kreutzer U, Bauer A. et al., (2008).Automatic home monitoring of implantable cardioverter defibrillators. *Europace,* 10:729-35.

Guevara-Valdivia ME. (2009). Monitoreo a distancia de los dispositivos automáticos implantables cardiovasculares (marcapasos, desfibriladores automáticos implantables y resincronizadores cardiacos). *Arch Cardiol Mex,* 79:221-225

Villar-Montini A.(2009). Tecnología de monitoreo remoto inalámbrico. *Arch Cardiol Mex,* 79(Supl 2):75-78

Wilkoff BL, Auricchio A, Brugada J, Cowie M, Ellenbogen KA, Gillis AM, et al.,(2008) "HRS/EHRA Expert Consensus on the Monitoring of Cardiovascular Implantable Electronic Devices (CIED): description of techniques, indications, personnel, frequency and ethical considerations: developed in partnership with the Heart Rhythm Society (HRS) and the European Heart Rhythm Association (EHRA); and in collaboration with the American College of Cardiology (ACC), the American Heart Association (AHA), the European Society of Cardiology (ESC), the Heart Failure Association of ESC (HFA), and the Heart Failure Society of America (HFSA). Endorsed by the Heart Rhythm Society, the European Heart Rhythm Association (a registered branch of the ESC), the American College of Cardiology, the American Heart Association . *Heart Rhythm* , 6:907-925.

Stuart Mendenhall G, Saba S,(2010).12-lead surface electrocardiogram reconstruction from implanted device electrograms. *Europace,* 12: 991-998

Part 3

Pacemaker Interactions with ICD and MRI

11

Interaction between the RF Field of MRI Apparatus and Pacemakers

Stefano Pisa, Paolo Bernardi, and Emanuele Piuzzi
Sapienza University of Rome
Italy

1. Introduction

Magnetic resonance imaging (MRI) is a tomography technique that measures the radio frequency (RF) field produced by the magnetic moments of hydrogen nuclei during their precession following the application of RF pulses, superimposed to a static magnetic field.
MRI is a widely accepted tool for the diagnosis of a variety of diseases. Nowadays, however, MRI is contraindicated for patients implanted with pacemakers (PM) due to possible adverse effects (ICNIRP, 2004). The most important of such effects seems to be the heating of the heart tissue around the catheter tip resulting from the high currents induced on the catheter by the RF field used in MRI technique (Nyenhuis, 2005).
In order to avoid thermal hazards resulting from MRI investigations, international agencies have issued guidelines reporting recommended limits. The International Commission on Non-Ionizing Radiation Protection (ICNIRP, 2004) considers that for whole-body exposures to MRI apparatus, no adverse health effects are expected if the increase in body core temperature does not exceed 1 °C. With regard to localized heating, ICNIRP assumes that adverse effects are avoided with a reasonable certainty if temperature remains lower than 38 °C in localized regions of the head, lower than 39 °C in the trunk, and less than 40 °C in the limbs. Accordingly, in ICNIRP (2004) limitations have been reported on the maximum power, expressed in terms of specific absorption rate (SAR), namely power per unit mass of tissue (W/kg), that can be dissipated inside the patient body during MRI investigations. More in detail, such limitations refer to whole body SAR (SAR_{WB}) and local SAR as averaged over 10 g of tissue (SAR_{10}). In particular, in normal conditions, the SAR_{WB} should not exceed 2 W/kg, while the SAR_{10} is limited to 20 W/kg in the extremities and 10 W/kg in the head and trunk.
The above reported SAR limitations should ensure safe MRI investigations for normal patients, but might not guarantee adequate protection for PM holders, mainly because of the previously mentioned catheter tip heating (Bernardi et al., 2009). To clarify this issue, the amount of heating in PM holders during MRI sessions has been investigated in several in vivo, in vitro, and numerical studies and reported temperature elevations spread from not significant values up to tens of degrees. Hence, in this Chapter, the studies available in the literature and concerning SAR distributions and temperature increments in PM holders, exposed to the field generated by MRI apparatus, will be described in order to evidence the main factors influencing the obtained SAR values and temperature increments. After a preliminary description of MRI apparatus in terms of field sources and distributions, the main in vitro (on phantoms), and numerical literature results will be presented. In

particular, the numerical literature survey will show that some authors used accurate models of the pacemaker, embedded in coarse body models, while other authors used anatomically correct body models, with crude pacemakers realizations. Both these approaches can overestimate or underestimate the actual temperature increases in pacemaker holders under MRI investigations. Hence, in the final part of this chapter, SAR distributions and temperature increments in PM holders, exposed inside an MRI apparatus, will be evaluated by using an anatomically based human body phantom together with fine pacemaker models equipped with different kinds of catheters, implanted following the vein path. This study will be performed by using a conformal FDTD code with graded mesh (C-GM-FDTD) for the solution of the electromagnetic (EM) problem, and a finite difference solution of the bioheat equation with graded mesh, for the evaluation of the corresponding temperature increments. This model will allow to investigate the influence of the PM and antenna geometry on the induced thermal increments, and to give some rules for the design of antenna or catheter geometries able to make MRI safe for PM holders.

2. MRI fields and coils

2.1 MRI apparatus

Magnetic resonance imaging technique is based on induced nuclear magnetic resonance of water molecules. For this reason MRI is the imaging technique of choice for pathologies where it is important to discriminate among different soft (well hydrated) tissues like brain, muscle, and tumors. MRI provides good spatial resolution (the ability to distinguish between two separate structures at an arbitrarily small distance from each other), and a high contrast resolution (the ability to distinguish the differences between two similar but not identical tissues). Unlike traditional X-rays and computer tomography (CT), MRI does not use ionizing radiation and it is generally a very safe procedure.

The human body is largely composed of water molecules. Each water molecule has two hydrogen atoms with a proton inside the nucleus. During an MRI examination of a person a static magnetic field B_0 produced by superconductive magnets (B_0 coil in Fig. 1) aligns the spin magnetic dipole moments of hydrogen protons in the direction of the applied field.

Each proton, or dipole moment, precesses about the static field, at the Larmor frequency $f_0 = \gamma B_0$ (where $\gamma \approx 42.58$ MHz/tesla). A radio frequency magnetic field that oscillates at f_0, is applied using an appropriate coil (RF tx/rx coil in Fig. 1) in the direction transverse to B_0 and by choosing the pulse duration of the excitation, the magnetic dipole moments can be rotated into the transverse direction. The decaying signal following the pulse excitation is detected using a RF receiving antenna. Spatially varying magnetic fields are applied during the scan in order to make the magnetic field strength dependent on the position within the patient, providing a straightforward method to control where the protons are excited by the RF field. These varying magnetic fields are generated by passing currents through solenoids, known as gradient coils (see Fig. 1). For an image of high quality, the applied RF magnetic field should be uniform over all regions of the body being imaged since a non uniform field introduces distortion into the image.

Moreover, for maximum energy coupling into the hydrogen nuclei it is necessary to have an antenna that can generate circularly polarized fields. Birdcage and TEM coils have been designed to satisfy both of these requirements and will be briefly described in the following.

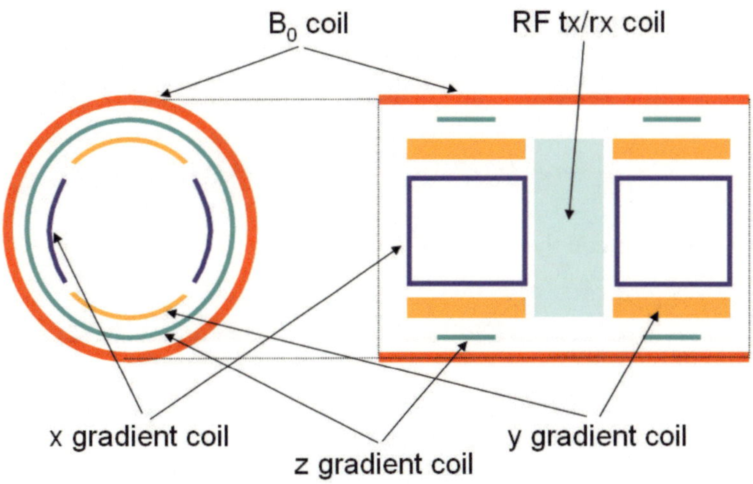

Fig. 1. MRI tomograph composed of five coils: one for the main static field B_0; three for the gradients and one for the RF transmission/reception

2.2 Birdcage coils

Birdcage coils are constituted by two conducting end-rings (ERs) connected by a number of conducting legs (rungs) distributed at equal spacing around the perimeter of the ERs (Jin, 1999). Capacitors are inserted into legs or ERs to achieve the tuning of the desired resonant mode. A low-pass (LP) coil has capacitors placed in the legs while a high-pass (HP) coil has the capacitors situated in ER segments. Fig. 2 shows a low-pass birdcage coil (a) and a high-pass birdcage coil (b) geometry modeled inside the commercial CAD Microwave Studio (MWS).

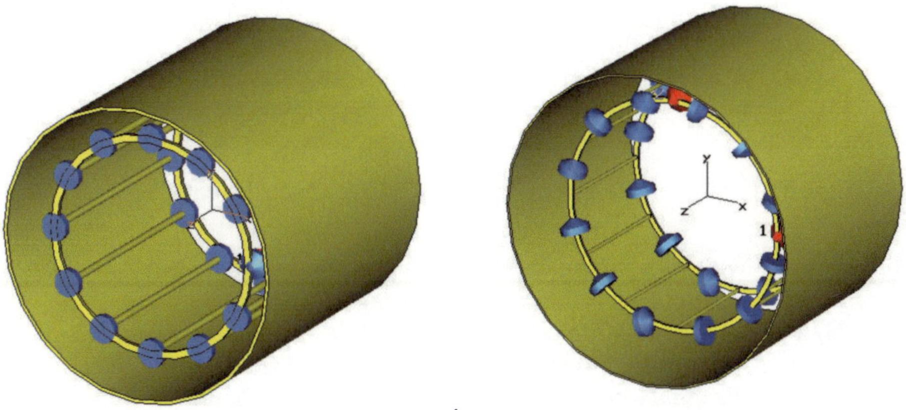

(a) (b)

Fig. 2. Low-pass birdcage coil (a); high-pass birdcage coil (b). Tuning capacitors are evidenced as blue disks

Capacitors are evidenced as blue disks and a cylindrical shield, that prevents the field from being radiated outside the coil, is added in the CAD model.

Birdcage coils are resonators characterized by more than one resonant mode: in fact, an N-leg coil has (N/2) + 1 distinct resonant modes (Jin, 1999). According to the theory reported in Giovannetti et al. (2002), the resonant frequencies for a low-pass birdcage are given by:

$$\omega_k = \left[C \left(Ler + Lleg / 2\sin^2 \frac{\pi k}{N} \right) \right]^{-1/2} \qquad (k = 0,1,2,....N/2) \tag{1}$$

Similarly, for a high-pass coil the resonant frequencies are:

$$\omega_k = \left[C \left(Ler + 2 \cdot Lleg \; 2\sin^2 \frac{\pi k}{N} \right) \right]^{-1/2} \qquad (k = 0,1,2,....N/2) \tag{2}$$

where *Lleg* represents the self-inductance of one leg, *C* the capacitance of the capacitor between two legs and *Ler* the self-inductance of the end-ring segments.
By applying a 50 Ω source between the leg and the ring (close to a capacitor) in the MWS model of the birdcage the reflection coefficient (S11) of the birdcage as a function of the frequency has been computed. Fig 3. shows the simulated magnitude of S11 for the low-pass birdcage coil (N = 12) shown in Fig. 2a. The seven resonances of the structure are evidenced in the figure as negative peaks in the spectrum. For the considered birdcage geometry the figure evidences a first resonance at about 128 MHz (B_0 = 3 T).

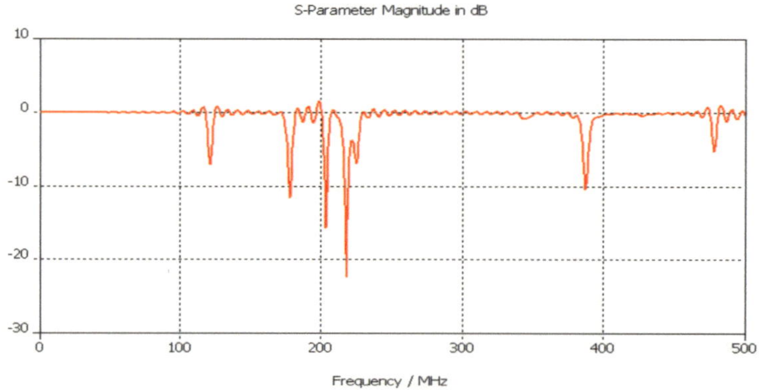

Fig. 3. Simulated S11 magnitude spectrum for the low-pass birdcage coil (N = 12) shown in Fig. 2a

For a birdcage coil with N legs, the current can be supposed to be constant along the legs with a co-sinusoidal amplitude variation among legs given by: I_k = cos 2 πk/N where k = 0,1,2,…N/2 is the mode order. Using the Biot-Savart equation, the magnetic field distribution can be computed from conductor currents associated with a given mode sustained by the birdcage. Note that the use of Biot-Savart equation implies a quasi-static magnetic field assumption, and it is valid when the coil dimensions are much smaller than the wavelength. For example, at 64 MHz (B_0 =1.5 T), the wavelength is 4.7 m; thus the quasi-static assumption holds for practical birdcage dimensions. This approximation also holds when increasing the static magnetic field strength, if the coil dimension decreases.
By using MWS the magnetic field inside the birdcage obtained by applying two excitation with 90° time phase shift in correspondence of two legs with 90° spatial shift has been

computed. This kind of excitation simulates the one usually adopted in real birdcages and produces a magnetic field with a circular clockwise polarization, with respect to the positive z-axis (see Fig. 2). A map of the computed magnetic field at 128 MHz (first resonance from the left in Fig. 3) on an axial (a) and a transversal (coronal) (b) section is reported in Fig. 4. The figure evidences a good uniformity of the field in the central region of the birdcage with the highest field values obtained in the region between the leg and the shield.

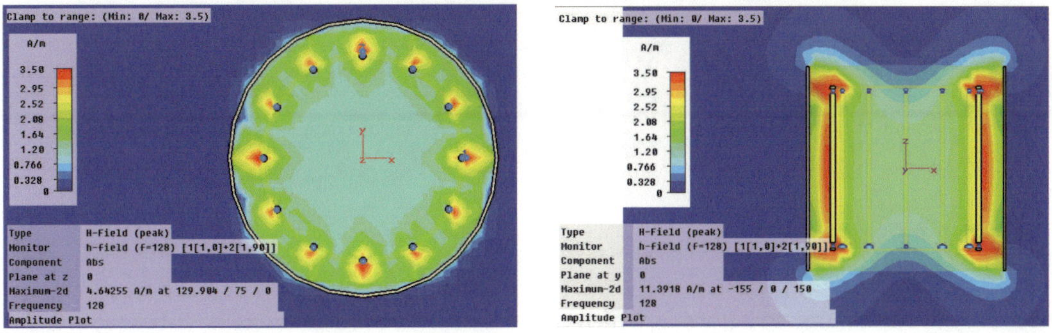

(a) (b)

Fig. 4. Maps of the computed magnetic field at 128 MHz inside the birdcage on axial (a) and transversal (coronal) (b) sections

2.3 TEM coils

The needs of using higher static magnetic fields B_0, and, consequently, higher Larmor frequencies for obtaining better MR images has introduced systems operating at 3 - 9.4 T (128 - 400 MHz). This development requires new types of antennas. One of the most commonly used is the transverse electromagnetic (TEM) coil proposed by Röschmann (1988) and Bridges (1988). These coils are based on TEM transmission lines with capacitive loads of various configurations, and have become known as "TEM resonators" (Röschmann, 1987).

The geometries of two TEM resonators are shown in Fig. 5. These resonators consist of multiple longitudinal conductors arranged in a circular cylindrical pattern and enclosed by a cylindrical shield with end-plates that form a cavity. Fig. 5 shows the most commonly used designs in which the inner conductors are metallic tubes (a) or strip conductors over a dielectric (b). The inner conductors connect to the end plates by tuning capacitors (blue disks in Fig. 5). These coils are driven by sources connected to the end of one or more conductors. Theoretical studies on TEM resonators have shown that they behave like loaded multiconductor transmission lines capable of supporting standing waves (Bogdanov & Ludwig 2002).

In the absence of excitation, and for symmetrically placed tubes, the condition for resonance results in:

$$\prod_{n=1}^{N}\left(1-\Gamma_n^{+}\Gamma_n^{-}e^{-2jk_n l}\right)=0 \qquad (3)$$

where Γ_n^+ and Γ_n^- are the modal decompositions of the reflection coefficients at the end of the lines and k_n is the wave number of mode n, which for TEM modes and lossless conductors is given by: $k_n = \omega_n/c$. The frequency response of the N = 12 element coil in Fig.

5a has been simulated by using MWS. The obtained return loss (S11 magnitude) at the input of this coil is shown in Fig. 6. It can be seen that N/2 + 1 = 7 modes are present.

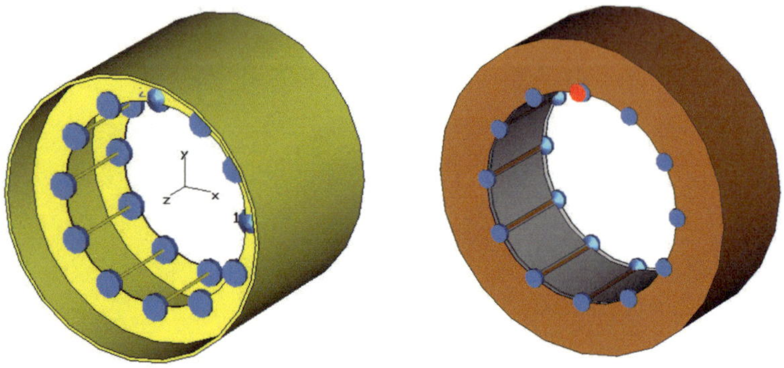

(a) (b)

Fig. 5. TEM resonators: structure in which the inner conductors are metallic tubes (a) or strip conductors over a dielectric (b). Capacitors are evidenced as blue disks.

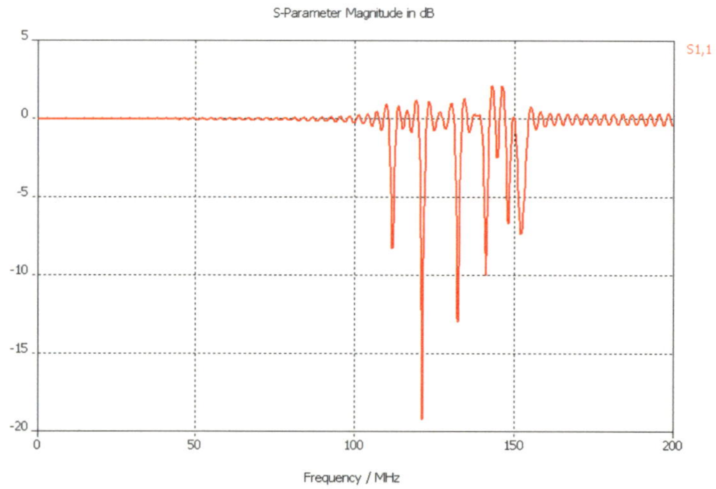

Fig. 6. Simulated S11 magnitude spectrum for the TEM resonator (N = 12) shown in Fig. 5a

The magnetic field distribution inside the coil can be determined by the conductor currents according to:

$$\underline{\mathbf{H}} = \sum_{n} \left[I_n^{m+} \underline{\underline{e^{-jk_n z}}} - I_n^{m-} \underline{\underline{e^{+jk_n z}}} \right] \underline{\mathbf{h}}_n(x, y) \tag{4}$$

where $\underline{\mathbf{h}}_n$ is the transverse vector mode function (Bogdanov & Ludwig 2002).
Because circular polarization is necessary to excite the MR signal, coils are commonly driven in quadrature so as to produce circularly-polarized fields. Fig. 7 shows a map of the magnetic field at 128 MHz (second resonance from the left in Fig. 6) computed by using MWS and the model reported in Fig. 5.a.

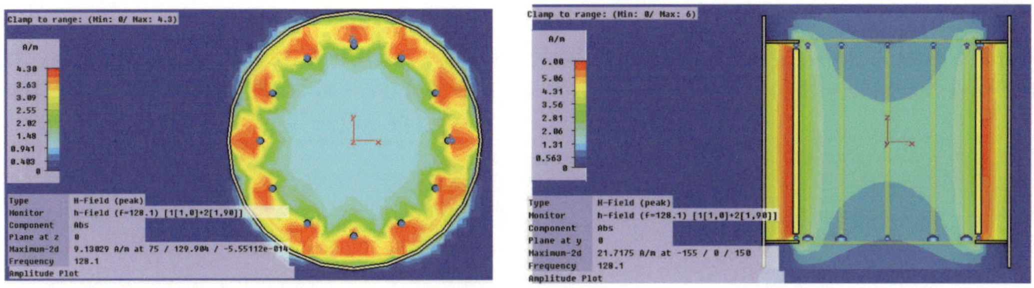

(a) (b)

Fig. 7. Maps of the computed magnetic field at 128 MHz inside the TEM coil on axial (a) and transversal (coronal) (b) sections

In particular, the figure shows maps on axial (a) and transversal (coronal) (b) sections. Similarly to the birdcage the figure evidences a good uniformity of the field in the central region, with the highest field values obtained in the region between the leg and the shield.

3. In vitro studies

In vitro studies are usually performed by using commercial MRI apparatus or dedicated experimental setups as the one shown in Fig. 8.

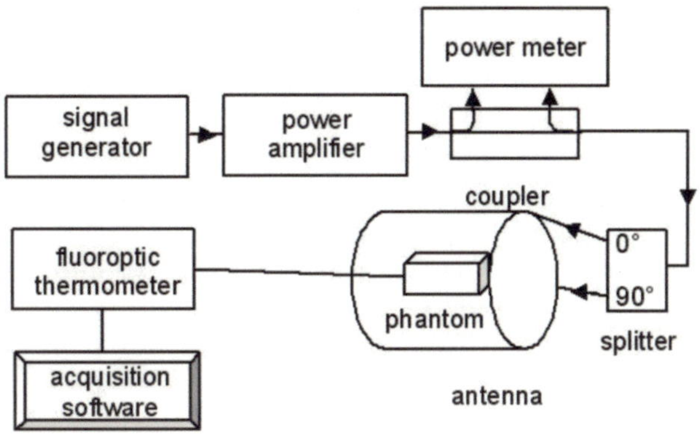

Fig. 8. Experimental setup

In the dedicated system of Fig. 8, the 64 MHz signal is first amplified and then sent to the antenna through a power splitter with 90° output shift. The applied RF power is monitored with a power meter. When commercial MRI systems are used, the pulse sequences used during regular clinical MR protocol are applied. The whole body SARs in a 80 kg body produced by the applied pulse levels and width are usually reported on the control display of the system.

Various human body models have been considered. During the experiments both with commercial MRI apparatus and dedicated experimental setup they are inserted inside the system antenna. The simplest phantom is constituted by a parallelepiped box (i.e 30 cm × 20 cm × 60 cm) filled with gelled saline material (i.e. HEC 2%, NaCl 0.36%) that mimics the electrical and thermal properties of an average human tissue at the considered frequency (for example at 64 MHz: ε_r = 78.2, σ = 0.6 S/m, K = 0.2 W/(m °C), C = 4178 J/(kg °C)) (Bassen et al., 2006; Pisa et al., 2008). A little bit more realistic is the phantom proposed by the American Society for Testing and Materials (ASTM) (ASTM 2007) in which a box model of the thorax (43.2 cm × 9 cm × 61 cm) is considered together with a head model, in the shape of a box (16.5 cm × 9 cm × 29.2 cm) (see Fig. 9.a).

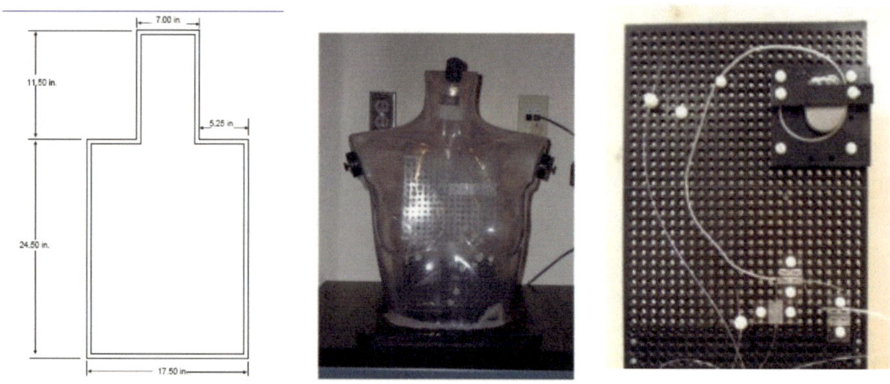

(a) (b) (c)

Fig. 9. ASTM phantom (a); human shaped trunk model (b); plastic grid with a PM (c)

Human shaped trunk models have been also realised by using torso-shaped transparent PVC phantoms (see Fig. 9b) (Mattei et al., 2008). Commercial PM and catheter are fixed to plastic grids (see Fig. 9c) and immersed in the phantom at a depth of about 1 cm inside the saline material.

Temperature increments are monitored via non perturbing thermometers. As an example, the Luxtron 3100 fluoroptic™ equipped with SMM probes can be cited. These sensors can reach an accuracy of 0.1 °C at the point of calibration.

Specific absorption rate (SAR) values are extrapolated from initial temperature rise rate through the equation:

$$SAR = C \left. \frac{dT}{dt} \right|_{t=0} \quad [\mathrm{W/kg}] \tag{5}$$

In order to reduce the thermal diffusion influence on SAR determination, the temperature variation is usually computed between 3 and 10 s from the beginning of the exposure. Moreover, the probe positioning close to the catheter must be accurately chosen in order to avoid strong errors in temperature and SAR evaluations (Mattei et al., 2007).

3.1 Experimental results

In order to investigate the amount of heating in the heart tissue around the catheter tip in patients implanted with pacemakers many in vitro (on phantom) studies have been performed.

Achenbach et al. (1997) exposed 11 PM inside a commercial MRI scan. For a particular PM lead, they reported a temperature increase of 63.1 °C after 90 s of exposure. In other seven electrodes the temperature increase exceeded 15 °C.

Sommer et al. (2000) exposed 21 PM models with 44 PM electrodes to MRI scanner using a pulse sequence that produces a whole body SAR of 1.3 W/kg. The PM catheters were inserted into the right ventricle of an isolate porcine heart, connected to a PM case and placed inside a box model of the thorax. The obtained temperature increases ranged from 0.1 to 23.5 °C, depending on the electrode type.

Roguin et al. (2004) applied to PMs placed in a box model of the thorax sequences with SAR less than 1.4 W/kg (regular clinical MR protocol) and 3.54 W/kg (non clinical protocol). Non clinical protocol gave rise to temperature increments at the catheter tip from 1.5 to 5.7 °C, while for clinical protocol the maximal heating was 0.9 °C.

Shellock et al. (2007) tested modern-day (manufactured after year 2000) pacemakers with an experimental set-up like the one shown in Fig. 8 and using the ASTM phantom. Temperature increments were lower than 0.5 °C for scan of the head and lumbar regions with SAR up to 3 W/kg. For the chest area temperature increases ranged between 0.4 to 3.6 °C at SAR of 2.0 W/kg.

Mattei et al., (2008) performed various measurements aimed at the identification of the major contributions involved in the heat generation. In particular they varied the position of the implant, inside box and human shaped phantoms, the length of the wire, the thickness of the insulation sheath, the wire geometries (shape) and the position of the implant including its lead with respect to the RF coil. They found that closer locations of the leads to the edge of the phantom and to the edge of the coil produce maximum heating. The lead length is the other crucial factor, whereas the implant area does not seem to have a major role in the induced temperature increase. Also the lead structure and the geometry of the phantom revealed to be elements that can significantly modify the amount of heating.

4. Numerical studies

Numerical studies on the interaction between RF field produced by MRI systems and PM can help in understanding the interaction mechanisms between the field and the PM and can be used to study SAR distributions and temperature increments produced by MRI apparatus inside realistic human body models (Pisa et al., 2010).

4.1 Human body models

In numerical studies the body models used in experiments (see Par. 3) can be used. For more realistic evaluations, anatomically heterogeneous body models have been realized. These models consist of large datasets obtained from MRI, CT, and anatomical images. To be used for computational electromagnetic dosimetry these digital data sets must be converted to a so-called "segmented" version. A segmented model is a model where every pixel, usually called in such models "voxel", contains a label which is uniquely associated to a given tissue. In such a way, it is possible to know which tissue fills each of the model voxels and hence assign the correct complex permittivity values to be used in numerical simulations.

In 1988, a high resolution human model has been obtained starting from the "Visible Human Project", developed by the National Library of Medicine (Ackerman, 1998). The Visible human is a 3-D digital image library representing an adult human male and female (see Fig. 10a).

The data sets for both the male and female include photographic images obtained through cryosectioning of human cadavers, and digital images obtained through computer tomography and magnetic resonance imaging of the same cadavers. The segmentation

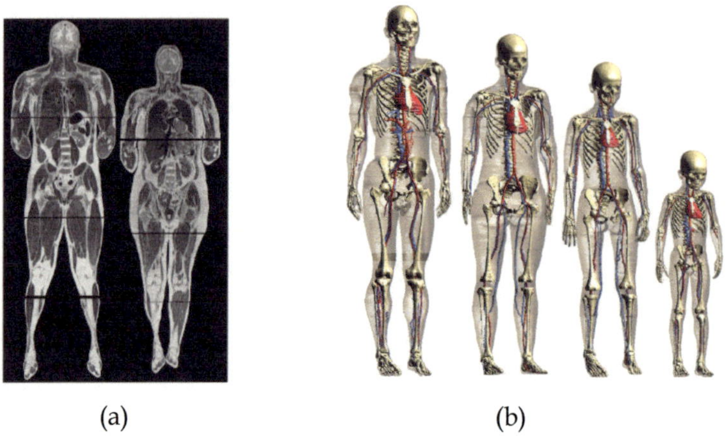

Fig. 10. Visible human male and female (a); virtual family (b)

procedure has been carried out for the male model by researchers at the Air Force Research Laboratory, Brooks Air Force Base, Texas, USA (Mason et al., 2000). The final segmented model comprises 586×340×1878 voxels with a resolution of 1×1×1 mm^3, and is segmented in about 40 different tissue types.

More recently Christ et al. (2010) have developed four anatomically correct whole body human models: an adult male (34 years old), an adult female (26 years old), and two children (an 11-year-old girl and a six-year-old boy) (see Fig. 10b). These four models are referred to as the Virtual Family and are based on high resolution magnetic resonance (MR) images of healthy volunteers. More than 80 different tissue types were distinguished during the segmentation.

4.2 Catheter models

Various catheter models have been proposed in literature. The most used is a simple bare cylindrical copper wire (see Fig. 11a) with various diameters and lengths (Ho, 2001; Golombeck & Dossel, 2004; Stuchly et al., 2006; Pisa et al., 2008), while a more realistic version is constituted by a copper wire covered with plastic (see Fig. 11b). This last catheter

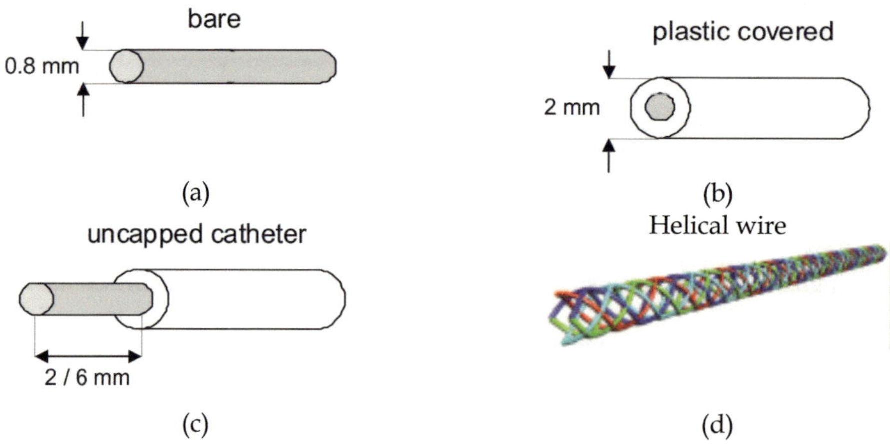

Fig. 11. Bare (a), plastic covered (b), uncapped (c), and helical wire (d), catheters

model has been further improved by removing between 2 and 6 mm of plastic from the tip (uncapped catheters) (see Fig. 11c) (Park et al., 2005; Pisa et al., 2010).
More recently, helical wire models have been proposed (see Fig. 11d) (Bassen et al. 2006; Neufeld et al., 2009). In particular Neufeld et al., (2009) realized their catheter staring from a 0.6 mm thick wire wound to form a helix and including a 10-mm long straight section. The helical wire is insulated by a thin coating (0.012 mm).

4.3 Pacemaker and body placement

The whole numerical set-up is made by a PM embedded inside a body model in turn inserted inside a coil. The PM is constituted by various lengths of the previously described catheters and by a metallic model of the casing. In the simplified models of the thorax the PM is inserted at a depth of about 1 cm inside the phantom following a planar geometry and the phantom is inserted inside the antenna (see Fig. 12a and 12b). When more realistic body models are considered the catheter follows the vein path with a placement approximating the clinical one from the casing to the heart and the anatomical model is inserted inside the coil (see Fig. 12c)

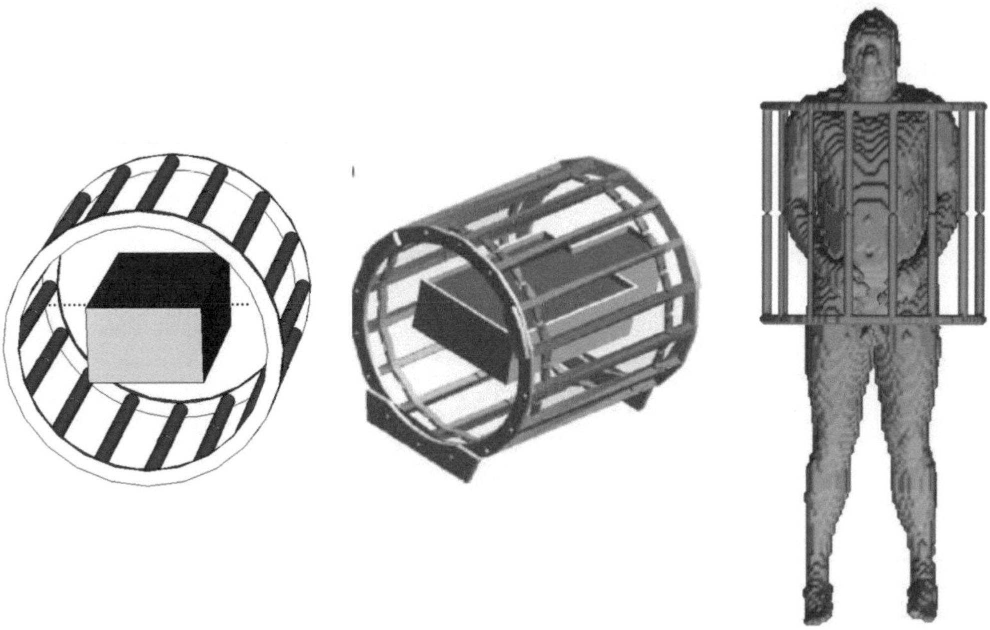

(a) (b) (c)

Fig. 12. Box (a), ASTM (b), and VH models inserted inside RF coils

4.4 Numerical results

The above cited human body and PM models have been used to study the interaction of the RF field produced by MRI antennas and pacemaker holders. These studies have been performed by using numerical technique for the solution of the EM and thermal problem, respectively. Among the EM solvers those based on the finite difference time domain (FDTD) technique are the most popular (Taflove & Hagness, 2000) but also the method of

moments (MoM) has been largely used (Burke & Poggio, 1981). For the solution of the thermal problem the Bio-heat equation (Pennes, 1948) has been solved by means of explicit or implicit (ADI) solutions (Bernardi et al., 2003; Pisa et al., 2003). In particular, the method of moments (MoM) (Park et al., 2005; Nyenhuis et al., 2005) and a conformal finite difference time domain (FDTD) method (Pisa et al., 2008) together with a finite difference solution of the bioheat equation have been used for studying the current along the catheter and the temperature distribution around the electrode tip produced by a realistic PM immersed in a homogeneous medium. For bare catheters, the obtained temperature rise ranges from 1 to 28 °C depending on the catheter length and position. Moreover, a commercially available computer aided design (CAD) has been used for evaluating the SAR distribution produced in a realistic human model by a coarse catheter model (1 cm diameter, 8 cm length) implanted in the heart region (Ho, 2001). With this model, a peak SAR averaged over 1 g of 2 W/kg near the metallic implant (compared to the value of 1.8 W/kg at the same location without the metallic implant) has been computed and no appreciable heating has been obtained. Similar results have been obtained in Golombeck & Dossel (2004) and Stuchly et al. (2006).
In order to investigate the effects of the PM geometrical parameters Pisa et al (2008) studied the exposure to a power of 100 W at 64 MHz of a box model of the thorax in the presence of a pacemaker with a unipolar catheter. A PM with a 60-cm long catheter (l_1 = 10 cm, l_2 = 26 cm, l_3 = 10 cm, l_4 = 14 cm in Fig. 13a) was placed inside the thorax. The PM was located in the left side in a typical operating position with the catheter tip 7.5 cm from the pacemaker.

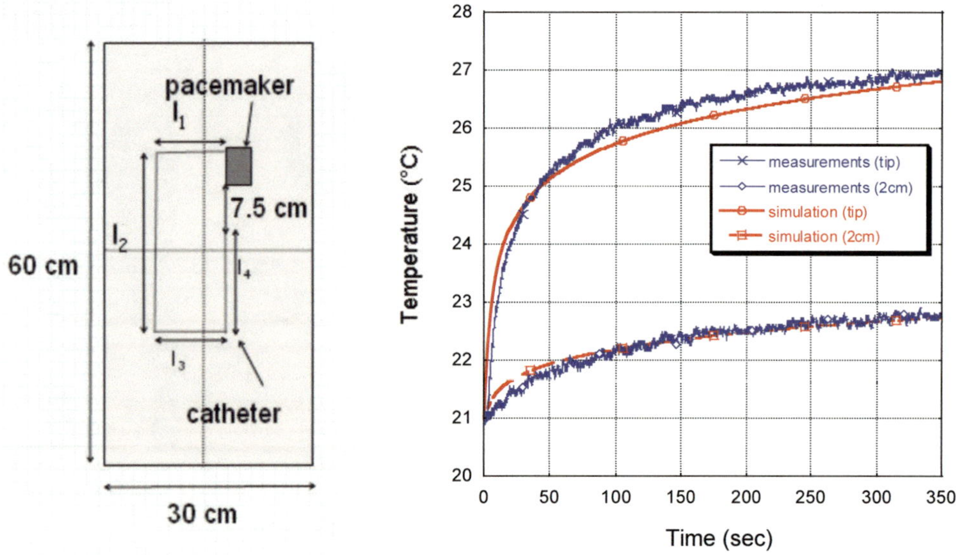

(a) (b)

Fig. 13. Section of the phantom model 1 cm below the phantom surface showing the geometry of the PM and catheter (a); time behaviour of the temperature on the experimental and numerical phantom at the catheter tip (b)

The exposure has been simulated by using the C-GM-FDTD code for the solution of the EM problem and the ADI-FD code for the solution of Fourier's equation. In the EM simulations the PM has been modeled as a copper box (40×10×50 mm^3) and the 60-cm long catheter has been modeled has a cylindrical wire of copper with a radius of 0.4 mm. This numerical setup simulates the one adopted in experiments (Pisa et al., 2006). Fig. 13b shows the time behavior of the simulated and measured temperature. After 6-min exposure, a temperature increment of 6 °C at a point just above the catheter tip and 1.8 °C at a point 2 cm below the catheter tip, can be observed, with a good agreement between measurements and simulations. SAR_{PEAK} of 2400 W/kg have been obtained at the catheter tip with a SAR_{WB} of about 1.0 W/kg.

The current distribution along the catheter has been computed as the circulation of the magnetic field around the catheter axis. Fig. 14a shows the obtained current distribution. The distance along the wire from the point in which the catheter is inserted in the pacemaker is reported on the horizontal axis (the catheter length is 60 cm).

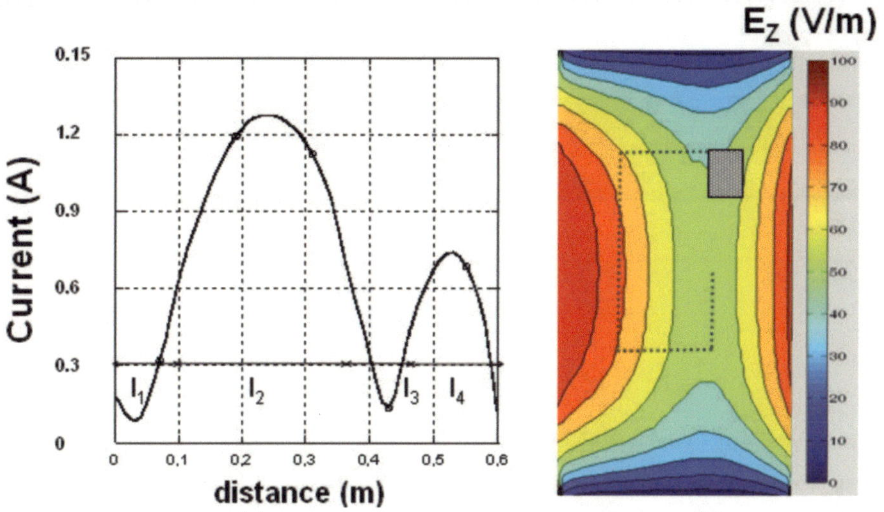

(a) (b)

Fig. 14. Current distribution along the catheter (a), maps of the computed unperturbed electric field in the coronal section passing through the catheter (b)

The obtained current distributions can be explained observing that at 64 MHz and in the presence of the dielectric phantom the wavelength is about 50 cm and hence comparable with the catheter length. Moreover the current inside the wire is mainly produced by the electric field component, obtained in the absence of the wire (unperturbed field in Fig. 14b), parallel to the wire axis. Correspondingly, in the considered exposure condition the strongest currents are produced by the E_z field along the l_2 and l_4 segments while lower currents are produced by the lower E_x component, acting on l_1 and l_3.

A further study has been performed in order to investigate the effect of the catheter cross-section on SAR. To this end, two more wires, of radius 0.2 and 0.8 mm, respectively, have been considered. The simulation results, for a circularly polarized magnetic field, have evidenced that the SAR values at the catheter tip increase when the wire section reduces. SAR_{PEAK} values of 2500 and 760 W/kg have been obtained for wire radius of 0.2 and 0.8 mm, respectively. It is worth noting that the increase of the wire radius determines an

increase of the current along the wire and at the tip. However, the corresponding increase of the section produces a reduction of the current density and hence the final effect is a reduction of the SAR at the catheter tip.
The effect of the catheter length has been also investigated by considering catheters with a 0.4-mm radius and different lengths. In the considered simulations the distance between the catheter tip and the pacemaker has been maintained equal to 7.5 cm while the length of the catheter has been changed. Fig. 15 shows the results obtained for a total length of 32 cm (l_1 = 7 cm, l_2 = 15 cm, l_3 = 7 cm, l_4 = 3 cm) and for a total length of 44 cm (l_1 = 10 cm, l_2 = 18 cm, l_3 = 10 cm, l_4 = 6 cm). In these simulations SAR_{PEAK} of 1000 and 1400 W/kg have been obtained for the two considered lengths.

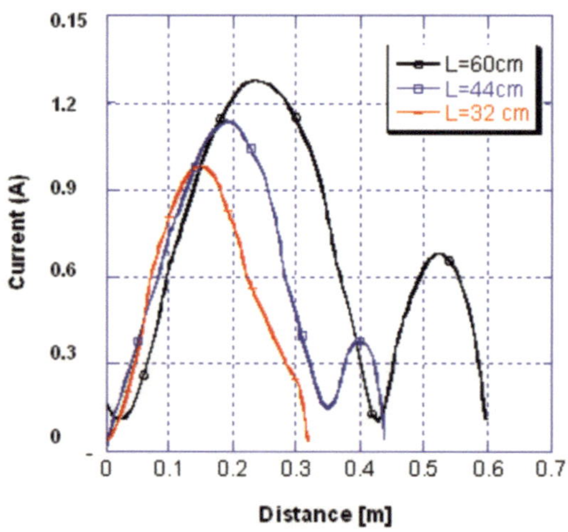

Fig. 15. Current distribution along the catheter for catheters of different lengths

In order to evaluate SAR and temperature distributions in a pacemaker holder in the presence of a more realistic model of the thorax and of the PM, a PM (see Fig. 16a) has been inserted inside the left part of the thorax of the VH model. The obtained model has then been inserted inside the birdcage (see Fig. 12c) and exposed to a 64 MHz left polarized field with a radiated power of 60 W.
Fig. 16b shows the current along the catheter, as a function of the distance from the point in which the catheter is inserted in the metallic box, obtained by considering a plastic covered (PC), a bare (BA), and two uncapped catheters (uncapped for 2 mm (M2) and uncapped for 6 mm (M6)).
The figure shows that for the bare catheter, the current distribution experiences strong variations with the position; these variations, as evidenced in (Pisa et al., 2008), are directly related to the distribution of the electric field parallel to the catheter axis. The presence of the plastic cover makes the current along the catheter smoother; moreover, in the M2 and M6 cases a strong reduction in the current is observed in correspondence of the tip where the catheter is uncapped.
The SAR_{PEAK} at the catheter tip is 15, 700, 2400, and 11900 W/kg for the bare, 6 mm uncapped, 2 mm uncapped, and plastic covered catheters, respectively. These results show that the PC catheter gives rise to the strongest SAR_{PEAK} value while the bare catheter

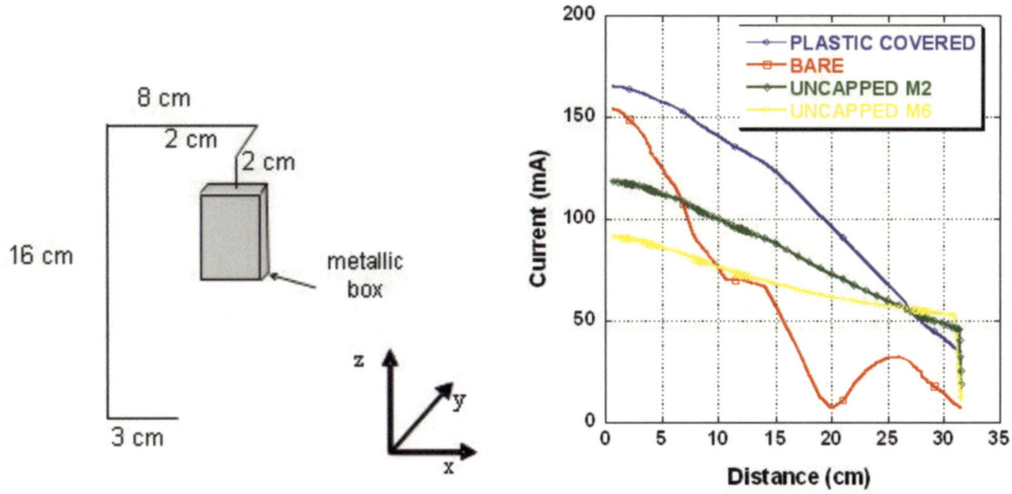

(a) (b)

Fig. 16. Metallic box equipped with a cylindrical catheter (a) and current along the catheter as a function of the distance from the point in which the catheter is inserted in the PM (b)

causes the lowest one with a SAR reduction factor of about 800. Intermediate SAR_{PEAK} values are obtained with the two partially capped catheters and the whole set of simulated data is within the range of experimental results reported in literature by considering various PM configurations (Mattei et a., 2008). The SAR_{10g} values grow from 0.8 W/kg for the BA to 9.7 W/kg for the PC catheter. Finally, the presence of the PM does not affect significantly the SAR_{WB}.

In order to assess the thermal risk associated with the computed SAR values, the graded mesh ADI solution of the bioheat equation has been applied considering the plastic covered catheter that, on the basis of our results, gives rise to the highest SAR. Fig. 17 shows temperature versus time at the catheter tip computed by neglecting the perfusion, in the presence of perfusion, and by adding the convection at the heart-blood interface. In the first case, temperature increments of more than 30 °C after 10 min exposure are obtained and the time behavior indicates an exponentially growing trend with a time constant of the order of hours. The presence of blood perfusion reduces temperature increments to 13.5 °C and, in this case, the steady state is reached in a few minutes. Finally, the presence of convection further reduces temperature increments to less than 13 °C and 12 °C for HB (blood convection coefficient) equal to 100 or 1000 W/($m^2 \cdot$°C), respectively. The results indicate that when blood perfusion is taken into account, a factor of three reduction of temperature increments is obtained with respect to the condition in which only the C and K terms are considered. However, the increments are still higher than those indicated as safe in the ICNIRP Statement (2004).

A further result of this study is that a thermal model considering only the K, C, B terms of the BHE and neglecting HB allows a worst case estimation of temperature elevations without significantly overestimating the real temperature distributions. Under these conditions, temperature increments of 0.2, 1.9, and 5.8 °C, after 10 min exposure, are obtained for the BA, UC-M6, and UC-M2 catheters, respectively.

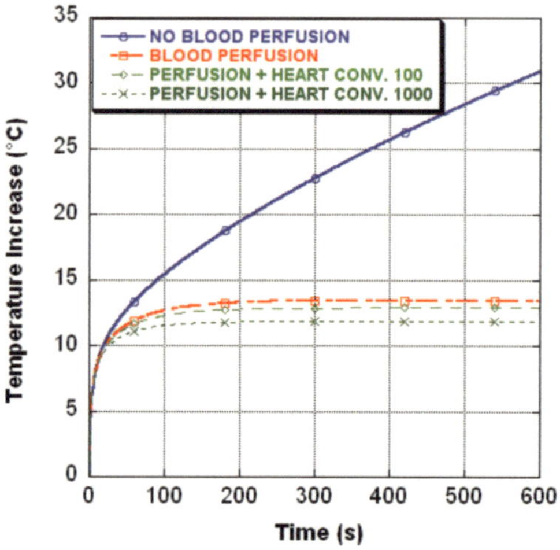

Fig. 17. Temperature increases at the catheter tip computed by neglecting the perfusion, and in the presence of perfusion

5. Conclusion

In this chapter the studies available in the literature and concerning SAR distributions and temperature increments in PM holders, exposed to the field generated by MRI apparatus, have been described in order to evidence the main factors influencing the obtained SAR values and temperature increments.

After a preliminary description of MRI apparatus in terms of field sources and distributions, the main in vitro (on phantoms), and numerical literature results have been presented. SAR distributions and temperature increments in PM holders, exposed inside an MRI apparatus, have been evaluated by using an anatomically based human body phantom together with fine pacemaker models equipped with different kinds of catheters, implanted following the vein path. This study has been performed by using a conformal FDTD code with graded mesh for the solution of the electromagnetic (EM) problem, and a finite difference solution of the bioheat equation with graded mesh, that includes blood perfusion in the tissues and convection at the heart-blood and skin-air interfaces, for the evaluation of the corresponding temperature increments.

The principal results of the study carried out are:

- The region with the highest SAR values is the one around the catheter tip where the current flowing along the catheter wire can induce strong current densities in the tissues.
- The current along the catheter is mainly induced by the electric field parallel to the catheter axis. Since strong E-field z-components are present, the highest currents are induced along vertical wires.
- Generally, shorter catheters with shorter vertical wires give rise to lower SAR at the catheter tip. Moreover, SAR values at the catheter tip increase when the wire section reduces. In fact, the increase of the wire radius determines an increase of the current

along the wire and at the tip. The corresponding increase of the section produces a reduction of the current density and hence the final effect is a reduction of the SAR at the catheter tip.

- The presence of a plastic cover increases the current along the catheter and, consequently, the SAR_{PEAK} at the catheter tip. In particular, the PC catheter gives rise to the strongest SAR_{PEAK} value, while the BA catheter causes the lowest one with an SAR reduction factor of about 800.
- In the VH model with the PC catheter, temperature increments of more than 30 °C after 10 min exposure are obtained and the time behaviour indicates an exponentially growing trend with a time constant of the order of hours. The presence of blood perfusion reduces temperature increments to about 13 °C and, in this case, the steady state is reached in a few minutes. The presence of convection further reduces temperature increments to less than 12 °C. These results indicate that when blood perfusion is taken into account, a three-fold reduction on temperature increments is obtained with respect to the case in which only the C and K terms are considered. However, the increments are still higher than those indicated as safe in ICNIRP (2004).
- In the worst case condition and after 10 min exposure, temperature increments in the 0.2 – 20 °C range are obtained on the heart muscle depending on the catheter and body model.
- Closer locations of the PM to the edge of the phantom and to the edge of the coil produce maximum heating.

A further result of this study is that in order to reduce temperature increments below safe levels and hence make MRI possible to PM holders, it is important to reduce the induced currents along the catheter wires. This can be accomplished, for example, by inserting lumped coils along the catheter or by using plastic insulating material with RF losses or, finally, by imaging only parts of the human body far from the PM, such as for example the head and lumbar regions.

6. References

Achenbach S., Moshage B., Diem W., Bieberle T., Schibgilla V. & Bachmann K. (1997), Effects of magnetic resonance imaging on cardiac pacemakers and electrodes, *Am. Heart. J.*, Vol. 134, No. 3, pp. 467-473.

Ackerman M. J. (1998), The Visible Human Project, Proc. IEEE, Vol. 86, pp. 504.

ASTM International Std F218202a (2007), Standard Test Method for Measurement of Radio Frequency Induced Heating Near Passive Implants During Magnetic Resonance Imaging, West Conshohocken, PA, 19428-2959 USA.

Bassen H., Kainz W., Mendoza G. & Kellom T. (2006), MRI-induced heating of selected thin wire metallic implants – laboratory and computational studies – findings and new questions raised. *Minim. Invasive Ther.*, Vol. 15, No 2, pp. 76-84.

Bernardi P., Cavagnaro M., Pisa S. & Piuzzi E. (2003), Specific absorption rate and temperature elevation in a subject exposed in the far-field of radio-frequency sources operating in the 10-900-MHz range, *IEEE Trans. Biomed. Eng.* , Vol. 50, No. 3, pp. 295-304.

Bernardi P., Cavagnaro M., Pisa S., & Piuzzi E. (2009), Safety aspects of magnetic resonance imaging for pacemaker holders, in Proceedings of ICEAA '09 (International Conference on Electromagnetics in Advanced Applications), Turin, Italy, pp. 869-872.

Bogdanov G. & Ludwig R. (2002), Coupled microstrip line transverse electromagnetic resonator model for high-field magnetic resonance imaging, *Magn Res in Med* Vol. 47, pp. 579–593.

Bridges J.F. (1988), Cavity resonator with improved magnetic field uniformity for high frequency operation and reduced dielectric heating in NMR imaging devices, U.S. Patent 4 751 464.

Burke J. & Poggio A. (1981), *Numerical electromagnetics code (NEC) – Method of moments*, Lawrence Livermore Nat. Lab., Livermore, CA, Tech. Rep. UCID-18834.

Christ A., Kainz W.,. Hahn E.G, Honegger K., Zefferer M., Neufeld E., Rascher W., Janka R., Bautz W., Chen J., Kiefer B., Schmitt P., Hollenbach H.P., Oberle M., Szerba D., Kam A., Guag J.W. & Kuster N. (2010), The virtual family - development of anatomical CAD models of twoadults and two children for dosimetric simulations, *Physics in Medicine and Biology*, Vol. 55, pp. 23-38.

Giovannetti G., Landini L., Santarelli M.F. & Postano V. (2002), A fast and accurate simulator for the design of birdcage coils in MRI. *Magn Reson Mat in Phys Biol and Med* , Vol. 15, pp. 36-40.

Golombeck M.-A. & Dossel O. (2004), MR-Tomography on patients with heart pacemakers - a numerical study, *Proc. 2004 IEEE EMBS Int. Conf.*, San Francisco USA, pp. 1076-1079.

Ho H.S. (2001), Safety of metallic implants in magnetic resonance imaging, *J. Magn. Reson. Imaging*, Vol. 14, No. 4, pp. 472–477.

ICNIRP (2004), Statement on: medical magnetic resonance (MR) procedures: protection of patients, *Health Phys.*, Vol. 87, No 2, pp. 197-216.

Jin J. (1999), Electromagnetic Analysis and Design in Magnetic Resonance Imaging, CRC Press, Boca Raton, FL, USA.

Mason, P.A., Hurt, W.D., Walters, T.J., D'Andrea, J.A., Gajsek, P., Ryan, K.L., Nelson, D.A., Smith, K.I. & Ziriax, J.M., 2000, Effects of frequency, permittivity, and voxel size on predicted specific absorption rate values in biological tissue during electromagnetic-field exposure, *IEEE Trans. Microwave Theory Tech.*, Vol. 48, ,pp. 2050-2058.

Mattei E., Triventi M., Calcagnini G., Censi F., Kainz W., Bassen H.I. & Bartolini P. (2007): Temperature and SAR measurement errors in the evaluation of metallic linear structures heating during MRI using fluoroptic probes. *Phys. Med. Biol.*, Vol. 52, No 6, pp. 1633-1646.

Mattei E., Triventi M., Calcagnini G., Censi F., Kainz W., Mendoza G., Bassen H.I. & Bartolini P. (2008): Complexity of MRI induced heating on metallic leads: Experimental measurements of 374 configurations, *BioMedical Engineering OnLine*, Vol. 7, No 11.

Neufeld E., Kuhn S., Szekely G. & Kuster N. (2009), Measurement, simulation and uncertainty assessment of implant heating during MRI, *Phys. Med. Biol.*, Vol. 54, pp. 4151-4169.

Nyenhuis J. A., Park S.M. & Kamondetdacha R. (2005), MRI and implanted medical devices: basic interactions with an emphasis on heating, *IEEE Trans. Dev. Mat. Reliab.*, Vol. 5, No 3, pp. 467-480.

Park S.M., Kamondetdacha R., Amjad A. & Nyenhuis J.A. (2005), MRI safety: RF induced heating on straight wires, *IEEE Trans. Magn.*, Vol. 41, No. 10, pp. 4197–4199.

Pennes H.H. (1948), Analysis of tissue and arterial blood temperatures in resting forearm, *J. Appl. Physiol.*, Vol. 1, pp. 93-122.

Pisa S., Cavagnaro M., Piuzzi E., Bernardi P. & Lin J.C. (2003), Power density and temperature distributions produced by interstitial arrays of sleeved-slot antennas for hyperthermic cancer therapy, *IEEE Trans. Microwave Theory Tech.*, vol. 51, No. 12, pp. 2418-2426.

Pisa S, Calcagnini G, Cavagnaro M, Piuzzi E, Triventi M, Bernardi P (2006). SAR and temperature elevations in pacemaker holders exposed to EM fields produced by MRI apparatus. in 2006 IEEE MTT-S International Microwave Symposium Digest, San Francisco: 1754-1757.

Pisa S., Calcagnini G., Cavagnaro M., Piuzzi E., Mattei E. & Bernardi P. (2008), A study of the interaction between implanted pacemakers and the radio-frequency field produced by magnetic resonance imaging apparatus, *IEEE Trans. Electromag. Compat.*, Vol. 50, No. 1, pp. 35-42.

Pisa S., Bernardi P., Cavagnaro M. & Piuzzi E. (2010), Power absorption and temperature elevation produced by magnetic resonance apparatus in the thorax of patients with implanted pacemakers, *IEEE Trans. Electromag. Compat.*, Vol. 52, No. 1, pp. 32-40.

Pisa S., Bernardi P., Cavagnaro M. & Piuzzi E. (2010), Interaction between the RF field of MRI apparatus and pacemaker Holders, Proc. ICEmB Conference, Genova, Italy, pp. 21-22.

Roguin A., Zviman M.M., Meininger G.R., Rodrigues E.R., Dickfeld T.M., Bluemke D.A., Lardo A., Berger R.D., Calkins H. & Halperin H.R. (2004), Modern pacemaker and implantable cardioverter/defibrillator systems can be magnetic resonance imaging safe. In vitro and in vivo assessment of safety and function at 1.5 T, *Circulation*, Vol. 110, No. 5, pp. 475-482.

Röschmann P. (1987), Radiofrequency penetration and absorption in the human body: Limitations to high-field whole-body nuclear magnetic resonance imaging. *Med Phys*, Vol. 14, pp. 922–932.

Röschmann P. (1988), High-frequency coil system for a magnetic resonance imaging apparatus, U.S. Patent 4 746 866.

Shellock F.G., Fischer L. & Fieno, S. (2000), Cardiac pacemakers and implantable cardioverter defibrillators: in vitro magnetic resonance imaging evaluation at 1.5-Tesla, *Journal of Cardiovascular magnetic resonance*, Vol. 9, pp. 21-31.

Sommer T., Vahlhaus C., Lauck G., von Smekal A., Reinke M., Hofer U., Bloch W., Traber F., Schneider C., Gieseke J., Jung W. & Schild H. (2000), MR imaging and cardiac pacemaker: in-vitro evaluation and in-vivo studies in 51 patients at 0.5 T, *Radiology*, Vol. 215, No. 3, pp. 869-879.

Stuchly M.A., Abrishamkar H. & Strydom M.L. (2006), Numerical evaluation of radio frequency power deposition in human models during MRI, *Proc. 2006 IEEE EMBS Int. Conf.*, New York City USA, pp. 272-275.

Taflove A. & Hagness S.C. (2000), Computational Electrodynamics: The Finite-Difference Time-Domain Method. Boston, MA: Artech House.

12

Adverse Interactions between ICD and Permanent Pacemaker Systems

Dirk Bastian and Klaus Fessele
Klinikum Nürnberg
Germany

1. Introduction

After the introduction of the implantable cardioverter defibrillator (ICD) in clinical practice by Mirowski in 1980 [Mirowski et al., 1980] the first available devices offered only a basic ventricular pacing option. Since approximately 5-20% of patients with an indication for ICD therapy following implantation criteria at that time (secondary prevention) needed antibradycardia pacing as well, the implantation of an additional pacemaker (PM) was often necessary up to the 1990s [Sticherling et al., 1997; Brooks et al, 1995; Geiger et al., 1997]. In contrast, the modern ICD systems offer all forms of antitachycardia and antibradycardia therapy integrated in one device. However in 1997 Sticherling et al. concluded in their review about combined ICD and antibradycardia pacing therapy, that even with the introduction of integrated devices the issue of interactions will stay clinically relevant, as many candidates for ICD implantation present with an already implanted pacemaker system [Sticherling et al., 1997]. In contrast to this prediction, today more than 10 years later, through the tremendous advances in device technology as well as in implantation and revision operation methods, the patients are rare, who are fitted with two separate active cardiac implantable electronic devices (CIED) for antibradycardia and antitachycardia therapy respectively. However these patients require extreme diligence at implantation, testing, programming and follow-up to avoid potentially dangerous interactions between the devices.

„Concomitant implantation of AICD and a permanent pacemaker requires an understanding of the functioning of both devices and their potential interactions" [Singer et al., 1988]

2. Indications and how to avoid simultaneous use of two active CIEDs

As mentioned above, the CIEDs available today offer all known antibradycardia and antitachycardia therapies including cardiac resynchronization therapy (CRT). Thus it is possible to provide each patient at first implantation with an adequate singular device according to his rhythmological indication. Today there is no indication for the primary simultaneous implantation of two separate CIEDs!

However the situation remains complex in patients, who were already treated with one CIED, but need a system upgrade in the further course due to different reasons. Currently typical clinical indications are the need for antitachycardia and/or cardiac resynchronization therapy in pacemaker patients.

In these particular cases careful preparation and planning of the operative procedure is extremely important. The pulse generator pocket and the scar need to be assessed. Before operation the function and position of old leads are reviewed and a decision is made regarding which leads will be continued to be used, be abandoned or extracted.

An essential requirement for ipsilateral implantation of new leads is an open vascular access route. In 25-33% of patients with an implanted device, a significant stenosis (> 50% stenosis) or even occlusion of the involved axillary, subclavian, brachiocephalic vein or superior vena cava (SVC) is encountered [Minden & Butter, 2008]. Therefore a periphereal phlebography should be performed before an upgrading procedure. Blood flow from the distal periphery, possible access sites, central draining into the SVC, valves and stenosis formation are evaluated. If there is a distal stenosis of the axillary or subclavian vein a more proximal entry into the vessel might be successful, although the long term risk of mechanical lead alteration is increased. If the subclavian vein or SVC show a central stenosis, but a proximal flow can still be seen, it is often possible to pass the stenosis using access to the axillary vein and a hydrophilic wire. A long sheath is introduced over the wire and the lead is positioned with the sheath still in place. Of course the risk of occlusion of the vessel is increased significantly after such a procedure, but the number of intravascular leads is reduced by the usage of old leads compared to performing a complete new implantation on the contralateral side. Leads that are implanted for less than two years can often be extracted by conventional means, thereby further decreasing the number of remaining leads.

In our institution an ipsilateral upgrade is pursued as general rule. Thus the contralateral side remains intact and is accessible for subsequent interventions, if needed, which is especially important for younger patients with expected long duration of implanted devices. If an ipsilateral upgrade is planned, the side of the old pulse generator needs to be taken into account as well. When upgrading a right sided pacemaker to ICD, a high-energy device should be used [Natale et al., 1997]. For upgrading to CRT different guiding catheters are needed for a right sided compared to a left sided approach.

If the patient already has an adequate antibradycardia PM it may seem to be a theoretical option to implant just a new ICD-system on the contralateral side. The pacemaker would keep up the antibradycardia therapy and the new ICD would act as antitachycardia system. The basic advantage would be to make the procedure a simpler one, equivalent in logistics and operation technique to the implantation of an ICD as first device. A right sided pacemaker combined with a new left sided ICD may offer the theoretical benefit of higher shock effectiveness, but that is of limited importance in view of the high energy-ICDs available today. However there is the disadvantage of potentially dangerous interactions. The elimination of these interactions cannot be guaranteed with 100% safety, even after extensive testing and meticulous programming. For this reason considering the up to date device and implantation technology, different solutions should be preferred and, if necessary, the patient should be transferred to a center with experience in this field.

With an ipsilateral occluded vein the following options can be discussed:

1. Preferably the contralateral implantation of a complete new system is done, followed by inactivation of the old device. The old generator is generally explanted and if the risk for lead removal is reasonable, the leads are extracted at the same time. Also functional deactivation of the old generator is possible (e.g. OOO, OVO or ODO mode) and should be made, if explantation is scheduled for a later time (fig. 1a to c). It has to be remembered that not all CIEDs allow complete deactivation (fig. 2). Principally deactivation by programming alone cannot be recommended as a permanent solution.

Firstly, an accidental reprogramming of the generator, e.g. at a later time in ignorance of the specific situation cannot be excluded. Secondly, battery depletion can cause automatic mode changes of the old generator leading to potential interactions [Bastian & Kirste, 2009].

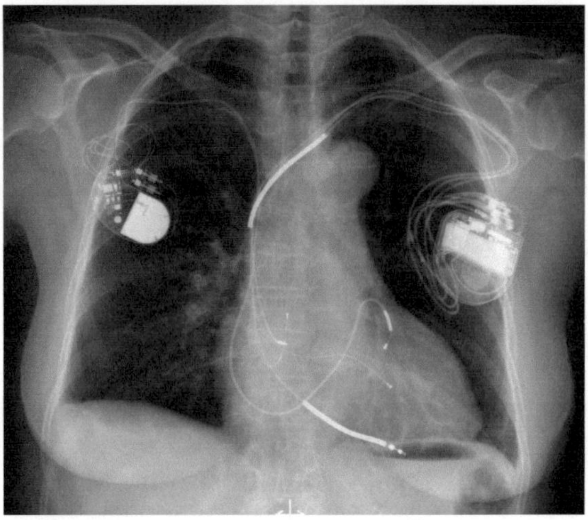

(a)

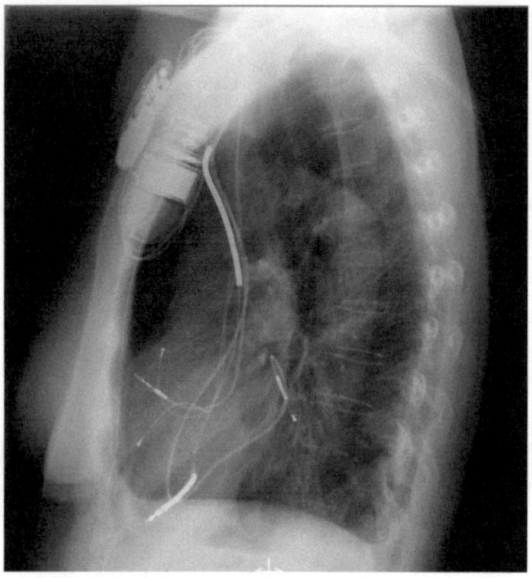

(b)

Fig. 1a and 1b. Chest x-ray PA and lateral. Female patient. DDDR-pacemaker on the right side (Affinity®DR 5330, St. Jude Medical, St. Paul, Minnesota, USA, unipolar leads). Implantation in 1994 cause of sick sinus syndrome. In 2008 indication for cardiac resynchronization therapy (chronic heart failure due to dilated cardiomyopathy, left bundle branch block): new implantation of a CRT-D system on the left side (Concerto C 174 AWK, Medtronic Inc., Minneapolis, MN, USA) because of an occluded right subclavian vein.

Standardparameter

	Initial	=>	[Change]	Aktuell	
Betriebsart	DDDR	=>	[Mode]	ODO	
Grundfrequenz	60		[Basic Rate]	60	min^{-1}
Hysteresefrequenz	Aus	=>		*	min^{-1}
Ruhefrequenz	50	=>		*	min^{-1}
Obere Grenzfrequenz (MTR)	125	=>		*	min^{-1}
2:1-Blockfrequenz	129	=>		*	min^{-1}
AV-Intervall	275			275	ms
PV-Intervall	225			225	ms
Frequenzabhängigkeit (AV-Int.)	Niedrig	=>		*	
Kürzestes AV-Intervall	70	=>		*	ms
V. Refraktärzeit	250			250	ms
Atriale Refraktärzeit (PVARP)	275			275	ms
Ventrikuläre Werte:			[Ventricular]		
V. AutoCapture	Aus	=>		*	
V. Impulsamplitude	2,00	=>	[Pulse Amplitude]	*	V
V. Impulsdauer	0,3	=>	[Pulse Width]	*	ms
V. Empfindlichkeit	3,0		[Sensitivity]	3,0	mV
V. Stimulationskonfiguration	Unipolar	=>	[Lead configuration]	*	
V. Wahrnehmungskonfig.	Unipolar (Spitze)			Unipolar (Spitze)	
Atriale Werte:			[Atrial]		
A. Impulsamplitude	2,00	=>	[Pulse Amplitude]	*	V
A. Impulsdauer	0,2	=>	[Pulse Width]	*	ms
A. Empfindlichkeit	0,75		[Sensitivity]	0,75	mV
A. Stimulationskonfiguration	Unipolar	=>	[Lead configuration]	*	
A. Wahrnehmungskonfig.	Unipolar (Spitze)			Unipolar (Spitze)	
Magnetreaktion	Batterietest			Batterietest	

Fig. 1c. Functional deactivated unipolar dual chamber pacemaker (Affinity® DR 5330, SJM) by programming the device to ODO mode after the CRT-D system has been implanted on the opposite side.

Parameter		Vorher	Aktuell
Batterie			OK
ERI, errechnet			5 J. 6 Mo.
Magneteffekt			AUTO
		Vorher	**Aktuell**
Mode			SSI
Grundfr. Tag/Nacht...	[Lower Rate limit]		30/30 ppm
Frequenzhysterese...			AUS ppm
Repetitiv			-----
Suc			-----
Nachtprogramm			AUS ppm
Nachtbeginn			-----
Nachtende			-----
Sensor			
Max.Sens.Freq			----- ppm
Sensorverstärkung			-----
Autom. Verstärkung			-----
Sensorschwelle			-----
Frequenzanstieg			----- ppm/s
Frequenzabfall			----- ppm/s
Obere Grenzfrequenz			----- ppm
Impulsamplitude	[Pulse Amplitude]		0.1 V
Impulsdauer	[Pulse Width]		0.10 ms
Ven. Empfindl.	[Ventricular Sensitivity]		1.0 mV
Atr. Empfindl.			0.8 mV
Refraktärzeit			300 ms
Polarität Pace			UNIP
Polarität Sense			UNIP
Elektroden-Check			AUS

Fig. 2. Functional deactivation of a unipolar single chamber pacemaker (Philos SR, Biotronik SE & Co. KG, Berlin, Germany). The programming is on SSI (VVI) with a basic rate of 30/min, minimal pacing output (impulse amplitude 0.1 V, pulse width 0.1 ms) and high ventricular sensitivity (1 mV). No interactions were observed until explantation 2 months later (same patient as in fig. 12).

2. Contralateral implantation of a functional additive system with continued use of the existing device. The obvious advantage would be the relative simplicity of the procedure. The intervention could be carried out in centers that have less experience with revision procedures. Considering the potential interactions this should be principally avoided.
3. Continued use of old leads with a contralateral new device could be achieved by subcutaneous tunneling over the sternum, but isn´t performed at our hospital anymore due to potential long term complications (especially mechanical lead alteration).
4. If the ipsilateral vein is occluded and the contralateral side cannot be used e.g. because of infection or radiation therapy, a remaining option is extraction of the old leads using a sheath, which serves as a tunnel for the new lead.
5. The final option is the implantation of epicardial leads.

The decision which procedure is finally chosen for a specific patient has to remain an individual one, of course.

3. Interactions

Inappropriate ICD therapy caused by oversensing of pacemaker signals

The problem was first described by Chapman and Troup in 1986 in a patient with recurrent ICD shocks after "double sensing" of bipolar DVI pacemaker actions [Sticherling et al., 1997; Chapman & Troup, 1986].

The underlying mechanism is the erroneous detection of ventricular tachyarrhythmias caused by the ICD oversensing atrial and/or ventricular pacemaker signals, as well as the ventricular response or intrinsic actions (double or triple counting) (fig. 5, 6, 20, 22b). To become an active oversensing problem the timing of the signals has to exceed the postventricular sense blanking period of the ICD, either due to programming of a long AV-delay or a significant local conduction delay, resulting in a delay between stimulus and locally evoked potential [Singer et al., 1988; Chapman & Troup, 1986; Calkins et al., 1990; Noguera et al., 1997]. The postventricular sense blanking period of an ICD is often around 120-150 ms and usually cannot be programmed. However, some devices allow significantly lower values. The blanking period should not be programmed shorter than 100 ms to avoid double counting (fig. 3 and 4)!

Clinical problem caused by interaction	Pathophysiology	=> Mechanism of interaction
ICD: Inappropriate therapy	PM: Pacing artifacts - unipolar - with high output - ineffective - high rate - asynchronous Noise from lead contact	ICD: Overcounting of PM artifacts + evoked / intrinsic potentials => erroneous VT/VF detection
ICD: Inadequate SVT/VT discrimination	PM: Pacing artifacts	ICD: oversensing of PM artifacts => - artifact as false intrinsic template - stable tachycardia classified as unstable
ICD: Delayed/inhibited VT/VF therapy	PM: VT/VF undersensing => - pacing during VT/VF	ICD: oversensing of PM artifacts => - VT/VF undersensing
ICD: Inhibited post-shock pacing	PM: Post shock ineffective pacing artifacts	ICD: oversensing of PM artifacts
PM: Post-shock dysfunction - device intact	ICD-shock => energy shunted over the PM-lead => thermal damage of endocardial tissue	PM: - increased stimulation threshold with loss of capture - impaired sensing function
PM: Post-shock dysfunction - device affected	ICD-shock - high energy, applicated near the PM	PM: damage or re-programming - e.g. fixed rate back-up-mode
PM: Inhibited pacing	Second CIED: ineffective pacing - Frequency > PM rate	PM: Inhibition by oversensing of artifacts

Table 1. Overview: potential interactions of 2 active implanted CIEDs. PM = pacemaker, ICD = implantable cardioverter defibrillator, VT = ventricular tachycardia, VF = ventricular fibrillation.

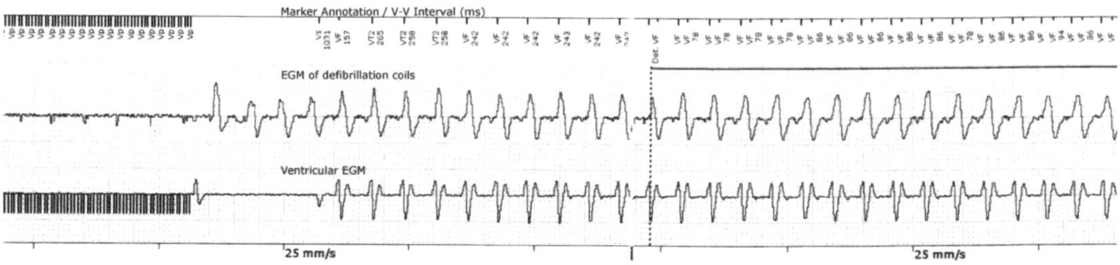

Fig. 3. Double counting of wide intrinsic QRS-complexes of an induced fast ventricular tachycardia (VT) due to the manufacturer preset ultra short hardware blanking period of only 8 ms/ noise blanking of 60 ms (ICD Lexos VR-T, Biotronik SE & Co. KG, Berlin, Germany). After extending the blanking period to 100 ms correct sensing was registered (not shown on this stripe).

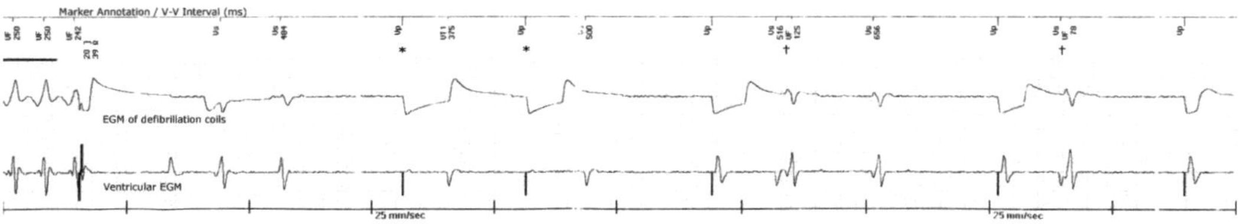

Fig. 4. Intermittent ineffective ventricular ICD pacing (*) and double counting of intrinsic QRS-complexes (†) after shock delivery. Postventricular sense blanking period (hardware blanking) 8 ms / noise blanking 60 ms (ICD Lexos VR-T, Biotronik SE & Co. KG, Berlin, Germany).

Double detection as cause of inappropriate ICD-therapy has been described also with a biventricular ICD with simultaneous right- and left ventricular sensing [Schreieck et al., 2001]. Additional factors that contribute to the problem of oversensing are leads that are located parallel or very close, unipolar pacer stimulation, high stimulation amplitude of the pacemaker and the use of epicardial or transvenous integrated bipolar ICD leads [Haffajee et al., 1996; Walker et al., 2000]. Inappropriate detection and following therapy are as well more likely to occur with a higher pacer stimulation rate, a lower VT/VF detection rate and shorter detection duration (VT/VF number of intervals to detect) of the ICD. Overall incidence of these interactions is very low. In 1990 a working group from Baltimore reported on a cohort of 30 patients with active pacemaker and ICD-systems with epicardial defibrillation leads [Calkins et al., 1990]. There was one case of double counting, however no inadequate shock was delivered. In another cohort consisting of 9 patients with epicardial ICD-systems, Cohen et al. showed oversensing in 5 cases, 4 patients had unipolar and 1 had bipolar pacemaker stimulation [Cohen et al., 1988]. In later studies with bipolar pacemakers and ICDs with true bipolar sensing no further cases with clinically relevant oversensing were described. [Sticherling et al., 1997]. However even with meticulous implantation, testing and best possible programming and the usage of modern systems, there is no safety guarantee that the interaction doesn´t show up in a particular case. In our own cohort we had one patient with implanted bipolar pacemaker (Kappa DR, Medtronic) and transvenous ICD (Marquis VR 7230, Medtronic; lead true bipolar) who had recurrent inadequate ICD-therapies due to double counting of the bipolar ventricular stimulation (fig. 5). Due to an increased stimulation threshold these stimuli were given with high energy after a long stimulated AV-delay of 240 ms. Many of the sensed pacer spikes were in the refractory period of the ICD, which was documented in the integrity counter of the ICD (fig. 5c). The stored frequent episodes of non sustained VTs were caused by overcounting (fig. 5d). Another example of device interaction is illustrated in fig. 6.

ICD Model: Marquis VR 7230
Serial Number:

9967 Software Version 7.0
Copyright Medtronic, Inc. 2002

VT/VF Episode #15 Report **Page 1**

ID#	Date/Time	Type	V. Cycle	Last Rx	Success	Duration
15	Oct 12 09:04:17	VF	280 ms	VF Rx 1	Yes	38 sec

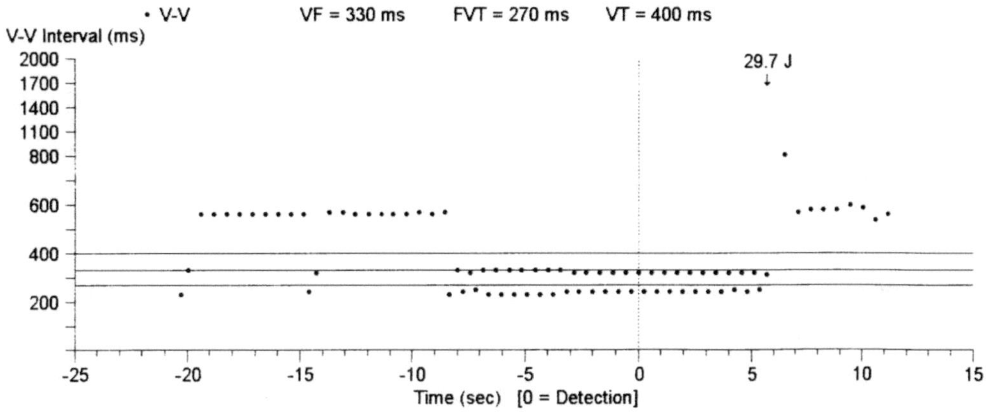

Fig. 5a. Inappropriate shock delivery caused by double counting. V-V interval plot.

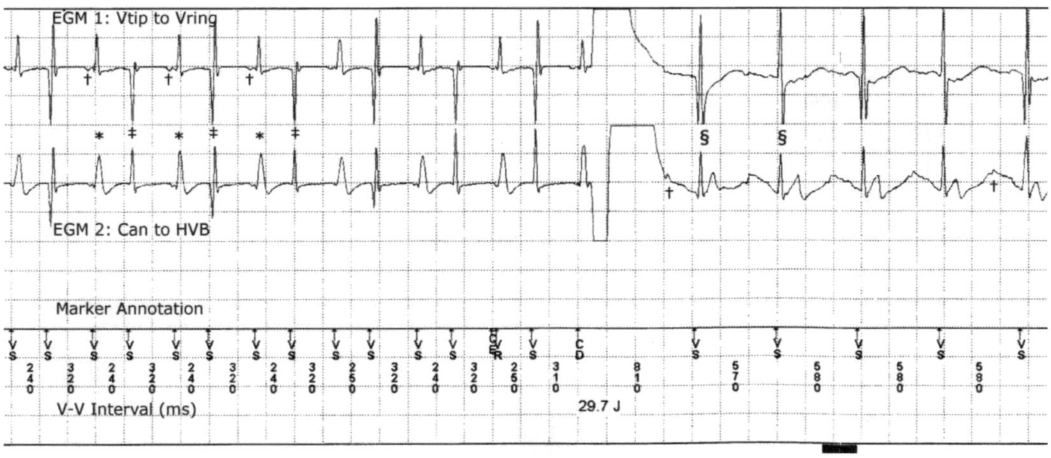

Fig. 5b. Inappropriate shock delivery caused by double counting. Intrinsic rhythm: sinus-arrest, considerable prolonged AV-conduction time (560 ms). * = intrinsic QRS-complex. PM rhythm: atrial pace-ventricular pace: † = paced p-Waves, ‡ = ventricular pacing artifact, prior to the shock ineffective due to pacing in the intrinsic ventricular refractory period. § = after shock delivery (CD) effective AV-sequential ventricular pacing by the PM, sensed by the ICD.

ICD Model: Marquis VR 7230
Serial Number:

9967 Software Version 7.0
Copyright Medtronic, Inc. 2002

Quick Look Report **Page 3**

Clinical Status: Since Sep 13, 2004

Episodes		**Pacing**	
VF	3	Sensed	100.0 %
FVT	0	Paced	<0.1 %
VT	9		
SVT	0		
NST	1581		

Observations (4)

- 42672 V-V intervals have been sensed at 120 or 130ms since Sep 13, 2004 16:19:59. Check for sensing issues (e.g. double counting of R-waves, lead fracture, loose set screw).
- 2 VF episodes were longer than 30 seconds. Most recent was Episode #15, Oct 12, 2004 09:04:17.
- 9 VT episodes were monitored. No VT therapies are delivered when VT Detection is set to Monitor. Most recent was Episode #19, Oct 27, 2004 09:37:26.
- 6 VT episodes were longer than 30 seconds. Most recent was Episode #19, Oct 27, 2004 09:37:26.

Fig. 5c. More than 42.000 ultra short V-V intervals sensed at 120 or 130 ms and some episodes with inadequate therapy delivery caused by double counting. 1581 episodes counted as non sustained VT (see fig. 8).

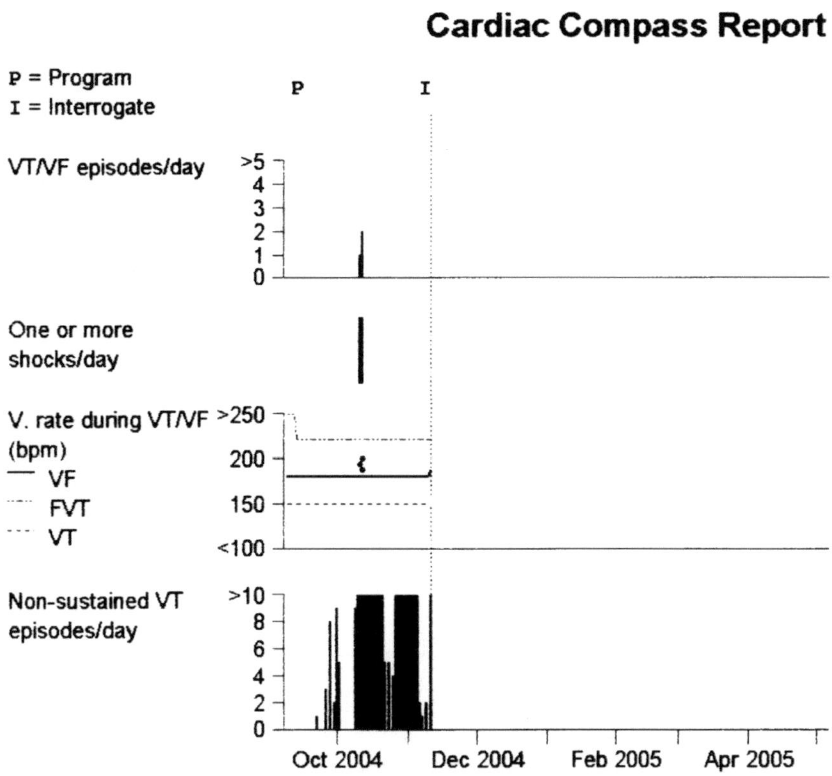

Fig. 5d. Frequent episodes of non sustained ventricular tachycardia: erroneous detection due to double counting.

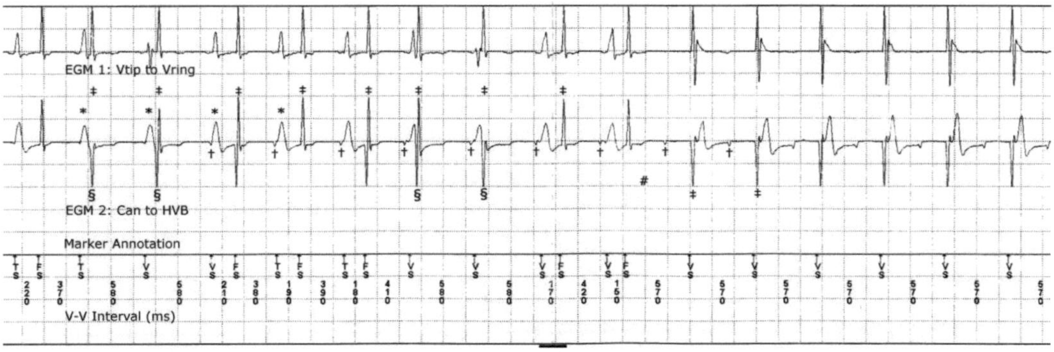

Fig. 5e. „Spontaneous termination“ of an inadequate detected non sustained VT episode (monitor zone). Intrinsic rhythm: sinus-arrest, considerable intrinsic AV-conduction delay. * = intrinsic QRS-complex. PM rhythm: atrial pace-ventricular pace: † = paced p-Waves, ‡ = ventricular pacing artifact. Intermittent double counting is caused by the ineffective ventricular pacing artifacts as explained in fig. 5b. Depending on the timing of the p-waves to the intrinsic QRS-complexes safety window pacing occurs without double counting (§). The overcounting is interrupted after the occurrence of a second degree type I AV block (Wenckebach) (#) followed by AV sequential PM pacing with the pacing artifact sensed by the ICD.

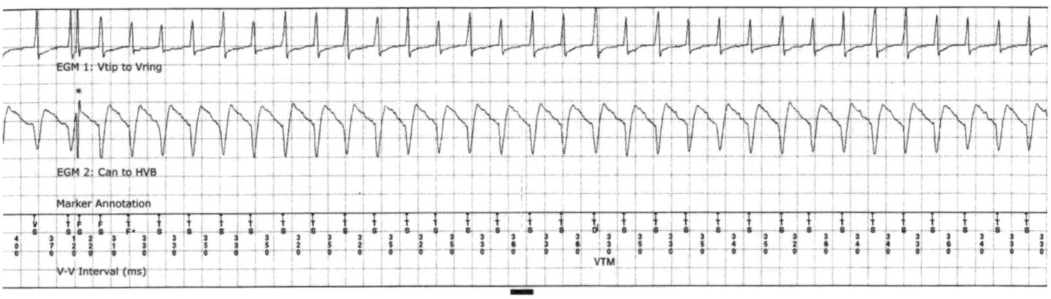

Fig. 6a. Detection of a VT in a programmed monitoring zone (marker TD VTM). Initially singular oversensing of a ventricular PM-spike (*). ICD: Marquis VR 7230, Medtronic, dual coil - true bipolar lead. ICD parameter settings for tachycardia detection: VT = Monitor 400-330 ms; FVT = via VF 270 ms; VF = 330 ms. Wavelet = auto. Pacemaker: Kappa DR, Medtronic, bipolar leads.

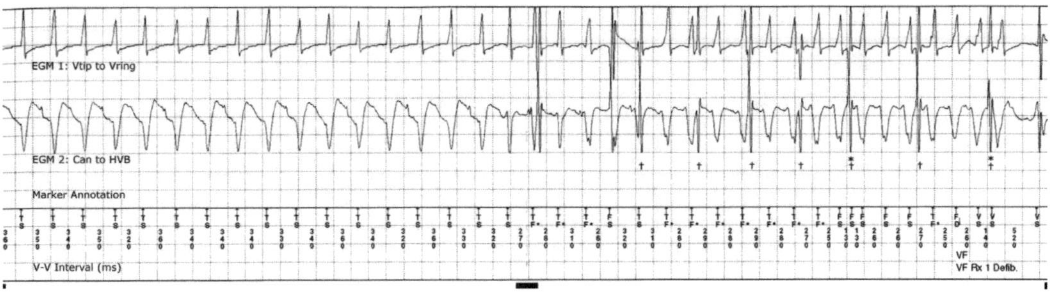

Fig. 6b. Detection of the VT in the VF-zone (marker FD VF) after spontaneous acceleration with change of morphology and intermitting overcounting (*) of ventricular PM actions (†).

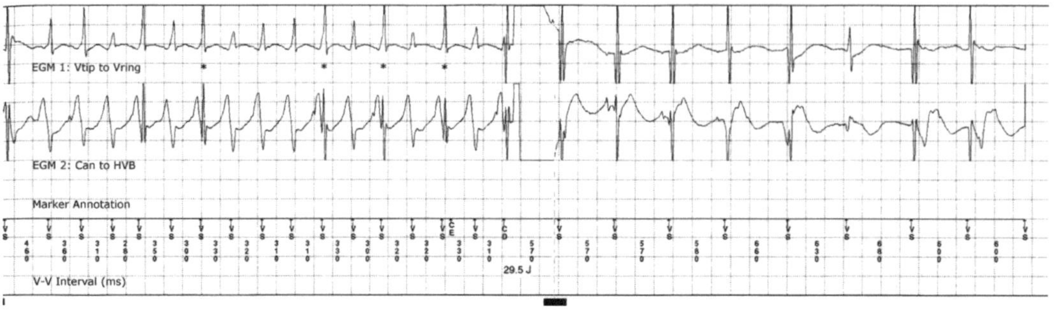

Fig. 6c. Termination of the VT by ICD shock (marker CD) after a second change of cycle length and morphology. The pacemaker artifacts (*) were not double counted.

Other situations where double counting can be encountered are ventricular sensing failure with asynchronous stimulation of the pacemaker in competition with the intrinsic rhythm [Singer et al., 1988], automatic or manual pacing threshold testing (fig. 27), asynchronous magnet testing [Brode et al., 1997; Epstein et al., 1989] as well as - independent of interactions-T-wave oversensing (fig. 7). Multiple counting can be caused by interference signals e.g. with a fractured lead (fig. 8) or mechanical lead-lead contact [Brode et al., 1997]. As a new, currently still experimental technology the combination of a device for cardiac contractility modulation (CCM) with an ICD, pacemaker or CRT-system is possible and useful [Seifert et al., 2008]. Of course it must be ensured that the CCM-signals are not being sensed by the second device.

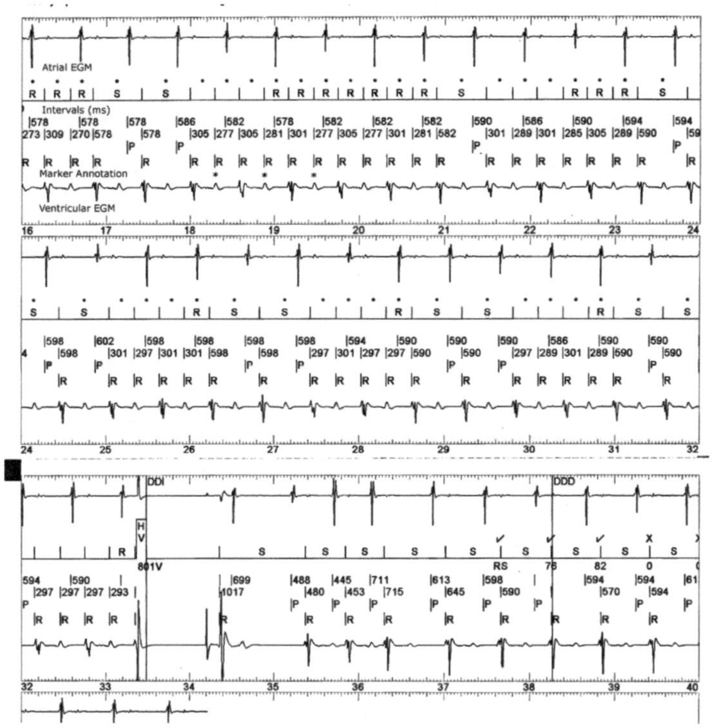

Fig. 7. Inappropriate ICD-therapy due to T-wave oversensing (*). ICD Atlas®DR V 240, SJM.

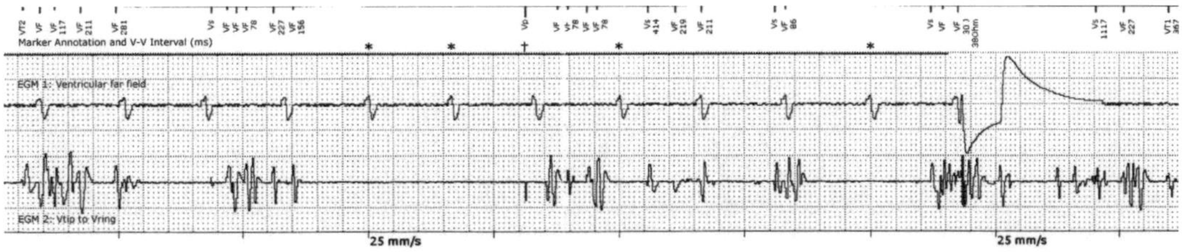

Fig. 8. Inappropriate ICD-therapy (30 J, ICD Lexos VR-T, Biotronik) due to ICD lead fracture (Sprint fidelis 6948, dual coil, Medtronic). Multiple artifacts in the pace-sense channel (bottom). The upper far field EGM shows no artifacts. Note that sensing (*) as well as ventricular pacing (†) function is also affected.

Another clinical interaction hasn´t been described in the literature so far: modern ICDs have different algorithms for differentiation of supraventricular and ventricular tachyarrhythmias. This includes taking a sample template of the normofrequent intrinsic chamber complex as a reference which is then compared to the morphology of a tachycardia. A match supports more a supraventricular tachyarrhthymia whereas in the case of a mismatch, the algorithm supports more the ventricular origin. Usually this template is automatically updated. With frequent oversensing of pacemaker stimulus artifacts by the ICD, such a stimulus may be erroneously recognized as ´intrinsic QRS complex` and saved as reference (Fig. 9). This could lead to misinterpretation of a supraventricular tachyarrhythmia as VT.

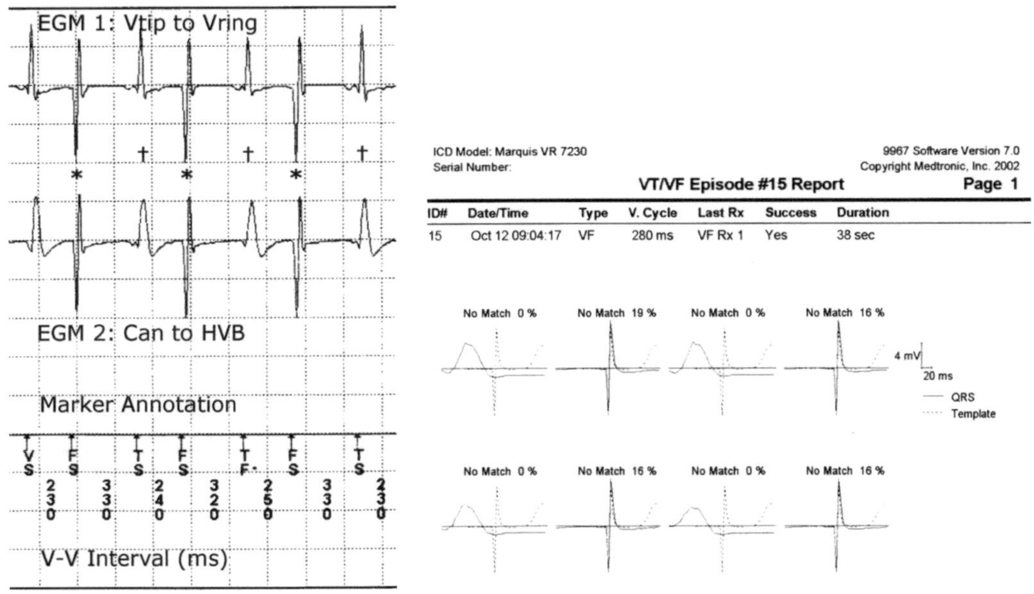

Fig. 9. Ventricular pacing artifact (*) erroneously saved as reference (template) for intrinsic chamber complex during automatic wavelet update (pacemaker Kappa DR, ICD Marquis VR 7230, Medtronic). † = true intrinsic QRS complex

Pro-arrhythmic effects of inadequate ICD-therapies have also been described [Sticherling et al., 1997; Epstein et al., 1989; Pinski & Fahy, 1995] (fig. 10).

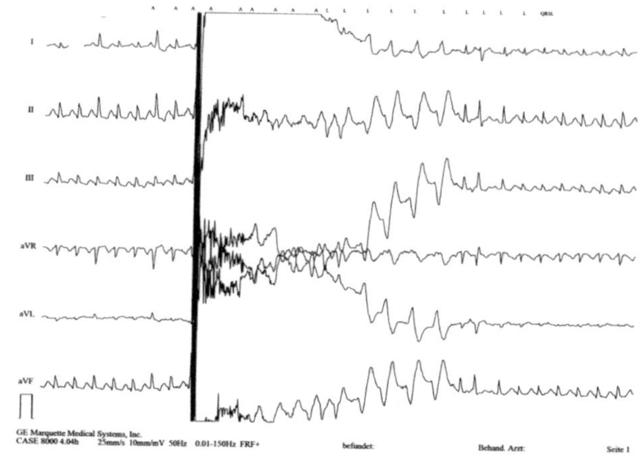

Fig. 10. Induction of non sustained VT by inadequate ICD-shock

Undersensing of ventricular tachyarrhythmia by the ICD

This problem is the most serious potential interaction. For safe recognition of VF with a low intrinsic amplitude today´s ICDs have high sensitivity, which adjust automatically to the perceived signal up to a programmed maximum value. The automatic adaptive sensing algorithms of different manufacturers have specific characteristics and are programmable to some extent. If a pacemaker programmed according to normal standards (e.g. with ventricular sensing of 2.5 mV with bipolar systems or less sensitive with an unipolar lead) doesn´t recognize VF because of the low amplitude, the pacemaker will stimulate with its basic rate or sensor rate (fig. 11a). This is also true for AAI-pacemakers, that usually don´t sense any signals from the ventricle, if they are not inhibited by far-field-signals [Singer et al., 1988] These stimulation artifacts can now be sensed by the highly sensitive ICD. Especially with unipolar pacing spikes with high amplitude, the automatic sensing threshold is changed to less sensitive values. The consequence may be undersensing of VF with the worst case scenario of the ICD withholding therapy (fig. 11b).

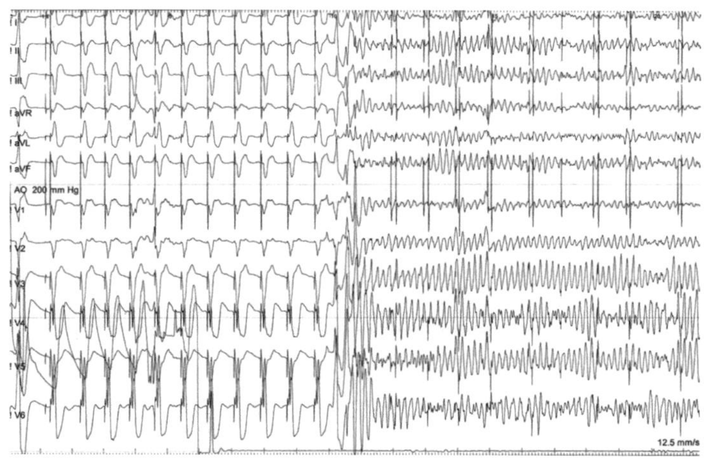

Fig. 11a. Undersensing of ventricular fibrillation during cardiac catheterization in a patient with unipolar DDD-pacemaker stimulation.

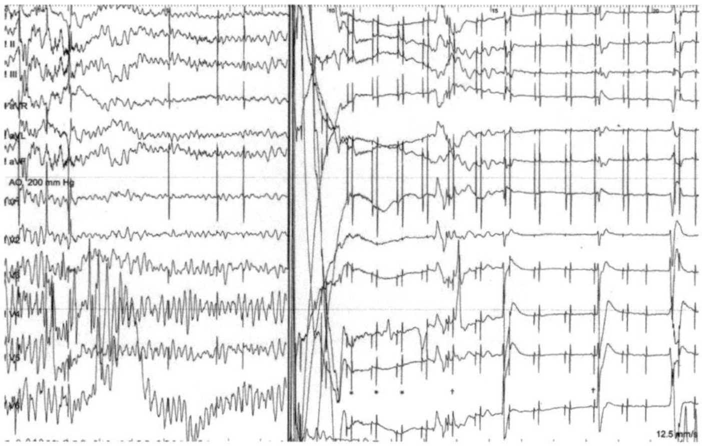

Fig. 11b. Effective ICD shock is delivered after a marked delay of 25 seconds. Subsequent loss of capture (*) and sensing failure of the implanted DDDR-pacemaker (†).

Although some authors think it is in principle possible to use unipolar pacemaker leads when careful implantation and testing are performed [Haffajee et al., 1996], the general opinion states a contraindication for unipolar pacemaker stimulation if there is a second active CIED present [Singer et al., 1988; Epstein et al., 1989; Mattke et al., 1997] (fig. 12). Although for many years there´s a predominant use of bipolar leads for conventional pacemakers, unipolar left ventricular leads are still used in implantation of CRT systems because of the venous anatomy. (fig. 13). The unipolar left ventricular stimulation generates a large pacing dipole [Le Franc et al., 1998].

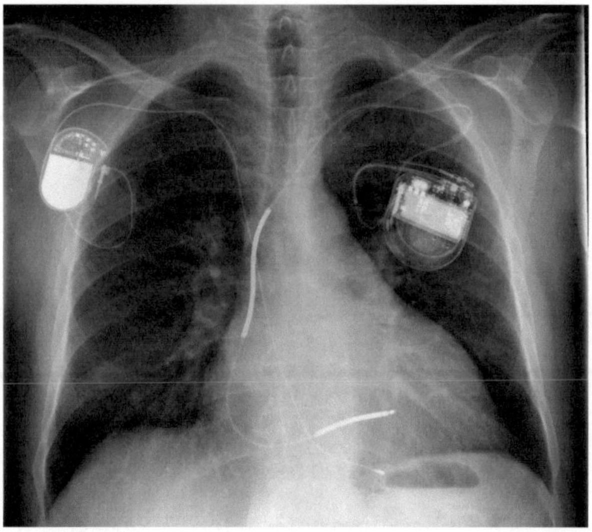

Fig. 12. Chest x-ray PA. Male patient, VVIR-pacemaker on the right side (Philos SR, Biotronik, implantation of unipolar lead 1975 cause of AV-Block III°). In August 2008: new implantation of a singular chamber ICD on the left side (Maximo VR, Medtronic) because of spontaneous VT with syncope, occluded right sided vein and permanent atrial fibrillation. Explantation of the pacemaker in October 2008.

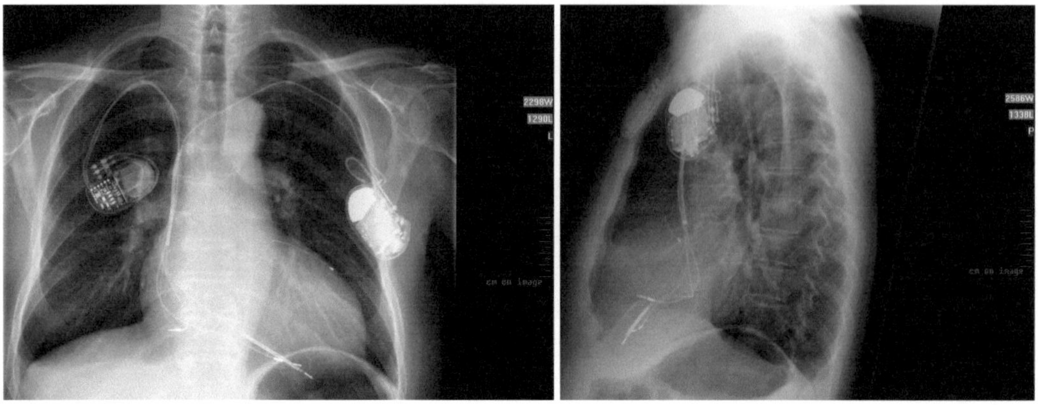

(a) (b)

Fig. 13 a and b. Chest x-ray PA and lateral. Implantation of a biventricular pacemaker CRT-P (Insync III 8042, Medtronic) in November 2005 in a patient with dilatated cardiomyopathy. The unipolar LV-lead is positioned in an unfavoured anterolateral way. 2 years later contralateral implantation of a singular chamber ICD (Lexos VR, Biotronik) as bridge to heart transplant. The bipolar right ventricular leads were placed very close together. However, testing showed no inhibition of the ICD dectecting induced ventricular fibrillation during pacemaker stimulation.

The problem was already described by Kim et al. in 1986 [Sticherling et al., 1997; Kim et al., 1986]. Among the 30 Baltimore patients inhibition of VF therapy was found in 2 patients with unipolar pacemakers and in one patient with a bipolar pacemaker under testing with high asynchronous output [Calkins et al., 1990]. Van Casteren et al. recently reported a case of temporary VF undersensing by a dual chamber ICD caused by oversensing of unipolar PM artifacts leading to delayed ICD therapy at defibrillation testing [Van Casteren et al., 2009]. So far there hasn't been a description of therapy inhibition of VF by oversensing in the clinical course of patients with bipolar pacemakers with standard programming and true bipolar transvenous ICDs and for example there was no occurence in the 4 patients observed by Sticherling et al. It has to be pointed out however that there might be the necessity to increase the stimulation energy due to future threshold increases, which will increase the possibility of interactions.

There are 3 further phenomena that were reported by Glikson et al. and resulted from asynchronous pacemaker stimulation during tachyarrhythmias while testing [Glikson et al., 1999]: 1. A fast VT was detected in a slower zone and therefore firstly treated with ATP ineffectively. 2. A VT was detected in the VF-zone due to oversensing of pacemaker-stimuli and VT-complexes (see fig. 6b). 3. A stable VT-cycle length was classified as instable and the VT detection prevented as the stability criterion was activated.

Inhibition of antibradycardia ICD-function

In the presence of 2 active CIEDs the stimulation of the pacemaker at the basic or sensor rate will inhibit the antibradycardia function of the ICD, which will work, as intended, only as the antitachycardia system. If the ventricular stimulation by the pacemaker should be ineffective, the ICD can act as a backup for antibradycardia stimulation with its (usually low) programmed basic rate. However, this ICD stimulation can be inhibited by oversensing of pacemaker stimuli resulting in a loss of the backup function. A clinical example is the inhibition of antibradycardia ICD back up stimulation by ineffective pacemaker artifacts after shock therapy (fig. 15, 24). The interaction can also be troublesome when e.g. a patient fitted with an AAI-pacemaker for sick sinus syndrome has received a VVI-ICD (fig 14). In case of a new AV-block the ICD could at least maintain ventricular stimulation - of course with loss of AV-synchronicity-, but there is the theoretical possibility of inhibition of ICD-stimulation by oversensing of atrial pacemaker spikes.

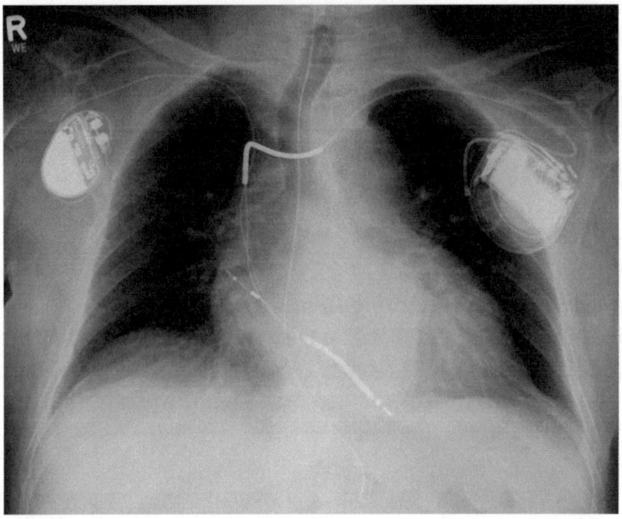

Fig. 14. Chest x-ray PA. Male patient, ICD implantation for secondary prevention (Marquis VR 7230, Medtronic, lead dual coil true bipolar). Three years later implantation of a bipolar AAIR pacemaker (Insignia I Ultra, Boston Scientific) on the right side because of sinus bradycardia with preserved atrioventricular conduction. The left subclavian vein was found to be occluded.

Shock-induced pacemaker dysfunction

Increase of stimulation and/or sensing threshold of pacemaker

Immediately after shock delivery there may be in rare cases an increase in stimulation threshold with loss of capture and/or impaired sensing function (fig. 11b, 15, 23b, 24).
The mechanism of these phenomena remains unclear. Either a shunting of current to the pacing lead by activation of zener diode and/or capacitive coupling of energy to the lead resulting in a local thermal damage at the electrode-myocardial interface are discussed [Sticherling et al., 1997; Calkins et al., 1990; Levine et al., 1983]. The dysfunction is generally only transient and is more common with external defibrillation than with internal shocks. Shocks with higher energy seem to cause a higher increase in stimulation threshold (compare fig. 22b and 23b) [Sticherling et al., 1997; Brode et al., 1997; Pinski & Fahy, 1995]. Among the 30 patients described by Calkins et al. there was a transient impairment of pacing and/or sensing in 7 cases with a duration of < 10 seconds in 4 patients, < 35 seconds in 2 patients and > 56 seconds in 1 patient. In another case with a unipolar pacemaker the sensing defect lasted > 10 minutes, the lead was changed to a bipolar one. [Calkins et al., 1990]. None of the dysfunctions had a clinical impact on the patients, 5 of the 7 patients had ICD therapies in the follow up without any noticeable adverse interactions. Mattke et al. reported 10 patients, with no one having transient or persisting loss of capture or sensing after ICD-shock delivery [Mattke et al., 1997].

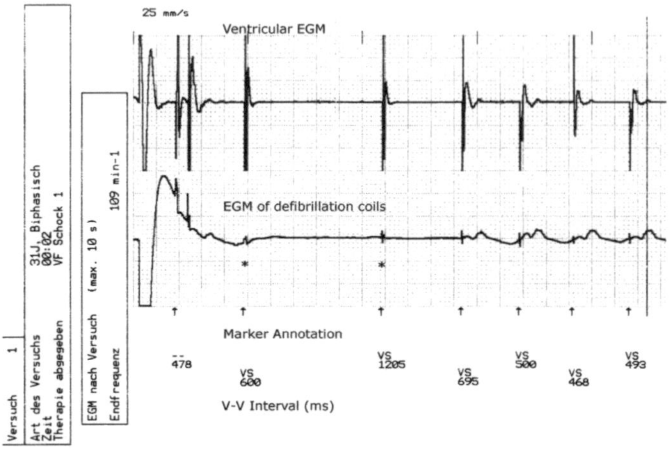

Fig. 15. Immediately after delivery of a 31 J-shock for termination of VF the transient ineffective ventricle stimulation (*) of the pacemaker (Kappa DR 401; Medtronic) can be seen in the ventricular pace-sense-channel (top) as well as in the ventricular electrogram of defibrillation coils (bottom) of the ICD (Ventak Prizm 2VR 1860; Guidant). The ICD detects the stimulation artifacts but not the following chamber complexes. ICD post shock pacing is inhibited by oversensing of the pacemaker stimuli.

Damage to or reprogramming of the pacemaker

This interaction is rarely described in the literature [Glikson et al., 1999; Gould et al., 1981]. Calkins et al. reported in 1990 three patients with reprogramming of the pacemaker to a back-up mode after ICD-shocks using epicardial high-voltage-electrodes [Calkins et al., 1990]. In contrast Geiger et al. published in 1997 5 patients out of 37 (13.5%) with a transvenous ICD, who showed on follow-up testing a reset of the pacemaker to baseline parameters (VOO bipolar) after shocks > 20 J [Geiger et al., 1997]. In the cohort of Mattke et al. one case of transient pacemaker-reprogramming was seen, the complication was never seen in pacemakers with a protective circuit [Mattke et al., 1997].
It is not known, if the current pacemaker generation can be damaged by shock delivery of high energy ICDs. If the subcutaneous ICDs, that are currently being developed, become available, the potential of interactions of these high energy shocks with additionally implanted pacemakers has to be considered.

4. Implantation

The prevention of potential interactions already starts with the implantation.

1. Only bipolar pacemaker leads and true bipolar ICD leads should be used [Brooks et al., 1995; Sheahan et al., 1997]. Unipolar pacemaker leads and ICD leads with pseudo-bipolar sensing increase the risk of interactions and are therefore contraindicated [Brooks et al., 1995; Cohen et al., 1988; Epstein et al., 1989; Mattke et al., 1997; Kim et al., 1986]. In addition it has to be pointed out, that during bipolar pacing the paced signal amplitude is directly related to the interelectrode separation on the pacing lead [Brode et al., 1997].
2. A parallel position of the leads increases far-field detection of pacemaker stimulus artifacts by the ICD lead and should therefore be avoided [Brooks et al., 1995]. A maximum lead distance of at least 2-3 cm and a 90° orientation of the pacemaker

dipoles should be pursued [Geiger et al., 1997; Sheahan et al., 1997]. For this reason it is mandatory to control the positioning of the leads in 2 planes. (fig. 16).

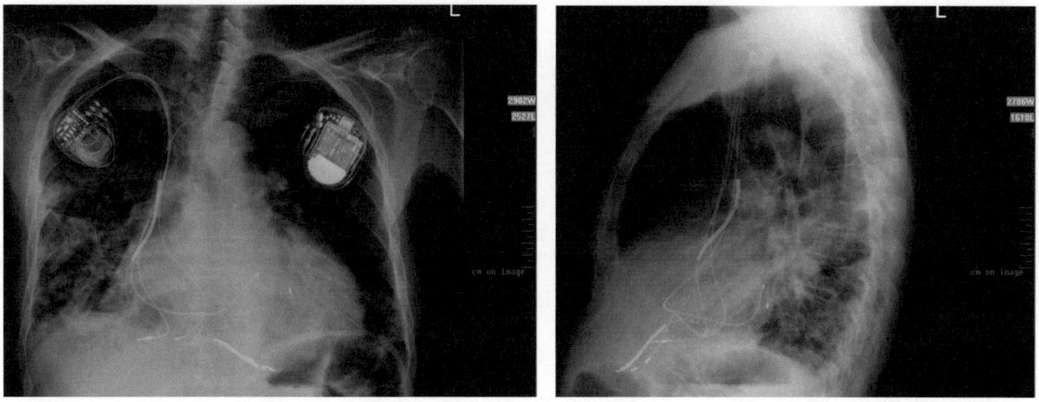

(a) (b)

Fig. 16 a and b. Chest x-ray PA and lateral: unfavourable positioning of ventricular electrodes to avoid oversensing: parallel position, very small distance < 1 cm. (Pacemaker/CRT-P: InSync, Medtronic. ICD: Lumax 300 VR-T, Biotronik)

To achieve a long distance e.g. the repositioning of a ventricle lead from the right ventricular apex (RVA) to a new position at the septum respectively in the right ventricular septal outflow tract (RVOT) seems reasonable (fig. 12) [Mattke et al., 1997]. However, an approach that is just guided by the anatomy is not sufficient on its own to prevent interactions [Brooks et al., 1995; Mattke et al., 1997]. Already at leads positioning the far-field-detection of pacemaker-spikes in the EGM and marker-channel of PSA, and after connection with the ICD should be watched. If necessary a different lead position has to be achieved [Cohen et al., 1988; Epstein et al., 1989] (fig. 17).

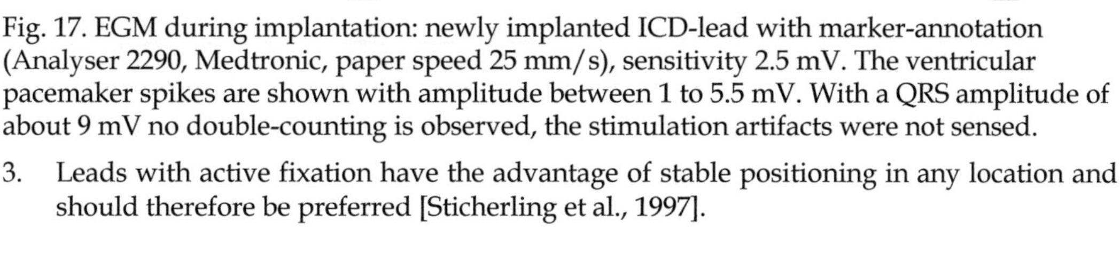

Fig. 17. EGM during implantation: newly implanted ICD-lead with marker-annotation (Analyser 2290, Medtronic, paper speed 25 mm/s), sensitivity 2.5 mV. The ventricular pacemaker spikes are shown with amplitude between 1 to 5.5 mV. With a QRS amplitude of about 9 mV no double-counting is observed, the stimulation artifacts were not sensed.

3. Leads with active fixation have the advantage of stable positioning in any location and should therefore be preferred [Sticherling et al., 1997].

5. Testing

Extensive testing for interactions is an essential part of the implantation procedure, if two CIEDs are left active [Sticherling et al., 1997; Walker et al., 2000; Cohen et al., 1988; Glikson et al., 1999; Blanck et al., 1994]. This is also necessary even if the explantation of one device is already planned and the presence of the two devices together is of limited duration. If a CCM device is to be combined with a second active CIED (e.g. CRT-D) testing for interactions is also mandatory [Seifert et al., 2008]. Real time telemetry is particularly helpful with its view of high resolution intracardiac electrogram (EGM) and marker annotations. In practice a structured step by step approach is helpful. An exemplary protocol was evaluated by Glikson et al. and was used by others in a modified form [Sticherling et al., 1997; Walker et al., 2000; Cohen et al., 1988; Glikson et al., 1999; Blanck et al., 1994]:

1. *Assessment of oversensing of pacemaker artifacts:* the predominant criterion to accept a newly positioned ventricular lead is the analysis of pacemaker spikes by the ICD. Therefore, the pacemaker is programmed for stimulation with maximum amplitude and pulse width for all connected leads. With dual or triple chamber leads a long AV delay is selected. Now under stimulation, the EGM of the ICD lead is analyzed using maximum sensitivity and watched for oversensing of pacemaker actions. If there is double or triple sensing it is suggested to first reduce the pulse width and then if necessary the amplitude of the pacemaker until no oversensing is seen any more [Sticherling et al., 1997]. If this setting is not sufficient for effective pacing with enough safety margins, then the lead has to be newly positioned. To avoid oversensing not only the absolute amplitude of the pacemaker - stimulation - artifact is of importance, but also the ratio of signal heights of spikes to the evoked potential respectively the intrinsic chamber complex (fig. 17, 18). The test protocol evaluated by Glikson et al. regarded stimulation artifacts > 2 mV or a ratio of stimulus artifact/evoked QRS > 1/3 as insufficient. [Cohen et al., 1988; Glikson et al., 1999]. The authors described a positive predictive value of 18% respective 14.4% for clinical relevant interactions and a negative predictive value of 100% respective 92.3%.

   If there is oversensing in the EGM of the ICD, the time interval from ventricular pacemaker spike to evoked QRS complex has to be shorter than the postventricular sense blanking period of the ICD (fig. 22b) [Cohen et al., 1988].

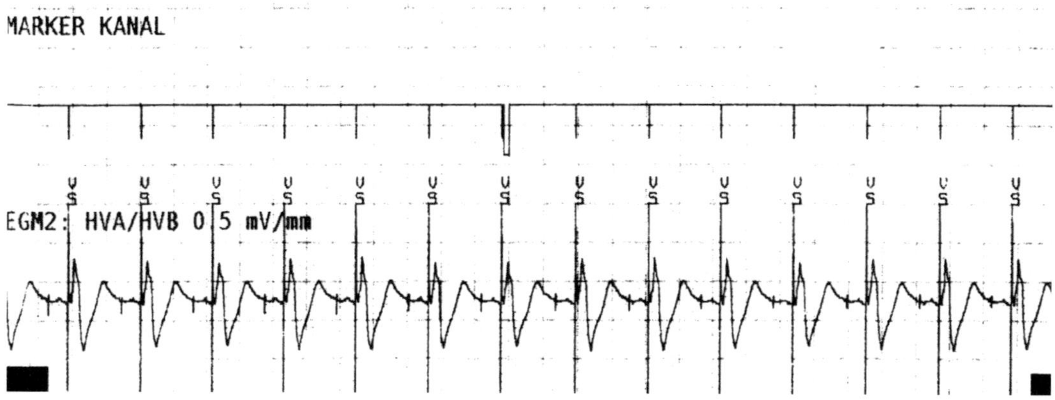

Fig. 18. Oversensig of the high ventricular pacing artifact (amplitude 12.5 mV) by the ICD. The stimulus artifact : evoked QRS ratio was inacceptably high (2.1). The atrial spikes as well as the QRS-complexes were not sensed.

2. *Rule out of VT/VF detection inhibition*: correct ICD-detection of induced VF has to be checked when there is asynchronous pacemaker stimulation. The pacemaker is set to a fixed rate mode (VOO or DOO) with - for each individual patient - the highest stimulation rate, maximum stimulation energy (with just no oversensing) and with 2- or 3-chamber devices with long AV–delay. During induced VF the EGM is analyzed, if ICD -detection and consecutive therapy of ventricular tachyarrhythmia are influenced by the pacemaker stimulation (Fig. 19). It´s recommended to test at least twice and with standard clinical as well as maximum ICD sensitivity.

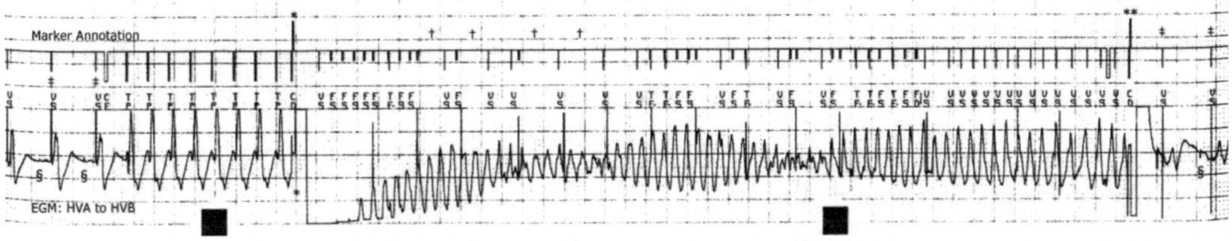

Fig. 19a. ICD testing. The ICD (Marquis VR 7230, Medtronic) was programmed to low sensitivity. The pacemaker (Kappa DR, Medtronic) with bipolar leads stimulates in DDD-mode with high pacing energy. Following induction of VF by t-wave shock (*) intermittend VF-undersensing occurs (†). However VF was detected and terminated by effective defibrillation (**). Before and after the test the ventricular pacing spike (not the QRS-complex) is sensed by the ICD (‡). Atrial pacing is to be seen in the EGM, but not sensed by the ICD. Paper speed 12.5 mm/s.

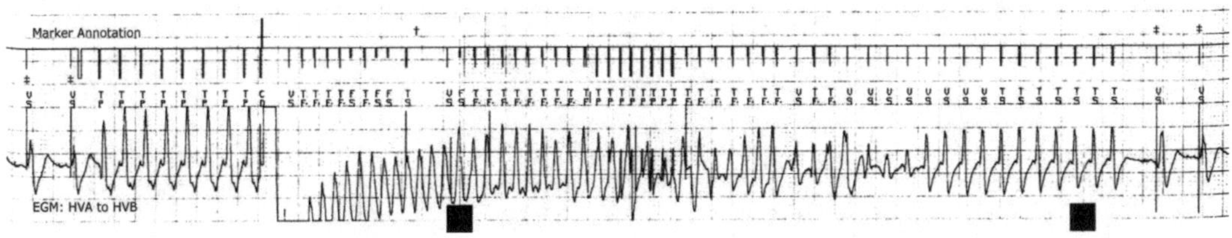

Fig. 19b. The pacemaker was programmed to higher sensitivity and lower pacing energy. Then the ICD was programmed to higher sensitivity and tested again. This time the induced VF showed higher amplitudes and terminated after ATP and organization to monomorphic VT. During the tachyarrhythmia oversensing of the pacing artifact and relevant VF-undersensing occurred only infrequently (†). The ventricular pacing spike was still sensed by the ICD before and after the test (‡). Paper speed 12.5 mm/s.

3. *Analysis of VF-detection by the pacemaker:* After completion of steps 1 and 2 testing of effectiveness of defibrillation e.g. as limited safety margin test can follow. The ICD is programmed to clinical sensitivity and e.g. to a shock energy with a safety margin of ≥ 10 J. At the same time the pacemaker is set to clinical parameters (see programming). Shock effectiveness is analyzed as well as the correct detection of induced VF by the pacemaker, to primarily avoid fixed rate pacemaker stimulation during ventricular tachyarrhythmias (Fig. 20 to 24). If there is asynchronous stimulation during VF, the event markers of the pacemaker are examined to distinguish undersensing from „noise reversion". According to the results, sensitivity and refractory periods of the pacemaker need to be adjusted.

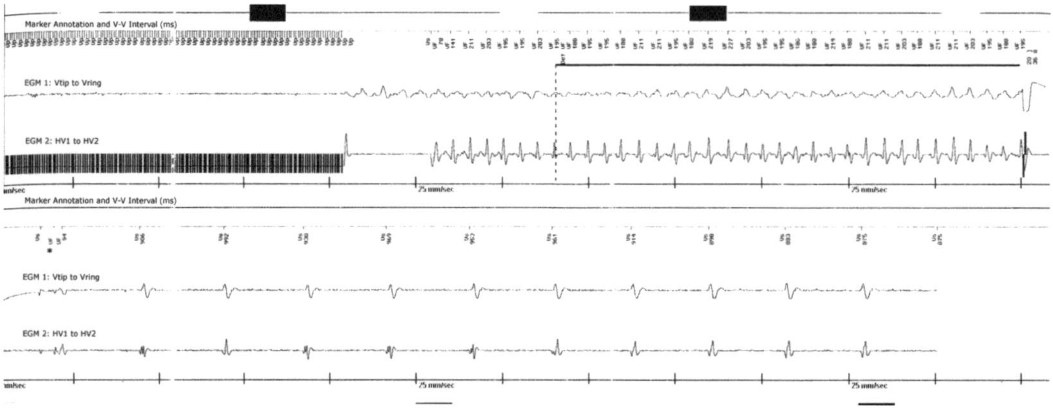

Fig. 20. Proper detection and termination of induced VF by a single chamber ICD (Lexos VR-T, Biotronik) in an patient with a combined CRT-P-system using an unipolar lead for left ventricular pacing (InSync III, Medtronic. Basic rate 60/min, paced AV-delay 170 ms, interventricular delay 4 ms). Only the first beat after the shock shows triple counting (*): the ICD sensed two pacing artifacts and the evoked QRS complex.

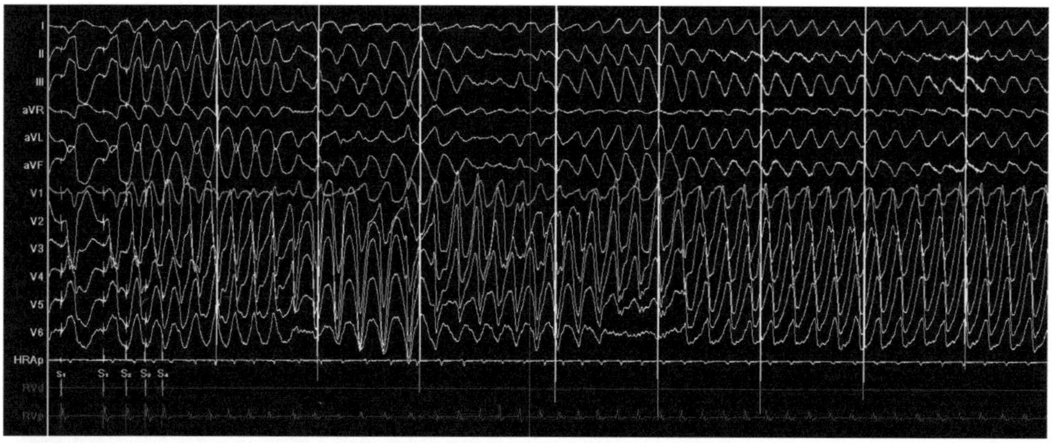

Fig. 21. Nearly continuous undersensing of ventricular flutter/fibrillation by an unipolar single chamber VVI pacemaker. (VF induced in the EP-laboratory. HRAp = high right atrium, RV = right ventricle)

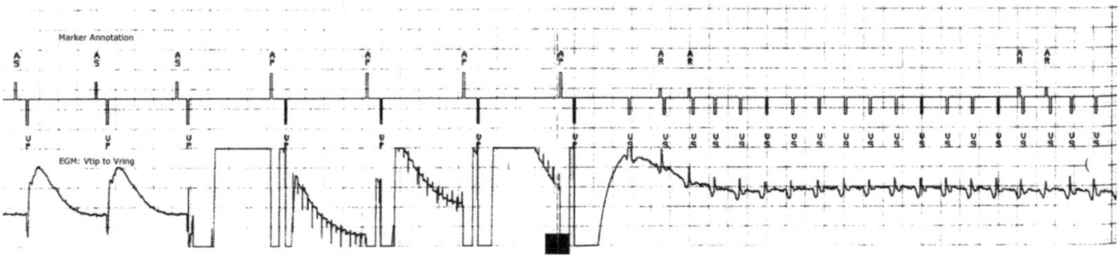

Fig. 22a. Correct ventricular sensing (VS) of an induced fast VT (CL 240 ms) by a dual chamber pacemaker (Kappa KDR 700, Medtronic). Paper speed 25 mm/sec.

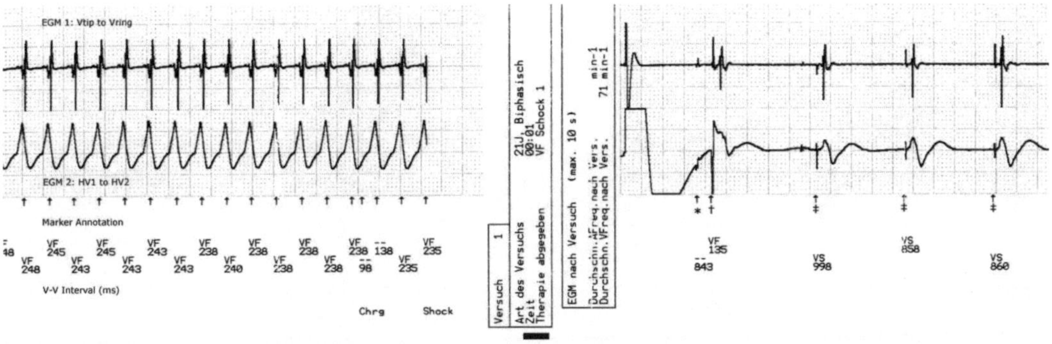

Fig. 22b. Same episode as fig. 22a. The EGM of the ICD (Ventak Prizm DR HE 1853, Guidant/BSCI) showed no oversensing of PM-actions during the VT, as the PM is inhibited. After correct termination with 21 J there is once double counting immediately after shock (atrial (*) and ventricular (†) pacing artifact). Thereafter the ventricular PM stimulus is detected by the ICD (‡), the evoked chamber complex falls into the blanking period.

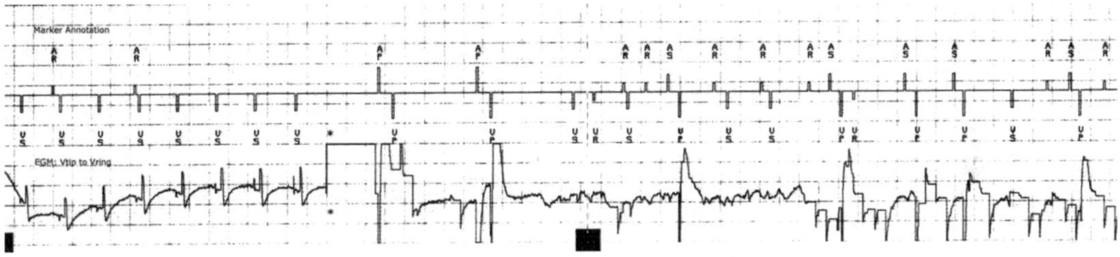

Fig. 23a. Complete undersensing of induced VF by the PM in the same patient as in fig. 22. * = t-wave shock for VF induction. Paper speed 25 mm/sec.

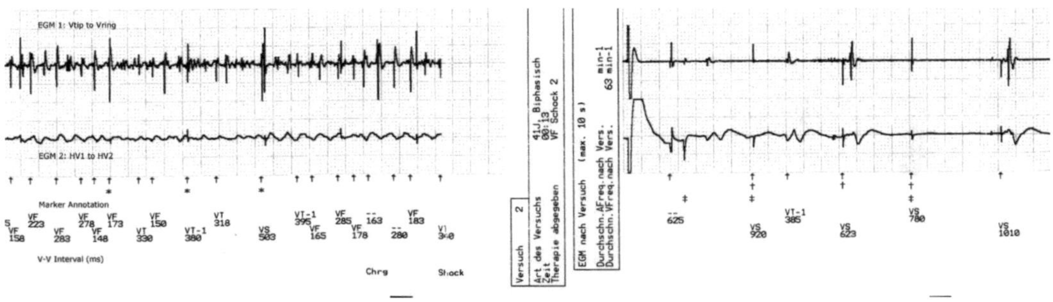

Fig. 23b. Intermitting undersensing of induced VF by the ICD resulting from oversensing of ventricular actions of the PM (*). After high energy shock (41 J) transient PM dysfunction († = defect of sensing, ‡ = ineffective pacing).

4. *Assessment of pacemaker function after shock delivery*: After all ICD-therapies sensing and effectiveness of PM stimulation are evaluated. Especially in patients who are permanently dependent on their pacemaker a loss of capture has to be looked out for and the programming of the ICD should include prolonged post-shock stimulation to increase the safety. Proper function of the programmed ICD post shock pacing has to be verified (fig. 4, 15). Finally, reprogramming or damage to the PM need to be excluded. [Pinski & Fahy, 1995].

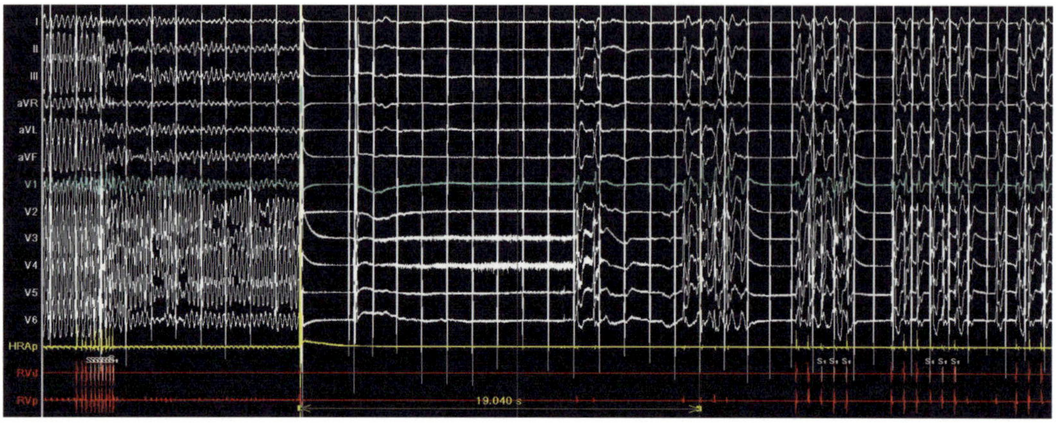

Fig. 24. Despite unipolar single chamber PM stimulation induced VF is correctly terminated by the ICD. However, after effective defibrillation there is continued ineffective PM stimulation as well as undersensing of intrinsic ventricular actions. (VF induced in the EP-laboratory. HRAp = high right atrium, RV = right ventricle)

"An absence of device interaction during implantation and testing procedures does not completely exclude the possibility of this occurring in the clinical setting…" [Blanck et al., 1994]

6. Programming and follow up

There are special points that need to be taken into account for the permanent programming of the two active devices to avoid future interactions.

1. As already emphasized, unipolar PM-stimulation has to be absolutely avoided. This also means that the commonly used practice to program bipolar sensing with unipolar stimulation for better visibility of PM-spikes in routine EKGs must not be done. Modern pacemakers have safety algorithms, which will switch permanently to unipolar stimulation, if there is a bipolar lead defect. This feature has to be deactivated (fig. 25).

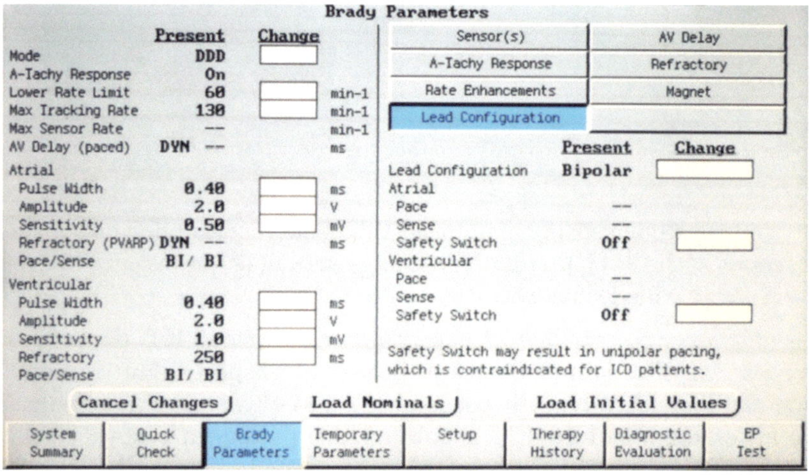

Fig. 25. Example of PM-programming for combined use together with a separate ICD to avoid interactions with bipolar lead configuration and high ventricular sensitivity.

The safety switch of the PM has to be deactivated to prevent automatic change to unipolar stimulation. In this demonstrated example of BSCI the lead configuration programming window shows the warning: "Safety Switch may result in unipolar pacing, which is contraindicated for ICD patients".

2. Increased sensitivity of the ventricular PM lead is programmed to guarantee pacemaker detection of ventricular tachyarrhythmias with low amplitude and therefore the occurrence of fixed rate stimulation is prevented, especially during VF [Cohen et al., 1988; Blanck et al., 1994]. However it is important to rule out oversensing of myopotentials by provocation testing especially in patients who are permanently dependent on their pacemaker. In our experience programming 1 mV is safe and effective with the modern leads. Automatic adaption of sensitivity should be deactivated (fig. 25).
3. Modern pacemakers feature algorithms to increase the stimulation rate if needed. Examples include sensor response or rate smoothing as well as algorithms for prevention and therapy of atrial tachyarrhythmias. The maximum rate of PM-stimulation must not exceed the detection rate of the ICD, as this could lead to inadequate detection of tachycardias and possible ICD-therapy [Brode et al., 1997; Blanck et al., 1994; Chamberlain-Webber et al., 1994].
4. In the presence of ICD-double counting, the first step is to analyze the EGM and see which signals are being detected by the ICD. Possible sources include atrial and/or ventricular PM-spikes, right- and if applicable left-ventricular evoked or intrinsic potentials, T-waves, and other different artifacts. Then the following questions need to be answered:
   a. How are the leads of the two devices positioned to each other? What kind of leads are in use?
   b. Is the PM-stimulation unipolar and/or with too high energy? Are any algorithms for automatic polarity switch or stimulation energy increase or impedance measuring active?
   c. Is the double-counting caused by too long conduction times, e.g. long AV-delay or long intra- respective interventricular disturbance of conduction or a long QT time? Are the programmed refractory periods too short?

   Depending on the cause of oversensing, changing the programming might solve the problem:
   a. Unipolar stimulation with high energy has to be avoided, automatic settings/changes deactivated (if necessary).
   b. It might help to increase the ventricular blanking period of the ICD and to adapt the automatic detection. The reliable detection of VF has to be ensured (fig. 26)!
   c. If there is oversensing of atrial or ventricular signals with long AV-delay of the PM, a shortening of the AV-delay is to be considered. However a short AV-delay may deteriorate the hemodynamic situation and the proportion of ventricular stimulation can be increased, which is usually not desired.
   d. In patients with an implanted 2-chamber PM or singular chamber-ICD and preserved AV-conduction, who have oversensing of ventricular spikes of the PM, the programming of a long AV-delay may be considered to promote intrinsic AV conduction and thereby avoid overcounting of ventricular stimulation artifacts [Sheahan et al., 1997].

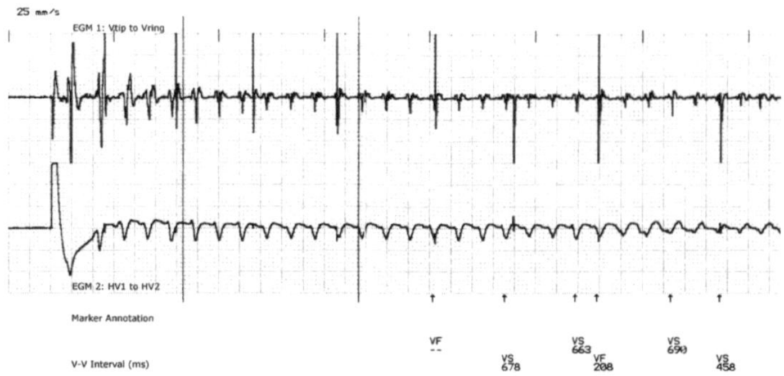

Fig. 26. Undersensing of a VT (induced by T-wave-shock) after reduction of ICD-sensitivity (Ventak Prizm 2VR 1860; Guidant) as reaction to overcounting of PM artifacts (Kappa KDR 401; Medtronic, bipolar leads!). The PM artifacts can be seen in the ventricular pace-sense-channel (top) as well as in the ventricular EGM of the defibrillation coils (bottom) and are being detected inconstantly by the ICD.

e. The reprogramming of a DDD(R)-pacemaker to AAI(R)-mode, if the AV-conduction is intact, was recommended by Brooks et al. and Chapman et al. to avoid interactions caused by oversensing of ventricular pacemaker stimuli [Brooks et al., 1995; Chapman & Troup, 1986].
f. Another last programming option with double-counting of PM spikes would be - if clinically possible in the individual patient - to limit the upper range of PM stimulation rate to less than half of the detection rate of the ICD [Chapman & Troup, 1986].

However, if oversensing with a clinical relevance can´t be avoided by programming, a revision of the system must be pursued.

5. The stimulation output of the PM should be minimized just ensuring an adequate safety margin for effective pacing [Blanck et al, 1994]. Thus the individual stimulation energy has to take the results of the threshold and interaction testing into account. In PM with automatic adaption of stimulation amplitude and pulse width the maximum value of adaptive stimulation energy has to be limited. Attention also needs to be paid to the fact that the automatic measurements of lead impedance are being conducted with higher energy (e.g. 5 volt). If there is oversensing with higher stimulation energies this automatic measurement has to be deactivated.
Caution is warranted in performing the pacemaker threshold testing in the presence of an active ICD. The stimulation with higher rates and energy can lead to inappropriate therapy due to oversensing of stimulation artifacts and of evoked and/or after loss of capture intrinsic QRS complexes [Cohen et al., 1988; Epstein et al., 1989; Azizi & Nägele, 2007]. This is particularly important for CRT-systems with a unipolar left ventricular (LV) lead (fig. 27). Principally the EGM of the ICD has to be watched for oversensing during testing. Some authors even recommend deactivation of the ICD during pacemaker testing [Singer et al., 1988], especially for CRT-PM-systems [Azizi & Nägele, 2007].
Depending on the testing results automatic threshold tests have to be turned off.
6. During programming of the detection criteria of the ICD, the avoidance of inadequate therapy deliveries have to be watched. Therefore - if clinical possible in the individual patient - a high VT/VF-detection rate and long detection durations should be programmed in the respective zones. The morphology as well as the stability criterion

for discrimination of SVTs should be used only, if an erroneous registration of PM artifacts by the ICD can be surely excluded (fig. 9). It is recommended to check the reference for intrinsic chamber complexes during device control and to deactivate automatic update. In patients with permanent high degree AV-Block the SVT-discrimination can be omitted.

7. In patients who are dependent on their pacemaker, the duration of post-shock pacing by the ICD with high stimulation energy should be extended. This will guarantee effective stimulation, if there is an increase of stimulation threshold of the antibradycardia pacemaker after the ICD shock [Singer et al., 1988; Pinsky & Fahy, 1995].
8. The specific details of programming have to be mentioned in the report and there must be references in the device card. As the combined use of two active CIEDs is rare, a lot of doctors might not be aware of all the problems and issues involved and therefore might change the programming to a more standard programming in ignorance of the specific situation.

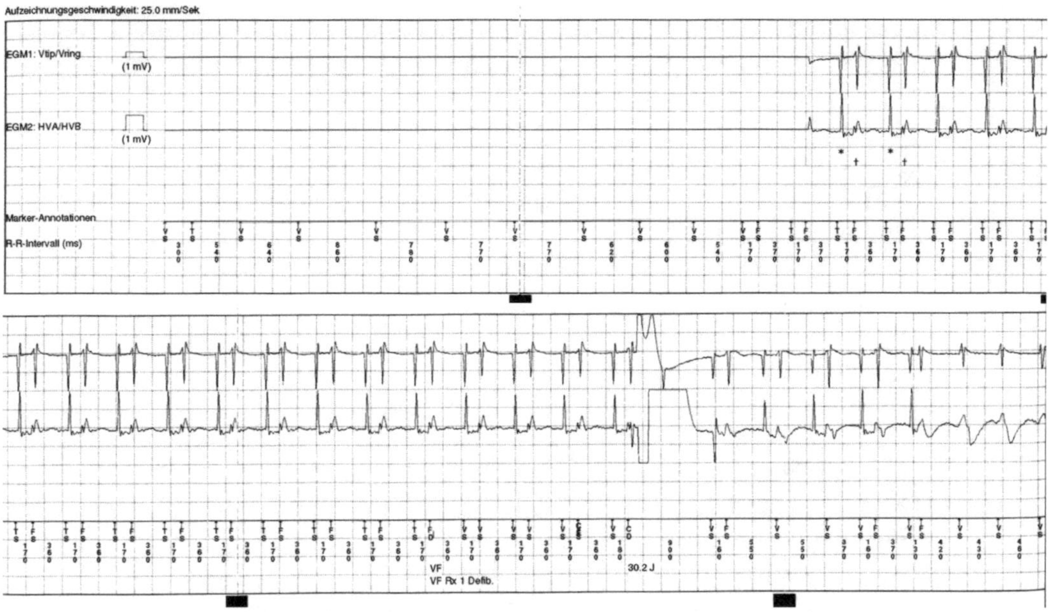

Fig. 27 a and b. Inappropriate shock (CD) due to double counting of stimulation artifacts of the unipolar LV lead (*) and the evoked potentials (†) at LV stimulation for threshold testing (ICD Marquis VR 7230; CRT pacemaker InSync III, Medtronic).

7. Conclusion

As there is no definitive guarantee for long term elimination of interactions and considering the modern technology, the combined use of two separate active CIEDs should be principally avoided. If in an individual case e.g. for a limited time after system upgrade the indication for a dual device therapy is seen, careful implantation, extensive testing and specific programming are essential to minimize the risk of possible dangerous adverse interactions.

There is a possibility that this currently rare problem will regain more clinical impact, when emerging new technologies, such as devices for cardiac contractility modulation, subcutaneous high energy ICDs without antibradycardia therapy or endocardial fixated "leadless pacemakers", are further developed and are used in clinical routine.

8. References

Azizi M, Nägele H. Inappropriate shock during left ventricular threshold measurement in a patient with coexisting ICD and a biventricular pacemaker. Herzschr Electrophys 2007; 18: 101-104.

Bastian D, Kirste W. Complex pacemaker dysfunction. Sometimes a problem does not come alone. Herzschr Electrophys 2009; 20: 185-190. [German]

Blanck Z, Niazi I, Axtell K, Sra J, Jazayeri MR, Dhala A, Deshpande S, Akhtar M. Feasibility of Concomitant Implantation of Permanent Transvenous Pacemaker and Defibrillator Systems. Am J Cardiol 1994; 74: 1249-1253.

Brode SE, Schwartzman D, Callans DJ, Gottlieb ChD, Marchlinski FE. ICD-Antiarrhyhtmic Drug and ICD-Pacemaker Interactions. J Cardiovasc Electrophysiol 1997; 8: 830-842.

Brooks R, Garan HG, McGovern A, Ruskin JN. Implantation of transvenous nonthoracotomy cardioverter-defibrillator systems in patients with permanent endocardial pacemakers. Am Heart J 1995; 129: 45-53.

Calkins H, Brinker J, Veltri EP, Guarnieri T, Levine JH. Clinical Interactions Between Pacemakers and Automatic Implantable Cardioverter-Defibrillators. J Am Coll Cardiol 1990; 16: 666-673.

Chamberlain-Webber R, Rankin I, Sutton R. Use of an implantable cardioverter defibrillator in a patient with a rate responsive pacemaker. Br Heart J 1994; 71: 191-192.

Chapman PD, Troup P. The automatic cardioverter-defibrillator: evaluating suspected inappropriate shocks. J Am Coll Cardiol 1986; 7: 1075-1078.

Cohen AI, Wish MH, Fletcher RD, Miller FC, McCormick D, Shuck J, Shapira N, Delnegro AA. The use and interaction of permanent pacemakers and the automatic implantable cardioverter defibrillator. PACE 1988; 11: 704-711.

Epstein AE, Kay GN, Plumb VJ, Shepard RB, Kirklin JR. Combined Automatic Implantable Cardioverter-Defibrillator and Pacemaker Systems: Implantation Techniques and Follow-Up. J Am Coll Cardiol 1989; 13: 121-131.

Geiger MJ, O'Neill P, Sharma A, Skadsen A, Zimerman L, Greenfield RA, Newby KH, Wharton JM, Kent V, Natale A. Interactions Between Transvenous Nonthoracotomy Cardioverter Defibrillator Systems and Permanent Transvenous Endocardial Pacemakers. PACE 1997; 20 [Pt. I]: 624-630.

Glikson M, Trusty JM, Grice SK, Hayes DL, Hammill SC, Stanton SS. A Stepwise Testing Protocol for Modern Implantable Cardioverter-Defibrillator Systems to Prevent Pacemaker-Implantable Cardioverter-Defibrillator Interactions. Am J Cardiol 1999; 83: 360-366.

Gould L, Patel S, Gomes GI, Chokshi AB. Pacemaker failure following external defibrillation. PACE 1981; 4 (5): 575-577.

Haffajee Ch, Casavant D, Desai P, Moon R, Voukydis P, Pacetti P. Combined Third-Generation Implantable Cardioverter Defibrillator with Permanent Unipolar Pacemakers: Preliminary Observations. PACE 1996; 19: 136-142.

Kim SG, Furman S, Waspe LE, Brodman R, Fisher JD. Unipolar pacer artefacts induced failure of an automatic implantable cardioverter/defibrillator to detect ventricular fibrillation. Am J Cardiol 1986; 57: 880-881.

Le Franc P, Klug D, Lacroix D, Jarwe M, Kouakam C, Kacet S. Triple Chamber Pacemaker for End-Stage Heart Failure in a Patient with a Previously Implanted Automatic Defibrillator. PACE 1998; 21: 1672-1675.

Levine PA, Barold SS, Fletcher RD, Talbot P. Adverse acute and chronic effects of electrical defibrillation and cardioversion on implanted unipolar cardiac pacing systems. J Am Coll Cardiol 1983; 8: 1413-1422.

Mattke S. Markewitz A. Müller D. Grünewald A. Fiek M, Schmöckel M, Hoffmann E, Steinbeck G. The Combined Tranvenous Implantation of Cardioverter Defibrillators and Permanent Pacemakers. PACE 1997; 20: 2775-2782.

Mirowski M, Reid PR, Mower MM, Watkins L, Gott VL, Schauble JF, Langer A, Heilman MS, Kolenik SA, Fischell RE, Weisfeldt ML. Termination of malignant ventricular arrhythmias with an implanted automatic defibrillator in human beings. N Engl J Med 1980; 303: 322-324.

Minden HH, Butter C. Upgrading to biventricular pacing: Indications and procedural challenges. Herzschr Electrophys 2008; 19 (Suppl.1): 38-43. [German]

Natale A, Sra J, Geiger MJ, Newby K, Akhtar M, Pacifico A. Right Side Implant of the Unipolar Single Lead Defibrillation System. PACE 1997; 20[Pt.I]: 1910-1912.

Noguera HH, Peralta AO, John RM, Venditti FJ, Martin DT. Combined use of non-thoracotomy cardioverter defibrillators and endocardial pacemakers. Heart 1997; 78: 50-55.

Pinski SL, Fahy GJ. The proarrhythmic potential of implantable cardioverter-defibrillators. Circulation 1995; 92: 1651-1664.

Schreieck J, Zrenner B, Kolb Ch, Ndrepepa G, Schmitt C. Inappropriate Shock Delivery Due to Ventricular Double Detection with a Biventricular Pacing Implantable Cardioverter Defibrillator. PACE 2001; 24: 1154-1157.

Seifert M, Hoffmann J, Meyhöfer J, Butter C. Improving left ventricular contractility by stimulation during the absolute refractory period - Cardiac contractility modulation (CCM). Herzschr Electrophys 2008; 19 (Suppl.1): 69-76. [German]

Sheahan RG, Dorian P, Poludnikiewicz M, Newman D. Dual Device Therapy in the Setting of Changing ICD Technology: Device-Device Interaction Revisited. PACE 1997; 20: 1704-1707.

Singer I, Guarnieri T, Kupersmith J. Implanted automatic defibrillators: effects of drugs and pacemakers. PACE 1988; 11: 2250-2262.

Sticherling Ch, Klingenheben T, Skupin M, Li YG, Hohnloser SH. Kombinierte Therapie mit transvenösen Kardioverter/Defibrillator- und antibradykarden Schrittmachersystemen. Z Kardiol 1997; 86: 105-112.

Van Casteren L, Huybrechts W, Willems R. Undersensing of ventricular fibrillation due to interference between a pacemaker and defibrillator in the same patient. Europace 2009; 11(10): 1390-1391.

Walker S, Levy T, Rex S, Brant S, Paul V. Preliminary Results with Simultaneous Use of Implantable Cardioverter Defibrillators and Permanent Biventricular Pacemakers: Implications for Device Interaction and Devolopment. PACE 2000; 23: 365-372.

13

Electromagnetic Interference of Pacemakers

Umashankar Lakshmanadoss MD[1], Priya Chinnachamy MD[2] and James P Daubert MD[3]

[1]*Johns Hopkins Medical Institutions, Baltimore, MD, USA;*
[2]*All India Institute of Medical Sciences, New Delhi,*
[3]*Duke University Medical Centre, Durham, NC,*
[1,3]*USA*
[2]*India*

1. Introduction

With expanding indications for device therapies for management of cardiovascular diseases, the number of patients receiving pacemaker implantations are increasing every year. These cardiac electronic devices rely on complex microcircuitry and use electromagnetic waves for their communication with the programmers. Therefore, they are susceptible to interference from the surrounding electromagnetic radiation. Electromagnetic interference (EMI) can be defined as any signal, either biologic or non-biologic, that falls within a frequency spectrum that are being detected by the sensing circuitry of the pacemaker. They can interfere with the optimal function of the pacemaker and is always a concern for the patients with a pacemaker, since the risk of EMI is greatest in pacemaker dependent patients.

EMI may potentially affect a pacemaker in one of three ways: Stopping the pacemaker from delivering the stimulating pulses that regulate heart's rhythm; causing the pacemaker to deliver the irregularly; and causing the pacemaker to ignore heart's own rhythm and deliver pulses at a fixed rate. EMI with pacemakers can be very complex, not only from the technical standpoint, but also from the view of public health issues. Pacemakers may be affected by various equipments in our daily life, varying from hospital equipments to security devices. Hospital procedures like electrocautery, cardioversion, defibrillation, magnetic resonance imaging, lithotripsy, radiofrequency ablation, diathermy etc., may interfere with the normal pacemaker function. Similarly other electromagnetic equipments like cell phones, digital media players (MP3, ipod etc.,) security devices, anti - theft devices, conduction heaters, microwave ovens, welding equipments may also interfere with the pacemaker. Complete avoidance of these equipments may not be practical for most of the patients with pacemaker and this may significantly affect the quality of life too. Hence, patients with these devices should be advised to employ certain recommended changes so that they can enjoy the full benefits of the pacemaker.

It is important that the clinician taking care of a patient with implanted device be aware of these resources and to provide appropriate education and protection to the patient. In this chapter, we will discuss about the various interferences with the pacemakers in day to day activities of the patients and the methods to tackle them.

2. Electro Magnetic Interference

There are three essential elements to any electromagnetic compatibility problem. There must be an electromagnetic source, a receptor (in our case the implanted cardiac device) that cannot function properly due to the electromagnetic phenomenon, and an environment between them that allows the source to interfere with the receptor. Each of these three elements must be present, although they may not be readily identified in every situation. Identifying at least two of these elements and eliminating (or attenuating) one of them generally solves electromagnetic compatibility problems.

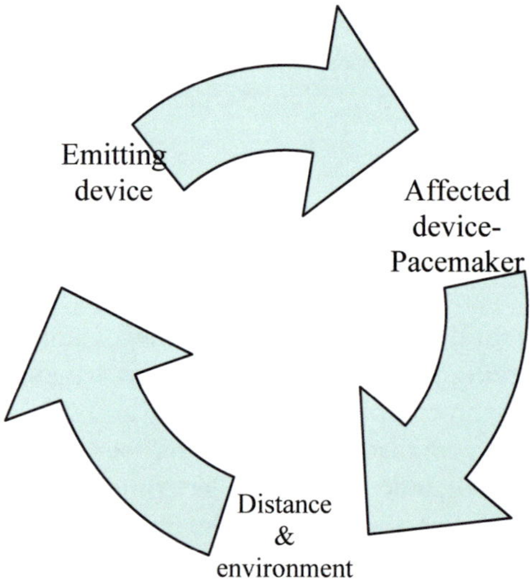

Fig. 1. Essentials of EMI.

The factors affecting EMI can be broadly classified into properties of the emitting device (i.e., frequency, which is inversely proportional to wavelength, and power of emissions); the physical relationship between the devices (i.e., distance); and the susceptibility of the affected device (i.e., electromagnetic shielding).

a. Emitting device

The frequency of electromagnetic radiation plays a role in relation to the length of various electric components in the susceptible device. These act as antennae to receive interfering signals. Long wavelengths (low frequencies) transfer minimal energy to small electronic components, and very short wavelengths (extremely high frequencies) are easily shielded. Frequencies between 10 kHz and 1 GHz are generally the most problematic. The amplitude (or power) influences the effect that the EMI has on the susceptible device. Handheld radios transmit at a constant power output of 2 to 5 W. Early analog cellular phones functioned at high power output levels, but more recent digital cellular phones can vary in their power output levels during use and function at less-problematic higher frequencies. The lowest power output occurs during standby operation, with variable power when the cellular phone is in use and maximal power when it is ringing (Shaw et al., 2004). Power output may be as low as 60 mW, with peaks to about 2 W, averaging 600 mW. Within hospitals, shielding from the base station may force cellular devices to operate at higher power. New cellular technologies introduce new variables that may affect EMI. Wireless local area networks (802.11) and Bluetooth function at a higher frequency and lower power as compared with cellular devices and are far less likely to produce EMI.

b. Affected device

Electromagnetic compatibility (EMC) refers to the ability of electronic devices of different types to operate in an electromagnetic environment without loss of intended function. The EMC of the affected device affects the degree of malfunction that may occur. Newer devices are designed according to more stringent standards, with attention to shielding and electromagnetic immunity, and are less susceptible to EMI. Equipment manufactured before 1993 are more susceptible to EMI as compared with more modern equipment, which are now subject to International Electrotechnical Commission Standard 60601-1-2. Even more higher standards are required for critical and life-support devices.

c. Distance and environment

For electromagnetic fields, the energy level falls rapidly as the distance from the source increases (proportional to the square of the distance). Clinically relevant EMI is very uncommon at distances greater than 1 m (Lawrentschuk, N 2004). Building structures and many other environmental factors may influence the degree of EMI. Electromagnetic radiation from multiple sources in a dense hospital environment may aggregate and produce more pronounced effects than anticipated. Although many factors affecting EMI are difficult to predict, the reduction in field strength with distance is generally predictable. According to Faraday's Law (Figure 2), the induced voltage is proportional to the induction area. Two important management variables are distance of the device from the EMI source and the duration of exposure. The intensity of an electric or magnetic field decreases with the square of the distance. Thus, if a patient doubles the distance from the source, he or she is exposed to only one fourth of the original field.

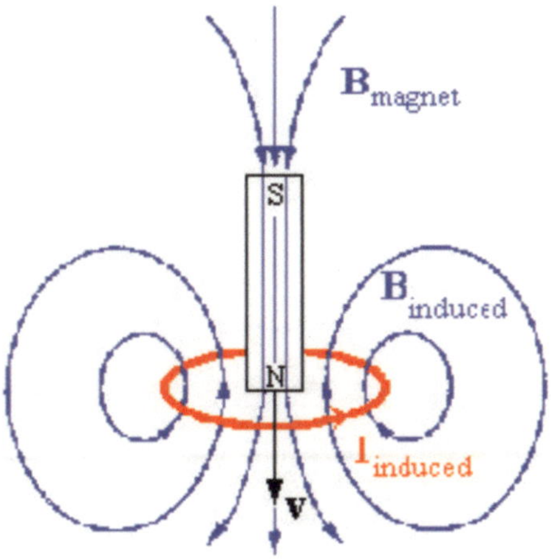

Fig. 2. Faraday's Law

EMI occurs when EM waves emitted by one electronic source or device impede the normal function of another electronic device. EM fields have both an electric field measured in volts per meter and a magnetic field measured in amperes per meter. Their sources can be broadly divided into radiofrequency waves with frequencies from 0.1 Hz to 100 MHz (eg, electric power, radio and television transmitter, electrocautery) and microwaves from 100 MHz to 12 GHz (eg, radar transmitters, cellular telephones, microwave ovens). EMI can be

galvanic, which requires direct contact with electrical current (eg, cautery), EM not requiring direct contact with the source (arc welding), or magnetic, that occurs from close contact with a strong magnetic field. eg, magnetic resonance imaging (MRI).
EMI signals in the 10 to 60 Hz frequency range can effect cardiac devices because they overlap the cardiac signal range. The amplitude and frequency of muscle potentials overlap the same range as the cardiac signals. Hence, oversensing of myopotential signals is common in unipolar sensing systems. (Figure 3). Myopotential signals commonly reach the 2 to 4 mV amplitude range. Bandpass filters permit only selected frequencies to pass through the sensing circuit. The typical ranges for P-waves are 20 to 40 Hz, R-waves 18 to 50 Hz, and T-waves 0 to 10 Hz (Figure 3)
Mechanical and electrical shielding designed into pacemakers and implantable cardioverter-defibrillators (ICDs), has, in most cases, enabled these medical devices to be immune to external electromagnetic interference (EMI) allowing the vast majority of patients to live their lives without the fear of EM device interactions. These device features include titanium casing, signal filtering, interference rejection circuits, feed through capacitors, noise reversion function, and programmable parameters. Bipolar leads sense less conducted and radiated interference because the electrode distance and the antenna are smaller than that of unipolar leads.

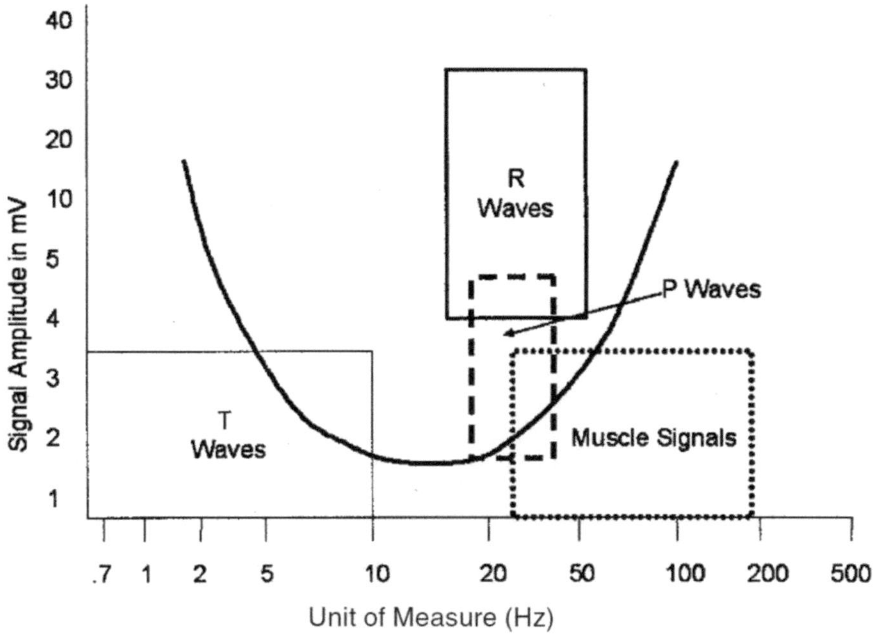

Fig. 3. Adapted from Sweesy MW et al. 2004

3. Factors influencing the response of the device

The programmed settings of the device (like sensitivity settings, polarity, mode, and refractory and blanking periods) can influence the response of the pacemaker to EMI. The more sensitive the setting, the more prone the device is to oversense the noncardiac signals. For example, an implantable cardioverter-defibrillator (ICD) and the atrial channel are most susceptible to EMI because they usually are set at highly sensitive settings. A left-sided unipolar system is more susceptible to EMI due to a larger loop for voltage induction between the lead and pulse generator.

Rarely, a device may receive permanent damage from high-output energy (i.e., Radiofrequency ablation, external defibrillation, or high-dose radiation therapy). The type of interaction depends on the frequency, field strength of the EMI, channel (Atrial {A} or Ventricular {V}) and portion of the timing cycle in which the signal is detected. The most commonly encountered response is oversensing. In a DDD (Table 1) pacing system, oversensing of EMI noise on the atrial channel will result in ventricular-triggered pacing, most often at or near the programmed upper tracking rate. In the DDD mode, anything sensed on the atrial channel will be interpreted as a P wave, and a sensed A-V delay will be initiated.

Position I (chamber(s) paced)	Position II (chamber(s) sensed)	Position III (response to sensing)	Position IV (rate modulation)	Position V (multisite pacing)
O - None	O = None	O = None	O = None	O = None
A = Atrium	A = Atrium	T = Triggered	R = Rate modulation	A = Atrium
V = Ventricle	V = Ventricle	I = Inhibited		V = Ventricle
D = Dual (A + V)	D = Dual (A + V)	D = Dual (T + I)		D = Dual (A + V)
S* = Single (A or V)	S* = Single (A or V)			

NASPE/BPEG = North American Society of Pacing and Electrophysiology and British Pacing and Electrophysiology Group.
*Manufacturers' designation only.

Table 1. Describing the nomenclature of the Pacemaker Modes

The A-V delay clock will time-out and the ventricle will be paced because no intrinsic conduction will have actually been initiated. Oversensing of EMI on the ventricular channel will be interpreted as an intrinsic R-wave and result in ventricular inhibition whether the device is operating in the DDD or VVI mode. Noise reversion will occur if the EMI is detected during the relative refractory period, or the noise sampling portion of the ventricular refractory period. Most devices will pace asynchronously at the programmed base rate when operating in the noise reversion mode. Back-up mode or power on reset pacing is automatically activated when the pacing system is subject to high energy EMI such as electrocautery or defibrillation. The back-up behavior is typically the same as the device's elective replacement behavior (ERI). The circuitry of cardiac devices implements a zener diode, which shunts energy away from the pacemaker circuitry. On occasion, this diode can be overwhelmed by electrical interference, resulting in permanent device damage. Although rare, it may be possible to induce rapid pacing when a device detects radiofrequency signals and amplifies that output, resulting in capture at rapid rates. This rapid pacing has been reported with magnetic resonance imaging and is potentially lethal whether or not the patient is pacemaker dependent. Various factors influencing EMI are described in Table 2.

One of the important features made by the manufacturers made over the past few decades to reduce the EMI is the change in lead polarity. In a unipolar system, the tip of the electrode acts as the negatively charged, current emitting cathode. The surface of the pulse generator

Factors influencing EMI
Controllable factors
1. Programmed parameters
Sensitivity settings
Sensing polarity
Pacing mode
Refractory periods
Blanking periods
Committed crosstalk detection window
Sensor settings
2. Distance and position of the patient
3. Duration of the exposure
Less Controllable Factors
1. Intensity of the EMI field
2. Nonprogrammable device characteristics and settings
3. Frequency of the signals
4. Zener diode
5. Lead configuration
6. Access codes, parity links, and reed switch closure

Table 2. Factors influencing EMI.

acts as the positively charged anode, to which electrons flow to complete the circuit. The case of the pulse generator must maintain contact with tissue and be at least partially uninsulated or else pacing cannot occur. This concept is important to consider during pulse generator implant or replacement. In these situations, pacing will not occur where the lead may be connected but the pulse generator may not be in contact in contact with the patient's skin or subcutaneous tissue. A bipolar lead places both electrodes within the heart, where the cathode is at the tip of the lead. The anode is a ring electrode that is located about 1-2 cm proximal to the tip. Bipolar leads are slightly thicker and may draw slightly more current than unipolar leads. Nevertheless, they offer a number of advantages including fewer incidences of EMI and are more commonly used in the United States. Because the electrodes in a bipolar system are close to each other and within the heart, there is less likelihood of extraneous signals being sensed as a cardiac event. This reduces the incidence of inappropriate pacemaker inhibition due to sensing of skeletal myopotentials. Bipolar sensing effectively has eliminated myopotential inhibition and crosstalk as pacemaker problems. Astridge PS et al., (1996) had shown that with bipolar sensing, there is considerably less sensing of external electric fields and less effect from electrocautery during surgery.

4. Pacemaker responses to EMI

4.1 Pacing Inhibition

This function normally allows the sensing of the electrical potential that is given off by the heart when it contracts. Sensing of the heart contractions causes the pacemaker to withhold the electrical stimulus (inhibit/standby). This response is limited to a heart rate range up to approximately 300 pulses per minute or 5 Hertz (Pinski et al. 2002). Radiated magnetic fields or conducted currents that are detected by the pacemaker in this rate range also cause the output of the pacemaker to erroneously withhold the electrical stimulus (inhibit/standby). Pacemaker will withhold pacing pulses, if electrical potentials are detected within the heart rate range. Sustained pacing inhibition is potentially catastrophic in pacemaker dependent patients. Depending on the duration of inhibition and emergence of escape rhythms, lightheadedness, syncope, or death could result. Prolonged inhibition is uncommon because of the protective algorithms available in pacemakers. The majority of patients currently undergoing pacemaker implantation are not completely dependent on pacemaker.

4.2 Triggering of rapid or premature pacing

Very strong electromagnetic fields could induce voltage in the lead(s) that may directly capture the myocardium. For example, 58-kHz acoustomagnetic Electronic article surveillance systems are capable of inducing 3.7 V in pacemaker leads leading to isolated premature paced beats (but no sustained rapid pacing) as observed by McIvor et al., (1998). Oversensing of EMI by the atrial channel of a pacemaker programmed to a tracking mode (DDD, VDD) can trigger ventricular pacing at or near the upper tracking rate limit. Alternatively, automatic mode switching may occur if this function is enabled. In some pacemakers, detection of noise in the atrial channel can trigger a noise reversion mode. Preferential detection of EMI is not uncommon because atrial sensitivity is usually programmed higher (more sensitive) than ventricular sensitivity. It is possible to observe rapid pacing due to atrial oversensing as the patient approaches an electromagnetic field, followed by a period of ventricular oversensing (inhibition or mode reversion) as the field becomes stronger. Patients who experience this problem are typically symptomatic and complain of rapid palpitations. If sustained, inappropriate pacemaker acceleration induced by atrial oversensing may cause palpitation, hypotension, or angina. Very rapid pacing could induce ventricular fibrillation.

4.3 Noise reversion mode

Pacemakers incorporate protective algorithms against prolonged inhibition from spurious signals. A common response is transient reversion to *asynchronous pacing*. These algorithms are based on the fact that rapid frequencies are unlikely to represent myocardial activation. In most pacemakers, a noise sampling or noise interrogation window (also known as relative refractory period) occupies the second part of the ventricular refractory period. Pacemakers do not respond to signals during the initial portion of the ventricular refractory period (i.e., ventricular blanking), which is usually nonprogrammable and fixed or adjusted automatically by the generator based on the strength and duration of the ventricular event. Signals recognized during the noise sampling window cannot reset the lower rate timer (therefore preventing inhibition), but can affect other timing intervals, most importantly, the ventricular refractory period. The pacemaker has a safety feature that identifies/classifies strong continuous radiated electromagnetic fields or conducted currents that occur outside of the cardiac rate range (i.e. > or = 300 Pulses per minute or 5 Hertz. Once a field or current is identified / classified, this safety feature allows a pacemaker to deliver pacing stimuli to the heart when sensing strong continuous radiated electromagnetic fields or conducted currents. Pacemaker reversion minimizes the types of continuous electromagnetic fields or conducted currents that can cause the pacemaker to be inhibited. Pacemaker will continuously pace the heart at the programmed low rate of the pacemaker in the presence of a strong continuous alternating magnetic field.

4.4 Electric (Power–On) reset

Momentary strong EMI, by inducing very high voltage within device circuits, or triggering special microprocessor timers, may cause reset of DDD and VVIR pacemakers to the VVI or VOO mode, a condition called power-on or electric reset. Electrosurgery and external or internal defibrillation are the most common causes of the reset phenomenon. In the reset mode, the pulse generator functions only with basic factory preset instructions (pacing mode and parameters) stored in the nonvolatile read-only memory, as communication between the random access memory (containing the programmable settings) and the microprocessor has been interrupted. In some pacemakers, the pacing mode and rate are similar during electrical reset and elective replacement indicator. In devices with different replacement and reset parameters, strong EMI may activate either one. In some pacemakers, two levels of electrical reset (partial and full) exist. Partial reset tends to occur with less intense interference, generally preserving the programmed pacing mode and rates. In some pulse generators, there will be no response to magnet application in the reset mode. The reset mode does not revert back when EMI is discontinued. A DDD(R) device reset to the VOO or VVI mode might cause hypotension, particularly in patients with pacemaker syndrome. Resolution of the problem requires a specific programmer command. Electric reset can be differentiated from battery depletion by telemetry of battery voltage and impedance. When reset is due to EMI, the battery voltage should be normal (approximately 2.8 V) and battery impedance normal or slightly rose according to battery age.

4.5 Damage to the generator or to the electrode-myocardial interface

In the overwhelming majority of cases, the effects of EMI are temporary, lasting only as long as the device is within range of the source. However, strong EMI (e.g., electrosurgery and external defibrillation) can cause permanent damage to an implanted device. Circuitry damage, (resulting in output failure, pacemaker runaway, and other malfunctions) can occur, requiring generator replacement (at times emergent). Increases in pacing thresholds secondary to local heat related injury at the myocardium lead interface are also possible.

4.6 Pacemaker magnet response

In the past, patients with a pacemaker in whom EMI was likely were frequently managed by placing a magnet over their device to produce asynchronous pacing. As device technology has expanded, it has become less clear how each individual device will respond to a magnet, and there appears to be no universal effect, even between two otherwise identical devices (Table 5). The response will depend largely on how the device has been programmed. For many pacemakers, the presence of a magnet will indeed induce continuous asynchronous pacing. For others, however, a very short period of asynchronous pacing might occur or there may be no effect at all. A static magnetic field of 10 Gauss or more will cause the pacemaker to deliver a continuous sequence of stimuli at 85 beats per minute for current pacemaker or other normal low rates specific to the older model pacemakers. Pacemaker will continuously pace the heart at the magnet rate (85 bpm for current pacemakers) while in the presence of a strong static magnetic field associated with either a permanent magnet or an electro-magnet. With the ICD, approximately 99% of them are programmed to have their anti-tachycardia function disabled in the presence of a magnet without affecting their bradycardia pacing. In the event of a magnet ever being applied to an implantable device, its function and programming should be checked at the earliest opportunity.

5. Sources of EMI:

Most of the common home and workplace items that can generate EMI typically do not interfere with normal operation of implantable medical devices.
Common electromagnetic sources are described in Table 3.

Electromagnetic fields
Daily life: 1. Cellular telephones 2. Electronic article surveillance devices 3. Metal detectors 4. Some home appliances (e.g., electric razor, toy remote controls)
Work and industrial environment: 1. High voltage power lines 2. Transformers 3. Welders 4. Electric motors
Medical environment: 1. Magnetic resonance image scanners 2. Electrosurgery 3. Defibrillation 4. Neurostimulators 5. TENS units 6. Therapeutic diathermy 7. Ionizing radiation 8. Radiotherapy 9. Lithotripsy

Table 3. Sources of EMI

6. EMI in daily life:

6.1 Household related exposures

6.1.1 Portable headphones

Portable headphones such as those used with portable digital music players (MP3 players) like iPods, generate powerful magnetic fields that have the potential to cause clinically relevant magnetic interference in pacemaker patients. Placement of portable headphones in a front shirt pocket in close proximity to a patient's pacemaker could temporarily deactivate the device and inhibit the delivery of a required therapy. Because magnetic field strength falls off quickly with distance, keeping the portable headphones even a short distance from the chest wall can effectively eliminate the potential for magnetic interference. Lee et al., (2009) noted that clinically significant magnetic interference can occur when portable headphones are placed in close proximity to implanted pacemakers (in 30% of study group). Patients are advised to keep portable the headphones at least 3 cm from their device.

Item	Low risk	Pacemaker Reversion	Pacemaker Inhibition	Remarks
Bingo Wand	X	X		Maintain 15cm distance
Casino slot machines	X			Low risk
Electric Guitars	X	X		Maintain 15cm distance
Electric Speakers	X	X		Maintain 15cm distance
Electric Toy Trains	X	X		Maintain 15cm distance
Electric Golf Cart	X	X		Maintain 15cm distance
Laser Tag	X	X		Maintain 15cm distance
Radio Controlled Model cars, Airplanes, Boats etc.,	X	X	X	Maintain 15cm distance
Rifle / Shot Guns	X			Low risk
Tatoo Machine	X	X		Maintain 15cm distance

Table 4. Electromagnetic Compatibility of devices involved in Hobbies

6.1.2 Cellular telephones and other wireless devices

Interference between pacemaker and cellular telephones were addressed by Hayes et al., (1997) They have investigated 980 device patients and 5533 cell phone exposures and found that interactions were highly variable by phone type, pacemaker manufacturer, and pacemaker model. Most interference was oversensing and occurred when the phone was placed directly over the implanted device. Modern digital cell phones generate strong, amplitude modulated fields with pulse repetition rates near the physiologic sensing range. Device manufacturers are advising to maintain a 10-15cm distance between the antenna of the cell phone and the implanted device. If using powerful cell phone, which is using greater than 3 watts, it is advisable to maintain a 30cm distance from the device.

Recently, third-generation mobile phones, UMTS (Universal Mobile Telecommunication System), were introduced in Europe. Ismail et al., 2010 conducted a study which included 100 patients, 23 with single-chamber and 77 with dual-chamber pacemakers. Two UMTS cellular phones (T-Mobile, Vodafone) were tested in the standby, dialing, and operating mode in this cohort of patients. Regardless of atrial and ventricular sensitivity settings, both UMTS mobile phones (Nokia 6650 and Motorola A835) did not show any interference with all tested pacemakers. In addition, both cellular phones did not interfere with the marker channels and the intracardiac ECGs of the pacemakers. Ismail et al. concluded that third-generation mobile phones are safe for patients with pacemaker. This is due to the high frequency band for this system (1,800–2,200 MHz) and the low power output between 0.01 and 0.25 W.

6.1.3 Hearing aids

Cochlear implant type of hearing aids is with low risk of having EMI with the pacemakers. Hearing Aids with transmitting necklace loops coupled into the ear piece Telcoil (T-coil) of the hearing aid emit magnetic fields. The transmitting antenna associated with this type of hearing aid system is incorporated into the necklace loop. This antenna radiates a magnetic field that is coupled into the T-coil in the earpiece of the hearing aid. Maintain a 6" (15cm) distance between the pacemaker and the portion of the hearing aid necklace radiating the magnetic field. If the transmitting antenna is closer than the noted distance, there is a potential for pacemaker reversion or inhibition. Individuals may want to reposition the loop so that it is located on the opposite shoulder from the implant site or look for an alternate transmitting antenna system that can also be worn in such a way to maintain the recommended distance of greater than 6" (15cm).

6.2 Work / environment related exposures

6.2.1 Electric shock

EMI from electric power can occur if patients come in proximity to high voltage overhead power lines (accidentally or by occupation) or it may be caused by electrical appliances held close or in direct contact with the chest. Implanted devices are susceptible to interference signals of 50–60 Hz, frequencies that lie within the bandwidth sampled for detection of intracardiac signals. A momentary shock from an electrical outlet (110 / 220 volts) or higher voltages, if in a commercial or industrial setting, will cause pacemaker inhibition or inhibition of the pacemaker portion of the ICD. A memorable momentary shock may cause some of the parameters of the pacemaker or ICD to be reset to nominal values. If any parameter changed, the physician can restore the original parameters in the office. Permanent damage to the pacemaker or ICD is unlikely to occur unless the shock is very severe. Prolonged external shocks greater than 2 seconds can cause reversion in the pacemaker. Prolonged external shocks greater than 8 seconds can cause inhibition in the pacemaker portion of the ICD and/or a shock therapy. As with momentary shocks, there is a low risk of permanent damage to the pacemaker or ICD from prolonged shocks associated with a 110 / 220 volt source. Bipolar sensing protects from EMI in all but the most extreme environmental conditions, like power generating stations, while with unipolar sensing inappropriate pacemaker behavior can occur during routine daily exposures. EMI from household appliances is more likely with improper grounding.

6.2.2 Magnets and pacemakers

Magnet responses vary widely among manufacturers and even among various models of a single manufacturer (Table 5). For example, magnet application in single-chamber systems may result in asynchronous pacing at the standard rate or the programmed rate, ventricular demand pacing at a fast rate, or ventricular triggered pacing. Magnet application in dual-chamber systems may result in dual-chamber asynchronous pacing at the programmed rate or at a standard rate, or at the programmed rate plus a fixed percent increment; or it may even result in asynchronous single-chamber ventricular pacing at a standard rate. Elective replacement indicators in some models may be elicited only in the magnet mode. In such instances, routine magnet application may be especially important for determining the need for replacement of a depleting pacer generator. The application of a magnet over the generator is rarely associated with adverse effects. On occasion ventricular ectopy may result from asynchronous ventricular pacing, but this is seldom sustained. Caution is warranted if the patient has both a pacer and an implantable cardioverter-defibrillator; some implanted defibrillators may have tachycardia therapy inactivated by prolonged magnet exposure. Because most devices respond to magnet application by asynchronous pacing, magnets may also be employed, both diagnostically and therapeutically, in cases where potential pacer malfunction is attributed to sensing problems. Magnet application can be therapeutic to terminate pacemaker mediated tachycardia or to restore pacing in cases of oversensing. In cases of pacemaker dependence, rapid magnet conversion to asynchronous pacing may be critical in preventing asystole due to oversensing or crosstalk inhibition (particularly if the appropriate pacemaker programmer is unavailable). In some contemporary pacemakers, however, magnet application may trigger specialized pacemaker functions such as threshold search or electrogram storage rather than asynchronous pacing.

Possible Responses to Magnet Application
1. Asynchronous pacing
2. Triggered Mode
3. Rate Change 4. Programmed rate 5. Faster rate than programmed
6. Threshold determination - Fixed percentage amplitude reduction over first few paced complexes
7. Trigger Electrogram storage
8. No change in pacer function - Programmable magnet response

Table 5. Responses to Magnet application

6.2.3 Electronic Article Surveillance Devices (EAS)

These are the scanners located on the the counter used to identify the items to be purchased and deactivate the anti-theft tags at checkout counters in stores. The transmitter in these devices emits an electromagnetic field designed to interact with a "tag" in a store item. As a result of the interaction, the tag emits back a signal that is then detected by the receiver. Customers are exposed to an electromagnetic field as they walk through the gate that consists of a pair of transmitter and receiver pedestals. EAS systems differ greatly in the frequency and strength of emitted fields. Electromagnetic fields from these devices have the potential to induce interference signals in the sensing circuit of implanted cardiac devices. McIvor et al. studied the effects of six EAS systems in 50 patients with pacemakers from seven different manufacturers. One exposure protocol mimicked the most common real-life situation, walking at a normal pace midway between the gates. A "worst-case scenario" protocol required the patients to lean against the transmitter gate with the body parallel and then perpendicular to the transmitter.

Interactions occurred with 48 pacemakers, almost exclusively with acoustomagnetic systems. No pacemaker reacted to the swept radiofrequency systems. Only two patients presented transient asynchronous pacing while exposed to an electromagnetic system. The frequency of interactions with the acoustomagnetic system increased with the duration and closeness of the exposure. It was 16% when walking through the gates and 96% when leaning against the pedestal. Transient asynchronous pacing was the most common response, followed by atrial oversensing with tracking, ventricular oversensing with inhibition, and "voltage-induced" paced beats.

Item	Low risk	Pacemaker Reversion	Pacemaker Inhibition	Remarks
Ab Stimulator			X	Not recommended to use
Badge with electronic circuit	X	X		Maintain 15cms from the wall unit
Bagde with magnetic clasp	X	X		Maintain 15cm distance
Body fat scale (Electronic)		X	X	Not recommended
Electric Blanket	X			Low Risk
Electric Fences	X		X	Momentary shock may change the settings
Elecric Tooth brush	X	X	X	Maintain 15cm distance
Electric grocery cart / personal sccoters	X	X		Maintain 15cm distance
Electric Shocks	X	X	X	A momentary shock will cause PM inhibition
Hair Dryer	X	X		Maintain 15cm distance
Home security System	X			Low risk
Home security system - Microwave	X	X		Maintain 15cm distance
Hot tub	X			Low Risk
Induction Stove Top	X	X		Maintain 60cm distance
Ionized air filter	X	X		Maintain 15cm distance
Magnetic back brace	X	X		Maintain 15cm distance
Massage Chair	X			Low Risk
Massager - handheld	X	X		Maintain 15cm distance
Medical alert Necklace / bacelet	X			Low risk
Microwave ovens	X			Low risk
Motor Cycle	X	X	X	Maintain 30cms distance from the ignition system
Pest control - Ultrasonic only	X	X		Maintain 15cm distance
Pest control - radiofrequency	X	X		Maintain 15cm distance
Sewing Machines	X	X		Maintain 15cm distance
Shaver with electrical cord	X	X		Maintain 15cm distance
Speakers	X	X		Maintain 15cm distance
TV Audio Headset	X	X		Maintain 15cm distance
TV Remote Infrared	X			Low risk

Table 6. Electromagnetic Compatibility of devices involved in daily Home Use.

Available evidence suggests that although severe interactions between EAS systems and implanted cardiac devices can occur, they are unlikely when patients walk through the gates at a normal pace. However, interactions are likely with prolonged, close exposure to acoustomagnetic or electromagnetic systems. Prolonged exposure may result in pacemaker reversion or inhibition. When scanning wands with deactivators are used, patients are advised to maintain a 60 cm distance between the wand and the implanted device.

6.2.4 House arrest anklets and bracelets:

House arrest anklets, worn by the individual, emit low level radio frequency signals at specific time intervals. These radio frequency signals are detected by a receiving unit connected to the telephone. The telephone periodically communicates with a central monitoring facility. As it is associated with low power transmission, the risk of affecting the pacemaker is very low. Patients with pacemaker should maintain a 6" (15cm) distance between pacemaker and the bracelet. If the device is closer than 6" (15cm), then, there can be a potential for pacemaker reversion or inhibition. The response is specific to the time interval and duration of the radio frequency transmission of the bracelet.

6.2.5 Metal detectors:

Metal Detectors or magnetometers are used in airports, government buildings and some schools. Metal detector archways or hand held wands in compliance with federal regulations are unlikely to affect Pacemaker. Walk through the archway metal detector is also considered as a low risk. If the archway detects metal in the device, patients should request a hand search. If hand held metal detector wand is to be used, patients should request that the wand not be placed directly over the device. If the security personnel insist on using the wand over the pacemaker, patients should be advised to request that the exposure of pacemaker to the magnetic field of the wand be limited to 1- 2 seconds every 10 seconds. X-ray radiation is also used in some airports for security check. Conpass-X-1280® is an X-ray body scanner that provides the detection of all dangerous objects within 10 seconds. (Detects metal & non metal weapons, explosives, dangerous liquids, diamonds, gold and illicit drugs (including swallowed). The amount of radiation used is lesser than the one used in diagnostic radiation. Other companies with similar systems are American Science & Engineering, Inc. & Rapiscan's Secure 1000®. These detection systems do not utilize an alternating magnetic field to detect metal as does the archway and wand metal detectors. Millimeter Wave Imaging Scanners are used in airports, courthouses and jails. They are otherwise called as 3D scanner, whole body imaging, or RF / Microwave scanner. These devices can emit a low magnetic radiation. Patients should keep their implanted heart device 6"(15cm) away from the walls of the scanner. If closer than 6"(15cm), there are chances for pacemaker reversion.

6.3 Hospital environment

Although patients with pacemakers usually spend less time in the hospital than in the outside environment, the hospital, ironically, is where the majority of patient encounters with EMI occur. Some interference sources, such as magnetic resonance imaging (MRI) and electrocautery devices, are encountered more frequently, whereas others, such as transcutaneous electrical nerve stimulation (TENS) units and dental equipment, although encountered frequently, are not routinely recognized as sources of electromagnetic radiation.

6.3.1 Direct Current Cardioversion (CV) and defibrillation in patients with pacemaker:

The use of CV in patients with implanted devices has long been a cause for concern with regard to the potential for adverse effects on the generator and/or leads, with the result that this simple and effective therapy may have been delayed or even denied to some patients. These concerns were largely fuelled by a number of reports in the 1970s and 1980s suggesting the potential for device interference or lead failure. Devices implanted within the last decade, however, are considerably more sophisticated, more likely to use bipolar lead configurations, and better protected against external interference than those of the period from which these reports arose, leaving the question of safety in patients with modern implantable devices open. In addition, CV has evolved over recent years with the development of equipment able to deliver biphasic shocks resulting in an increased efficacy and lower energy requirements. Manegold et al., 2007 studied 29 patients with pacemaker undergoing elective external cardioversion for atrial fibrillation, using an anterior-posterior shock electrode orientation with a distance to the implanted device ≥ 8 cm. He noted that there is reduction of the pacing impedance immediately after the cardioversion. However there was no device or lead dysfunction noted in any of those patients. Waller et al., recommended that the defibrillator paddles be placed ≥15cm from the pulse generator and be oriented in an anterior-lateral, anterior-posterior or left pectoral-right hypochondrial (for right sided generators) positions in order to place the electric field perpendicular and not parallel to the course of the leads. Some manufacturers recommend use of VOO or AOO modes during cardioversion in order to switch off the amplifier. Additionally, the time between two successive shocks ought to be about ≥ 5 min in order to allow cooling of the diodes. After defibrillation, the pacemaker should be interrogated and the program confirmed. Expected pacing threshold rise should be managed by increasing the output and any change in sensing threshold should similarly be corrected by reprogramming.

6.3.2 Electro Convulsion Therapy (ECT):

ECT is used to treat depression, anxiety and other mental disorders. ECT usually delivers measured electrical stimuli over a brief period of time (1-2 seconds). These briefly applied electrical stimuli induce a seizure that may last for several minutes. As a result the pacemaker may respond by either pausing (inhibiting) or delivering 1-2 pacemaker stimuli. The pacemaker portion of the ICD will be inhibited for as long as the current is present (1-2 beats). If ECT is used for longer than 8 seconds, there may be a potential for pacemaker reversion. The activity detected during the seizure period may affect the rate response circuit. If the rate response circuit is programmed "on", there is the potential to elevate the rate of the pacemaker portion of the ICD or the pacemaker rate. It is recommended that individuals considering this procedure consult the cardiologist to evaluate any possible risks associated with these responses in conjunction with their medical condition.

6.3.3 Electrocautery

Electrocautery is used in surgeries to cut tissue and stop the bleeding of blood vessels. Several electrosurgical techniques can generate EMI. During electrosurgery in monopolar modes, the electric current spreads out and penetrates the entire body of the patient. This stray current may be interpreted by an implanted device as an intracardiac signal. Casavant D et al., 1998, described that pacing inhibition, pacing triggering, automatic mode switching, noise reversion or spurious tachyarrhythmia detection can occur, depending on the type of device, the programmed settings, the duration of EMI, and the channel in which the current is oversensed. It is recommended to apply the magnet over the pacemaker during the surgical procedure. When cautery performed less than 6" (15cm) or grounding electrode is placed less than 6"(15cm) from device, damage can occur and/or the output of the device can be affected even when the magnet is applied. Damage may occur to the tissue at the lead tissue interface. Currents induced into the lead system may initiate an arrhythmia. Magnet application in the pacemaker causes the pacemaker to deliver a sequence of stimuli at a normal low rate (usually 85 bpm magnet rate). If magnet is not placed over the pacemaker, application of electrosurgery should be limited to 1-2 seconds every 10 seconds. If these timing intervals are restrictive, reprogramming of the pacemaker should be considered, especially for individuals that are dependent on the pacemaker.

6.3.4 Extracorporeal Shock Wave Lithotripsy

Extracorporeal shock wave lithotripsy (ESWL) is a noninvasive technique that uses electrohydraulic waves to disintegrate renal calculi. An underwater electrical spark causes rapid expansion of water vapor, which generates an electrohydraulic wave directed toward a semielliptical housing that diverts the wave toward a focal point in the bath. The patient is positioned in the bath so that the renal calculi are at the focal point. Potential causes of pacemaker dysfunction inherent in the use of this technique include EMI and mechanical disruption of the pulse generator and its casing. In vivo and in vitro studies have evaluated the extent of EMI and the mechanical disruption of pacemakers, when the pacemakers were placed at various distances from the electrohydraulic wave source. The extracorporeal shock wave is capable of producing extrasystoles and therefore is delivered a few milliseconds after the R-wave. The extracorporeal shock wave is delivered after the atrial spike in patients with dual-chamber pacemakers who are atrially paced. The number of chambers paced and/or sensed and the pacemaker settings largely influence the effect that ESWL has on pacemakers. ESWL, triggered synchronously after the ventricular pacing spike, exhibited no interference on single chamber pacemaker function. Rate-responsive pacemakers increased their pacing rate to the upper pacing limit when exposed to synchronous ESWL. Dual-chamber pacemakers programmed to DDD settings exhibited inhibition because they oversensed the electromagnetic ESWL wave. Reprogramming the pacemaker to VVI or VOO mode resulted in normal pacemaker function. Piezoelectric crystals in rate responsive pacemakers may shatter, when placed at the electrohydraulic wave focal point but remain intact when placed 5 centimeters from the focal point. Patients with a rate-responsive pacemaker that contains piezoelectric crystals should not undergo ESWL if the device is implanted in the abdomen, but this procedure may safely be performed in such a patient if the device is located in the thorax. Careful pacemaker follow-up monitoring should continue for at least several months after the procedure to ensure that no damage was sustained to the reed switch. In addition to continuous electrocardiographic monitoring, the following guidelines should be followed in treating patients with pacemakers who have ESWL (Cooper et al., 1988):

1. Single-chamber pacemakers generally do not require sensing and/or pacing changes.
2. Reprogram dual-chamber devices to VVI mode.
3. The piezoelectric activity-sensing, rate-responsive, and single-chamber function should be turned off.

6.3.5 Radiofrequency catheter ablation

Radiofrequency catheter ablation is first-line therapy for a variety of supraventricular and ventricular arrhythmias. The interaction between radiofrequency current and implantable devices has been studied most thoroughly during palliative ablation of the atrioventricular junction for drug-refractory atrial fibrillation. Patients with atrial fibrillation often receive pacemakers for associated spontaneous (i.e., bradycardia-tachycardia syndrome) or drug-induced bradycardia. Radiofrequency current (delivered as an unmodulated sine wave at 500 to 1000 kHz) is an intense source of pulsed interference that interacts unpredictably with permanent pacemakers. Energy delivery may result in asynchronous pacing, rapid tracking, electric reset, and premature triggering of the elective replacement indicator. It is impossible to predict (with the exception of some device-specific effects) the type of interaction that will be seen. Different interactions may be seen (in the same patient) during consecutive energy applications. Most of the interactions are transient and terminate with cessation of energy delivery.

Chang et al (1994) studied 19 pulse generators implanted in 12 dogs. They found that interactions depended on proximity of current application to the pacing leads. Interactions were frequent at 1 cm and absent at greater than 4 cm. The most dangerous interaction was *runaway* pacing with possible induction of ventricular fibrillation. Ellenbogen et al reported on the acute effects of radiofrequency ablation on pacemakers in 35 patients. They observed normal function in 14 patients. The most common interaction was asynchronous pacing because of noise reversion, followed by oversensing resulting in refractory period extension and *functional undersensing* of pacemaker. The clinical incidence of acute interaction between radiofrequency current application and permanent pacemakers has ranged from 7% to 100%. (Chang et al., 1994)

6.3.6 Radiotherapy

Radiotherapy can induce different responses in implanted devices. EMI produced by the radiotherapy machine can result in pacing inhibition, tracking, noise reversion, or inappropriate ICD discharges. Usually, the effects are mild and observed only while the machine is switched on or off. Interference may be more severe with betatrons or with linear accelerators that misfire and hence best avoided. Maintain a 6" (15cm) distance from electronic cabinetry associated with radiating device. If the device is closer than 6" (15cm) to the cabinetry, there may be a potential for pacemaker reversion or ICD shock. In 1991, Rodriguez and colleagues showed severe malfunctions of pacemakers and ICDs: of the 17 pacemakers exposed to photon radiation eight failed before 50 Gy, whereas four of the six pacemakers exposed to electron radiation failed before 70 Gy. Direct radiation of pacemakers or ICDs at therapeutic levels should be strictly avoided. Furthermore, pacemaker and ICDs have to be controlled in short periods during and after radiation therapy, and pacemakers or ICDs should be exchanged after the radiotherapy when the accumulative dose on the pacemaker exceeds 5 Gy.

6.3.7 Transcutaneous Electrical Nerve Stimulation (TENS)

TENS units are external, noninvasive devices that are used for the treatment of patients with chronic pain. A TENS unit consists of electrodes placed on the skin and connected to a generator that applies 20 ms rectangular pulses of up to 60 mA at a frequency of 20–110 Hz. Although they are deceptively harmless in appearance, when used with the pacemaker-dependent patient, the patient may experience clinically significant ventricular pacing inhibition caused by EMI. Chen et al., 1990 published a case report documenting EMI from TENS devices in pacemakers. The resultant inappropriate ventricular inhibition was corrected by reprogramming the pacemaker's sensitivity setting. In situations in which substantial clinical benefit of using a TENS unit may exist, prolonged telemetry monitoring is required, and sensitivity settings may require adjustment. TENS can be used safely in patients with modern implanted bipolar pacemakers and in patients with unipolar pacemakers if sensitivity is reduced. It has been recommended that TENS electrodes not be placed parallel to the lead vector.

6.3.8 Transurethral Resection of the Prostate (TURP)

This procedure introduces electrical current into the body that may affect the implanted devices of individuals. Currents induced into the lead system may initiate an arrhythmia. If the grounding electrode is placed less than 6" (15cm) from device, damage can occur and/or the output of the device can be affected even when the magnet is applied. Magnet application in the pacemaker causes the pacemaker to deliver a sequence of stimuli at a normal low rate (usually 85 bpm magnet rate). If no magnet is present over the pacemaker, limiting the application of TURP electrosurgery to 1-2 seconds every 10 seconds may reduce the risk of symptoms in individuals who are dependent on the pacemaker. If these timing intervals are restrictive, reprogramming of the pacemaker should be done.

6.3.9 Dental devices

The modern dental office comprises a variety of electromagnetic devices that can interfere with pacemaker function. Miller et al., (1998) evaluated cardiac pacemaker function in proximity to contemporary electric dental equipment. A dual-chamber pacemaker with bipolar leads programmed to DDD mode and a single-chamber pacemaker with a unipolar lead programmed to VVI mode were set to maximum sensitivity, and then their function while in proximity to dental equipment was evaluated. Pacemaker inhibition was noted while the pacemaker was near an electrosurgical unit, the ultrasonic bath cleaner, and the ultrasonic scaler. EMI was absent with standard operations of the amalgamator, the electric pulp tester, a composite curing light, dental hand pieces and/or drills, the electric toothbrush, the dental chair and light, ultrasonic instruments, a radiography unit, and a sonic scaler. The non-pacemaker-dependent patient who has a dental procedure should not experience clinical symptoms from pacemaker inhibition. If the pacemaker-dependent patient cannot avoid interaction with interference-causing dental equipment, the patient's pacemaker should be programmed to asynchronous pacing mode before the dental procedure is initiated.

6.3.10 Medical procedures

Item	Low risk	PM Reversion	PM Inhibition	Remarks
Acupuncture - No electrical stimulus	X			Low risk
Acupuncture AC - Alternating Current	X	X	X	For use on torso - AC can cause pacemaker reversion. Lower risk of device detecting AC when used on extremities.
Acupuncture DC - Direct Current	X			Low risk
Diathermy		X		Diathermy is NOT recommended.
EEG Electroencephalography	X			Scan brain wave activity. Low risk of affecting PM
EMG Electromyography	X		X	Low risk If the stimuli are separated by more than 10 seconds. If it is necessary to apply stimuli at a rate faster than once every 10 seconds, magnet application is recommended.
Laser Surgery	X			Low risk
Lasik Eye Surgery	X			Low risk
Lie Detector Test	X			Lie detector tests introduce only direct current into the body. This direct current poses a low risk of affecting a pacemaker. If pacemaker or pacemaker portion of ICD is delivering stimuli, the heart rate variation parameters of the test may not be valid.
Magnetic therapy	X	X		Maintain a 6" (15cm) distance between all therapy magnets and an implanted device.
Mammogram	X			Low risk

Medical Helicopter	X			Low risk of affecting pacemaker. The vibration may increase pacing rate if the rate response function is programmed "on". Recommended to put patient on extra padding.
Radiation Therapy (External X-ray or Gamma knife)	X	X		Maintain a 6" (15cm) distance from electronic cabinetry associated with radiating device. **The Maximum cumulative gamma exposure levels for pacemaker is 500 rads**

Table 6. Electromagnetic Compatibility of devices involved in Medical Procedures.

6.3.11 MRI in patients with pacemaker

It has been estimated that each patient with a pacemaker or ICD has a 50% to 75% likelihood of having a clinical indication for MRI over the lifetime of their device. MRI tests have long been considered a contraindication for cardiac device patients.

In vitro analysis of modern permanent pacemakers (manufactured after 1996) revealed that maximal force acting upon devices was less than 100 g in a 1.5-T MRI scanner (Roguin A et al., 2004). This amount of force is unlikely to dislodge a chronic device that is anchored to the surrounding tissue. Pacemakers have the potential for receiving electromagnetic interference in the MRI environment, resulting in radiofrequency noise tracking, asynchronous pacing, inhibition of demand pacing, programming changes, or loss of function. The static magnetic field of the MRI scanner can alter device function by inducing unexpected reed switch opening or closure. Such potential risks have led to concerns from device manufacturers and MRI authorities regarding the performance of MRI procedures in cardiac implantable device recipients. However, several studies have assessed techniques to safely perform MRI in recipients of implanted cardiac devices.

Nazarian et al., (2009) from our institution (author UL), after a extensive research, recommended avoiding MRI in patients with less than 6 weeks' time since device implant or patients with no fixation (superior vena cava coil) leads. To reduce the risk of inappropriate inhibition of pacing due to detection of radiofrequency pulses, Nazarian et al., also recommended device programming to an asynchronous, dedicated pacing mode in pacemaker-dependent patients. To avoid inappropriate activation of pacing due to tracking of radiofrequency pulses, they suggest device programming in patients without pacemaker dependence to a nontracking ventricular or dualchamber inhibited pacing mode. In our institution, we typically deactivate tachyarrhythmia monitoring to avoid battery drainage that results from recording of multiple radiofrequency pulse sequences as arrhythmic episodes.

Potential Effects of Magnetic Resonance Imaging on Pacemakers
1. Strong Static magnetic field
Reed switch closure resulting in asynchronous pacing
2. Radiofrequency field
Alterations of pacing rate (leads detecting the RF signals and pace the heart in rapid rates)
Spurious tachyarrhythmia detection
Heating
3. Time-varying magnetic gradient field
Induction voltage (resulting in pacing)
Heating
Reed switch closure

Table 7. Effects of MRI on Pacemakers. (Pinski et al., 2002)

Finally, to reduce the risk of thermal injury and changes in lead threshold and impedance, the estimated whole-body averaged specific absorption rate of MRI sequences should be limited to <2.0 W/kg when possible. At the end of the examination, all device parameters should be checked, and programming should be restored to pre-MRI settings. MRI of pacemaker-dependent patients should not be performed unless there are highly compelling circumstances and when the benefits clearly outweigh the risks.

Recommendations for the Performance of MRI in Patients With Pacemakers
1. Only be performed at extremely experienced centers
2. Obtain written and verbal informed consent.
specifically list risks, including (1) pacemaker dysfunction (2) Pacemaker damage (3) Arrhythmia (4) Death.
3. A physician with ACLS and pacemaker/ICD expertise should decide whether it is necessary to reprogram the pacemaker before the MRI and should be in.
4. A person with expertise in MR physics and safety should be involved (use lowest RF power levels, weakest/slowest necessary gradient magnetic fields)
5. Appropriate personnel and a "crash cart," including defibrillator, must be available throughout the procedure to address an adverse event.
6. Maintain visual and voice contact with the patient throughout the procedure.
7. After MRI, interrogate the pacemaker function reprogram as needed

Table 8. Recommendations for the Performance of MRI in Patients With Pacemakers (Adapted from Lavine et al., 2007)

7. Discussion with the patients

Most of the patients can be reassured that they can conduct their regular lives normally without fear of EMI, especially if their device utilizes bipolar sensing. In almost all cases in the home and daily living environment, the device reverts back to normal function as soon as the patient increases distance from the EMI source. Extra precaution with EMI should be exercised with pacemaker- dependent patients. It may be necessary to test the questionable EMI source in a medical facility while the patient is being monitored. Stored electrograms provide a useful tool for verifying EMI interference. To minimize EMI interactions or reduce the chance of a serious device response in the medical environment, one should assess the need for the procedure or test, the dependency status of the patient, and optimal device reprogramming (such as temporarily reprogramming to asynchronous mode). Cardiac device function should be evaluated once the procedure is complete, especially if EMI interactions were noted. Patients in specialized industrial environments should be assessed individually, and the manufacturers too are usually willing to offer specific guidelines or recommendations for device patients in that environment. Emerging technologies continue to create new challenges and raise new questions concerning EMI and patients with implantable cardiac devices.

8. Conclusions

Clear instructions and guidance are required to ensure that an EMI safe area is identified before proceeding with remote device handling. Advances in electronic technology, including hermetic shielding, filtering, bipolar sensing, and algorithms designed to reject sources of EMI have been of great help in returning patients with pacemakers to active lives in their communities after pacemaker implantation. New technologies have increased concern about interference with pacemaker function. It is important for physicians to remain vigilant about the potential risks of EMI from external sources with regard to pacemaker function.

9. References

Astridge, P. S., G. C. Kaye, S. Whitworth, P. Kelly, A. J. Camm, and E. J. Perrins. 1993. The response of implanted dual chamber pacemakers to 50 Hz extraneous electrical interference. *PACE - Pacing and Clinical Electrophysiology* 16 (10) (1993/): 1966-74.

Casavant, D., C. Haffajee, S. Stevens, and P. Pacetti. 1998. Aborted implantable cardioverter defibrillator shock during facial electrosurgery. *Pacing and Clinical Electrophysiology : PACE* 21 (6) (Jun): 1325-6.

Chang, A. C., D. McAreavey, D. Tripodi, and L. Fananapazir. 1994. Radiofrequency catheter atrioventricular node ablation in patients with permanent cardiac pacing systems. *Pacing and Clinical Electrophysiology : PACE* 17 (1) (Jan): 65-9.

Chen, D., M. Philip, P. A. Philip, and T. N. Monga. 1990. Cardiac pacemaker inhibition by transcutaneous electrical nerve stimulation. *Archives of Physical Medicine and Rehabilitation* 71 (1) (Jan): 27-30.

Cooper, D., B. Wilkoff, M. Masterson, L. Castle, K. Belco, T. Simmons, V. Morant, S. Streem, and J. Maloney. 1988. Effects of extracorporeal shock wave lithotripsy on cardiac pacemakers and its safety in patients with implanted cardiac pacemakers. *Pacing and Clinical Electrophysiology : PACE* 11 (11 Pt 1) (Nov): 1607-16.

Ellenbogen, K. A., M. A. Wood, and B. S. Stambler. 1996. Acute effects of radiofrequency ablation of atrial arrhythmias on implanted permanent pacing systems. *Pacing and Clinical Electrophysiology : PACE* 19 (9) (Sep): 1287-95.

Hayes, D. L., P. J. Wang, D. W. Reynolds, M. Estes 3rd, J. L. Griffith, R. A. Steffens, G. L. Carlo, G. K. Findlay, and C. M. Johnson. 1997. Interference with cardiac pacemakers by cellular telephones. *The New England Journal of Medicine* 336 (21) (May 22): 1473-9.

Ismail, M. M., A. M. A. Badreldin, M. Heldwein, and K. Hekmat. 2010. Third-generation mobile phones (UMTS) do not interfere with permanent implanted pacemakers. *Pacing and Clinical Electrophysiology* 33 (7): 860-4.

Lawrentschuk, N., and D. M. Bolton. 2004. Mobile phone interference with medical equipment and its clinical relevance: A systematic review. *The Medical Journal of Australia* 181 (3) (Aug 2): 145-9.

Lee, S., K. Fu, T. Kohno, B. Ransford, and W. H. Maisel. 2009. Clinically significant magnetic interference of implanted cardiac devices by portable headphones. *Heart Rhythm : The Official Journal of the Heart Rhythm Society* 6 (10) (Oct): 1432-6.

Levine PA (1985) in Modern Cardiac Pacing, Effect of cardioversion and defibrillation on implanted cardiac pacemakers, ed Barold SS (Futura Publ. Co, Mount Kisco, NY), pp p875–886.

Levine, G. N., A. S. Gomes, A. E. Arai, D. A. Bluemke, S. D. Flamm, E. Kanal, W. J. Manning, et al. 2007. Safety of magnetic resonance imaging in patients with cardiovascular devices: An american heart association scientific statement from the committee on diagnostic and interventional cardiac catheterization, council on clinical cardiology, and the council on cardiovascular radiology and intervention: Endorsed by the american college of cardiology foundation, the north american society for cardiac imaging, and the society for cardiovascular magnetic resonance. *Circulation* 116 (24) (Dec 11): 2878-91.

Manegold, J. C., C. W. Israel, J. R. Ehrlich, G. Duray, D. Pajitnev, F. T. Wegener, and S. H. Hohnloser. 2007. External cardioversion of atrial fibrillation in patients with implanted pacemaker or cardioverter-defibrillator systems: A randomized comparison of monophasic and biphasic shock energy application. *European Heart Journal* 28 (14) (Jul): 1731-8.

McIvor, M. E., J. Reddinger, E. Floden, and R. C. Sheppard. 1998. Study of pacemaker and implantable cardioverter defibrillator triggering by electronic article surveillance devices (SPICED TEAS). *Pacing and Clinical Electrophysiology : PACE* 21 (10) (Oct): 1847-61.

Miller, C. S., F. M. Leonelli, and E. Latham. 1998. Selective interference with pacemaker activity by electrical dental devices. *Oral Surgery, Oral Medicine, Oral Pathology, Oral Radiology, and Endodontics* 85 (1) (Jan): 33-6.

Mortazavi, S., E. Park, J. Florio, J. Poore, G. Bornzin, P. A. Levine, and J. Sholder. 1996. Effect of pentaphasic pulse sequence as an impedance sensor on standard electrocardiographic recordings. *PACE - Pacing and Clinical Electrophysiology* 19 (11 II) (1996/): 1678-81.

Nazarian, S., and H. R. Halperin. 2009. How to perform magnetic resonance imaging on patients with implantable cardiac arrhythmia devices. *Heart Rhythm : The Official Journal of the Heart Rhythm Society* 6 (1) (Jan): 138-43.

Rodriguez, F., A. Filimonov, A. Henning, C. Coughlin, and M. Greenberg. 1991. Radiation-induced effects in multiprogrammable pacemakers and implantable defibrillators. *Pacing and Clinical Electrophysiology : PACE* 14 (12) (Dec): 2143-53.

Roguin, A., M. M. Zviman, G. R. Meininger, E. R. Rodrigues, T. M. Dickfeld, D. A. Bluemke, A. Lardo, R. D. Berger, H. Calkins, and H. R. Halperin. 2004. Modern pacemaker and implantable cardioverter/defibrillator systems can be magnetic resonance imaging safe: In vitro and in vivo assessment of safety and function at 1.5 T. *Circulation* 110 (5) (2004/08): 475-82.

Shaw, C. I., R. M. Kacmarek, R. L. Hampton, V. Riggi, A. El Masry, J. B. Cooper, and W. E. Hurford. 2004. Cellular phone interference with the operation of mechanical ventilators. *Critical Care Medicine* 32 (4) (Apr): 928-31.

Sweesy, M. W., J. L. Holland, and K. W. Smith. 2004. Electromagnetic interference in cardiac rhythm management devices. *AACN Clinical Issues* 15 (3) (Jul-Sep): 391-403.

Waller, C., F. Callies, and H. Langenfeld. 2004. Adverse effects of direct current cardioversion on cardiac pacemakers and electrodes is external cardioversion contraindicated in patients with permanent pacing systems? *Europace : European Pacing, Arrhythmias, and Cardiac Electrophysiology : Journal of the Working Groups on Cardiac Pacing, Arrhythmias, and Cardiac Cellular Electrophysiology of the European Society of Cardiology* 6 (2) (Mar): 165-8.

14

Magnetic Resonance Imaging with MR Conditional Cardiac Pacemakers

Josef Vymazal, Aaron Rulseh, Miloš Táborský and Radovan Žáček
Na Homolce Hospital, Prague
Czech Republic

1. Introduction

1.0.0.1

The emergence and rapid development of Magnetic Resonance Imaging (MRI) in recent years has made MRI competitive with, and in many cases preferable to, many existing invasive and non-invasive imaging technologies. Primarily a neuroradiologic tool when introduced, MRI has quickly become the method of choice in many clinical fields, including cardiovascular imaging. In detecting the extent and precise location of myocardial ischemia, or in the diagnosis of arrhythmogenic right ventricular cardiomyopathy, MRI is the preferred investigative method. In general, MRI can currently be applied in the examination of almost all organs and systems, with the exception of those that have a low density of protons, such as the flat bones of the calvarium or the lungs. MRI is non-invasive, and since the electromagnetic energy applied in MRI is relatively weak, it carries no radiation burden. Furthermore, it is highly improbable that this energy is able to break chemical or biological bonds. Therefore, after almost thirty years of the clinical use, MRI is considered a safe technique.

1.0.0.2

There are approximately 60 million MRI scans performed worldwide every year (Sutton et al., 2008), and approximately two million Europeans currently have a cardiac pacemaker. It is estimated that between 50-75% of patients with a cardiac implant will be indicated for an MRI (Nazarian & Halperin, 2009), and every five seconds a patient is denied an MRI because of an implantable cardiac device (Medtronic, 2010). The increase in both indications for MRI and the prevalence of implanted cardiac pacemakers has necessitated the development of an MR conditional cardiac pacemaker system. As mentioned, MRI is preferable to other imaging methods in many cases, and the advent of MR conditional pacemaker systems allows the clinician to take advantage of this imaging modality (Figures 1, 2).

2. Magnetic resonance imaging

2.1 Basic principles

2.1.0.3

A thorough exposition of the principles governing magnetic resonance imaging is beyond the scope of this text, and we refer those interested readers to any of the excellent resources available on this subject (McRobbie et al., 2007). It is however important to explain some of the basic principles of the modality as they relate to the safety of implanted cardiac pacemakers and related devices. An MR system unsurprisingly uses magnetic fields to induce and detect subtle changes in the imaging subject, transforming this information into images. The system is able to accomplish this feat using three cooperating fields: a static magnetic field, gradient magnetic fields, and radio frequency (RF) fields.

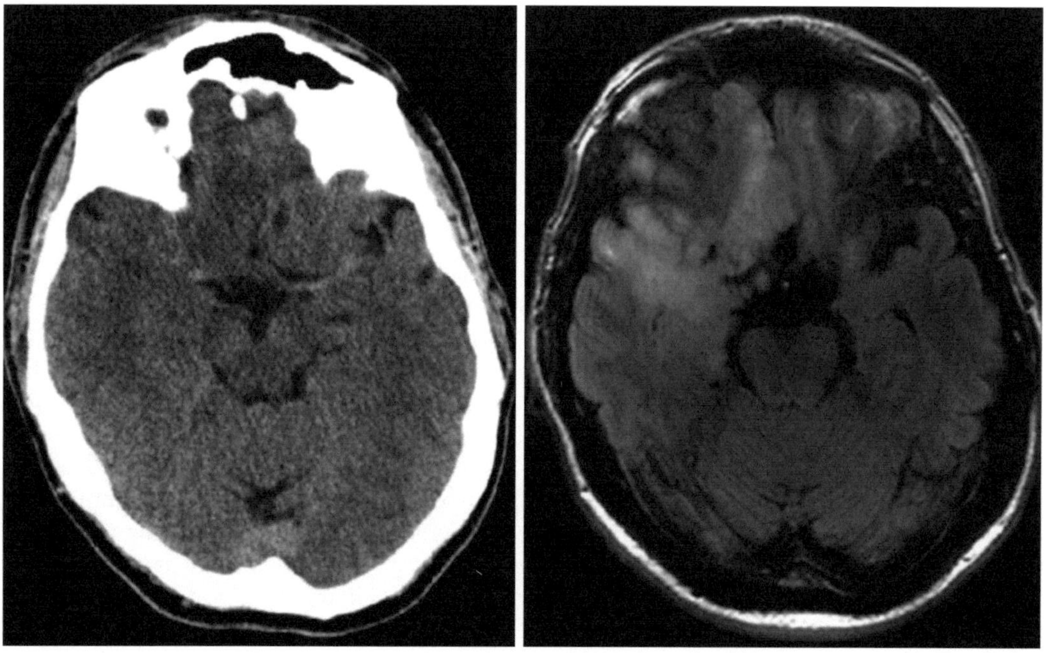

(a) CT (b) FLAIR

Fig. 1. Computerized tomography (CT) image and fluid-attenuated inversion recovery (FLAIR) MR image in the same patient with an EnRhythm MRI SureScan MR conditional pacemaker system. The images illustrate the advantages of MRI in some pathologies. In this patient, only slight hypodensity in the frontal region is visible in the CT image. The FLAIR image shows the extent and character of the pathology with greater precision – in this case, low grade astrocytoma.

2.1.0.4

The static magnetic field (B_0) of an MR system, as the name implies, remains constant and is present at all times, even when no examination is taking place. The magnetic flux density (magnitude) of this field is denoted in Tesla (T) (1T = 10,000 gauss), with most clinical scanners in use today being 1.5T or 3T. As a comparison, the magnetic flux density of the earth is approximately 50 μT (0.5 gauss). The source of this field is a coil, made of a specific alloy that when cooled to a temperature close to absolute zero loses nearly all electrical resistance. This condition is called superconductivity, and it enables the static magnetic field to remain on at all times, without the requirement of an external electric current to maintain the field. Another advantage of superconductive coils is their ability to provide a very homogeneous field, which is necessary for MR imaging.

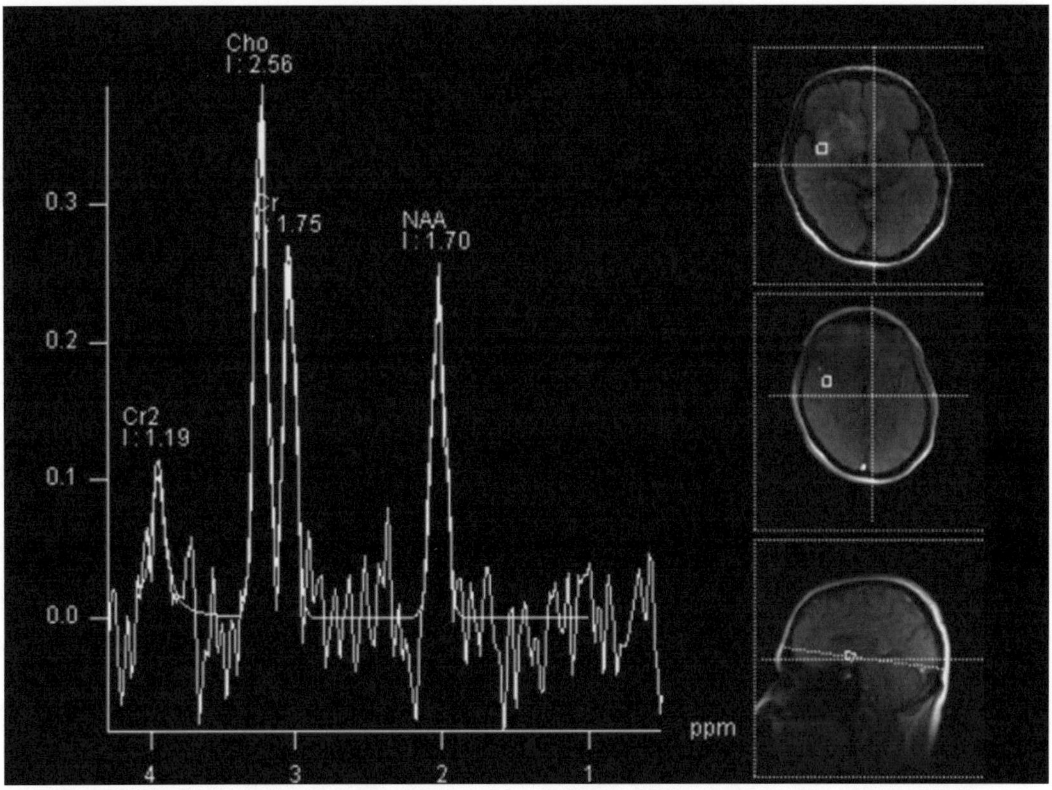

Fig. 2. MR conditional pacemaker systems also enable NMR spectroscopic studies of the brain, where individual brain metabolites are visualized. This spectroscopic examination was performed in the same patient as presented in Figure 1, and here an increased choline peak suggests the presence of brain tumor. This technique is especially sensitive to the homogeneity of the magnetic field, and the presence of the MR conditional cardiac pacemaker system did not negatively influence the results.

2.1.0.5

Clinical MRI is proton imaging, and only hydrogen nuclei in different local magnetic environments and conditions are imaged. Protons have a property called spin, which is the total angular momentum of its constituent parts (in fact many MR-related texts use spins synonymously with protons), as well as a magnetic dipole moment. When the subject is placed in the B_0 field, the protons tend to align with the B_0 field, and their magnetic dipole moments begin to precess. The usual analogy given to help visualize precession is the wobble of a spinning top. Precession results from torque when a magnetic dipole is placed in an external field. This is termed Larmor precession, and the frequency of precession is proportional to the magnetic field magnitude as stated by the Larmor equation (see Equation 1, where ω is precessional frequency, γ is gyromagnetic ratio (a constant for a given nucleus), and B_0 is the magnitude of the magnetic field). This alignment of protons in the B_0 field is the first step in creating MR images.

$$\omega = \gamma B_0 \quad (1)$$

2.1.0.6

Magnet field gradients are provided by the three paired orthogonal gradient coils, being superimposed on the static (B_0) field. The gradients are applied in short pulses and vary in amplitude, time and direction, allowing slice selection, frequency encoding, and phase encoding. To state this more simply, the linear gradients produced by the gradient coils allow spatial encoding of the imaging data (the gradient coils also serve an important role in many pulse sequences). Two critical properties of gradient coils that affect image quality and have important safety implications are the gradient strength and the gradient slew rate. Gradient strength (amplitude) is the change in field strength per unit distance, and is given in mT/m. The gradient slew rate is the rate of ascent or descent of a gradient from zero to its maximum amplitude, and is given in mT/m/msec, or more often in T/m/s.

2.1.0.7

Radio frequency pulses, in the most simplistic sense, are used to excite the protons so that meaningful data can be captured and used for image reconstruction. An RF pulse is a magnetic field oscillating at the Larmor frequency. When these pulses are applied for specific short durations, they are able to transfer energy to protons, or more accurately to change the spin state of protons, which are precessing at the same frequency. This is termed nuclear magnetic resonance, and is the process after which this modality is named. The result of the process is a change in energy state in the same direction as the B_0 field (a decrease in longitudinal magnetization), and the development of precessional phase coherence (development of transversal magnetization). Transversal magnetization is an essential process for MRI (Figure 3). Precessional phase coherence results in a vector of magnetization transverse to the B_0 field that, in the absence of phase coherence, is canceled out. Since this vector is not in the same plane as the B_0 field, it is not obscured by the B_0 field and can be detected. The protons quickly return to a lower energy state after cessation of the RF pulse in a process called relaxation. Longitudinal relaxation results in the transfer of thermal energy to the surrounding environment (spin-lattice relaxation), and is the basis for an important safety consideration, the specific absorption rate (SAR), which will be discussed shortly.

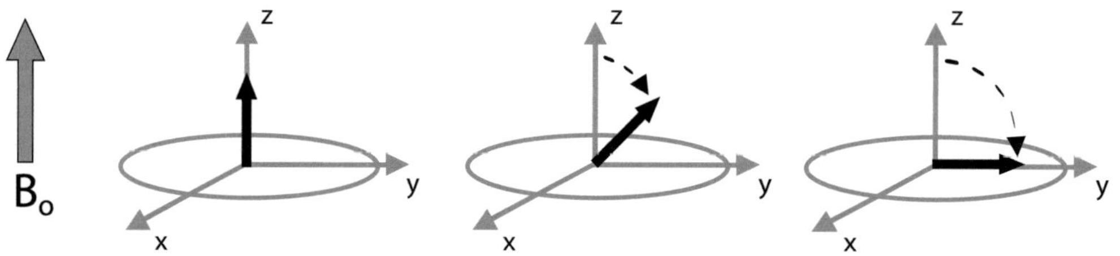

Fig. 3. The development of transversal magnetization.

2.1.0.8

An important point to note about the magnetic field produced by an MR system is that it extends beyond the bore of the magnet—this is call the fringe field. The fringe field produced by the superconductive coils of an MR system is analogous to the magnetic flux lines that can visualized by placing iron shavings around a permanent magnet (Figure 4). The magnetic flux density of the fringe field decreases by the squared distance from the magnet, and this attenuation of magnitude is enhanced by the active magnetic shielding present in all modern scanners. The "5 gauss line" is clearly marked around the scanner, generally being a line painted on the floor of the scanner room, which denotes the point at which the field is 5 gauss (0.5 mT). Five gauss is considered the maximum safe level of exposure for the general public, and access between this line and the bore of the magnet is strictly controlled.

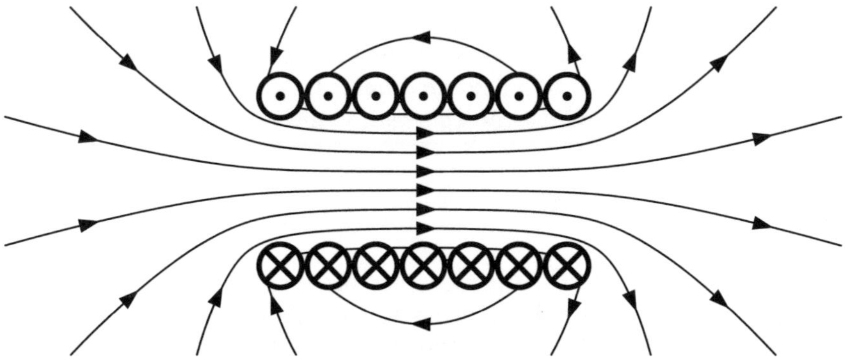

Fig. 4. Diagram illustrating the magnetic flux lines of a solenoid.

2.2 Safety

2.2.0.9

MRI is remarkable in that it can deliver images with superb soft tissue contrast while exposing the patient to very little risk. Nevertheless, there are important safety concerns that must be considered when performing an MR examination. In contrast to the stochastic effects of ionizing radiation used in many radiological modalities, e.g., X-ray or computerized tomography (CT) examinations, the effects of the magnetic fields used in MR systems on biological tissues follow a deterministic model. Therefore, the magnitude of the effect is dependent on parameters relating to exposure and can be predicted to a large extent, allowing the establishment of appropriate safety thresholds.

2.2.0.10

Several international organizations provide valuable safety recommendations for MRI. The International Electrotechnical Commission (IEC) and the International Commission on Non Ionizing Radiation Protection (ICNIRP) are two such organizations that provide guidance to manufacturers, regulatory bodies, and the public. As our discussion on MRI safety will primarily focus on implanted devices, we encourage readers interested in more detailed safety information to consult the documentation provided by the commissions mentioned above, or any of the excellent texts available on this subject (ICNIRP, 2009; IEC, 2010; Shellock, 2009).

2.2.0.11

The response of matter to an applied external field can be classified as diamagnetic, paramagnetic, or ferromagnetic (superparamagnetism, antiferromagnetism, and other types of magnetism may also be described, but are omitted here for the sake of simplicity). Diamagnetism is present in all materials and is the weakest property of the three. When para- and ferromagnetism are not present, diamagnetism is the dominant property and the material is said to be diamagnetic. The electrons in these materials are covalently bound, balanced in magnetic moment, and tend to align in a way that opposes the applied external field. Most biological tissues are diamagnetic. In paramagnetic materials, the magnetic moments of electrons do not balance completely, and these materials exhibit a magnetization that is proportional to the applied external field. Paramagnetism is stronger than diamagnetism, and when present in a material it overpowers its inherent diamagnetic properties. Finally, ferromagnetic materials have domains in which the magnetic moments of unpaired electrons align parallel to each other. The domains are arranged in random orientations, but in the presence of an external field the domains become aligned and the material is said to be magnetized. Ferromagnetism is several orders of magnitude stronger than paramagnetism.

2.2.1 Magnetic field safety

2.2.1.1

The magnetic fields used in MRI can interact with implanted devices in several ways. Para- and ferromagnetic materials, provided they are not spherical in shape, will attempt to align themselves with the external B_0 and gradient fields to minimize free energy. This magnetomechanical interaction may exert force, torque or vibrational effects on the implanted device, which if significant could lead to tissue damage, lead displacement, or device malfunction. The B_0 field may intermittently affect reed switch activity, leading to asynchronous pacing or inhibition of pacing. Current may be induced in the leads by the gradient magnetic fields, this in turn may cause over- or under-sensing resulting in pacing inhibition or acceleration. Restrictions in the maximum gradient slew rate help to minimize induced current. RF fields may also induce current in the leads leading to inappropriate pacing. Furthermore, RF fields may cause significant heating of the leads due to induction, with lead temperatures increasing up to 20°C (Luechinger et al., 2005). Lead heating is an important safety consideration as it may lead to tissue necrosis. The SAR, the energy absorbed per unit of tissue mass and time, is restricted to minimize temperature gains. The SAR is calculated by the MR system, and more restrictive SAR limits must be observed when imaging patients with MR conditional pacing systems.

2.2.2 Device Safety

2.2.2.1

ASTM International (formally, the American Society for Testing and Materials) is a voluntary standards development organization responsible for the development of medical device safety standards in the MR environment recognized by the FDA (ASTM, 2008). The standard stipulates that device testing evaluate magnetically induced displacement force, magnetically induced torque, heating by RF fields, and MR image artifacts from passive implants. After testing, the device may be classified into one of three categories: MR safe, MR conditional, and MR unsafe.

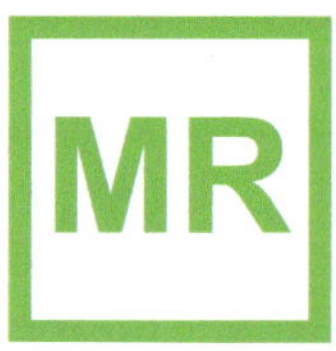

Fig. 5. MR safe symbol

2.2.2.2

MR Safe – MR safe items pose no known hazards in all MR environments (Figure 5). Items in this category include diamagnetic materials known to be MR safe, or if determined to be MR safe from product testing, must include the highest static field strength that the item was tested in.

Fig. 6. MR conditional symbol

2.2.2.3

MR Conditional – MR conditional items have been demonstrated to pose no known hazards in a specified MRI environment with specified conditions of use (Figure 6). Field conditions that define the MRI environment include static magnetic field strength, spatial gradient, dB/dt (time varying magnetic fields), radio frequency fields, and specific absorption rate. Additional conditions, including specific configurations of the item may be required. Conditions for safe operation must be defined and observed.

Fig. 7. MR unsafe symbol

2.2.2.4

MR Unsafe – MR unsafe items are known to pose hazards in all MR environments (Figure 7). The presence of an MR unsafe item is obviously a contraindication to MR examination. Implantable cardiac pacemakers usually belong to this category.

3. MR conditional cardiac pacemaker systems

3.1 Introduction

3.1.0.5

The same need to perform MRI examinations in some patients with implanted cardiac pacemakers that spurred the development of MR conditional devices, also led some clinicians and researchers to attempt MRI examinations in non-pacemaker dependent patients with nonapproved devices. In each instance, the benefit of performing the examination was determined to out-weigh any associated risks. There have been some publications detailing the results of such endeavors, and in general they report satisfactory results (Luechinger et al., 2005; Nazarian et al., 2006; Sommer et al., 2006). However, one cannot generalize from these studies that all non-dependent patients with nonapproved cardiac pacemakers can safely undergo an MRI examination, even when implementing stringent safety precautions, as these studies are limited by small sample sizes and the variety of implanted pacemakers, leads, and combinations thereof that were investigated. At least ten deaths have been attributed to MRI procedures in patients with cardiac pacemakers (Kanal et al., 2007; Martin et al., 2004). In light of these documented events, the clinician must be aware of potentially fatal outcomes when a standard implanted cardiac pacemaker is exposed to the strong magnetic fields of an MR system. These studies can however provide valuable guidance in those situations when a patient would benefit greatly from an MRI but has an MR unsafe device.

3.1.0.6

One response to the limited sample size in the studies mentioned previously has been the creation of the MagnaSafe Registry (MagnaSafe, 2010). The MagnaSafe Registry is a prospective multi-center study designed to determine the risk of non-thoracic 1.5T MRI scanning for patients with implanted cardiac devices, and aims to collect data from 1500 MRI examinations (1000 cardiac pacemakers, 500 implantable cardioverter-defibrillators). The data collected should help to refine safe scanning protocols and allow relatively better informed consent in those instances when an MRI is warranted and the patient does not enjoy the benefit of an MR conditional device. Some critics however have voiced concern over the utility of the registry, correctly pointing out that the study will likely lack the necessary power to establish the safety of any one device/lead combination.

3.1.0.7

With the vast number of cardiac pacemakers on the market, a great number of leads, and an overwhelming number of component combinations, device manufacturers have turned their attention to developing cardiac pacemaker systems designed specifically to minimize the safety concerns relevant to MRI examinations. MR conditional pacemaker systems are specific pacemaker/lead combinations that have undergone rigorous testing to establish their safety.

3.2 General principles shared by MR conditional pacemaker systems

3.2.0.8

Two manufacturers have been award CE approval to market their MR conditional pacemaker systems in the European Economic Area (EEA). Medtronic currently has CE approval for three systems: the EnRhythm, Advisa, and Ensura MRI SureScan pacing systems. Biotronik currently has CE approval for two systems: the Evia and the Entovis ProMRI MR conditional pacing systems.

3.2.0.9

These devices differ in some aspects from standard cardiac pacemakers. First, the amount of ferromagnetic parts is minimized, therefore the static magnetic field does not induce significant torque or vibration. Second, the leads of the pacemaker are isolated, therefore increases in temperature are also minimized. Third, the gradient and RF fields do not interfere with the pacing regime of the device on the condition that an MR conditional mode is activated. These features enable MR scanning in closed bore 1.5 Tesla systems.

3.2.0.10

MR scanners at 1.5 Tesla currently represent the gold standard of clinical MR imaging. A common sense rule that usually applies in MR imaging is that if a metallic implant is safe at a field strength of 1.5 Tesla, it is automatically safe for lower external fields. In the case of MR conditional cardiac pacemakers, this common sense rule does not apply. These devices have been constructed to be safe at a resonance frequency of approximately 64 MHz that corresponds to the external field of 1.5 Tesla. Different resonance frequencies, lower or higher, may interfere with the pacemaker system and thus be dangerous.

3.2.0.11

Our institution has practical experience with MRI in patients with MR conditional cardiac pacemakers as part of routine clinical practice, and also as participants in the EnRhythm SureScan clinical study (Vymazal et al., 2009). Over thirty patients with this device have been scanned at 1.5 Tesla in our hospital, and we have experienced no adverse events to date.

3.3 MRI in patients with MR conditional pacemaker systems

3.3.0.12

In a certain sense, the emergence of these medical devices complicates what has been, until now, a relatively straightforward situation. While until recently the presence of any implanted cardiac pacemaker was an absolute contraindication to MRI, now a radiological technician or radiologist has to ensure that several pre-MRI scanning conditions are met. First, it is important to ascertain that the patient does not have any other implanted devices, and that there are no abandoned, broken or intermittent leads, lead extensions or lead adapters present. This should be verified by chest X-ray, which also serves to identify the system as MR conditional. A standard chest X-ray reveals radiopaque markers on the device, unique for the specific type of pacemaker (Figure 8). Specific radiopaque markers are also present in the leads of Medtronic systems (Figure 9). The pacing system must be implanted for at least six weeks, and must in the left/right pectoral region. The six week period after the system has been implanted is an arbitrary period that also applies for most stents, metallic prosthesis, and other implants. The patient must also bring printed confirmation that specific MR pacing parameters have been activated. This includes activation of the MR conditional mode, and selection of an MRI pacing mode and rate. The printed confirmation is generated by a programming device and should be signed by the cardiologist or cardiovascular technician (Figure 10). Finally, suitable equipment for the MRI environment must be used for patient monitoring during the scanning procedure. An external defibrillator must also be available. Pre-MRI requirements are given in Table 1.

	Medtronic	Biotronik
Time since implantation	>6 weeks	>6 weeks
Radiopaque marker	PVX/PTA	SF
IPG position	L/R pectoral	Chest area
Activate MR Mode	✓	✓
Capture threshold <2.0 V at 0.4 ms	✓	✓
Lead impedance 200-1500 Ω	✓	✓

Table 1. Pre-MRI requirements for patients with MR conditional cardiac pacemaker systems. IPG, implantable pulse generator

3.3.0.13

After the pre-MRI scanning conditions have been met, the patient may undergo an MRI at 1.5 Tesla. Specific rules and limitations for imaging in patients with MR conditional systems are quite similar between systems and manufacturers, and are summarized in Table 2. Of note, the lateral decubitus position is contraindicated, and Biotronik further restricts patient position to only dorsal. Transmit coils cannot be used with Biotronik systems, only receive-only coils may be used. Biotronik systems also have a scan exclusion zone which must be observed (Figure 11). No coils, including receive-only coils, may be positioned within the scan exclusion zone. The result of this limitation is that no imaging data may be collected for this zone. The total scan time is also restricted to thirty minutes in Biotronik systems.

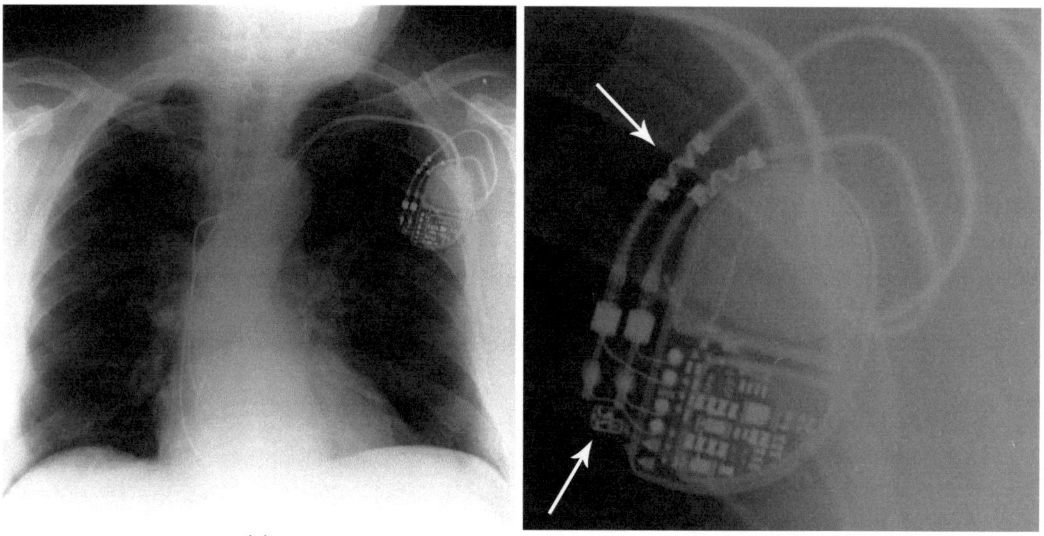

(a) (b)

Fig. 8. Plain film chest X-ray allows visual confirmation of lead placement and integrity, implantable pulse generator (IPG) position, and MR conditional radiopaque markers (arrows).

	Medtronic	Biotronik
B_0 field	1.5T	1.5T
GSR	≤ 200 T/m/s	≤ 200 T/m/s
SAR – head	≤ 2W/kg	≤ 2W/kg
SAR – body	< 3.2W/kg	< 3.2W/kg
Patient position	No lateral decubitus	only dorsal
Patient monitoring	ECG/PO/BP	ECG+PO/ECG+BP
Scanning	Whole body	Scan exclusion zone
Coils	Transmit/receive	Only receive
Min. patient height	–	1.4 m

Table 2. Specific rules and limitations for MR scanning in patients with MR conditional cardiac pacemaker systems. SAR, specific absorption rate; GSR, gradient slew rate; ECG, electrocardiogram; PO, pulse oximetry; BP, blood pressure

3.3.0.14

After the MR examination is finished, the integrity of the pacemaker system should be evaluated by the programming machine, and it should be returned to normal operating mode.

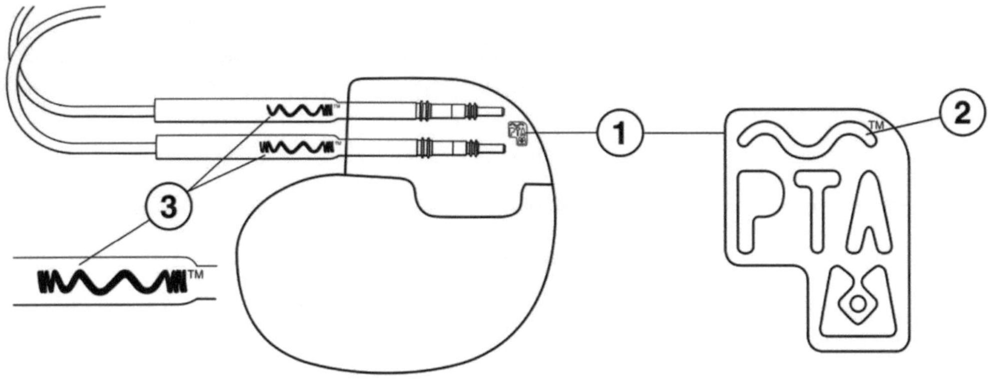

Fig. 9. Radiopaque symbols on the Medtronic EnRhythm MRI SureScan system. ① – Location of the device radiopaque symbol, ② – Device radiopaque symbol, ③ – Lead radiopaque symbol.

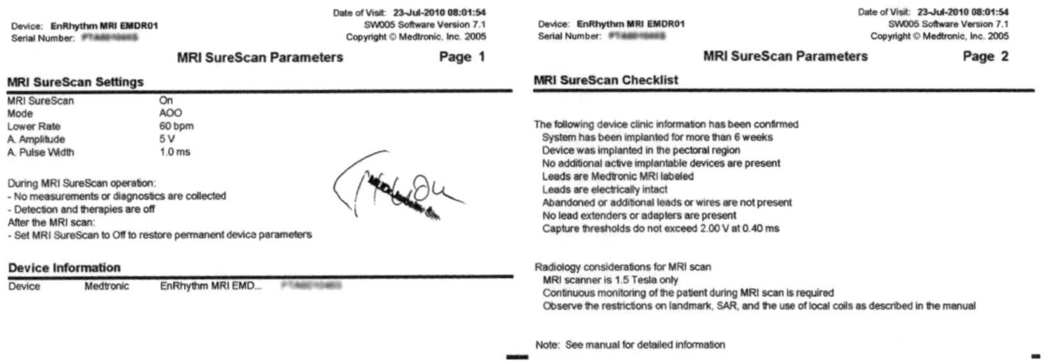

Device: EnRhythm MRI EMDR01
Serial Number: [redacted]

Date of Visit: 23-Jul-2010 08:01:54
SW005 Software Version 7.1
Copyright © Medtronic, Inc. 2005

MRI SureScan Parameters Page 1

MRI SureScan Settings

MRI SureScan	On
Mode	AOO
Lower Rate	60 bpm
A. Amplitude	5 V
A. Pulse Width	1.0 ms

During MRI SureScan operation:
- No measurements or diagnostics are collected
- Detection and therapies are off

After the MRI scan:
- Set MRI SureScan to Off to restore permanent device parameters

Device Information

Device	Medtronic	EnRhythm MRI EMD...	[redacted]

Device: EnRhythm MRI EMDR01
Serial Number: [redacted]

Date of Visit: 23-Jul-2010 08:01:54
SW005 Software Version 7.1
Copyright © Medtronic, Inc. 2005

MRI SureScan Parameters Page 2

MRI SureScan Checklist

The following device clinic information has been confirmed
System has been implanted for more than 6 weeks
Device was implanted in the pectoral region
No additional active implantable devices are present
Leads are Medtronic MRI labeled
Leads are electrically intact
Abandoned or additional leads or wires are not present
No lead extenders or adapters are present
Capture thresholds do not exceed 2.00 V at 0.40 ms

Radiology considerations for MRI scan
MRI scanner is 1.5 Tesla only
Continuous monitoring of the patient during MRI scan is required
Observe the restrictions on landmark, SAR, and the use of local coils as described in the manual

Note: See manual for detailed information

Fig. 10. Example pre-MRI report documenting activation of the MR conditional mode, and selection of an MRI pacing mode and rate.

3.4 Currently approved MR conditional pacemaker systems

3.4.0.15 EnRhythm MRI™ SureScan™ pacing system

Medtronic's EnRhythm MRI SureScan pacing system received CE approval in November, 2008, and was the first MR conditional pacing system commercially available. The EnRhythm MRI SureScan pacing system consists of the EnRhythm MRI SureScan implantable pulse generator (IPG) and the CapSureFix MRI SureScan pacing leads. When the EnRhythm MRI SureScan pacing system was introduced, an isocenter landmark exclusion zone was stipulated between the superior surface of C1 and the inferior surface of T12, with respect to the position of the patient within the scanner bore, relative to the isocenter landmark of the bore. Recently this restriction has been lifted, and the EnRhythm MRI SureScan pacing system is now approved for full body imaging (Burrows, 2010).

3.4.0.16

The EnRhythm MRI SureScan pacing system can be identified on chest X-ray by specific radiopaque markers (Figure 12). The device radiopaque marker found on the IPG features the Medtronic company symbol, with a tilde (~) symbol above designating the device as MR conditional. Between these two symbols three letters are visible, in this case "PTA", which identifies this as a first generation SureScan device. Radiopaque markers on the leads are seen as a set of wavy lines close to the lead/IPG junction. This identifies the leads as MR conditional SureScan pacing leads.

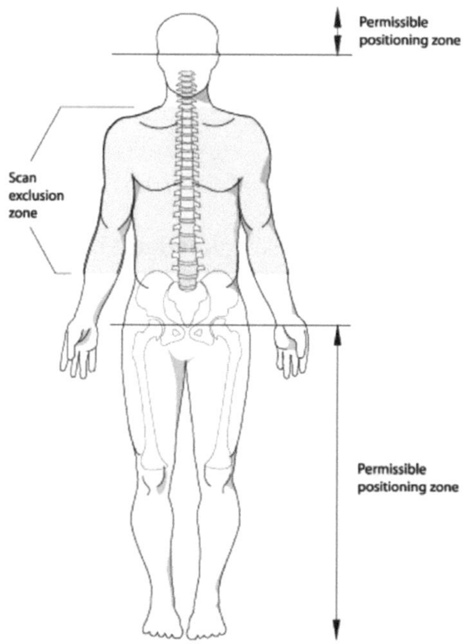

Fig. 11. Permissible positioning zone and scan exclusion zone for Biotronik Evia and Entovis ProMRI pacemaker systems. Starting from the foot end, the maximum allowed positioning mark for the isocenter is at the hip bone level. Starting from the top of the skull, the maximum allowed positioning mark for the isocenter is at the level of the eyes.

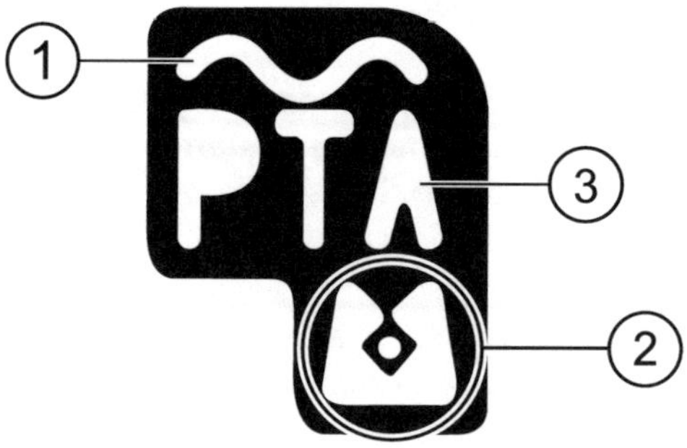

Fig. 12. Figure demonstrating the EnRhythm radiopaque device marker. ① – Marker identifying the device as MR conditional, ② – Medtronic identifer, ③ – Specific device identifier.

3.4.0.17
The EnRhythm MRI SureScan pacing system is no longer commercially available, having been supplanted by the company's next generation MR conditional pacing systems.

3.4.0.18 Advisa DR MRI™ SureScan™ pacing system
The Advisa DR MRI SureScan pacing system received CE approval in June, 2009, and is one of Medtronic's second generation MR conditional pacing systems. The Advisa DR MRI SureScan pacing system consists of the Advisa MRI SureScan IPG and the MRI SureScan leads.

3.4.0.19
The Advisa DR MRI SureScan pacing system can also be identified on chest X-ray by specific radiopaque markers (Figure 13). The device radiopaque marker found on the IPG features the Medtronic company symbol, with a tilde (~) symbol above designating the device as MR conditional. Between these two symbols three letters are visible, in this case "PVX", which identifies this as a second generation SureScan device. Radiopaque markers on the leads are seen as a set of wavy lines close to the lead/IPG junction. This identifies the leads as MR conditional SureScan pacing leads.

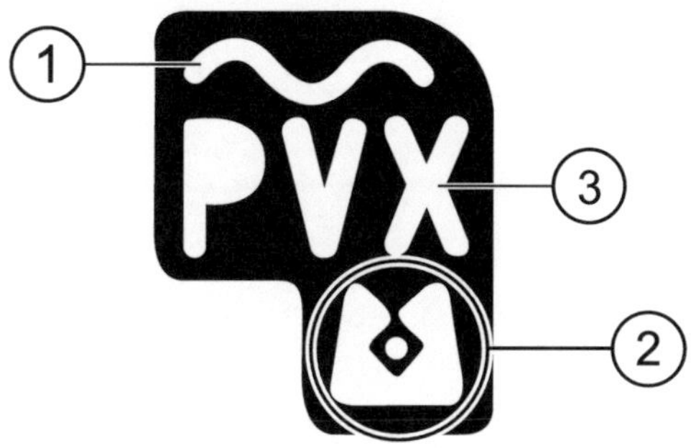

Fig. 13. Figure demonstrating the Advisa/Ensura radiopaque device marker. ① – Marker identifying the device as MR conditional, ② – Medtronic identifer, ③ – Specific device identifier.

3.4.0.20 Ensura MRI™ SureScan™ pacing system
The Ensura MRI SureScan pacing system was awarded CE approval in June, 2010, and is also a second generation MR conditional pacing system produced by Medtronic. The Ensura MRI SureScan pacing system is closely related to the Advisa MRI SureScan pacing system, and from the perspective of MRI safety they are the same. The Ensura system does differ in the pacing options available, being essentially a less featured and more affordable version of Advisa.

3.4.0.21
The radiopaque markers of the Ensura MRI SureScan pacing system are identical to the Advisa system described above (Figure 13).

3.4.0.22 Evia ProMRI® MR conditional pacing system
Biotronik received CE approval for the Evia ProMRI MR Conditional Pacing System in April, 2010. The Evia ProMRI system consists of the Evia SR/DR ProMRI IPG and Safio MR

conditional leads. A "-T" following the IPG model designation indicates that the device is equipped for Home Monitoring® service. Specific limitations with respect to MRI are summarized in Table 2, of note, a scan exclusion zone and permissible positioning zones within the MRI bore must be observed for safe operation (Figure 11).

3.4.0.23
The Evia ProMRI IPG can be identified by radiopaque markers on the device (Figure 14). The Biotronik logo is visible on the left, followed by two letters, in this case "SF", which identify the device family. No radiopaque markers are present on the leads, necessitating that the investigating physician carefully review the patient documentation to ensure approved Safio leads are present.

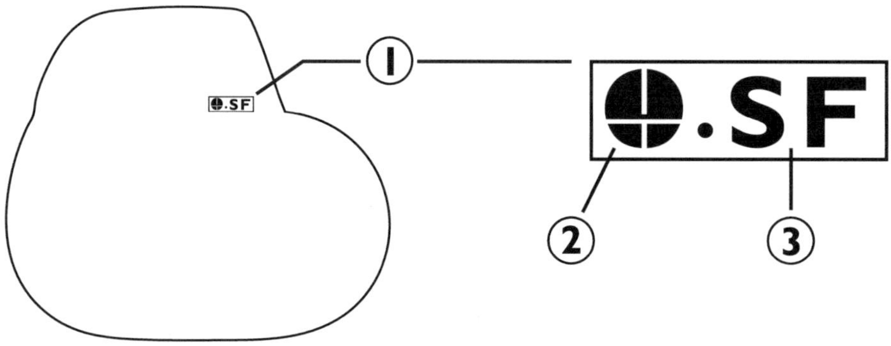

Fig. 14. Figure demonstrating the Biotronik radiopaque device marker. ① – Radiopaque device marker, ② – Biotronik identifier, ③ – Specific device identifier.

3.4.0.24 Entovis ProMRI® MR conditional pacing system
3.4.0.25
The Entovis ProMRI MR Conditional Pacing System produced by Biotronik also received CE approval in April, 2010. The Entovis ProMRI MR Conditional Pacing System consists of the Entovis DR/SR ProMRI IPG and Safio MR conditional leads. Like the Evia ProMRI IPG, a "-T" following the model designation indicates that the device is equipped for Home Monitoring® service. The Entovis ProMRI IPG is identical to the Evia ProMRI IPG from the perspective of MRI safety and radiopaque markers, as the two devices differ only in feature set and price point (Figures 11, 14).

4. Conclusion

4.0.0.26
MR conditional pacing systems are being actively developed, tested and refined by many cardiac pacemaker manufacturers. Currently, there are no FDA-approved MR conditional pacemaker systems, although several companies are actively pursuing this. The Revo MRI SureScan pacemaker system produced by Medtronic is expected to be the first system to gain FDA approval, after receiving unanimous recommendation from the FDA Circulatory System Devices Advisory Panel in March, 2010. The Revo MRI SureScan pacemaker system is a second generation Medtronic pacemaker system like the Advisa and Ensura. If approved, this system will have the same isocenter landmark exclusion zone that the

EnRhythm system launched with. No transmit coils may be used in this zone, but receive only coils are permitted, allowing off-center imaging of thoracic and abdominal organs (Figure 15). In other respects the Revo system is not expected to differ significantly from other second generation Medtronic systems.

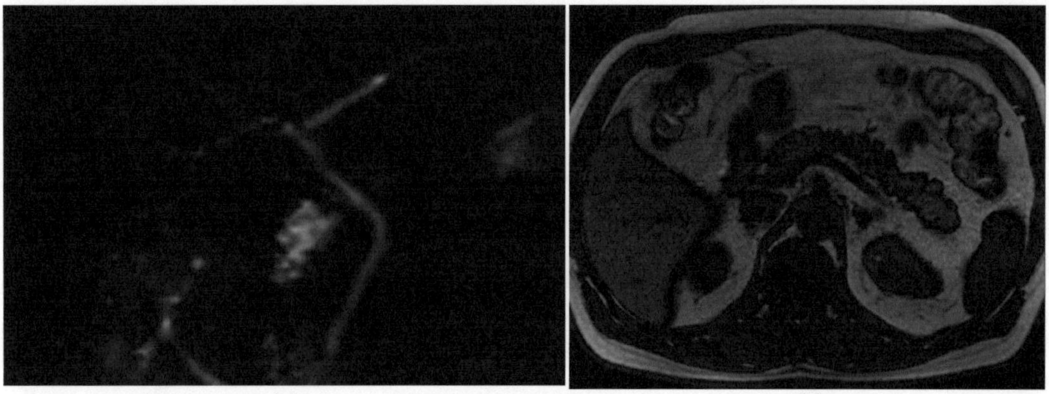

(a) (b)

Fig. 15. (a) Magnetic resonance cholangiopancreatography (MRCP) examination in a patient with an EnRhythm MRI SureScan MR conditional pacemaker system using an off-center scanning approach. (b) True fast imaging with steady-state precession (TrueFISP) image of the abdomen in the same patient, also performed using an off-center scanning approach.

4.0.0.27

In the future we expect to see more of these devices gaining approval and appearing in our daily practice. As indications for MRI and the prevalence of implanted cardiac pacemakers increase, MR conditional cardiac pacemakers will do our patients a great service by giving them access to a powerful imaging modality while exposing them to a minimum of risk.

5. References

ASTM (2008). ASTM f2503-08 (2008) standard practice for marking medical devices and other items for safety in the magnetic resonance environment, *Technical report*, American Society for Testing and Materials (ASTM) International. doi: 10.1520/F2503-08.

Burrows, J. (2010). Updated information on enrhythm surescan pacemaker system. Personal communication.

ICNIRP (2009). Guidelines on limits of exposure to static magnetic fields, *Health Physics* 96(4): 504–514. PMID: 19276710.

IEC (2010). Particular requirements for the basic safety and essential performance of magnetic resonance equipment for medical diagnosis. IEC 60601-2-33 (3rd edn.), *Technical report*, International Electrotechnical Commission (IEC).

Kanal, E., Barkovich, A. J., Bell, C., Borgstede, J. P., Bradley, W. G., Froelich, J. W., Gilk, T., Gimbel, J. R., Gosbee, J., Kuhni-Kaminski, E., Lester, J. W., Nyenhuis, J., Parag, Y., Schaefer, D. J., Sebek-Scoumis, E. A., Weinreb, J., Zaremba, L. A., Wilcox, P., Lucey,

L., Sass, N. & the ACR Blue Ribbon Panel on MR Safety (2007). ACR guidance document for safe MR practices: 2007, *Am. J. Roentgenol.* 188(6): 1447–1474.

Luechinger, R., Zeijlemaker, V. A., Pedersen, E. M., Mortensen, P., Falk, E., Duru, F., Candinas, R. & Boesiger, P. (2005). In vivo heating of pacemaker leads during magnetic resonance imaging, *European Heart Journal* 26(4): 376–383.

MagnaSafe (2010). The MagnaSafe registry, web. URL: *http://www.magnasafe.org*

Martin, E. T., Coman, J. A., Shellock, F. G., Pulling, C. C., Fair, R. & Jenkins, K. (2004). Magnetic resonance imaging and cardiac pacemaker safety at 1.5-Tesla, *Journal of the American College of Cardiology* 43(7): 1315–1324. PMID: 15063447.

McRobbie, D. W., Moore, E. A., Graves, M. J. & Prince, M. R. (2007). *MRI from Picture to Proton*, 2 edn, Cambridge University Press.

Medtronic (2010). MRI safety must be proven for cardiac devices, web. URL: *http://www.medtronic.com*

Nazarian, S. & Halperin, H. R. (2009). How to perform magnetic resonance imaging on patients with implantable cardiac arrhythmia devices, *Heart Rhythm: The Official Journa of the Heart Rhythm Society* 6(1): 138–143. PMID: 19121814.

Nazarian, S., Roguin, A., Zviman, M. M., Lardo, A. C., Dickfeld, T. L., Calkins, H., Weiss, R. G., Berger, R. D., Bluemke, D. A. & Halperin, H. R. (2006). Clinical utility and safety of a protocol for noncardiac and cardiac magnetic resonance imaging of patients with permanent pacemakers and Implantable-Cardioverter defibrillators at 1.5 tesla, *Circulation* 114(12): 1277–1284.

Shellock, F. G. (2009). *The Reference Manual for Magnetic Resonance Safety, Implants, and Devices: 2009 Edition*, 1 edn, Biomedical Research Publishing Company.

Sommer, T., Naehle, C. P., Yang, A., Zeijlemaker, V., Hackenbroch, M., Schmiedel, A., Meyer, C., Strach, K., Skowasch, D., Vahlhaus, C., Litt, H. & Schild, H. (2006). Strategy for safe performance of extrathoracic magnetic resonance imaging at 1.5 tesla in the presence of cardiac pacemakers in Non-Pacemaker-Dependent patients: A prospective study with 115 examinations, *Circulation* 114(12): 1285–1292.

Sutton, R., Kanal, E., Wilkoff, B. L., Bello, D., Luechinger, R., Jenniskens, I., Hull, M. & Sommer, T. (2008). Safety of magnetic resonance imaging of patients with a new Medtronic EnRhythm MRI SureScan pacing system: clinical study design, *Trials* 2(9): 68–68.

Vymazal, J., Taborsky, M. & Zacek, R. (2009). Magnetic resonance imaging with implanted cardiac pacemaker enrhythm MRI surescan with MR compatible electrodes capsurefix MRI - first experience, *Ces Radiol* 63(1): 9–12.

Part 4

Complications of Pacemaker Implant

15

Complications of Pacemaker Implantation

Michele Schiariti, Mariateresa Cacciola and Paolo Emilio Puddu
University of Rome "La Sapienza" and Ospedali Riuniti, Reggio Calabria, Italy

1. Introduction

The use of permanent pacemakers (PM) and implantable cardioverter-defibrillators (ICD) continues to grow worldwide (Birnie et al., 2006; Goldberger & Lampert, 2006) with over 3 million PM and 250000 ICD in use by the end of last century (Chua et al., 2000). The rate of device implantations is increasing with aging of the general population and expanding indications. Despite the relative ease of device implantation, the complication risk is still present and sometimes underestimated. The proposal for this chapter is at addressing the most common intra-operative and delayed complications with a special eye to the surgical complications. We will also address electromagnetic interference and psychological problems.

2. Complications related to the location type

Depending on the location type (venous access, pocket, lead and generator) it is possible to dissect several different clinical presentations of complications related to PM implantation which occur, more frequently, in the immediate post-operative course.

2.1 Venous access-related complications

Pneumothorax. This complication occurs uncommonly and is directly related to operator experience, the difficulty of the subclavian puncture, and is almost eliminated using the cephalic cut-down technique. However, these traditional comparisons may become obsolete as the axillary vein cannulation technique (Martin et al., 1996) threatens to eliminate this controversy. Pneumothorax is often asymptomatic and noted on routine follow-up plain chest radiograph, but occasionally it requires active medical treatment including intercostal chest drain and aspiration. Aggarwal et al. (1995, 1996) reported a large series of 1088 consecutive patients; pneumotorax represented an overall rate of 1.9% of subclavian insertions. There was no significant difference in the pneumothorax rate between dual chamber (n = 12, 2.1%) and single chamber (n=7, 1.4%). Pneumothorax required active medical treatment in 8 patients (0 8%); 5 patients had an intercostal chest drain inserted and 3 were treated by aspiration. A further 11 patients (1.0%) developed an insignificant pneumothorax (< 10% of pulmonary field in chest x-ray film with no symptoms or progression in subsequent chest radiograph). More recently, Zhan et al. (2008) collected over 67000 patients and presented similar rates. Finally, Pakarinen et al. (2010) also concluded, in a retrospective 1-year single-centre survey, that short-term implantation-related

complications of contemporary device therapy are still frequent, and occur much more frequently when trainees rather than experienced cardiologists are the operators.
Hemothorax. This complication results from trauma to the great vessels rather than the lung. The risk can be minimized by direct inward and outward passes of the puncture needle rather than a side-to-side, potentially "lacerating" movement. If an arterial puncture is performed, recognition, withdrawal, and digital pressure are important. It is important to remember that the artery needs not be cannulated with the introducer. It is essential to always check the fluoroscopic path of the guidewire into the inferior vena cava before introducer insertion. In the Aggarwal et al. (1995) series, the inadvertent arterial puncture was the most common intra-operative complication which occurred in 27 patients (2.7% of subclavian insertions): no serious sequelae ensued.
Air embolism. Deep inspiration at the time of central venous access may cause significant air to be drawn into the venous system due to the physiological negative pressure developed. It can be prevented through operator care and using introducers with haemostatic valves. The diagnosis is obvious because it is heralded by a hissing sound as the air is sucked in and with the fluoroscopic confirmation that follows. Patients are surprisingly tolerant of this occurrence. Usually no therapy is required, as the air is filtered and consequently absorbed in the lungs. The real incidence of this occurrence is not clearly defined in the Literature. However, several cases are reported (Ninio & Hii, 2006; Ostovan & Aslani, 2007; Turgeman et al., 2004): respiratory distress, hypotension, and arterial oxygen desaturation were the most frequent consequences, which was related to the size of the embolus. It is then appropriate to administer 100% oxygen along with inotropic support in some cases. Aspiration of the embolus from the right heart has also been successfully reported (Ostovan & Aslani, 2007).

2.2 Pocket-related complications

Hematoma. Pocket hematoma is an acute, relatively common complication after PM or ICD implantation. It was estimated that 14 to 17% of early reoperations were due to this complication (Aggarwal et al., 1995; Chauhan et al., 1994). The site of bleeding may be the pocket or back-bleeding around the lead venous entry site. The use of electro-cautery is useful to minimize pocket related bleeding. Bleeding from the venous entry site usually subsides during the procedure but ongoing bleeding is controlled by a firm suture placed through and around the lead entry/pectoral muscle interface (Pavia & Wilkoff, 2001). Usually, hematomas are managed conservatively unless expanding in size, tense or painful. In these occasions, reoperation to evacuate the hematoma and identify and arrest the site of bleeding is required. Evacuation was required in 1 to 2% of implant cases in a recent series (Kiviniemi et al., 1999). The risk is increased in anticoagulated patients. The large number of patients receiving coumarin for atrial fibrillation or valve replacement management of anticoagulation might be a major determinant of hematoma development. On the other hand, the complete avoidance of perioperative anticoagulation therapy might promote thromboembolic events and, in particular, cerebral stroke. Intravenous heparinization has been shown to be associated with an increased risk of hematoma development (Michaud et al., 2000) while oral anticoagulation therapy with warfarin did not increase the rate of pocket hematoma in two small series (al-Khadra, 2003; Goldstein et al., 1998). The increasing use of low-molecular-weight heparin and more effective inhibition of platelet aggregation with ticlopidine/clopidogrel also may affect the susceptibility to intra-operative bleeding and pocket hematoma. It has been shown that long-term warfarin with an international normalized ratio of about 2.0 is safe over a 15-year experience (Belott & Reynolds, 2000), although anticoagulation is in general discontinued for at least the duration of the procedure. Wiegand et al. (2004) investigated the influence of patient comorbidity, implantation strategy, operator experience, antiplatelet therapy, and anticoagulation therapy on hematoma rate on a large series of 3164 devices (2792 pectoral PM and 372 ICD). Predictors of hematoma occurrence were determined prospectively and were analyzed by multivariate regression analysis. According to the results of this important investigation (Wiegand et al., 2004) the following recommendations were given: a) implantation, with the patient receiving combined ASA and clopidogrel treatment, should be performed only by very experienced implanters soon after coronary stenting has been performed (i.e. less than 1 month after) in patients who are highly symptomatic or in whom PM or ICD implantation is vitally indicated; b) in all remaining patients, either therapy with thienopyridine should be discontinued or implantation should be performed when drug treatment can be safely stopped; c) perioperative high-dose heparinization should be reserved for patients with artificial valves (particularly those in the mitral position) and those who have recently experienced arterial embolism, cardioversion, and deep venous thrombosis or pulmonary embolism. Continued oral anticoagulation therapy might be a suitable alternative in the latter patients. All remaining patients who are in need of anticoagulation therapy should receive low-dose heparinization post-operatively until oral anticoagulation therapy is re-established.

Erosion and wound dehiscence. It is a sub-acute complication after device implantation caused by a progressive skin erosion. If the subcutaneous pocket fashioned at the time of initial implantation is too small for the device, undue tension on the overlying skin may cause gradual subcutaneous tissue, and possible eventual skin erosion. Care should also be taken when fashioning the pocket to create the pocket plane on the surface of the muscle. If the pocket is too superficial, erosion may also occur. In the event of erosion, the associated potential for infection is high and therefore extraction of the total device-lead system is usually advised.

Wound pain. Minor wound pain is expected after device implantation, almost always controlled with simple analgesia. In general, the pre-pectoral site is extremely well-tolerated. Continuing pain will usually improve or manifest an obvious infection eventually. However, pain that initially improves then recurs or occurs temporarily remote from the implant may suggest infection even in the absence of any outward localizing signs, and consequently may necessitate surgical exploration or even empirical removal and reimplant at another site. Alternatively, mechanical trauma from the device location adjacent to anterior chest wall structures may be the culprit. In this situation, device relocation or pocket revision may be indicated.

Infection. Similar to other prosthetic materials, infections complicate a small proportion of patients with these devices. Along with the increase in device implantation, the incidence of device infections has also been increasing, but at a faster rate. (Voight et al., 2006). In the USA, data from Medicare recipients from 1990 to 1999 showed an increase in the number of device infections from 0.94 per 1000 recipients to 2.11 per 1000 recipients, an increase of 124%; the estimated rate of infection of endocardial leads being between 1 and 2%, but varying from 0.13 to 12.6%. (Cabell et al., 2004; Voight et al., 2006). Grimm et al. (1993) reported an incidence of ICD system infection ranging from 2 to 8%. The exact reason for a time-related increase of infections remains unexplained, but it is hypothesized to be due to increasing co-morbidities in device recipients, improved surveillance and detection of cardiac device infection, and improving survival of patients with devices (Uslan & Baddour, 2006). The mortality of persistent infection when infected leads are not removed can be as high as 66% (Rettig et al., 1979). The physical manifestations range from mild systemic symptoms with no local reaction to fulminant life-threatening sepsis. Early infections (no more than 60 days from implant) tend to be more clinically evident as opposed to the more indolent course of late onset infections. These infections can present with only pain at the implant site. When infection is present, complete device removal with transvenous lead extraction is followed by antimicrobial therapy with the device reimplanted at a later date. In the Chua et al. (2000) experience including both PM and ICD leads, the median time for device reimplantation was 5 days with no subsequent evidence of recurrent or new infection at a mean follow-up period of 46 weeks. Partial system removal is associated with high recurrence rate and should be reserved for very selected cases. Once a strong clinical suspicion for infection is established, the whole system should be considered contaminated. The time of onset of the infection is extremely variable. Margey et al. (2010) reported a median duration from device implant or revision to presentation with confirmed cardiac device infection of 150 days (range 5–2920 days, with an interquartile 25% of 35 days and an interquartile 75% of 731 days). Fever, chills and malaise were the most common presenting symptoms. Evidence of generator site inflammation was present in 90%. Frank erosion or purulent discharge could be identified in 66%. A third of cases met diagnostic criteria for cardiac device related endocarditis. The majority had non-specific laboratory abnormalities, including elevation in leukocyte count, anaemia, elevated erythrocyte sedimentation rate, or C-reactive protein level. Therefore, the clinical diagnosis of device infection is very easy.

Microbiological findings. It is not always possible to define the agent of infection: in a very recent report (Margey et al., 2010) out of 39 cardiac device infection cases, a causative organism was identified only in 62%. The most frequent causative organism was methicillin sensitive *Staphyloccoccus aureus* (30.8%), followed by coagulase negative *Staphylococcus* (20.5%), and *Streptococcus* species (7.7%). Blood cultures were performed in 84% of the cardiac device infection group, and were positive in 54% of these cases. Cultures of generator site tissue and lead tips were performed in those undergoing device extractions (82%) and were positive in 38 and 18%, respectively. In cases where all 3 swabs were positive, the same causative organism was identified in each case. Of those patients in whom blood cultures were negative, all had already received antibiotic therapy by the time cultures were drawn.

Echocardiographic findings. Cardiac ultrasound does not seem to have an high diagnostic sensitivity. In the Margey et al. (2010) series 87% of the patients underwent transthoracic echocardiography during their admission and 36% also underwent transoesophageal echocardiography. In those in whom echocardiography was performed, vegetations were identified on the lead in 18%, and involving the heart valves in 5%. The tricuspid valve was the only valve involved. On the other hand, patients with intracardiac vegetations identified on transesophageal echocardiogram can safely undergo complete device extraction using standard percutaneous lead extraction techniques. Permanent devices can safely be reimplanted provided blood cultures remain sterile. The presence of intracardiac vegetations identifies a subset of patients at increased risk for complications and early mortality from systemic infection despite device extraction and appropriate antimicrobial therapy (Grammes et al., 2010).

2.3 Lead-related complications

Cardiac perforation. Permanent PM implantation may be complicated by cardiac perforation, which can lead to longer hospital stays, tamponade, or even death (Aizawa et al., 2001; Ellenbogen et al., 2002; Garcia-Bolao et al., 2001; Gershon et al. 2000). The incidence of perforation after permanent PM reportedly is between 0.5% and 2%, but the predictors of perforation have not been defined (Hill, 1987; Sivakumaran et al., 2002). Lead perforation is a less-recognized delayed complication of device implantation. Delay in recognition may prove fatal. Careful evaluation of pacing and sensing thresholds and follow-up echocardiographic evaluation is mandatory to remain vigilant for this potentially fatal complication. The clinical manifestations of significant perforations are variable and include chest pain, dyspnoea, and hypotension. These signs, in conjunction with a new pericardial effusion immediately following permanent PM implantation, suggest PM-related cardiac perforation. Predictors of post implantation pericardial effusion, which serves as a marker of perforation, include concomitant use of trans-venous PM, steroid use within 7 days, and older age. Perforation of the right ventricle as a late complication of device implantation is rare and requires a high suspicion for prompt recognition and intervention. Routine chest radiography may not be diagnostic, and further testing such as CT scan and echocardiography are essential, combined with PM interrogation, for evaluation of high thresholds. A higher clinical suspicion should be maintained in the elderly, in whom perforation occurs more frequently (Mahapatra et al., 2005). In addition, consideration should be given in the elderly to implant the lead in sites other than the right ventricular apex, such as the right ventricular septum or outflow tract, in an attempt to minimize the risk of this complication later during the follow-up. Acute perforation of the right atrium or right ventricle has been reported in up to 1% of patients (Chauhan et al., 2005).

Malposition. There have been several reports of inadvertently lead malposition during PM implantation. Some of those are related to cardiac structural abnormalities. In patients with an atrial septal defect lead could be erroneously implanted in the left ventricle. The presence of a right bundle branch block configuration during ventricular pacing should induce the suspect of a malposition that can be confirmed by a lateral chest x-ray or by ultrasound. The malposition could be discovered years after the implantation and pacing (Vanhercke et al., 2008). There are not recommendations about the removal of lead if there are not concomitant complications such thrombus, embolism or the posterior mitral leaflet perforation causing an acute mitral incompetence (Seki et al., 2009; Van Gelder et al., 2000). In any case, if timely removal of a malpositioned lead in the left ventricle, through a patent foramen ovale or atrial septal defect is not performed, life-long anticoagulation with warfarin should be recommended. Cases are reported too of a malpositioned lead, which had inadvertently been inserted into the left subclavian artery and passed through the aortic valve into the left ventricular apex (Reising et al., 2007), despite the finding of an apparently elevated "venous" pressure at the time of insertion. The error was not detected despite the anterior–posterior chest radiography (no lateral view), electrocardiograms, and a computed tomography scan of the chest with contrast during which the lead was said to be in the right ventricle. Careful analysis of post-procedure electrocardiograms and lateral chest x-ray film images can minimize the chance that such an error will go undetected There is no consensus as to how to proceed in cases such as this because few are reported in the Literature, which may also be related to publication bias. Recently, it was suggested that transcatheter lead removal should not be performed because of an inability to detect the presence of thrombi on the lead wires (Van Gelder et al., 2000). To our knowledge, the risk of trauma to the valve leaflets has not yet clarified. However, cases of endocarditis have been reported, including one with a large aortic valve vegetation (Schulze et al., 2005).

Lead dislodgement. Lead dislodgement is a clinically relevant and possibly dangerous occurrence. It typically occurs either early (within the first 6 weeks of implantation) or late (beyond the first 6 weeks of implantation), occasionally very late dislodgments were also described (Tokano et al., 2004). Early dislodgements are more common then late dislodgements. Atrial lead dislodgment occurs more commonly than ventricular dislodgements in the early period (Chauhan et al., 2005). The incidence of early dislodgement of a ventricular lead in a DDD PM was 0.5 to 2.5% (Aggarwal et al., 1995; Fortescue et al., 2004). Lead dislodgment occurs less commonly as a consequence of advancements in pacing lead placement and lead design. After dislodgement, the lead usually remains intracardiac but cases are described where leads were completely pulled out (Von Bergen et al., 2006), as in the lead dislodgement secondary to a "ratchet-like" mechanism through the sewing sleeve. Fluoroscopy is occasionally needed to identify the location of the lead tip. However, some mechanisms of PM lead dislodgement involve retraction of the lead toward the generator. This includes Twiddler's syndrome, which refers to lead dislodgement due to conscious or unconscious manipulation of the pulse generator causing it to rotate around its long axis (Abrams & Peart, 1995; Bracke et al., 2005; Chauhan et al., 1994; Higgins et al., 1998; Newland & Janz, 1994; Solti et al., 1989). Typically, placement beneath the pectoral muscle and suturing the generator to the underlying fascia is thought to preclude the patient from manipulating the device. Additionally, "Reel syndrome" (Carnero-Varo et al., 1999; Vural et al., 2004) has been described, which entails the generator rotating around its transverse axis "reeling" in the lead. In certain adult populations, such as in patients with a history of significant weight loss, the "Sagging Heart syndrome" may represent a previously unrecognized cause of acute lead dislodgment (Iskos et al., 1999). It is a rare form of lead dislodgment that may occur due to an unexpected and marked postural descent of the heart after permanent PM implantation. Iskos et al. (1999) described this, in 2 patients, which was related to a history of morbid obesity followed by weight loss of over 40 kilograms. Lead replacement with active fixation leads was required in both cases.

2.4 Generator-related complications

Set screw loose. Set screw could be a cause of complication: although PM infections that were apparently localized at set screw site were reported (Henrikson & Brinker, 2006), the most important complications are related to the loose of set screw and of electrical contact. Inappropriate mode switching in a dual chamber PM due to oversensing of a high frequency signal from a conductor/ring discontinuity (loose set screw) was reported by Kuruvilla et al. (2002). A retrospective review of complications with connectors and lead-to-header interfaces was performed (Tyers et al., 1992) years following 649 pacing procedures between 1980 and 1990. There were 88 lead revisions (13.6%), 81 device replacements or modifications (12.5%), and 480 new implants (74%) using devices of 5 manufacturers. Two basic connector types were studied, one utilizing a set screw and the other using a side-lock compression fitting. The set screw makes electrical contact and mechanically secures the lead connector pin with a set screw insulated by a self-sealing grommet or an integral or separate set screw cover. The side-lock makes electrical contact with an automatic spring mechanism while the plastic lead terminal is secured in the connector block of the pacemaker by a Delrin side-lock compression fitting. The follow-up during at most 12 years of 459 set screw connector devices gave 14 complications (3.1%) whereas 82 side-lock connector devices were followed for up to 5 years with 1 complication (1.2%). The set screw and side-lock connectors were reliable over the period of follow-up. Although the complication rate appeared lower with the side-lock, follow-up was shorter and the number of implants smaller. With the leads used in this study (Tyers et al., 1992), the side-lock proved to be a desirable feature due to simplicity, speed, safety, and ease of use. One limitation is the requirement for a precise IS-1 connector terminal diameter.

3. Complications unrelated to the location site

There are a series of complications after PM or ICD implantation, more frequently occurring late after insertion, which do not recognize a clear-cut relation with the location site and rather present as a more generalized syndrome.

3.1 Superior vena cava syndrome

Superior vena cava syndrome (SVCS) is characterized by gradual, insidious compression/obstruction of the superior vena cava. Although the syndrome can be life-threatening, its presentation is often associated with a gradual increase in symptomatology. For this reason, diagnosis is often delayed until significant compression of the superior vena cava has occurred. Initially, there are few symptoms, however, over time, symptoms of superior vena cava compression/obstruction gradually develop. As the compression becomes more severe, the patient may develop shortness of breath and swelling of the arms and face. SVCS is chiefly associated with malignancy. Currently, more than 90% of patients with SVCS have an associated malignancy as the cause. Of the nonmalignant causes of SVCS, thrombosis from central venous instrumentation (catheter, PM, guidewire) is an increasingly common event, especially as these procedures become more common. PM-induced SVCS is a rare complication of permanent PM insertion, with an estimated prevalence ranging from 1:40000 to 1:250, and usually occurring more than 1 month after implantation (Bolad et al., 2005; Gilard et al., 2002; Spittel & Hayes, 1992). The obstruction is internal and composed of thrombus, fibrosis, or a combination of the two, typically involving the pacing wires within the superior vena cava (Spittel & Hayes, 1992). Although the mortality associated with benign causes of SVCS is low, those patients who become symptomatic are often debilitated by it, necessitating intervention. Various therapies have been used to treat PM-related SVCS. The various treatment modalities used to relieve SVCS symptoms may be summarized under the following categories: a) anticoagulation (heparin, warfarin, acenocoumarol, phenprocoumon, dicumarol); b) thrombolysis, either systemic or catheter-directed (tissue plasminogen activator, urokinase, alteplase, or streptokinase); c) surgical, intervention on superior vena cava using a spiral saphenous vein conduit, or reconstruction using a pericardial patch, or a thrombectomy; d) balloon venoplasty alone; and e) stenting of the lesions (usually preceded by venoplasty) using wallstents, SMART stents, Palmaz stents, or Z stents. There is no current consensus about their relative efficacy and merits. Riley et al. (2010) recently reviewed and summarized all of the reported cases of this complication that were treated in order to aid clinical decision making and spur future research in this area. It was recognized from the outset of this venture that any attempt at a pooled analysis of results could be significantly hampered by the small number of cases in each treatment group and publication bias, particularly the underreporting of treatment failures and of SVCS recurrences after initially successful interventions. The poor efficacy of anticoagulation and thrombolysis is not surprising given that histological studies in cases of lead-induced SVCS have shown that only a minority of cases are due to thrombosis without concomitant fibrosis; these types of lesions usually present relatively soon after device implantation. The majority are due to fibrotic narrowing and superimposed thrombosis, particularly if symptoms develop after more than a year (Gilard et al., 2002); among patients reported in this survey, the median interval between implantation and onset of SVCS symptoms was 48 months. Therefore, residual superior vena cava stenosis after successful thrombolytic therapy is likely a factor in re-thrombosis and short symptom-free periods (Leonelli et al., 2000). The disappointing results of venoplasty alone may also reflect high rates of restenosis. For example, patency rates as low as 30% have been reported at 1-year following balloon dilations of benign axillary and subclavian vein stenoses (Bolad et al., 2005; Frances et al., 1995; Gilard et al., 2002; Spittel & Hayes, 1992). The short-term results of surgery and stenting are more encouraging but the paucity of data on long-term efficacy and outcomes is a matter of concern. Even though surgical reconstruction has been practiced for over three decades, adequate follow-up data were only available for 17 patients over a median period of 16 months. Given that surgical reconstruction is a highly invasive and expensive undertaking, it is not surprising that percutaneous intervention employing venoplasty plus stenting has become the most commonly reported treatment for SVCS.

3.2 Pericarditis

The first reported case of pericarditis following permanent PM implantation was published in 1975 (Kaye et al., 1975). Pericarditis should be distinguished from acute or delayed lead perforation in which a migration of the electrode tip is observable. In pericarditis there are no changes in the tip position at x-ray examination and no changes in pacing or sensing thresholds (Ellenbogen et al., 2002). To date only a few cases of pericarditis related to PM implantation have been published (Ellenbogen et al., 2002; Kaye et al., 1975; Kono et al., 2008; Levy et al., 2004; Snow et al., 1987; Vinit et al., 2007;). Clinical manifestation of pericarditis resembled the classic post-pericardiotomy syndrome with pleuritic chest pain, dispnoea, and the presence of pericardial and pleurical effusion, raised erythrocyte sedimentation rate without polyarthopathy. Usually, effusion does not require pericardiocentesis because of the small size of effusion that responds to non steroid drugs or to steroids. Large effusion volumes could requires pericardiocentesis when tamponade is present. In the Greene et al. (1994) and Levy et al. (2004) series a higher incidence of pericarditis was found when active fixation leads were used overall for atrial stimulation. Several reported cases were related with an atrial active-fixation lead (Schiariti et al., 2009; Sivakumaran et al., 2002). Generally, pericarditis after permanent PM implantation has a benign and self-limited course. However, replacement of an active-fixation lead with a passive one has also been reported in order to prevent recurrence of pericarditis (Schiariti et al., 2009).

3.3 Undersensing

Loss of ventricular sensing could be caused by dislodgment or mechanical damage to the lead connected to the system, as perforation of the insulating sheath. Sometimes undersensing could be resolved after repositioning the lead, restoring its integrity with silicone adhesive as described by Costeas & Schoenfeld (1991), or reprogramming the device. In the past the ability to attach an unprotected unipolar lead to a bipolar connector, shared by the Voluntary (VS-1) and International (IS-1) designs, invited the possibility of injury to the insulating sheath by accidental tightening of the proximal screw. Sensing in PM and ICD is crucial to normal device behaviour. Since both devices treat different arrhythmias, the technical approach to signal detection is also completely different. A PM has a fixed threshold of sensing, above which events are sensed and therapy of the device withheld. On the other hand, the defibrillator has a variable threshold of sensing to detect tachyarrhythmias, with sometimes very small and changing electrogram amplitudes. Van Casteren et al. (2009) described undersensing of ventricular fibrillation due to interference between a PM and defibrillator in the same patient. The R-on-T phenomenon is a well-known entity that predisposes to dangerous arrhythmias. Typically, a premature ventricular complex occurring at the critical time during the T wave of the preceding beat precipitates ventricular tachycardia and fibrillation. This phenomenon can occur not only in asynchronous ventricular PM, but also in synchronous PM, if loss of sensing of the intrinsic rhythm becomes evident (Chemello et al., 2010).

3.4 Oversensing

Oversensing is a phenomenon potentially leading to ICD malfunctioning by interfering with intracardiac signals and usually is related to myopotentials, T-waves, electrical spikes of an additionally implanted PM or other technical devices i.e. microwaves, stimulation therapy in physiotherapy, and electric coagulation (Lin et al., 2004; Schulte et al., 2001; Secemsky et al., 1982; Weretka et al., 2003). The ICD system often misinterprets these cardiac/non-cardiac potentials as a malignant arrhythmia and delivers inappropriate shock therapy, which in many patients is an extremely uncomfortable event and greatly affects quality of life. In some cases, inappropriate therapy delivery is described as potentially life-threatening (Kiviniemi et al., 1999), especially when the shock falls in the vulnerable phase of QRS complex, triggering ventricular tachycardia or ventricular fibrillation (VF). Rauwolf et al. (2007) evaluated in a large cohort of 518 ICD patients the incidence and various types of ventricular oversensing (VO), the occurrence of inappropriate shock deliveries as well as the frequency of complications requiring invasive procedures to solve VO during a long-term follow-up. The most frequent oversensing mechanism was observed as T-wave oversensing in 10 patients, 8 (1.5%) patients were noticed with VO due to myopotentials; 5 patients suffered from VO due to electrode failure and consecutive noise sensing with inadequate therapy delivery. Double-counting was recorded in 4 patients, leading to 8 inadequate shocks in 2 patients and short episodes without therapy delivery; 3 patients experienced VO according to electromagnetic field interference with the ICD device by inducing an alternating current in the sensing electrode or to alternating current. In 1 patient, microwave energy was applied for pain relief at the skin close to the ICD pocket. The signals from electromagnetic field transmitter were detected from the atrial and ventricular channel of the ICD, misinterpreted as VF inducing an inappropriate shock delivery. The second patient had VO while swimming through an electrically opening pool door. In another case, the inadequate shock was due to an alternating current application during physiotherapy session using electric stimulation of the skin. There were 6 patients who had an ICD and an additionally implanted PM. There were different reasons for these double device implantations: a) first ICD generation with large volume were implanted abdominally; b) first ICD generation were only available as single-chamber devices; c) pre-existing biventricular pacemaker for CHF therapy; and d) insurance requirements (Geiger et al., 1997; Shivkumar et al., 2000).

3.5 Crosstalk

The oversensing of an atrial pacing pulse in the ventricular channel, has been described primarily in patients with unipolar PM and high atrial outputs (Helguera & Pinski, 2005). Although their high operating ventricular sensitivity could make ICD prone to cross-talk inhibition, this complication has been very uncommon. Crosstalk is one of the serious complications occurring with dual-chamber PM and ICD and it is defined as the inappropriate detection of a spontaneous or PM-generated event in one channel by the other channel, which can cause the inhibition of the second channel's output. There are two functions designed to prevent the crosstalk inhibition. One is the ventricular blanking period that coincides with the atrial stimulus. This prevents the detection of the atrial spike or activation that could cause the inhibition of the ventricular channel output. An additional backup system is the ventricular-safety-pace, which prevents asystole if crosstalk occurs due to atrial far-field activity sensed after the blanking period of the ventricular electrode.

3.6 Pacemaker syndrome

The PM syndrome consists of the cardiovascular signs and symptoms of heart failure and hypotension induced by the loss of both A-V and V-V synchrony that is associated with right ventricular apical pacing. It was first described by Mitsui et al. (1969) and occurs with single o dual chamber pacing mode. The clinical adverse effect are most severe when intact ventriculo-atrial conduction is present. Atrial contraction can coincide with ventricular systole against closed atrioventricular valve. This situation may lead to raised mean pressures in both atria, to atrial dilatation and retrograde blood flow into vena cava and pulmonary veins and contributes to decreased cardiac output. Nishimura et al. (1982) showed a great decrease in blood pressure more than 20 mmHg is suggestive of PM syndrome. When ventricular function is normal, estimates of atrial contribution to cardiac output vary from 15-20%. In elderly patients, in hypertensive cardiomyopathy, hypertrophic cardiomyopathy, and restrictive cardiomyopathy, the atrial kick contributes as much as 50%. The reduction in cardiac output associated with non physiologic pacing and loss of atrioventricular synchrony triggers changes in vascular tone. The autonomic nervous system enhances sympathetic activity modulated by arterial baroceptors which are triggered by low blood pressure (Alicandri et al., 1978; Ellenbogen et al., 1990; Pehrsson et al., 1988). The increase in left atrial, pulmonary and left ventricular filling pressures result in inhibitory reflexes mediated by vagal nerve and in increased production of atrial natriuretic peptide, a potent arterial and venous vasodilator (Theodorakis et al., 1992). The opposing reflexes may cause an inadequate vasoconstrictor response and decrease vascular tone. The dual chamber pacing does not ensure that pacemaker syndrome will not develop (Travill & Sutton, 1992). When the leads stimulate the myocardium to depolarize, paced depolarization of both atria and ventricles occurs cell to cell fashion rather than via usual conduction pathways. This depolarization is slower and less efficient and can result in dyssyncrony of atria and ventricles and of the right and left sides of the heart. It is necessary to program an appropriate atrioventricular delay between 120 and 200 ms. Too much short a delay reduces filling of the ventricles in diastole and of the atria during systole; too much a long one may produce asynchrony. In presence of atrio-ventricular block a rapid atrial pacing (AAI or AAIR) prevents the regular atrial filling and reduce cardiac output. Many patients cannot tolerate the rapid pacing associated with activity mode (Ellenbogen et al., 1997; Ellenbogen et al., 2007). An inappropriate mode switching of DDDR pacing in response to interference noise or dying battery, then rhythm change, can also cause PM syndrome. The retrograde depolarization of the atria which occurs with dual- o single–chamber devices can cause endless-loop tachycardia or PM-mediated tachycardia (Pioger et al., 2007).

The majority of symptoms of PM syndrome are likely attributable to the reduction in cardiac output that is associated with right ventricular pacing. It induces a contraction similar to that caused by left bundle branch block, asynchronous ventricular contraction leading to altered diastolic filling time, increase in mitral regurgitation and reduction in left ventricular ejection fraction (Lamas & Ellenbogen, 2004). The cardiac output is greater during AAI pacing than with dual-pacing DDD. Wigger (1925) showed that ventricular pacing results in reduced ventricular-pump function in mammals. Ventricular desyncronization imposed by pacing results in chronic left ventricular remodeling, including asymmetric hypertrophy and dilatation. Ventricular pacing increases atrial pressure and size, as well as to favor the development of electrophysiological proprieties that could facilitate the development of atrial fibrillation. In patients with an ICD, dual-chamber pacing paradoxically led to increased risks of heart failure, hospitalization and death by a factor of 1.6 by inducing ventricular pacing (Wilkoff et al., 2002). Bordachar et al. (2004) showed an increase in cardiac output from 2.2 l/min at baseline to 3.8 l/min with institution of biventricular pacing in patients with heart failure.

Symptoms of PM syndrome are nonspecific and diagnosis depends heavily on correlation between onset of symptoms and onset of pacing or change in pacing mode. The PM interrogation plays a crucial role in determining PM mode contribution to symtoms: dyspnoea on exertion, paroxysmal nocturnal dyspnoea, orthopnoea, hypotension, pre-syncope and syncope (Furman, 1994). Physical examination can often reveal elevated neck veins, rales, and pedal oedema. Syncope is uncommon and usually associated with systolic blood pressure declines of greater than 20 mmHg. The other symptoms attributed to PM syndrome include easy fatigability, malaise, headache, and sensation of fullness and pulsations in the head and neck. A diagnosis can be confirmed by placing a magnet over the PM, converting the system to VOO mode at predetermined rate to induce ventriculo-atrial conduction and symptoms (upright) (Ross & Kenny, 2000). ECG, Holter monitor or event recorder may reveal a prolonged PR interval, ventriculo-atrial conduction, or atrio-ventricular dissociation. Echocardiogram may show decreased cardiac output with ventricular pacing versus conduct sinus activity or atrio-ventricular synchronous pacing. Symptoms usually resolve after reprogramming PM parameters, such atrio-ventricular delay, postventricular atrial refractory period, sensing level, and pacing threshold voltage or using hysteresis to help maintain atrio-ventricular synchrony in patients with VVI PM and intact sinus node function or addition of an atrial lead.

The incidence of PM syndrome in various studies ranges from 25% (Travill & Sutton, 1992) to 83% (Heldman et al., 1990), depending to large degree on diagnostic criteria and to the therapy used for diagnosis. When surgical revision is required to upgrade a patient from VVIR pacing, the incidence has been low, 2.7% in the Canadian trial of Physiolgic Pacing (Connolly et al., 2000). In the PASE (Lamas et al., 1998) and MOST (Lamas et al., 2002) studies in which devices could be easily upgraded to DDDR mode by simple reprogramming, the incidence of PM syndrome was higher. The PM syndrome may also be underestimated or it may be subclinic. The symptoms often have been ascribed to the aging process, to the worsening of heart failure or to coronary artery disease. Memory deficit in elderly patients complicate reporting of symptoms. Therefore, up to 75% of patients who have felt generally well for many years with single-chamber PM have noted improvement in their quality of life after upgrading to dual–chamber PM at the time of a pulse-generator change (Sulke et al., 1992).

Atrio-ventricular dyssynchrony is associated with atrial fibrillation and, therefore, thromboembolic complications, and also heart failure. The investigators have assumed the same complications for PM syndrome. The results of completed randomized clinical trials of PM mode selection have been somewhat conflicting. Andersen et al., (1994) compared AAI with VVI pacing in 225 patients with sinus node dysfunction and demonstrated persistent reduction in primary endpoints of atrial fibrillation, thromboembolic events, chronic atrial fibrillation , and all cause mortality in AAI paced group. In the PASE study 407 patients in sinus rhythm and bradycardia were randomized to VVIR or DDDR. There was a 26% crossover rate due to the development of PM syndrome but no difference in quality of life, death, stroke, first hospitalization for heart failure, development of atrial fibrillation were observed. Also larger trials, the Canadian Trail of Physiologic Pacing and MOST performed to randomizing 2568 and 2020 patients to atrial-based or ventricular pacing failed to show differences in the endpoints, stroke or death. Only the incidence of atrial fibrillation was lower with dual-chamber pacing. In subsequent analyses of MOST data the percentage of ventricular pacing correlated with risk of congestive failure. This percentage was greater in DDR versus VVIR mode (90% versus 58%). The ventricular dyssyncrony induced by pacing even when atrio-ventricular synchrony is preserved increases the risk of PM syndrome, heart failure hospitalization and atrial fibrillation. The benefit derived from atrio-ventricular sequential pacing is likely counterbalanced by detrimental effects of frequent and unnecessary right ventricular pacing. These observations have led to renewed interest in single-chamber atrial pacing (Pioger et al., 2007) for sinus node dysfuncition and the development of new dual-chamber PM algorithms designed to minimize right ventricular pacing (Sweeney et al., 2007a) and additional research will determine if different forms of ventricular pacing, such as biventricular or ventricular-septal pacing, will improve outcome in patients who require ventricular stimulation.

3.7 ICD-specific complications

After the first clinical implantation (Mirowski et al., 1980), numerous primary and secondary prevention trials resulted in rapid expansion of indication for use of ICD. In the successive 15 years, the annual ICD insertion has increased by 20-fold (Maisel et al., 2006). Consequently, the number of implanted ICD system and the number of patients with longer follow-up has continuously increased. Despite advances in system design and manufacturing to answer to any different clinical situation, device malfunctions and software glitches will continue to occur. The increasing complexity in ICD hardware with significant proportion of biventricular resynchronization devices may result in higher

complications rates. The surgical complications, infection or erosion, hematoma, pneumothorax, are similar in type and frequency to those seen with routine PM implantation (DiMarco, 2003). The other generator–related complications are defined as early generator depletion (less than 4 years after implantation), recalls, power reset and lead connector problems (an average of 1.4% per patient-year) (Ezekowitz et al., 2007). The lead is a life-line whose purpose is to convey critical information about heart's rhythm to the ICD generator and, in turn, to deliver life-sustaining therapy when needed. The long-term reliability of the leads is the main problem. ICD leads are significantly more complex than PM leads and must allow high voltage energy delivery for defibrillation when necessary and, may be inherently more susceptible to failure. The mechanical stress can cause fracture in a lead or failure in insulation by chronic excessive pressure on the body of the lead by the ligature used for fixation (Dorwarth et al., 2003) or the subclavian crush syndrome (Antonelli et al., 1998) or the higher activity patients or the multiple leads or the anatomic reasons in females. The insulation degradation by breakdown of polyurethane polymers due, in most cases, to metal ion oxidation like in the Medtronic models 6936 and 6966. This lead failure can produce oversensing following appropriate shocks (Ellelbogen et al., 2003). It is likely that this problem remains clinically silent until a high-voltage shock is delivered. Detection of a ring-to-coil impedance drop and a high short interval counter may be a useful indicator of middle insulation breach. The newer lead models have multi-lumen design with steroid elution: each conductor is individually insulated by silicon rubber, which should prevent the lead injury. Silicone leads also seem to be prone to insulation failure (Mewis et al., 1997). More than half of lead defects (56%) results from insulation failure (Kleemann et al., 2007). The lead defect depends mainly on follow-up time after implantation. The lead survival rates at 5 and 8 years are 85% and 60%, respectively (Kleemann et al., 2007). The annual lead failure rate, defined as lead-related problem requiring surgical revision, reaches 2.5% in 5 years (Eckstein et al., 2008) and 20% in 10 years old leads (Kleemann et al., 2007).
The great variation observed in ICD lead survival is due to variety of factors including variable study definitions of lead malfunction, variable performance of models and patient characteristics and implantation techniques (Maisel & Kramer, 2008). The lead dislocation and exit block tend to occur early, while the other problems are more evenly distributed over time (Duray et al., 2009). The left ventricular lead dislocation reaches rate varied between 0%, 4.7% and 7.5% for increased complexity to implant procedure in the coronary sinus (Duray et al., 2009). The dislocation can be observed on x-ray combined with significant changes in sensing/pacing performance. The exit block is a failure to capture at reasonable device output without change in impedance and lead position. The lead fracture results in changes in impedance (more than 2000 Ohm), in changes in sensing/pacing performance (intermittent o permanent) and is confirmed by fluoroscopy. The oversensing is sensing of artifacts (chaotic, far field, T-wave, myopotential, noise from contact with another lead) without significant change in lead impedance o position, similar to what seen with PM. The other recorded problems are: unstable impedance measurements, R-wave reduction and loss of capture (Eckstein et al., 2008).
The tools available to detect impending ICD lead failure are limited. At implantation, all ICD systems are tested including determination of sensing, lead and shock impedances, pacing thresholds, and defibrillation thresholds after repetitive induction of ventricular fibrillation. Follow-up, every 3-6 months or early as needed, consisted of interrogation and retrieval of all stored data since last visit, as well determination of sensing, impedance

measurements, and pacing thresholds. The need for increased surveillance of patients with older leads should include test for oversensing during provocative maneuvers and measurement of high voltage coil and pace/sense impedances and defibrillation underthreshold testing. A big help could have come from wireless home monitoring of device than can immediately detect any abnormality thus reducing the risk for patients (Corrado et al., 2009). Anyway electrical testing, x-ray, fluoroscopy, or direct visualization may be used to detect lead abnormalities but are imprecise.

ICD dysfunction may result in failure to deliver therapy for ventricular tachycardia and thus result in syncope or sudden death. Pooled data of randomized clinical trials that involve around 3500 patients indicate an ICD-unresponsive sudden-death rate of nearly 5% (Anderson, 2005). Primary ventricular arrhythmia detection is based on the tachycardia detection rate which is usually programmed with a safety margin of 20 beats/min below the clinical arrhythmia. But there is high (30%) slow ventricular tachycardia incidence (less than 150 beats/min) in ICD recipients without prior history of slow ventricular tachycardia (Sadoul et al., 2005). The patients could exhibit symptoms such as syncope, palpitations, and congestive heart failure, leading to hospital admission and sometimes death. A low detection rate may lead to inappropriate therapy during supraventricular tachycardia. Most ICD can be programmed to enhance the discrimination between supraventricular and ventricular arrhythmias by additional criteria such sudden onset, stability, ventricular electrogram morphology or vector timing and correlation, and relationship between the atrium and ventricle. For terminating monomorphic tachycardias, antitachycardia pacing is standard technique and is painless for patient. But is not always effective and can accelerate ventricular tachycardia or, if applied during a supraventricular rhythm, induce a ventricular arrthymia and following shock. Trappe et al (1995) reported an acceleration rate of only 3% in selected patients with recurrent inducible ventricular tachycardia that had been successfully terminated during predischarge test. Inappropriate delivery of ICD therapy, triggered by artefacts due to lead dysfunction, extraneous noise interference, or rapid atrial rates, mainly during atrial fibrillation or sinus tachycardia, remains a major clinical challenge.

Clinical trial experience has revealed that up to 25% of patients receive inappropriate shocks (Germano et al., 2006). ICD shocks reduce the physical functioning and mental well-being and increase anxiety of patients while obligating strict driving restrictions. The risk of death with inappropriate shocks in SCD-HeFT was increased by a factor of 2, while for an appropriate shock the risk was increased by a factor of more than 5. The arrhythmia much likely signaling a meaningful change in patient's clinical status, including a worsening of heart failure and myocardial ischemia with abnormalities in the levels of electrolytes. An examination of randomized trials for primary and secondary prevention has shown that the number of appropriate shocks exceed the sudden death and overall mortality rate in the control group (Germano et al., 2006). Many episodes may have been nonsustianed nonfatal events. Therefore, there are appropriate shocks and necessary shocks. Alternatively the ICD proarrhytmic effect may be considered (Tung et al., 2008). The pacing–associated short-long sequences were found at the onset of 21% to 35% of all episodes of ventricular tachycardia and fibrillation (Sweeney et al., 2007b). Device malfunction or local lead effect with mechanical irritation and late fibrosis may be potential mechanism for ventricular arrhythmias. The reversal activation wavefronts from epicardial resynchronization increases dispersion of refractoriness with demonstrated improvement of ventricular arrhythmias and sudden death after implantation (Basu et al., 2007). Nevertheless, ICD is clinically proven to improve survival in selected patients at risk for sudden cardiac death, but monitoring of this device remains critical to inform physicians and patients about device performance and to identify underperforming products as early as possible. The last highly publicized recall of Sprint Fidelis (Medtronic Inc., Minneapolis, Minnesota) lead was issued October 2007 (Food and drug Administration, 2007). The higher rates of lead fracture (2.3% to 6.7% at 30 months) led to more media-provoked mass hysteria as about 268000 patients were at risk in the world. The lead failure produced inappropriate shocks and ICD storm due to sensing of electrical noise: 5 deaths were reported in initial advisory (Catanchin et al., 2008). To overcame the problems of lead insertion and of lead failure an entirely subcutaneous implantable cardioverter-defibrillator was designed and tested. A report of the initial evaluation was recently published (Bardy et al., 2010).

Any effort to development ICD technology should be mainly directed to reliability of the system and to patient safety. Electrical storm is defined as a state of cardiac electrical instability manifested by several episodes of ventricular tachyarrythmias over a short period of time, there or more appropriate ventricular detection in 24 hours, usually requiring antitachycardia pacing or the delivery of multiple electrical shocks. It occurs in approximately 25% of ICD patients within 3 years, with typically 5-55 individual ventricular tachyarrythmias within one storm (Israel & Barold, 2007). The majority of episodes are ventricular tachycardias. Electrical storm consists of monomorphic ventricular tachycardia by reentry but ventricular fibrillation indicating acute ischemia is rare. The aetiology of electric storm is not clearly understood. The factors contributing to storm onset are: worsening of cardiac function, electrolyte disturbance, autonomic imbalance, drug proarrhythmia, a context with other illness, psychological stress, excess ethanol consumption and cardiac resynchronization therapy (Kantharia et al., 2006). In 35% of the patients storms represent their first event. The majority of storms occurred during winter (Greene et al., 2000). The immediate mortality is low, but the re-admission to hospital are frequent (50-80%). The prognosis is relatively good with an overall survival at 2 years of 95% and at 6 years of 77.5%. These patients could be treated with amiodarone i.v., and with reprogramming high rate pacing. The key intervention is reduction of elevated sympathetic tone by beta blockers and frequently benzodiazepines. Substrate mapping and radio frequency ablation may be useful in treatment and prevention.

3.8 Removal of devices

The value of extraction of infected or hazardous epicardial and endocardial PM or ICD leads is well established (Rusanow & Spotnitz, 2010) by open or percutaneous techniques including all lead types and indications. PM and ICD infections generally respond to antibiotics, complete hardware removal, and a hardware free interval. However, these principles cannot always be invoked, and the risk of complications is likely to increase when hardware cannot be completely removed or when a hardware-free interval is unsafe or inadvisable. Percutaneous lead extraction is superior to open extraction in terms of safety and comfort, but epicardial extraction techniques remain critically important in selected patients. Lead extraction is performed in the operating room under general anesthesia, with pump standby. Temporary transvenous pacing wires are placed when indicated despite presence of vegetations until a permanent system can safely be implanted.

Recommendations for extraction of chronically implanted transvenous pacing and defibrillator lead were published by Love et al. (2000). The percutaneous techniques should be attempted first in all patients except those presenting with large vegetations, atrial thrombus, epicardial leads, or ICD patches. After endocardial leads are dissected free at their venous entry site, anchoring collars are removed. A gentle traction is applied and if failed, a locking stylet could be inserted into the lead, and traction should be again attempted. If this too failed, telescoping sheaths could be advanced over the lead, maintaining countertraction with the locking stylet. Techniques described by Byrd et al. (1985; 1990) and electrosurgical dissection by means of an equipment manufactured by Cook Medical Inc (Bloomington, IN) or Excimer laser (Spectranetics Corp., Colorado Springs, CL) are used to extract heavily fibrotic leads. More recently, a new extraction tool, the Evolution mechanical dilator sheath (Cook Medical, Bloomington, IN), was introduced. It uses a rotational mechanism with a stainless-steel bladed tip to overcome fibrosis and cut adherences. Its rotational mechanism allows the sheath to advance down the lead body while cutting fibrotic attachments. The outer sheath covers the cutting edge when cutting activity is not desired so that venous walls are protected from damage. In addition, a shorter Evolution dilator sheath (Shortie) has been designed with a sharper and tougher blade to facilitate venous access in cases with extensive calcification under the clavicle. Initial experience with the Evolution mechanical dilator sheath for lead extraction has been reported recently (Hussein et al., 2010). Extensive surgical debridement of the pocket is performed using electrocautery and blunt dissection. Timing of device reimplantation is based primarily on sterility of blood cultures, but also on resolution of vegetations. Reimplantation is usually performed on the contralateral side. In select cases, an ipsilateral lateral sub-pectoral location may be used depending on the extent of pocket infection. Persistent inability to extract the lead prompted conversion to an open technique, when indicated. The commonest open technique after failed endocardial extraction was pursestring or snare-controlled right atriotomy through a median sternotomy (Byrd et al., 1990). Median sternotomy with cardiopulmonary bypass are used in the presence of atrial or superior vena cava thrombi, or large vegetations on the leads or on the tricuspid valve. Epicardial leads and patches were removed through a median sternotomy or left, right, or subxiphoid thoracotomy. The surgical approach is based on lead and patch location according to the the North American Society of Pacing and Electrophysiology Guidelines (Love et al., 2000).

4. Electromagnetic interference (EMI)

Electrical devices generate electromagnetic fields that may interfere with PM and ICD. The incidence of that interference is still controversial and only partially explored because the plenty of new electronic devices that are continuously introduced. These facts forced physicians to adopt very restrictive rules for use of electronic devices by patients who had cardiac implantable devices, on the other hand industries paid more attention to project safe devices. Nowadays third-generation mobile phones, Universal Mobile Telecommunication System (UMTS), were recently introduced in Europe. The safety of these devices with regard to their interference with implanted devices was studied among 100 patients by Ismail et al. (2010) who concluded that third-generation mobile phones are safe for patients with permanent PM regardless of atrial and ventricular sensitivity settings. This is due to the high-frequency band for this system (1800-2200 MHz) and the low power output between

0.01 W and 0.25 W. Also media players cause telemetry interference with PM, but it is not known whether they cause direct interference with them. Thaker et al. (2009) studied the interaction between PM and 3 different media players. PM interference was categorized as type I, II, or III. Types I and II interferences described telemetry interference and type III interference was defined as any direct interference with PM function or programmed parameters. It was concluded that media players cause telemetry interference with PM, but they do not directly interfere with PM function. Recently Lee et al. (2009) published the evidence that interferences could be generated by magnetic field of portable headphones. PM or ICD function was assessed in 100 patients during exposure to 8 different models of portable headphones to determine the incidence of clinically relevant magnetic interference. The magnetic field strength of the headphones was also measured in vitro. They concluded that clinically relevant magnetic interference from portable headphones occurred in 30 (30%) of 100 patients and more commonly affected ICD than PM patients (21/55, 38.2% versus 9/45, 20.0%; P = .048). All patients affected by magnetic interference experienced a magnet response, characterized by asynchronous pacing in PM patients and by inhibition of tachyarrhythmia detection in ICD patients. In all but one of the 30 cases of magnetic interference, removal of the headphones from the patient's chest immediately restored normal device function. Headphones with a measured magnetic field strength more or equal to 10 Gauss at 2 cm were much more likely to cause magnetic interference than were those with lower magnetic field strength (30/100 patients versus 0/100 patients; p <0.0001). Magnetic interference was not observed when headphones were placed more than 3 cm apart from the skin surface. It was concluded that clinically significant magnetic interference can occur when portable headphones are placed in close proximity to implanted PM and ICD. Patients with such a device should be advised to keep portable headphones at least 3 cm distant from their device.

5. Psychological problems

All studies concerning the quality of life in patients instrumented with PM or ICD are limited by the inability to mask therapy. The recorded effects can reflect the beliefs and expectations of patients. The patients may perceive the device as an electronic security or as a source of physical and emotional discomfort. Introducing a foreign body into the heart may cause a change in body image, cause problems in psychosocial adaptation and contribute to development of affective disorders. There are differences in intrusiveness of the two devices: ICD shocks are often painful and are delivered at unpredictable times, while pacing is unlikely felt by the patients. The interval between follow-up visit is closer for ICD patients who are encouraged to contact the clinic when they experience some problems and they can feel more dependent. Over 70% of the PM recipients are at least 70 years old (Ross & Kenny, 2000). It is difficult to examine the quality of life in the elderly because of age-related cardiovascular and cerebrovascular physiological changes, including reduced cardiac output, blunted autonomic compensatory responses and altered cerebral autoregulation. The aging and the development of the other conditions may overwhelm the moderate improvements in cardiovascular functional class and minimize the long-term effect on general quality of life. Depression and anxiety are more common in patients with permanent PM than in the general population. In one trial the quality of life was found to be similar to that of patients who require long-term hemodialysis (Lamas et al., 2002). Aydemir et al. (1997) reported that 19.1% of PM patients warranted a psychiatric diagnosis, and 10.7%

were clinically depressed. Pycha et al. (1990) identified depression of moderate severity in 35% of ICD patients, Heller et al. (1998) in 20-58%. In other studies the prevalence of affective disturbance is relatively low (Duru et al., 2001). There are important methodological differences that may account for divergent results: some studies have used short-term design and have measured quality of life with non standard instruments. In PASE study, in which the primary end-point was quality of life, no overall benefit from dual-chamber pacing as compared with single-chamber ventricular pacing was found (Lamas et al., 1998). Only patients with sinus-node dysfunction did appear to benefit from dual-chamber pacing, but those with PM implanted because of heart block did not. In individual patient the quality of life appeared to improve after upgrading to dual-chamber (Sulke et al., 1992), while it was lower at time of PM syndrome than at time of implantation. PM implantation improved health-related quality of life. The mode select was associated with much smaller, but significant, improvements in several domains, particularly physical function (Fleischmann et al., 2006). Atrioventricular synchronous pacing has a beneficial effect on most domains of quality of life in patients with hypertrophic obstructive cardiomyopathy refractory to drug treatment (Gadler et al., 1999). In a large primary-prevention population with moderately symptomatic heart failure ICD therapy was not associated with adverse quality effects during 30 months of follow-up (Mark et al., 2008). The occurrence of ICD shocks was associated with increased psychological distress in both patients and their families. The quality of life of patients in the month after a shock was significantly decreased in perceived general health, physical and emotional functioning, social functioning, and self-rated health. This result did not persist however, because the shock experience remembers the patients have a device with a life preserving function. They report limitations in their activities and admit anxiety about battery depletion and technical problems. The most distressing aspects of receiving a shock are the lack of warning, multiple shocks, nervousness, fear of sudden death, dizziness, weakness and chest soreness. Educational interventions and support group might incorporate knowledge about the effects of devices, to facilitate anticipatory guidance and preparation of patient and family members for ICD shocks.

6. Conclusion

Strict adherence to the widely accepted guidelines and recommendations, awareness of potential complications, and a meticulous approach to the implant and post implant techniques and follow-up may certainly reduce the incidence of complications after implantation of PM and ICD, more than often life-saving devices. To be aware of PM and ICD complications is an essential first step for good clinical practice in this area.

7. References

Abrams, S. & Peart, I. (1995). Twiddler's syndrome in children: an unusual cause of pacemaker failure. *Br Heart J*, 73, 190–192

Aggarwal, R.K.; Connelly, D.T.; Ray, S.G.; Ball, J. & Charles, R.G. (1995). Early complications of permanent pacemaker implantation: no difference between dual and single chamber systems. *Br Heart J*, 73, 571-575

Aggarwal, R.K.; Connelly, D.T.; Ray, S.G. & Charles, R.G. (1996). Acute and early complications of permanent pacing: A prospective audit of 926 consecutive patients from a UK center. *Int J Angiol,* 5, 78–81

Aizawa, K.; Kaneoko, Y.; Yamagishi, T.; Utsugi, T.; Suzuki, T.; Ishikawa, S.; Otaki, A.; Morishita, Y.; Hasegawa, A.; Kurabayashi, M. & Nagai R. (2001). Oozing from the pericardium as an etiology of cardiac tamponade associated with screw-in atrial leads. *Pacing Clin Electrophysiol,* 24, 381–383

Alicandri, C.; Fouad, F.M.; Tarazi, R.C.; Castle, L. & Morant, V. (1978). Three cases of hypotension and syncope with ventricular pacing: possible role of atrial reflexes. *Am J Cardiol,* 42, 137-142

al-Khadra, A.S. (2003). Implantation of pacemakers and implantable cardioverter defibrillators in orally anticoagulated patients. *Pacing Clin Electrophysiol,* 26, 511–514

Andersen, H.R.; Thuesen, L.; Bagger, J.P.; Vesterlund, T. & Thomsen, P.E. (1994). Prospective randomised trial of atrial versus ventricular pacing in sick-sinus syndrome. *Lancet,* 344, 1523-1528

Anderson, K.P. (2005). Sudden cardiac death unresponsive to implantable defibrillator therapy: an urgent target for clinicians, industry and government. *J Interv Card Electrophysiol,* 14, 71-78

Antonelli, D.; Rosenfeld, T.; Freedberg, N.A.; Palma, E.; Gross, J.N. & Furman, S. (1998). Insulation lead failure: is it a matter of insulation coating, venous approach, or both? *Pacing Clin Electrophysiol,* 21, 418-421

Aydemir, O.; Ozmen, E.; Küey, L.; Kültür, S.; Yeşil, M.; Postaci, N. & Bayata, S. (1997). Psychiatric morbidity and depressive symptomatology in patients with permanent pacemakers. *Pacing Clin Electrophysiol,* 20, 1628-1632

Bardy, G.H.; Smith, W.M.; Hood, M.A.; Crozier, I.G.; Melton, I.C.; Jordaens, L.; Theuns, D.; Park, R.E.; Wright, D.J.; Connelly, D.T.; Fynn, S.P.; Murgatroyd, F.D.; Sperzel, J.; Neuzner, J.; Spitzer, S.G.; Ardashev, A.V.; Oduro, A.; Boersma, L.; Maass, A.H.; Van Gelder, I.C.; Wilde, A.A.; van Dessel, P.F.; Knops, R.E.; Barr, C.S.; Lupo, P.; Cappato, R. & Grace, A.A. (2010). An entirely subcutaneous implantable cardioverter-defibrillator. *N Engl J Med,* 363, 36-44

Basu R.I.; Fendelander, L. & Singh, J.P. (2007). Cardiac resynchronization therapy and its potential proarrhythmic effect. *Clin Cardiol,* 30, 498-502

Belott, P. & Reynolds, D. (2000). Permanent pacemaker and implantable cardioverter defibrillator implantation. In: *Clinical cardiac pacing and defibrillation,* Ellenbogen, K.A.; Kay, G. & Wilkoff, B. (Eds), pages 573-644, WB Saunders, Philadelphia

Birnie, D.; Williams, K.; Guo, A.; Mielniczuk, L.; Davis, D.; Lemery, R.; Green, M.; Gollob, M. & Tang, A. (2006). Reasons for escalating pacemaker implants. *Am J Cardiol,* 98, 93-97

Bolad, I.; Karanam, S; Mathew, D.; John, R.; Piemonte, T. & Martin, D. (2005). Percutaneous treatment of superior vena cava obstruction following transvenous device implantation. *Cath Cardiov Int,* 65, 54–59

Bordachar, P.; Lafitte, S.; Reuter, S.; Sanders, P.; Jaïs, P.; Haïssaguerre, M.; Roudaut, R.; Garrigue, S. & Clementy, J. (2004). Echocardiographic parameters of ventricular dyssynchrony validation in patients with heart failure using sequential biventricular pacing. *J Am Coll Cardiol,* 44, 2157-2165

Bracke, F.; van Gelder, B.; Dijkman, B. & Meijer, A. (2005). Lead system causing Twiddler's syndrome in patients with an implantable cardioverter-defibrillator. *J Thorac Cardiovasc Surg*, 129, 231–232

Byrd, C.L.; Schwartz, S.J.; Hedin, N.B.; Goode, L.B.; Fearnot, L.E. & Smith, H.J. (1990). Intravascular lead extraction using locking stylets and sheaths. *Pacing Clin Electrophysiol*, 13, 1871–1875

Byrd, C.L.; Schwartz, S.J.; Sivina, M.; Yahr, W.Z. & Greenberg J.J. (1985). Technique for the surgical extraction of permanent pacing leads and electrodes. *J Thorac Cardiovasc Surg*, 89, 142–144

Cabell, C.H.; Heidenreich, P.A.; Chu, V.H.; Moore, C.M.; Stryjewski, M.E.; Corey, G.R. & Fowler, V.G.Jr. (2004). Increasing rates of cardiac device infections among Medicare beneficiaries: 1990-1999. *Am Heart J*, 147, 582-586

Carnero-Varo, A.; Perez-Paredes, M.; Ruiz-Ros, J.A.; Gimenez-Cervantes, D.; Martinez-Corbalan, F.R.; Cubero-Lopez, T. & Jara-Perez, P. (1999). "Reel Syndrome": a new form of Twiddler's syndrome? *Circulation*, 100, e45–e46

Catanchin, A.; Anderson, L.; Jones, S. & Ward, D. (2008). When life-saving devices terminate life. *J Cardiovasc Electrophysiol*, 19, 316-318

Chauhan, A.; Grace, A.A.; Newell, S.A.; Stone, D.L.; Shapiro, L.M.; Schofield, P.M. & Petch, M.C. (1994). Early complications after dual chamber versus single chamber pacemaker implantation. *Pacing Clin Electrophysiol*, 17, 2012-2015

Chemello, D.; Subramanian, A. & Kumaraswamy, N. (2010). Cardiac arrest caused by undersensing of a temporary epicardial pacemaker. *Can J Cardiol*, 26, e13-e14

Chua, J.D.; Wilkoff, B.L.; Lee, I.; Juratli, N.; Longworth, D.L. & Gordon, S.M. (2000). Diagnosis and management of infections involving implantable electrophysiologic cardiac devices. *Ann Intern Med*, 133, 604-608

Connolly, S.J.; Kerr, C.R.; Gent, M.; Roberts, R.S.; Yusuf, S.; Gillis, A.M.; Sami, M.H.; Talajic, M.; Tang, A.S.; Klein, G.J.; Lau, C. & Newman, D.M. (2000). Effects of physiologic pacing versus ventricular pacing on the risk of stroke and death due to cardiovascular causes. Canadian Trial of Physiologic Pacing Investigators. *N Engl J Med*, 342, 1385-1391

Corrado, A.; Gasparini, G. & Raviele, A. (2009). Lead malfunctions in implantable cardioverter defibrillators: where are we and where should we go? *Europace*, 11, 276-277

Costeas, X.F. & Schoenfeld, M.H. (1991). Undersensing as a consequence of lead incompatibility: case report and a plea for universality. *Pacing Clin Electrophysiol*, 14, 1681-1683

DiMarco, J.P. (2003). Implantable cardioverter-defibrillators. *N Engl J Med*, 349, 1836-1847

Dorwarth, U.; Frey, B.; Dugas, M.; Matis, T.; Fiek, M.; Schmoeckel, M.; Remp, T.; Durchlaub, I.; Gerth, A.; Steinbeck, G. &, Hoffmann, E. (2003). Transvenous defibrillation leads: high incidence of failure during long-term follow-up. *J Cardiovasc Electrophysiol*, 14, 38-43

Duray, G.Z.; Schmitt, J.; Cicek-Hartvig, S.; Hohnloser, S.H. & Israel, C.W. (2009). Complications leading to surgical revision in implantable cardioverter defibrillator patients: comparison of patients with single-chamber, dual-chamber, and biventricular devices. *Europace*, 11, 297-302

Duru, F.; Büchi, S.; Klaghofer, R.; Mattmann, H.; Sensky, T.; Buddeberg, C. & Candinas, R. (2001). How different from pacemaker patients are recipients of implantable cardioverter-defibrillators with respect to psychosocial adaptation, affective disorders, and quality of life? *Heart,* 85, 375-379

Eckstein, J.; Koller, M.T.; Zabel, M.; Kalusche, D.; Schaer, B.A.; Osswald, S. & Sticherling, C. (2008). Necessity for surgical revision of defibrillator leads implanted long-term: causes and management. *Circulation,* 117, 2727-2733

Ellenbogen, K.A.; Gilligan, D.M.; Wood, M.A.; Morillo, C. & Barold, S.S. (1997). The pacemaker syndrome : a matter of definition. *Am J Cardiol,* 79, 1226-1229

Ellenbogen, K.A.; Kay, G.N.; Lau, C.P. & Wilkoff, B.L. (Eds.). (2007). *Clinical cardiac pacing, defibrillation and resynchronization therapy.* 3rd, pages 291-335. WB Saunders, Philadelphia

Ellenbogen, K.A.; Thames, M.D. & Mohanty, P.K. (1990). New insights into pacemaker syndrome gained from hemodynamic, humoral and vascular responses during ventriculo-atrial pacing. *Am J Cardiol,* 65, 53-59

Ellenbogen, K.A.; Wood, M.A. & Shepard, R.K. (2002). Delayed complications following pacemaker implantation. *Pacing Clin Electrophysiol,* 25, 1155–1158

Ellenbogen, K.A.; Wood, M.A,; Shepard, R.K.; Clemo, H.F.; Vaughn, T.; Holloman, K.; Dow, M.; Leffler, J.; Abeyratne, A. & Verness, D. (2003). Detection and management of implantable cardioverter defibrillator lead failure: Incidence and clinical implications. *J Am Coll Cardiol,* 41, 73-80

Ezekowitz, J.A.; Rowe, B.H.; Dryden, D.M.; Hooton, N.; Vandermeer, B.; Spooner, C. & McAlister, F.A. (2007). Systematic review: implantable cardioverter defibrillators for adults with left ventricular systolic dysfunction. *Ann Intern Med,* 147, 251-262

Fleischmann, K.E.; Orav, E.J.; Lamas, G.A.; Mangione, C.M.; Schron, E.; Lee, K.L. & Goldman, L. (2006). Pacemaker implantation and quality of life in the Mode Selection Trial (MOST). *Heart Rhythm,* 3, 653-659

Food and Drug Admistration. (2007). Statement on Medtronic's voluntary market suspension of their Sprint Fidelis defibrillator leads. October 15

Fortescue, E.B.; Berul, C.I.; Cecchin, F.; Walsh, E.P.; Triedman, J.K. & Alexander, M.E. (2004). Patient, procedural, and hardware factors associated with pacemaker lead failures in pediatrics and congenital heart disease. *Heart Rhythm,* 1, 150–159

Frances, C.M.; Starkey, I.R.; Errington, M.L. & Gillespie, I.N. (1995). Venous stenting as treatment for pacemaker-induced superior vena cava syndrome. *Am Heart J,* 129, 836–837

Furman, S. Pacemaker syndrome. (1994). *Pacing Clin Electrophysiol,* 17, 1-5

Gadler, F.; Linde, C.; Daubert, C.; McKenna, W.; Meisel, E.; Aliot, E.; Chojnowska, L.; Guize, L.; Gras, D.; Jeanrenaud, X. & Kappenberger, L. (1999). Significant improvement of quality of life following atrioventricular synchronous pacing in patients with hypertrophic obstructive cardiomyopathy. Data from 1 year of follow-up. PIC study group: Pacing In Cardiomyopathy. *Eur Heart J,* 20, 1044-1050

Garcia-Bolao, I.; Teijera, R. & Diaz-Dorronsoro, I. (2001). Late fatal right ventricular perforation as complication of permanent pacing leads. *Pacing Clin Electrophysiol,* 24, 1036–1037

Geiger, M.J.; O'Neill, P.; Sharma, A.; Skadsen, A.; Zimerman, L.; Greenfield, R.A.; Newby, K.H.; Wharton, J.M.; Kent, V. & Natale, A. (1997). Interactions between transvenous nonthoracotomy cardioverter defibrillator systems and permanent transvenous endocardial pacemakers. *Pacing Clin Electrophysiol,* 20, 624-630

Germano, J.J.; Reynolds, M.; Essebag, V. & Josephson, M.E. (2006). Frequency and causes of implantable cardioverter-defibrillator therapies: is device therapy proarrhythmic? *Am J Cardiol,* 97, 1255-1261

Gershon, T.; Kuruppu, J. & Olshaker, J. (2000). Delayed cardiac tamponade after pacemaker insertion. *J Emerg Med,* 18, 355–359

Gilard, M.; Perennes, A.; Mansourati, J.; Etienne, Y.; Fatemi, M.; Blanc, J.J. & Boschat, J. (2002). Stent implantation for the treatment of superior vena cava syndrome related to pacemaker leads. *Europace,* 4, 155–158

Goldberger, Z. & Lampert, R. (2006). Implantable cardioverter–defibrillator: expanding indications and technologies. *J Am Med Assoc,* 295, 809–818

Goldstein, D.J.; Losquadro, W. & Spotnitz, H.M. (1998). Outpatient pacemaker procedures in orally anticoagulated patients. *Pacing Clin Electrophysiol,* 21, 1730–1734

Grammes, J.A.; Schulze, C.M.; Al-Bataineh, M.; Yesenosky, G.A.; Saari, C.S.; Vrabel, M.J.; Horrow, J.; Chowdhury, M.; Fontaine, J.M. & Kutalek, S.P. (2010). Percutaneous pacemaker and implantable cardioverter-defibrillator lead extraction in 100 patients with intracardiac vegetations defined by transesophageal echocardiogram. *J Am Coll Cardiol,* 55, 886-894

Greene, M.; Newman, D.; Geist, M.; Paquette, M.; Heng, D. & Dorian, P. (2000). Is electrical storm in ICD patients the sign of a dying heart? Outcome of patients with clusters of ventricular tachyarrhythmias. *Europace,* 2, 263-269

Greene, T.O.; Portnow, A.S. & Huang, S.K. (1994). Acute pericarditis resulting from an endocardial active fixation screw-in atrial lead. *Pacing Clin Electrophysiol,* 17, 21-25

Grimm, W.; Flores, B.F. & Marchlinski, F.E. (1993). Complications of implantable cardioverter defibrillator therapy: follow-up of 241 patients. *Pacing Clin Electrophysiol,* 16, 218-222

Heldman, D.; Mulvihill, D.; Nguyen, H.; Messenger, J.C.; Rylaarsdam, A.; Evans, K. & Castellanet, M.J. (1990). True incidence of pacemaker syndrome. *Pacing Clin Electrophysiol,* 13, 1742-1750

Helguera, M.E. & Pinski, S.L. (2005). Cross-talk inhibition and asystole resulting from postshock high-output pacing: a new form of implantable cardioverter-defibrillator proarrhythmia. *Heart Rhythm,* 2, 310-312

Heller, S.S.; Ormont, M.A.; Lidagoster, L.; Sciacca, R.R. & Steinberg, S. (1998). Psychosocial outcome after ICD implantation: a current perspective. *Pacing Clin Electrophysiol,* 21, 1207-1215

Henrikson, C.A. & Brinker, J.A. (2006). A pacemaker infection that was apparently localized to the atrial set screw. *J Cardiovasc Electrophysiol,* 17, E3

Higgins, S.L.; Suh, B.D.; Stein, J.B.; Meyer, D.B.; Jons, J. & Willis, D. (1998). Recurrent Twiddler's syndrome in a nonthoracotomy ICD system despite a Dacron pouch. *Pacing Clin Electrophysiol,* 21, 130–133

Hill, P.E. (1987). Complications of permanent transvenous cardiac pacing: a 14-year review of all transvenous pacemakers at one community hospital. *Pacing Clin Electrophysiol,* 10, 564–570

Hussein, A.A.; Wilkoff, B.L.; Martin, D.O.; Karim, S.; Kanj, M.; Callahan, T.; Baranowski, B.; Saliba, W.I. & Wazni, O.M. (2010). Initial experience with the Evolution mechanical dilator sheath for lead extraction: Safety and efficacy. *Heart Rhythm*, 7, 870-873

Iskos, D.; Lurie, K.G.; Shultz, J.J.; Fabian, W.H. & Benditt, D.G. (1999). "Sagging heart syndrome": a cause of acute lead dislodgment in two patients. *Pacing Clin Electrophysiol*, 22, 371-375

Ismail, M.M.; Badreldin, A.M.; Heldwein, M. & Hekmat, K. (2010). Third-generation mobile phones (UMTS) do not interfere with permanent implanted pacemakers. *Pacing Clin Electrophysiol*, 33, 860-864

Israel, C.W. & Barold, S.S. (2007). Electrical storm in patients with an implanted defibrillator: a matter of definition. *Ann Noninvasive Electrocardiol*, 12, 375-382

Kantharia, B.K.; Patel, J.A.; Nagra, B.S. & Ledley, G.S. (2006). Electrical storm of monomorphic ventricular tachycardia after a cardiac-resynchronization-therapy-defibrillator upgrade. *Europace*, 8, 625-628

Kaye, D.; Frankl, W. & Arditi, L.I. (1975). Probable postcardiotomy syndrome following implantation of a transvenous pacemaker: report of the first case. *Am Heart J*, 90, 627-630

Kiviniemi, M.; Pirnes, M.; Eranen, H.J.; Kettunen, R.V. & Hartikainen, J.E. (1999). Complications related to permanent pacemaker therapy. *Pacing Clin Electrophysiol*, 22, 711–720

Kleemann, T.; Becker, T.; Doenges, K.; Vater, M.; Senges, J.; Schneider, S.; Saggau, W.; Weisse, U. & Seidl, K. (2007). Annual rate of transvenous defibrillation lead defects in implantable cardioverter-defibrillators over a period of >10 years. *Circulation*, 115, 2474-2780

Kono, K.; Todoroki, M.; Karasawa, T.; Ito, I.; Tadokoro, K. & Shinbo G. (2008). Delayed pericarditis associated with an implantable cardioverter defibrillator implantation using an active-fixation lead. *Pacing Clin Electrophysiol*, 31, 621–623

Kuruvilla, C.; Voigt, L.; Kachmar, K.; Reddy, C.V. & Kassotis, J. (2002). Inappropriate mode switching in a dual chamber pacemaker due to oversensing of a high frequency signal from a conductor/ring discontinuity (loose set screw). *Pacing Clin Electrophysiol*, 25, 115-117

Lamas, G.A. & Ellenbogen, K.A. (2004). Evidence base for pacemaker mode selection: from physiology to randomized trials. *Circulation*, 109, 443-451

Lamas, G.A.; Lee, K.L.; Sweeney, M.O.; Silverman, R.; Leon, A.; Yee, R.; Marinchak, R.A.; Flaker, G.; Schron, E.; Orav, E.J.; Hellkamp, A.S.; Greer, S.; McAnulty, J.; Ellenbogen, K.A.; Ehlert, F.; Freedman, R.A.; Estes, N.A.3rd.; Greenspon, A. &, Goldman, L. (2002). Mode Selection Trial in Sinus-Node Dysfunction. Ventricular pacing or dual-chamber pacing for sinus-node dysfunction. *N Engl J Med*, 346, 1854-1862

Lamas, G.A.; Orav, E.J.; Stambler, B.S,; Ellenbogen, .K. A.; Sgarbossa, E.B.; Huang, S.K.; Marinchak, R.A.; Estes, N.A.3rd.; Mitchell, G.F.; Lieberman, E.H.; Mangione, C.M. & Goldman, L. (1998). Quality of life and clinical outcomes in elderly patients treated with ventricular pacing as compared with dual-chamber pacing. Pacemaker Selection in the Elderly Investigators. *N Engl J Med*, 338, 1097-1104

Lee, S.; Fu, K.; Kohno, T.; Ransford, B. & Maisel, W.H. (2009). Clinically significant magnetic interference of implanted cardiac devices by portable headphones. *Heart Rhythm,* 6, 1432-1436

Leonelli, F.M.; Pisano, E.; Requarth, J.A.; Potenza, D.; Tomassoni, G.; O'Conner, W. & Natale, A. (2000). Frequency of superior vena cava syndrome following radiofrequency modification of the sinus node and its management. *Am J Cardiol,* 85, 771–774

Levy, Y.; Shovman, O.; Granit, C.; Luria, D.; Gurevitz, O.; Bar-Lev, D.; Eldar, M.; Shoenfeld, Y. &, Glikson M. (2004). Pericarditis following permanent pacemaker insertion. *Isr Med Assoc J,* 6. 599-602

Lin, D.; Dixit, S.; Russo, A.M. & Hsia, H.H. (2004). Total failure to sense ventricular fibrillation with inappropriate defibrillator sensitivity adjustment. *Pacing Clin Electrophysiol,* 27, 1321–1323

Love, C.J.; Wilkoff, B.L. & Byrd, C.L. (2000). Recommendations for extraction of chronically implanted transvenous pacing and defibrillator leads: indications, facilities, training. *Pacing Clin Electrophysiol,* 23, 544–551.

Mahapatra, S.; Bybee, K.A.; Bunch, T.J.; Espinosa, R.E.; Sinak, L.J.; McGoon, M.D. & Hayes, D.L. (2005). Incidence and predictors of cardiac perforation after permanent pacemaker placement. *Heart Rhythm,* 2, 907-911

Maisel, W.H. & Kramer, D.B. (2008). Implantable cardioverter-defibrillator lead performance. *Circulation,* 117, 2721-2723

Maisel, W.H.; Moynahan, M.; Zuckerman, B.D.; Gross, T.P.; Tovar, O.H.; Tillman, D.B. & Schultz, D.B. (2006). Pacemaker and ICD generator malfunctions: analysis of Food and Drug Administration annual reports. *J Am Med Assoc,* 295, 1901-1906

Margey, R.; McCann, H.; Blake, G.; Keelan, E.; Galvin, J.; Lynch, M.; Mahon, N.; Sugrue, D. & O'Neill, J. (2010). Contemporary management of and outcomes from cardiac device related infections. *Europace,* 12, 64-70

Mark, D.B.; Anstrom, K.J.; Sun, J.L.; Clapp-Channing, N.E.; Tsiatis, A.A.; Davidson-Ray, L.; Lee, K.L. & Bardy, G.H. (2008). Sudden cardiac death in heart failure trial investigators. Quality of life with defibrillator therapy or amiodarone in heart failure. *N Engl J Med,* 359, 999-1008

Martin, C.; Auffray, J.P.; Saux, P,; Albanese, J. & Gouin, F. (1996). The axillary vein: An alternative approach for percutaneous pulmonary artery catheterization. *Chest,* 90, 694–697

Mewis, C.; Kühlkamp, V.; Dörnberger, V.; Mermi, J. & Seipel, L. (1997). High incidence of isolator fractures in transvenous implantation of cardioverter defibrillators. *Z Kardiol,* 86, 85-94

Michaud, G.F.; Pelosi, F.Jr.; Noble, M.D.; Knight, B.P.; Morady, F. & Strickberger, S.A. (2000). A randomized trial comparing heparin initiation 6 h or 24 h after pacemaker or defibrillator implantation. *J Am Coll Cardiol,* 35, 1915–1918

Mirowski, M.; Reid, P.R.; Mower, M.M.; Watkins, L.; Gott, V.L.; Schauble, J.F.; Langer, A.; Heilman, M.S.; Kolenik, S.A.; Fischell, R.E. & Weisfeldt, M.L. (1980). Termination of malignant ventricular arrhythmias with an implanted automatic defibrillator in human beings. *N Engl J Med,* 303, 322-324

Mitsui, T., Hori, M.; Suma, K.; Wanibuchi, Y. & Saigusa, M. (1969). The "pacemaker syndrome". In: *Proceedings of Eighth Annual International Conference on Medical and*

Biological Engineering, pages 29-33, Jacobs, J.E. (Ed.), Association for the Advancement of medical Instrumentation Chicago

Newland, G.M. & Janz, T.G. (1994). Pacemaker-twiddler's syndrome: a rare cause of lead displacement and pacemaker malfunction. *Ann Emerg Med,* 23, 136–138

Ninio, D.M. & Hii, J.T. (2006). Wind-iatrogenic air embolus around pacing leads during defibrillator implant with coexisting pulmonary fibrosis. *Pacing Clin Electrophysiol,* 29, 213-214

Nishimura, R.A.; Gersh, B.J.; Vlietstra, R.E.; Osborn, M.J.; Ilstrup, D.M. & Holmes, D.R.Jr. (1982). Hemodynamic and symptomatic consequences of ventricular pacing. *Pacing Clin Electrophysiol,* 5, 903-910

Ostovan, M.A. & Aslani, A. (2007). A life-saving procedure for treatment of massive pulmonary air embolism. *J Invasive Cardiol,* 19, 355-356

Pakarinen, S.; Oikarinen, L. & Toivonen, L. (2010). Short-term implantation-related complications of cardiac rhythm management device therapy: a retrospective single-centre 1-year survey. *Europace,* 12, 103-108

Pavia, S. & Wilkoff, B. (2001). The management of surgical complications of pacemaker and implantable cardioverter-defibrillators. *Curr Opin Cardiol,* 16, 66-71

Pehrsson, S.K.; Hjemdahl, P.; Nordlander, R. & Aström, H. (1988). A comparison of sympathoadrenal activity and cardiac performance at rest and during exercise in patients with ventricular demand or atrial synchronous pacing. *Br Heart J,* 60, 212-220

Pioger, G.; Leny, G.; Nitzsché, R.; Ripart, A. (2007). Safe limits of ventricular pacing in unselected patients. *Pacing Clin Electrophysiol,* 30 (Suppl 1), S66-S70. Erratum in: *Pacing Clin Electrophysiol,* 30, 1424

Pycha, C.; Calabrese, J.R.; Gulledge, A.D. & Maloney, J.D. (1990). Patient and spouse acceptance and adaptation to implantable cardioverter defibrillators. *Cleve Clin J Med,* 57, 441-414

Rauwolf, T.; Guenther, M.; Hass, N.; Schnabel, A.; Bock, M.; Braun, M.U. & Strasser, R.H. (2007). Ventricular oversensing in 518 patients with implanted cardiac defibrillators: incidence, complications, and solutions. *Europace,* 9, 1041-1047

Reising, S.; Safford, R.; Castello, R.; Bosworth, V.; Freeman, W. & Kusumoto, F. (2007). A stroke of bad luck: left ventricular pacemaker malposition. *J Am Soc Echocardiogr,* 20, e1-e3

Rettig, G.; Doenecke, P.; Sen, S.; Volkmer, I. & Bette, L. (1979). Complications with retine transvenous pacemaker electrodes. *Am Heart J,* 98 587-594

Riley, R.F.; Petersen, S.E.; Ferguson, J.D. & Bashir, Y. (2010). Managing superior vena cava syndrome as a complication of pacemaker implantation: a pooled analysis of clinical practice. *Pacing Clin Electrophysiol,* 33, 420-425

Ross, R.A. & Kenny, R.A. (2000). Pacemaker syndrome in older people. *Age Ageing,* 29, 13-15

Rusanov, A. & Spotnitz, H.M. (2010). A 15-year experience with permanent pacemaker and defibrillator lead and patch extractions. *Ann Thorac Surg,* 89, 44-50

Sadoul, N.; Mletzko, R.; Anselme, F.; Bowes, R.; Schöls, W.; Kouakam, C.; Casteigneau, G.; Luise, R.; Iscolo, N.; Aliot, E. & Slow VT Study Group. (2005). Incidence and clinical relevance of slow ventricular tachycardia in implantable cardioverter-defibrillator recipients: an international multicenter prospective study. *Circulation,* 112, 946-953

Schiariti, M.; Cacciola, M.T.; Pangallo, A.; Ciancia, F. & Puddu, P.E. (2009). Delayed pericarditis and cardiac tamponade associated with active-fixation lead pacemaker in the presence of mitochondrial myopathy and Ockham's razor. *J Cardiovasc Med (Hagerstown),* 10, 879-882

Schulte, B.; Sperzel, J.; Carlsson, J.; Dürsch, M.; Erdogan, A.; Pitschner, H.F. & Neuzner, J. (2001). Inappropriate arrhythmia detection in implantable defibrillator therapy due to oversensing of diaphragmatic myopotentials. *J Interv Card Electrophysiol,* 5, 487-493

Schulze, M.; Ostermaier, R.; Franke, Y.; Matschke, K.; Braun, M. & Strasser, R. (2005). Aortic endocarditis caused by inadvertent left ventricular pacemaker lead placement. *Circulation,* 112: e361-e363

Secemsky, S.I.; Hauser, R.G.; Denes, P. & Edwards, L.M. (1982). Unipolar sensing abnormalities: incidence and clinical significance of skeletal muscle interference and undersensing in 228 patients. *Pacing Clin Electrophysiol,* 5, 10–19

Seki, H.; Fukui, T.; Shimokawa, T.; Manabe, S.; Watanabe, Y.; Chino, K. & Takanashi, S. (2009). Malpositioning of a pacemaker lead to the left ventricle accompanied by posterior mitral leaflet injury. *Interact Cardiovasc Thorac Surg,* 8, 235-237

Shivkumar, K.; Feliciano, Z.; Boyle, N.G. & Wiener, I. (2000). Intradevice interaction in dual chamber implantable cardioverter defibrillator preventing ventricular tachyarrhythmia detection. *J Cardiovasc Electrophysiol,* 11, 285–258

Sivakumaran, S.; Irwin, M.E.; Gulamhusein, S.S. & Senaratne, M.P.J. (2002). Postpacemaker implant pericarditis: incidence and outcomes with active fixation leads. *Pacing Clin Electrophysiol,* 25:833–837

Snow, M.E.; Agatston, A.S.; Kramer, H.C. & Samet, P. (1987). The postcardiotomy syndrome following transvenous pacemaker insertion. *Pacing Clin Electrophysiol,* 10, 934-936

Solti, F.; Moravcsik, E.; Renyi-Vamos, F.Jr. & Szabo, Z. (1989). Pacemaker Twiddler's syndrome (rotation of the pacemaker around the electrode cable, a rare complication of pacemaker therapy). *Acta Chir Hung,* 30, 231–236

Spittel, P.C. & Hayes, D.L. (1992). Venous complications after insertion of a transvenous pacemaker. *Mayo Clin Proc,* 67, 258–265

Sulke, N.; Dritsas, A.; Bostock, J.; Wells, A.; Morris, R. & Sowton, E. (1992). "Subclinical" pacemaker syndrome: a randomised study of symptom free patients with ventricular demand (VVI) pacemakers upgraded to dual chamber devices. *Br Heart J,* 67, 57-64

Sweeney, M.O.; Bank, A.J.; Nsah, E.; Koullick, M.; Zeng, Q.C.; Hettrick, D.; Sheldon, T.; Lamas, G.A. & Search AV Extension and Managed Ventricular Pacing for Promoting Atrioventricular Conduction (SAVE PACe) Trial. (2007a). Minimizing ventricular pacing to reduce atrial fibrillation in sinus-node disease. *N Engl J Med,* 357, 1000-1008

Sweeney, M.O.; Ruetz, L.L.; Belk, P.; Mullen, T.J.; Johnson, J.W. & Sheldon, T. (2007b). Bradycardia pacing-induced short-long-short sequences at the onset of ventricular tachyarrhythmias: a possible mechanism of proarrhythmia? *J Am Coll Cardiol,* 50, 614-622

Thaker, J.P.; Patel, M.B.; Shah, A.J.; Liepa, V.V.; Brunett, J.D.; Jongnarangsin, K.; Gardiner, J.C. & Thakur, R. (2009). Do media players cause interference with pacemakers? *Clin Cardiol,* 32, 653-657

Theodorakis, G.N.; Kremastinos, D.T.; Markianos, M.; Livanis, E.; Karavolias, G. & Toutouzas, P.K. (1992). Total sympathetic activity and atrial natriuretic factor levels in VVI and DDD pacing with different atrioventricular delays during daily activity and exercise. *Eur Heart J*, 13, 1477-1481

Tokano, T.; Nakazato, Y.; Sasaki, A.; Yamashita, H.; Iida, Y.; Kawano, Y.; Mineda, Y.; Nakazato, K.; Yasuda, M.; Sumiyoshi, M.; Nakata, Y. & Daida, H. (2004). Dislodgment of an atrial screw-in pacing lead 10 years after implantation. *Pacing Clin Electrophysiol*, 27, 264-265

Trappe, H.J., Pfitzner, P.; Heintze, J.; Kielblock, B.; Wenzlaff, P.; Fieguth, H.G. & Klein, H. (1995). Die Bedeutung der antitachykarden Stimulation bei Patienten mit Defibrillatoren der 3 Generation. *Z Kardiol*, 84, 35-43

Travill, C.M. & Sutton, R. (2007). Pacemaker syndrome: an iatrogenic condition. *Br Heart J*, 68, 163-166

Tung, R.; Zimetbaum, P. & Josephson, M.E. (2008). A critical appraisal of implantable cardioverter-defibrillator therapy for the prevention of sudden cardiac death. *J Am Coll Cardiol*, 52, 1111-1121

Turgeman, Y.; Antonelli, D.; Altar, S. & Rosenfeld, T. (2004). Massive transient pulmonary air embolism during pacemaker implantation under mild sedation: an unrecognized hazard of snoring. *Pacing Clin Electrophysiol*, 27, 684-685

Tyers, G.F.; Sanders, R.; Mills, P. & Clark, J. (1992). Analysis of set screw and side-lock connector reliability. *Pacing Clin Electrophysiol*, 15, 2000-2004

Uslan, D.Z. & Baddour, L.M. (2006). Cardiac device infections: getting to the heart of the matter. *Curr Opin Infect Dis*, 19, 345–348

Van Casteren, L., Huybrechts, W. & Willems, R. (2009). Undersensing of ventricular fibrillation due to interference between a pacemaker and defibrillator in the same patient. *Europace*, 11, 1390-1391

Van Gelder, B.M.; Bracke, F.A.; Oto, A.; Yildirir, A.; Haas, P.C.; Seger, J.J.; Stainback, R.F.; Botman, K.J. & Meijer, A. (2000). Diagnosis and management of inadvertently placed pacing and ICD leads in the left ventricle: a multicenter experience and review of the literature. *Pacing Clin Electrophysiol*, 23, 877-883

Vanhercke, D.; Heytens, W. & Verloove, H. (2008). Eight years of left ventricle pacing due to inadvertent malposition of a transvenous pacemaker lead in the left ventricle. *Eur J Echocardiogr*, 9, 825-827

Vinit, J.; Sagnol, P.; Buttard, P.; Laurent, G.; Wolf, J.E. & Dellinger A. (2007). Repeated delayed pericarditis after pacemaker surgery: a post-pericardiotomy like syndrome? *Rev Med Interne*, 28, 137–140

Voight, A.; Shalaby, A. & Saba, S. (2006). Rising rates of cardiac rhythm management device infections in the United States: 1996 through 2003 [letter]. *J Am Coll Cardiol*, 48, 590–591

Von Bergen, N.H.; Atkins, D.L.; Gingerich, J.C. & Law, I.H. (2007). "Ratchet" syndrome, another etiology for pacemaker lead dislodgement: a case report. *Heart Rhythm*, 4, 788-789

Vural, A.; Agacdiken, A.; Ural, D. & Komsuoglu, B. (2004). Reel syndrome and pulsatile liver in a patient with a two-chamber pacemaker. *Jpn Heart J*, 45, 1037–1042

Weretka, S.; Michaelsen, J.; Becker, R.; Karle, C.A.; Voss, F.; Hilbel, T.; Osswald, B.R.; Bahner, M.L.; Senges, J.C.; Kuebler, W. & Schoels, W. (2003). Ventricular oversensing: a study of 101 patients implanted with dual chamber defibrillators and two different lead systems. *Pacing Clin Electrophysiol,* 26, 65–70

Wiegand, U.K.; LeJeune, D.; Boguschewski, F.; Bonnemeier, H.; Eberhardt, F.; Schunkert, H.; & Bode, F. (2004). Pocket hematoma after pacemaker or implantable cardioverter defibrillator surgery: influence of patient morbidity, operation strategy, and perioperative antiplatelet/anticoagulation therapy. *Chest,* 126, 1177-1186

Wigger, C. (1925). The muscular reactions of mammalian ventricles to artificial surface stimuli. *Am J Physiol,* 73, 346-378

Wilkoff, B.L.; Cook, J.R.; Epstein, A.E.; Greene, H.L.; Hallstrom, A.P.; Hsia, H.; Kutalek, S.P. & Sharma, A. (2002). Dual chamber and VVI implantable defibrillator trial investigators. Dual-chamber pacing or ventricular backup pacing in patients with an implantable defibrillator: the dual chamber and VVI implantable defibrillator (DAVID) Trial. *J Am Med Assoc,* 288, 3115-3123

Zhan, C.; Baine, W.B.; Sedrakyan, A. & Steiner, C. (2008). Cardiac device implantation in the United States from 1997 through 2004: a population-based analysis. *J Gen Intern Med,* 23(Suppl 1), 13-19

16

Common Pacemaker Problems: Lead and Pocket Complications

Enes Elvin Gul and Mehmet Kayrak
Selcuk University,
Meram School of Medicine,
Cardiology Department Konya,
Turkey

1. Introduction

Pacemakers may cause undesirable complications during and after implantation. Complications associated with the implantation procedure are uncommon, but include bleeding, infection, or collapsed lung. Generally, each of these problems can be treated quite effectively. Though rare, ***pacemaker*** problems can occur long after the implantation procedure. These "late" complications include generator failure (extremely rare), and lead failure (less rare). Most of these complications are uncommon, and can be prevented by simple manoeuvres. Nonetheless, there are some complications related to pacemaker system disfunctions which may cause life-threatening complications. Pacemaker malfunctions may be corrected with accurate, timely diagnosis, but will not be discussed in this chapter.

Pacemaker complications can be divided into acute (immediate) or chronic according to implantation time (or date); lead or pocket complications according to the site of complication; and implantation or system failures, according to aethiology (Table 1). The most common and frequent complications are those related to implantation. Pacemaker implantation is a safe procedure in experienced hands, but these complications can be caused even by experienced operators. By following the suggested maintenance schedule, physicians usually detect pacemaker problems before they become serious. However, it remains important for patients to be aware of the symptoms of bradycardia, symptoms that might indicate a pacemaker malfunction. Once again, these symptoms include weakness, easy fatigability, lightheadedness, dizziness, and loss of consciousness. Patients experiencing any of these symptoms should notify their doctor. Especially following complications such as lead dislodgment, pnemothorax, lead indection, and cardiac tamponade, the patients must be informed about these symptoms.

The frequency of complications varies between 10% and 59% for the procedures. This wide range exists due to the common problem of defining complications. In some papers, a localized infection or rib fracture is defined as a minor complication. However, in other papers, these complications are not even recorded. If the pacemaker lead becomes dislodged on day 4, is this a complication or not? Some authors say yes; others no. This ambiguity leads to a great challenge when trying to compare papers. In this chapter, we will try to discuss these problems systematically and transparently.

Significant reductions in frequency of complications related to pacemakers have been noted due to emerging technological developments, ever increasing experience and patient education.

Complications	
Pocket complications	*Lead complications*
Pocket hematoma	Acute perforation
İnfection	Dislodgement
Erosion	Infection
Migration of pacemaker	Vein thrombosis
Twiddler's syndrome	Migration

Table 1. Classification of pacemaker complications.

2. Complications related to the implantation procedure

Several lead-related complications deserve attention, including lead dislodgement, pneumothorax, loose connector pin, conductor coil (lead) fracture, and insulation break.

2.1 Lead dislodgement

Pacing lead displacement and dislodgement is a relatively common problem and can occur in 5-10 % of the patients (National Pacemaker and ICD database, 2001). Historically, the most common complication of transvenous pacing has been lead dislodgement. The leads can displace within chambers or out of chambers and should be suspected if the wire appears too taut or too redundant. Leads may dislodge from the initial implant site in the first few days to few weeks following the implantation. Active and passive fixation mechanism of leads help prevent this complication. Atrial lead dislogement is slightly more common than it is for venrricular leads. Acceptable dislodgmenet rates should be probably be less than 1% for ventricular leads and no more than 2-3% for atrial leads (Braunwald). Although passive fixation leads are stable in the atrial appendage, active fixation leads are necessary to prevent dislodgement in patients with prior cardiac surgery. Lead dislodgement may result in an increase in pacing thresholds, failure to capture, or failure to sense. Lead dislodgement may be radiographically visible or it may be microdislodgement, where there is no radiographic change in position, but there is significant increase in pacing threshold and/or decline in the electrocardiogram amplitude (Figure 1). Also migration of a dislodged lead out of the heart may be associated with thromboembolic complications if it is not detected acutely.

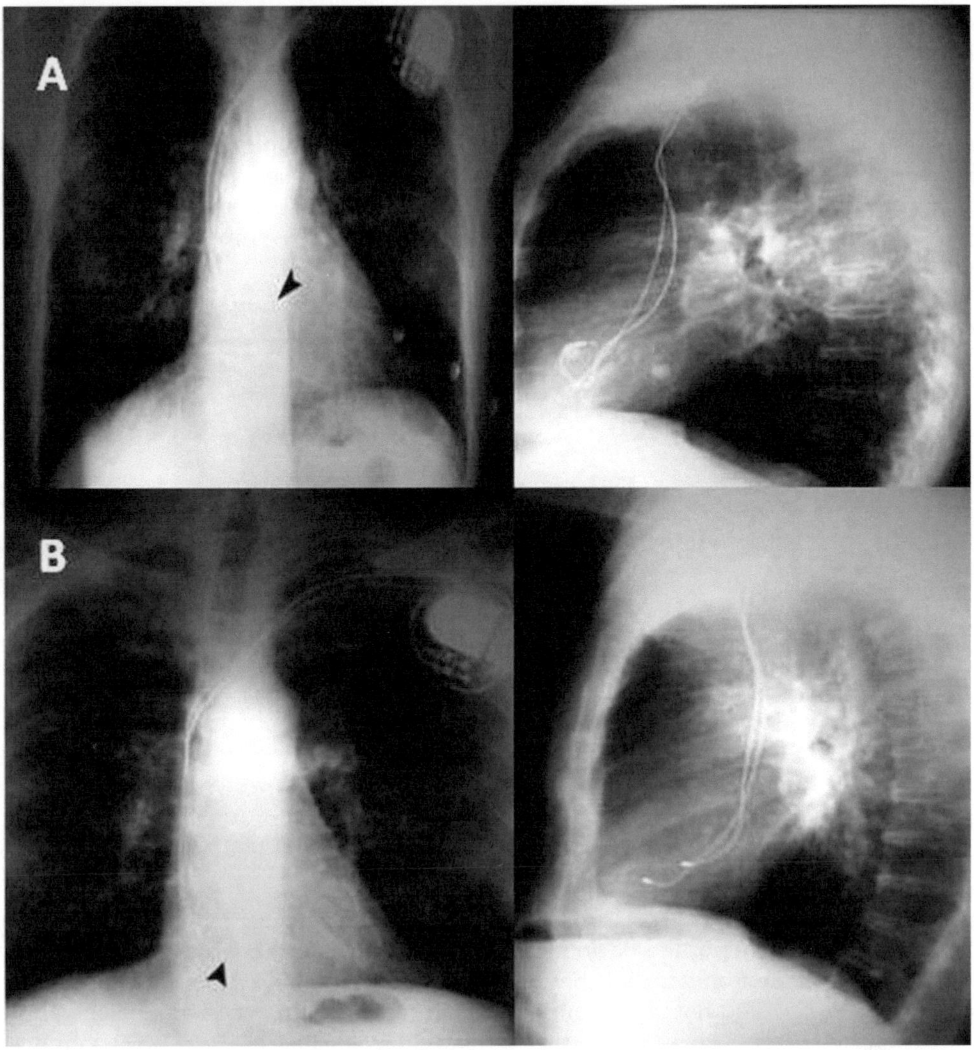

Fig. 1. Top (A): Postero-anterior and lateral chest X-ray films obtained 24 hours after pacemaker implantation showing atrial lead tip (arrow head) inside the right atrial appendage; Bottom (B): Radiograph obtained three months later showing displacement of atrial lead (arrow head) towards tricuspid annulus.

2.2 Pneumothorax, hemothorax, and air embolism

This complication occurs uncommonly and is directly related to operator experience, the difficulty of the subclavian vein puncture, and is almost eliminated using the cephalic cut-down technique. The incidence of pneumothorax ranges from 1.6 to 2.6 % with 80 % of thesecases requiring chest tube placement if > 10 % of the lung is involved, the patient has continued repiratory distress, or hemo-pneumothorax is present (Grier et al., 1990). A pneumothorax estimated to involve < 10 % of the pleural space can probably be observed without chest tube placement. This can occur from inadvertent puncture and laceration of the subclavian vein or the subclavian artery or the lung.

If a pneumothorax develops, it may manifest during the pacemaker procedure or as late as 48 hours after implantation (Figure 2). However, these traditional comparisons may become obsolete as the axillary vein cannulation technique (Martin et al., 1996) threatens to eliminate this controversery. To minimize the risk of pneumothorax, fluoroscopic guidance of the subclavian puncture should be used together with careful technique, or to use safe sheats with one-way mechanism which also reduces risk of other potential complications (hemothorax, inadvertent arterial puncture, air embolism, arteriovenous fstula, thoracic duct injury, and brachial plexus injury). Often pneumothorax is asymptomatic and noted on routine follow-up plain chest radiograph.

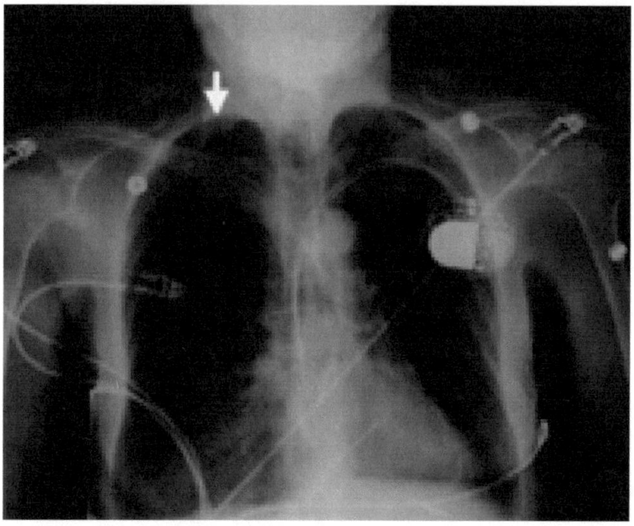

Fig. 2. Chest X-ray showing right pneumothorax (arrow) 8 h after placement of a left-sided permanent dual chamber pacemaker.

Location of pneumothorax, i.e. ipsilateral or contralateral was reported. Contralateral pneumothorax to the site of the pacing system has been reported, which was secondary to an unsuccessful attempt on that side (Sebastian et al., 2005).

In the setting of pneumothorax, pneumopericardium can occur when air dissects through the pulmonary parenchyma along the perivascular sheats back to the hilum. The pericardium is weakest at its reflection surrounding the ostia of the pulmonary veins and air can leak into the pericardial space at this location. In haemodynamically stable patients, CT scan of the chest is investigation of choice (Figure 3). In unstable patients emergency echocardiography may be useful to identify pericardial effusion (Burney et al., 2004).

Deep inspiration at the time of central venous access may cause significant air to be drawn into the venous system due to the physiological negative pressure developed. Three obligatory conditions need to coexist for pulmonary air embolism to occur: (1) there must be a source of gas/air; (2) an open access to the venous system; and (3) a pressure gradient between the source of gas/air and the venous sytem (Yeakel, 1968). It can be prevented through operator care and using introducers with hemostatic valves. The diagnosis is obvious because it is heralded by a hissing sound as the air is sucked in and with the fluoroscopic confirmation that follows (Figure 4). 100% oxygen should be administered along with ionotropic support in some cases. Aspiration of the embolus from the right heart has also been successful. However, usually no therapy is required, as the air is filtered and consequently absorbed in the lungs.

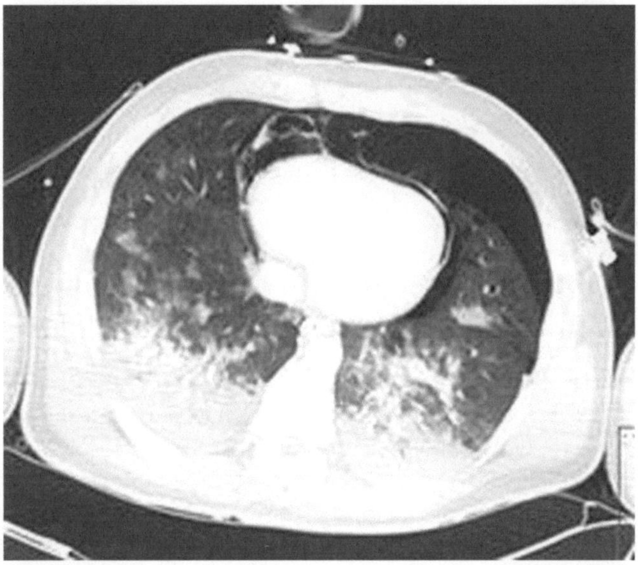

Fig. 3. CT scan of the chest showing massive hemothorax, pneumothorax, and pneumopericardium.

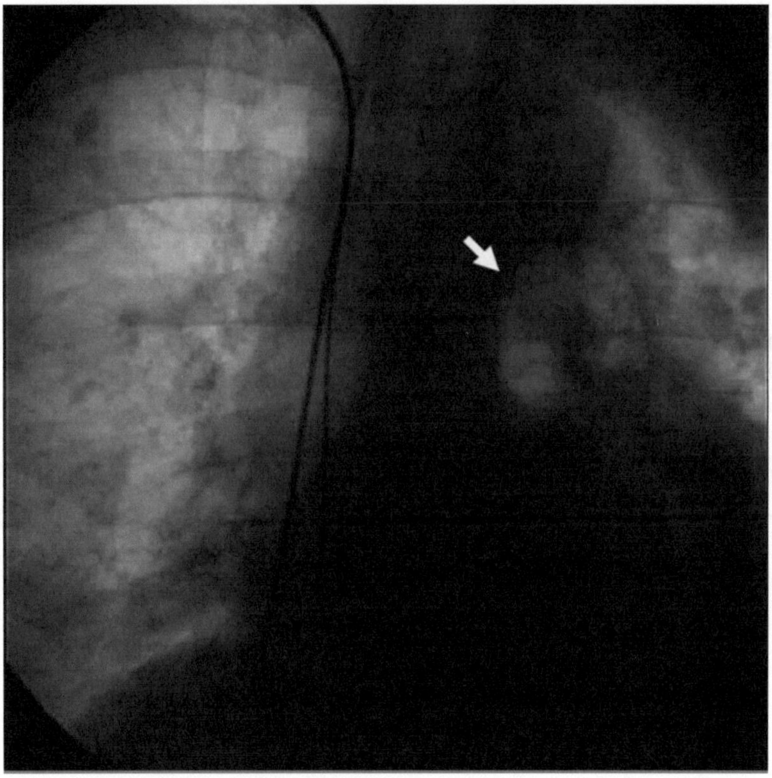

Fig. 4. Chest X-ray showing a large air embolus (arrow) in the main pulmonary artery bifurcation during permanent pacemaker implantation.

Three main issues are important in diagnosis and management of this problem: (1) deep inspiration should be avoided in the presence of an open intravenous route; (2) when using a peal-away sheath, temporarily close the intravenous entrance route before inserting the lead; and (3) snoring may be an alarm sound! (Turgeman et al., 2004).

2.3 Lead perforation

Myocardial perforation during lead placement is an uncommon but potentially serious complication. The published incidence of this complication varies from 0.4 to 5.2%, but nowadays it is usually lower than 1% (Danik et al., 2007; Carlson at al., 2008). The use of active fixation leads is associated with higher rate of cardiac perforations (Geyfman et al., 2007). Recently, several reports on increased rate of cardiac perforations with both active and passive defibrillation leads of one model have published (Satpathy et al., 2008).

The definition of a subacute and delayed myocardial perforation is normal X-ray and electrical parameteres (R-wave sensing, pacing threshold, impedance) 24 hours after implantation without clinical signs of perforation and the diagnosis of lead perforation by X-ray (Figure 5), echocardiography, or computed tomography 5 days to 1 month (subacute) or ≥ 1 month (delayed) after implantation. Delayed lead perforation (occuring more than 1 month after implantation) is a rare complication. Its pathophysiology and optimal management are currently unclear. Delayed lead perforations are fewer in number than acute lead perforations in the literature (Velavan et al., 2003; Khan et al., 2005). Delayed lead perforations have caused chest pain, hemopneumothorax and pneumothorax, but no cases of cardiac tamponade or death have been documented (Trigano & Caus, 1996). One of the distinguishing features of delayed lead perforation as opposed to acute lead perforation is the decrease or absence of cardiac tamponade or death.

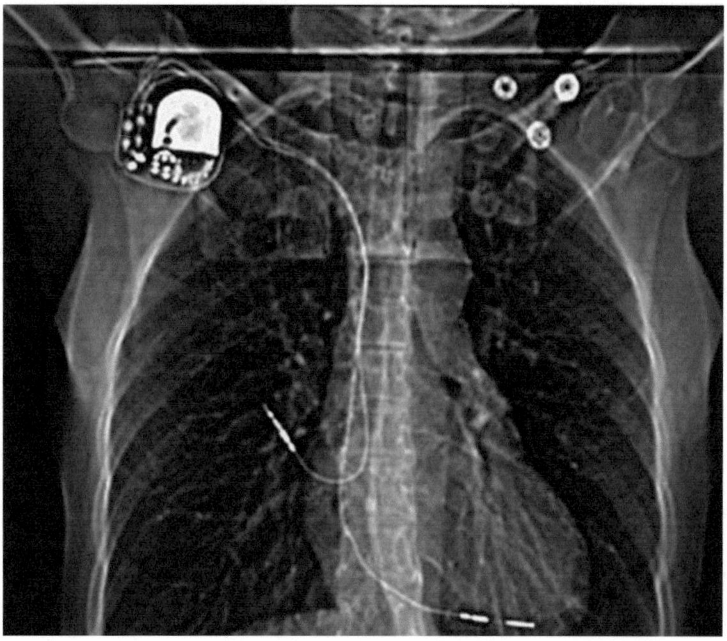

Fig. 5. Chest X-ray demonstrating severe lead perforation due to implantable cardioverter-defibrillator implantation.

Surprisingly, the perforation rate did not differ significantly between the pacemaker and ICD implantation. Hirschl et al. found that atrial leads perforated more frequently than ventricular leads, and ICD leads perforate more frequently than ventricular pacemaker leads (Hirschl et al., 2007). The factors that may influence the perforation ratio rate could be divided into three groups:

1. Lead design (diameter, fixation mechanism, construction of the lead tip, pre-shaped J-curve),
2. Physicians' experience and training level,
3. Patient-related factors

Clinical presentations of late perforation may vary widely from asymptomatic patients to sudden cardiac death. This highlights the importance of a high degree of suspicion and the need of proper diagnostic methods. Diagnosis of a perforation is usually based on clinical findings. Echocardiographic imaging may suggest perforation, but unless the lead is completely through the myocardium, the study may be inconclusive. More recently, CT has been reported as a method of diagnosing myocardial perforation (Figure 6). Diagnosis of perforation is made using four signs:

1. Decrease in arterial blood pressure without any other explanation,
2. Decrease in pulsatility of the cardiac silhouette as monitored by fluoroscopy,
3. Increased size of the cardiac silhouette,
4. Abnormal position of the transvenous lead too far out toward the left ventricle along the pericardial outline

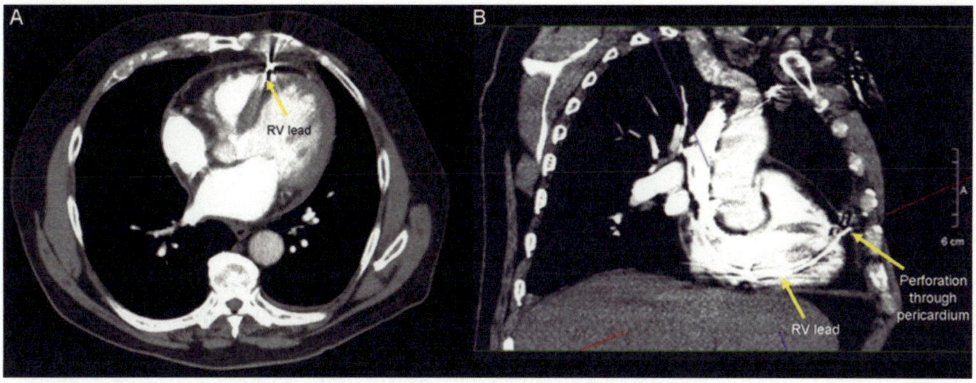

Fig. 6. CT images of the thorax emonstrating right ventricular (RV) lead position and cardiac perforation by RV electrode.

Currently, approprate management of lead perfroration is uncertain. Perforation associated with hemodynamic compromise must be dealt with as an emergency. The lead may perforate any of the great veins, the atria, or ventricle during the implant procedure. This complication almost always occurs in the cardiac chamber on lead manipulation or fixing a screw in lead, and consequently bleeds into the pericardial space. A most devastating manifestation is cardiac tamponade, which requires prompt diagnosis and percutaneous pericardiocentesis, possibly followed by surgical intervention if the bleeding persists. Rarely, trauma to the great veins above the pericardial reflection may cause bleeding directly into the mediastinum. This is much more of a concern when extracting leads than implanting them and is an emergent indication for open chest surgery. Furhermore, the management described in the literature depends on the lead type.

Another late complication of lead perforation occurs at the time of lead extraction if required. While active fixation leads have mostly been extracted transvenously after retraction of the coil, extraction of passive fixaton leads causes concern because of the bulky tip of the lead may cause tissue damage during removal. Khan and colleagues recommend that lead extraction should be done in the operating room under TEE observation with cardiac surgery backup (Khan et al., 2005).

Overall, our experience with delayed lead perforations with lead perforations has provided a management scheme as outlined above that incorporates clinical history, chest X-ray, and device interrogation among other diagnostic tools (echocardiography, CT etc.).

2.4 Extracardiac stimulation

Extracardiac stimulation usually involves the diaphragm or pectoral or intercostal muscles. Diaphragmatic stimulation may be caused by direct stimulation of the diaphragm (usually stimulation of the left hemidiaphragm) or stimulation of the phrenic nerve (usually stimulation of the right hemidiaphragm). Diaphragmatic stimulation occuring during the early postimplantation period may be caused by microdislodgment of the pacing lead. This phenomenon is most commonly in patients with LV coronary vein branch lead placement for biventricular stimulation. During implant, high-output pacing at maximal voltage and pulse width should be tested routinely to avoid diaphragmatic stimulation. Stimulation can be minimized or alleviated by decreasing the voltage output or pulse width, or both, but an adequate pacing margin of safety must be maintained after the output parameters are decreased. If the problem cannot be resolved by reprogramming the pacemaker output, lead repositioning will be required at the moment.

Pectoral stimulation may be due to incorrect orientation of the pacemaker with its active surface in contrast with the muscle or a current leak from a lead insulation failure or exposed connector.

2.5 Venous thrombosis and superior vena cava syndrome (SVCS)

Venous thrombosis occurs early or late after pacemaker implantation in 30% to 50% of patients and may remain asymptomatic because of the development of venous collaterals (Oginosawa et al., 2002). Manifestations vary from usually asymptomatic, acute symptomatic thrombosis, and even SVCS (Mazzetti et al., 1993). Venous complications of pacemaker/ICD system implantation rarely cause immediate clinical problem. Only a few percent (1-3%) of patients with severe stenosis or occlusion of the deep veins of an upper extremity become symptomatic (Stoney et al., 1976; Crook et al., 1977).

A few factors were proposed as predictors of severe venous stenosis/occlusion: a) presence of multiple pacemaker leads (compared to a single lead), b) use of hormone therapy, c) personal history of venous thrombosis, d) the presence of temporary wire before implantation, e) previous presence of a pacemaker (ICD as an upgrade) and f) the use of dual-coil leads. The presence of arm swelling, collateral veins on the arm, thorax or abdomen and possible associated facial suffision, cyanosis or edema with head and neck discomfort are classical symptoms. Routine preoperative venography to detect has been advocated before all device lead revision cases, so as alternative access can be considered (Spittell & Hayes, 1992).

Different management approaches should be used, depending on the time since onset of stenosis/thrombosis, its location, and the presence of symptoms. Asymptomatic patients are usually not treated because their disease is silent and often undetected. Symptomatic patients who develop venous thrombosis should be treated promptly. Specific treatment depends on thrombosis or fibrosis being causative and varies from heparin followed by warfarin or thrombolysis to percutaneous angioplasty or an open surgical procedure. Surgery is always the last resort, reserved for patients with symptomatic occlusions that do not respond to treatment with anticoagulation or have contraindications to endovascular procedure (Rozmus et al., 2005).

A rare associated complication is pulmonary thromboembolism that is potentially life-threatening. The presence of pulmonary embolism in a patient with a device should be arouse the suspicion of thromboic pacemaker (or ICD) lead source (Phibbs & Marriott, 1985).

2.6 Twiddler syndrome

Displacement of pacemaker leads due to twisting of the box on part of the patient is called Twiddler's syndrome, first described in 1968 (Nicholson et al., 2003).Twiddler syndrome that causes device malfunction is a rare complication in patients with an implantable cardioverter defibrillators (ICD) (Fahraeus & Höijer, 2003). Twisting of the pulse generator within the device pocket may cause the dislocation of the lead, diaphragmatic stimulation, and loss of capture (Figure 7). The prevelance of this syndrome is 0.07% (Gungor et al., 2009). Classically, Twiddler syndrome occurs in obese women with loose, fatty subcutaneous tissue and is characterized by rotation of pulse generator on its long axis with subsequent coiling of pacemaker leads (Bhatia et al., 2007). Other risk factors are mental disorders, female sex, and the small size of the implanted generator with a large pocket (Cardall et al., 1999). This disorder may induce lead dislodgement or lead fracture and cause life-threatening symptoms in case of pacemaker dependency. When the pulse generator is rotated along the transverse axis it is referred by us as the Reel sundrome, a variant of Twiddler syndrome (Camero-Varo et al., 1990).

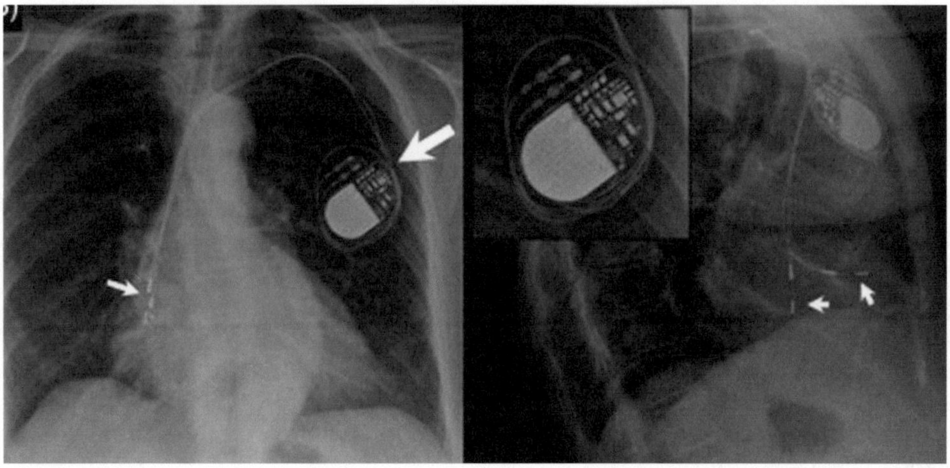

Fig. 7. Pacemaker Twiddler syndrome. Postero-anterior and lateral chest X-ray showing displacement of both leads, especially the ventricle one, retracted and floating in the right atrium (arrows).

In Twiddler syndrome, electrocardiography shows failure of capture and the chest radiography reveals the dislodged and twisted leads (Pereira et al., 1999). Hypoperfusion symptoms such as fatigue, tiredness, confusion, presyncope, and syncope may be observed (Cardall et al., 1999). If the problem has occured because of pacemaker migration or poorly fashioned pacemaker pocket, the pocket should be revised. As an inappropriate ICD therapy may be proarrhythmic and may lead to sudden cardiac death, Twiddler syndrome should be considered in patients with ICD who had resistant ventricular arrhythmias and abdominal pulsation. To avoid this life-threatening complication of ICD implantation, we should take care to limit the pocket size, suture the device to the fascia, and instruct the patients not to manipulate their device pockets.

2.7 Postpacemaker implant pericarditis

Pericarditis is an uncommon but potentially serious complication following a pacing system implantation. Pericarditis has been reported as a complication of pacemaker implantation associated with the use of active- and passive-fixation leads (Greene et al., 1994). It appeared to occur significantly more often when active-fixation atrial leads were used, affecting 5% of implants in this study. Active-fixation atrial leads have lower early dislodgement rates and are easier to remove after chronic placement. However, because the atrial wall is thin, these leads may be more likely to perforate the myocardium and cause pericarditis. Perforation through the right ventricular wall is also possible though the wall thickness is greater than in the atrium, and thus presumably less likely to occur. Alternatively, traumatic inflammation extending from the lead screw and traversing through the myocardium to the pericardium is also possible mechanism (Sivakumaran et al., 2002). Patients developing pericarditis postpacemaker implantation should be followed closely due to the risk of cardiac tamponade. If there is no evidence of tamponade or symptomatic pericardial effusion, it is reasonable initially to treat the patient conservatively, i.e., observation and pain medications. Anti-inflaammatory medications, e.g., nonsteroidal or steroids, may relieve symptoms. However, if the medications cannot be withdrawn without symptom recurrence, it may be necessary to remove and reposition the leads.

3. Pocket-related complications

3.1 Pocket hematoma

Hematomas occuring at the pacemaker pocket site can vary from a small ecchymosis to large and tense swelling (Figure 8). The risk of haematoma is increased in patients taking antithrombotic or anticoagulant drugs (Goldstein et al., 1998). Most small hematomas can be managed conservatively with cold compress and withdrawal of antiplatelet or antithrombotic agents. In patients requiring oral anticoagulants (warfarin), to take INR of about 2.0 at the time of implantation is safe (Belott & Reynolds, 2000). Unfractionated heparin or low-molecular-weight heparin are always discontinued prior to device implant and ideally avoided for a minimum of 24 hours post implantation. Administration of anticoagulants can be resumed within 48-72 h after implantation if there is no evidence of substantial hematoma formation. Occasionally, large hematomas that compromise the suture line or skin integrity may have to be surgically evacuated. Evacuation of the hematoma is very rarely needed (<0.5% of cases). Needle aspiration increases risk of infection and should not be done. Aspiration should be considered only if there is continued bleeding, potential compromise of the suture line or skin integrity, or pain refractory analgesics (Pavia & Wilkoff, 2001).

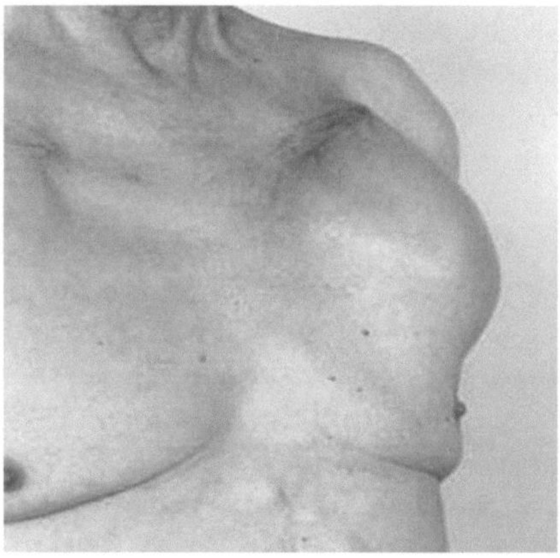

Fig. 8. Pocket hematoma

In patients who require therapeutic anticoagulation, heparin should be delayed for at least 24 to 48 hours after implantation to avoid bleeding complications.

3.2 Wound pain

Patients should be told to expect some local discomfort at the pacemaker implantation site. For several reasons, a patient could experience a painful pacemaker site, commonly called ''painful pocket'', and the complaint should be taken seriously. The diferential diagnosis includes:

- Infection
- Pacemaker implanted too superficially
- Pacemaker implanted too laterally
- Pacemaker allergy

Minor wound pain is expected after device implantation, almost always controlled with simple analgesia. In general, the pre-pectoral site is extremely well-tolerated, i.e., the pacemaker pocket should be formed in the prepectoralis fascia. If it is placed anterior to the adipose layer, i.e., within subcutaneous tissues, significant pain may result. If the pacemaker is positioned too laterally, impingement on the axillary space may cause discomfort. Continuing pain will usually improve or manifest an obvious infection eventually. However, pain that initially improves then recurs or occurs temporarily remote from the implant may suggest infection even in the absence of any outward localizing signs, and consequently may necessitate surgical exploration or even empirical removal and reimplant at another site. If a painful pocket is explored for any reason, specimens for culture should be obtained.

3.3 Skin erosion

Skin erosion is caused by the underlying pacemaker generator has been reported several times as a complication of pacemaker implants (Kiviniemi et al., 1999). This is the most common late complication of pacemaker implantation abd its incidence has been estimated around 0.8% (Harcombe et al., 1998).

Factors predisposing skin erosion are the tissue fragility in old-age patients, the presence of a thin subcutaneous fat layer and abrasive action exerted on the skin from external agents (Figure 9). Other common causes of skin erosion are possible infections of the site and the pressure exercised from the device on the subcutanous tissue (Harcombe et al., 1998). Griffith et al. concluded that if pacemaker erosion is not caused by infection it can be successfully managed by ipsilateral re-implantation, i.e., revision and this is a financially advantageous solution (Griffith et al., 1994). If true eroison occurs, the system is considered contaminated and current opinion favors removal of the generator and leads to the clean site (Shapiro et al., 2004; Guiseppe et al., 2009). It is crucial to identify early signs of erosion before the hardware breaks the skin. If the skin is intact, surgical revision of the pocket is often all that is needed to protect the hardware from contamination and infection.

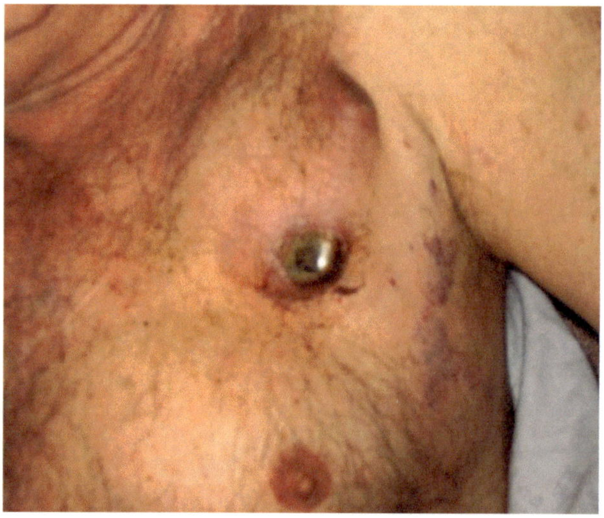

Fig. 9. Erosion of the automated implantable cardioverter-defibrillator (AICD).

3.4 Allergic reactions to the pacemaker component

Pacemaker component allergy is a relatively uncommon cause of erithema and pain at the site of an implanted pacemaker. Diagnosis is often postponed and/or misinterpreted as a skin infection. Allergies to multiple pacemaker components have been well described (Hayes & Loesl, 2002). Most reactions occur between several weeks to a few months after implantation. The diagnosis should be suspected in cases of skin reaction following pacemaker implantation that does not respond promptly to antibiotic treatment. When infection has been ruled out, it may still be difficult to make a diagnosis of a pacemaker component allergy, for several reasons. Because a true allergic reaction to a pacemaker component is rare, the clinician may simply fail to include it in the differential diagnosis. Also, the allergy testing required is sophisticated and must be done correctly. Important, corticosteroid use can result in skin anergy and in a false-negative skin test.

Allergies to various pacemaker components have been reported, including titanium (Peters et al., 1984; Yamauchi et al., 2000), polychloroparaxylene (Iguchi et al., 1997), nickel (Landwehr & van Ketel, 1983), polyurethane (Abdallah et al., 1994), epoxy (Andersen, 1979), mercury (Brun & Hunziker, 1980), cadmium (Laugier et al., 1975), chromate (Laugier et al., 1975), silicone (Raque & Goldschmidt, 1970), and cobalt (Tilsey & Rotstein, 1980).

Once an allergy has been demonstrated, it is imperative that the component either be eliminated from subsequent pacing systems or be completely coated. The only definitive treatment is removal of the allergens. Some patients may respond to topical corticosteroids

(Viraben et al., 1995). But replacement of the device for one that is free of allergenic components or wrapped with an inert coating is the treatmnet choice (Déry et al., 2002).

3.5 Device-related infections

Despite improvements in the design and implantation techiques, infection of the cardiac devices remain a serious problem. The first reports on infective complications after permanent endocardial stimulation were published in the 1960s. The reported incidence of pacemaker-related infection ranges from 0.5% to 6% in early series (Hill, 1987; Kearney et al., 1994). Recently, Uslan et al. reported the overall incidence of device-related infection to be 1.9 per 1000 device-years (Uslan et al., 2007). In the study by Aggarwal et al (Aggarwal et al., 1995), the incidence of infections in patients with dual-chamber (1%) compared with single-chamber devices (0.82 %) was similiar, whereas in the study by Chauan et al. (Chauan et al., 1994), wound infections developed in 0.6% of patients with single-chamber versus 2.1% of patients with dual-chamber devices. This infection is associated with substantial morbidity, mortality, and financial cost (Sohail et al., 2007). The mortaility of persistent infection when infected leads are not removed can be as high as 66% (Rettig G, Doenecke et al. Complications with retained transvenous pacemaker electrodes. Am Heart J 1997; 98:587-594). In a study by Sohail et al (Sohail et al., 2007) generator pocket infection (69%) and device-related endocarditis (23%) were the most common clinical presentations of infection.
Several factors have been anecdotally reported (Eggimann et al., 2000) to be associated with an increased the risk of PPM infection, inckuding diabetes mellitus, malignancy, operator inexperience, advanced age, corticosteroid use, anticoagulation, recent device manipulation, chronic renal failure, and bacteremia from a distant focus of infection. Pacemaker endocarditis is most commonly complicated by tricuspid valve vegetations (Bortolotti et al., 1993), tricuspid regurgitation, and occasionally by secondary pulmonary embolism (Klug et al., 1997). Also, the presence of multiple leads is a potential cause for central venous thrombosis, and has been thought to increase the risk of device infection by serving as a nidus for seeding of bacteria (Howarth et al., 1998).
Device infection is defined as either: (a) deep infection - infection involving the generator pocket and/or the intravenous portion of the leads, with or without bacteremia, requiring device extraction or (b) superficial infection - characterized by local inflammation, involving the skin but not the generator pocket, and treated with oral antibiotics. Also Charles Byrd divided pacemaker-related infections into the following groups (Ellenbogen et al., 2007)

- endocarditis;
- inflammation of myocardial tissue;
- infected vegetations;
- infected implanted foreign bodies;
- bacteremia without signs of endocarditis;
- local infections of subcutaneous tissue;
- chronic infections limited to the pocket area;
- superinfection of pacemaker pocket area;
- chronic pocket infection with granulation tissue

Early infections are most commonly caused by Staphylococcus aureus and late infections most commonly by Staphylococcus epidermidis, although infections by Staphylococcus lugudensis (Anguera et al., 2005), streptococcus bovis, mitis, and sanguis, pseudomonas (Laguno et al., 1998), enterococci and fungi and even Mycobacterium fortuitum (Sharma et al., 2005) have been described (Figure 10).

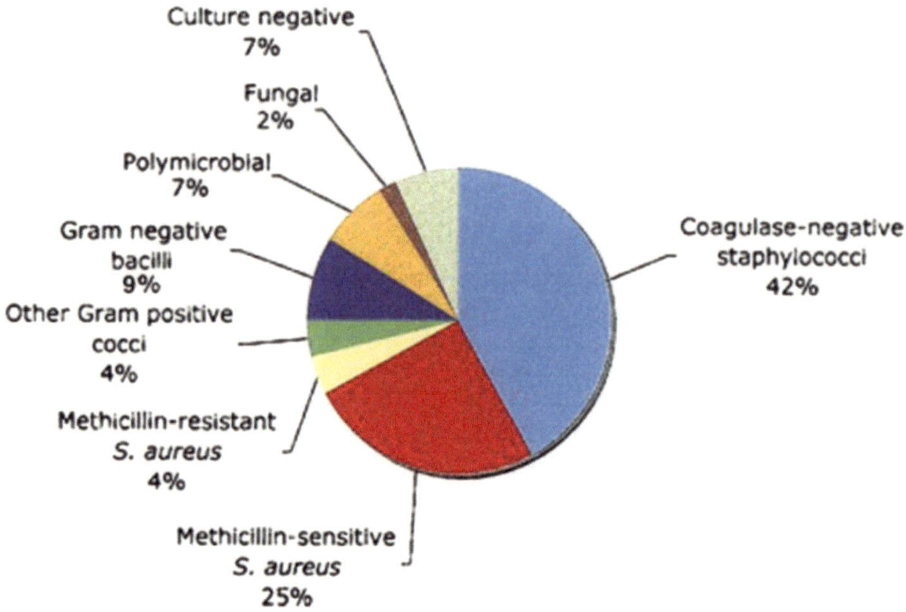

Fig. 10. Microbiology of permanent pacemaker/ICD infections (With permission of: Sohail MR, Uslan DZ, Khan AH et al. Management and Outcome of Permanent Pacemaker and Implantable Cardioverter-Defibrillator Infections. J Am Coll Cardiol 2007; 49:1851-9).

Pacemaker infection must be recognized and be treated properly. It may appaer as:

- Local inflammation and abscess formation in the area of the pulse generator pocket
- Erosion of part of the pacing system through the skin with secondary infection
- Fever associated with positive blood cultures with or without a focus of infection elsewhere

The most common clinical presentation is infection around the generator; septicemia is uncommon mode of presentation.

There is general consensus that once there is pacemaker pocket or lead infection, removal of the whole pacemaker systme followed by a course of appropriate antibiotics results in the best prospect for long term eradication of infection. Antibiotic prophylaxis has been routinely prescribed to prevent the occurence of this complication; however, there is insufficient evidence that this strategy is benefical. In a study by de Oliveira et al (de Oliveira et al., 2009) found that antibiotic prophylaxis (single dose of 1 g of cefazolin) significantly reduces infectious complications in patinets undergoing pacemaker or cardioverter-defibrillators. When pacemaker lead or pocket infection is complicated by vegetations on the leads, heart valves or chamber endocardium or when there is secondary pulmonary embolism, removal of the entire device is more urgently indicated. The main recommendation is in favor of if there is vegetations that might obstruct main pulmonary artery should have removal under cardiopulmonary bypass (Tascini et al., 2006; Ruttman et al., 2006; Kaul et al., 2009).

The duration of antimicrobial treatment for cardiac device infections (CDI) depended on the clinical presentation and the causative agent. In a large case series from the Cleveland Clinic Foundation (Chua et al., 2000), the median duration of antibiotic treatment in CDI cases with pocket infection and those with bacteremia was 26 days and 41 days, respectively. An algorithm for management of the patient with an infected pacing or ICD system is shown in (Figure 11). This algorithm also demonstrates the timing and need of a replacement device. Guidelines suggested by Mayo Clinic for diagnosis and management of device infections are listed in (Table 2).

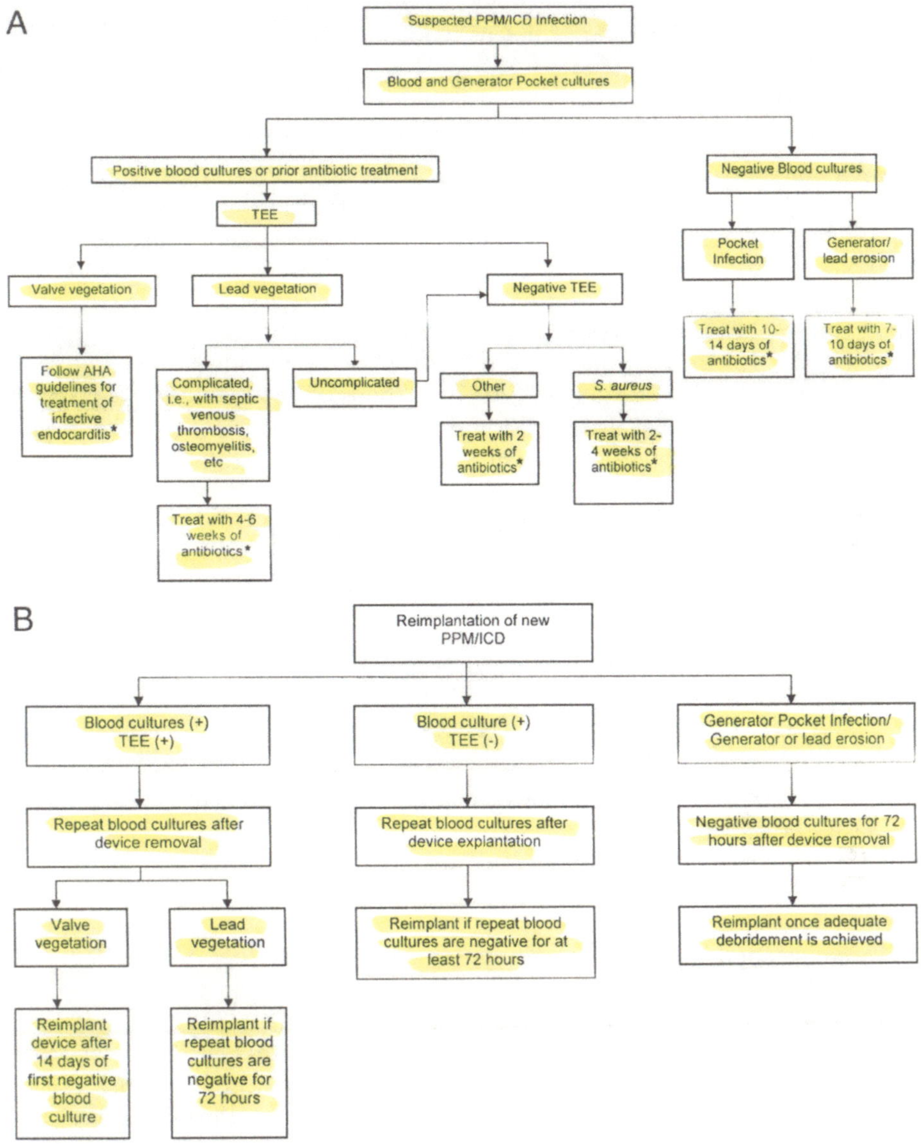

Fig. 11. Mayo Clinic algorithm of cardiac device infection management. (A) Treatment algorithm based on blood and generator pocket cultures. This algorithm applies only to the patients with complete explanation of the implanted system. (B) Algorithm for reimplantation of new pulse generator. (With permission from Sohail MR, Uslan DZ, Khan AH, et al. Management and outcome of permanent pacemaker and implanted cardioverter-defibrillator infections. JACC 2007; 49:1851-9).

1.	All patients should have at least 2 sets of blood cultures drawn at initial evaluation.
2.	Generator tissue Gram stain and culture and lead tip culture should be obtained.
3.	Patients who either have positive blood cultures or have negative blood cultures but had recent antibiotics before obtaining blood cultures should have a transesophageal echocardiogram (TEE) to assess for device-related endocarditis.
4.	Sensitivity of TTE is low and is not recommended to evaluate for devvice-related endocarditis.
5.	Patients with negative blood cultures and recent prior antibiotics and valve vegetations on TEE should be managed in consultation with an infectious diseases expert.
6.	All patients with device infection should undergo complete device removal, regardless of clinical presentation.
7.	A large (>1 cm) lead vegetation is not a stand alone indication for surgical lead removal.
8.	Blood cultures should be repeated in all patients after device explantation. Patients with persistently positive blood cultures should be treated for at least 4 weeks with antimicrobial even if TEE is negative for vegetations or other evidence of infection.
9.	Duration of antimicrobial therapy should also be extended to ≥4 weeks in patients with complicated infection (endocarditis, septic venous thrombosis, osteomyelitis, metastatic seeding).
10.	Adequate debridement and control of infection should also be achieved at all sites before reimplantation of a new device.
11.	Reevaluation for continued need of the device should be performed before new device placement.
12.	If an infected cardiac device cannot be removed, than long-term suppressive antibiotic therapy should be administered after completing an initial course of treatment and securing a clinical response to therapy. Infectious diseases expert opinion should be sought.

Table 2. Guidelines for diagnosis and management of cardiac device infections (Modified from Mayo Clinic Guidelines).

4. References

National Pacemaker and ICD database. UK and Ireland. Annual Report 2001 Braunwald

Grier D, Cook PG, Hartnell GG. Chest radiographs after permanent pacing. Are they really necessary? Clin Radiol 1990; 42:244-9

Martin C, Auffray JP, Saux P, et al. The axillary vein: An alternative approach for percutaneous pulmonary artery catheterization. Chest 1996; 90:694-697

Sebastian CC, Wu WC, Shafer M, Choudhary G, and Patel PM. Pneumopericardium and Pneumothorax After Permanent Pacemaker Implantation. PACE 2005; 28:466-468

Burney K, Burchard F, Papouchado M, Wilde P. Cardiac pacing systems and implantable cardiac defibrillators (ICDs): a radiological perspective of equipment, anatomy and complications. Clin Radiol 2004; 59:699-708

Yeakel AE. Lethal air embolism from plastic blood-storage container. JAMA 1968; 204:175-177

Turgeman Y, Antonelli D, Atar S, and Rosenfeld T. Massive Transient Pulmonary Air Embolism during Pacemaker Implantation under Mild Sedation: An Unrecognized Hazard of Snoring. PACE 2004; 27:684-685

Danik SB, Mansour M, Singh J, Reddy VY, Ellinor PT, Milan D et al. Increased incidence of subacute lead perforation noted with one implantable cardioverter-defibrillator. Heart Rhythm 2007; 4:439-42

Carlson MD, Freedman RA, Levine PA. Lead perforation: incidence in registries. Pacing Clin Electrophysiol 2008; 31:13-5

Geyfman V, Storm RH, Lico SC, Oren JW. Cardiac tamponade as complication of active-fixation atrial lead perfrorations: proposed mechanism and management algorithm. Pacing Clin Electrophysiol 2007; 30:498-501

Satpathy R, Hee T, Esterbrooks D, Mohiuddin S. Delayed defibrillator lead perforation: an increased phenomenon. Pacing Clin Electrophysiol 2008; 31:10-2

Velavan P, Chauman A. An unusual presentation of delayed cardiac perforation caused by atrial screw-in lead. Heart 2003; 89:364

Khan M, Joseph G, Khaykin Y, Zrada K, Wilkoff B. Delayed lead perforation: A disturbing trend. Pacing Clin Electrophysiol 2005; 28:251-253

Trigano AJ, Caus T. Lead explanation late after atrial perforation. Pacing Clin Electrophysiol 1996; 19:1268-1269

Hirschl DA, Jain VR, Spindola-Franco H, Gross JN, and Haramati LB. Prevelance and Characterization of Asymptomatic Pacemaker and ICD Lead Perforation on CT. PACE 2007; 30:28-32

Oginosawa Y, Abe H, Nakashima Y. The incidence and risk factors for venous obstruction after implantation of trabsvenous pacing leads. Pacing Clin Electrophysiol 2002; 25:1605-1611

Mazzetti H, Dussaut A, Tentori C, et al. Superior vena cava occlusion and/or syndrome related to pacemaker leads. Am Heart J 1993; 125:831-837

Stoney WS, Addlestone RB, Alford WC Jr, Burrus GR, Frist RA, Thomas CS Jr. The incidence of venous thrombosis following long-term transvenous pacing. Ann Thorac Surg 1976; 22:166-170

Crook BR, Gishen P, Robinson CR, Oram S. Occlusion of the subclavian vein associated with cephalic vein pacemaker electrodes. Br J Surg 1977; 64:329-331

Spittell P, Hayes D.Venous complications after insertion of a transvenous pacemaker. Mayo Clin Proc 1992; 67:258-265

Rozmus G, Daubert JP, Huang DT, Rosero S, Hall B, and Francis C. Venous Thrombosis and Stenosis After Implantation of Pacemakers and Defibrillators. Journal of Interventional Cardiac Electrophysiology 2005; 13:9-19

Phibbs B, Marriott H. Complications of permanent transvenous pacing. N Engl J Med 1985; 22:1428-1432

Nicholson WJ, Touhy KA, Tikemeier P. Twiddlers syndrome. N Engl J Med 2003; 348:1726-7

Fahraeus T, Höijer CJ. Early pacemaker Twiddler syndrome. Europace 2003; 5:279-281

Gungor H, Duygu H, Yildiz BS, Gul I, Zoghi M, and Akin M. Twiddler syndrome as a rare cause of implantable cardioverter defibrillator malfunction. J Cardiovasc Med 2009; 10:352-353

Bhatia V, Kachru R, Parida AK, Kaul U. Twiddlers syndrome. Int J of Cardiol 2007; 116:e82

Cardall TY, Brady WJ, Chan TC, Perry JC, Vilke GM, Rosen P. Permanent cardiac pacemakers: issues relevant to the emergency physician; part II. J Emerg Med 1999; 17:697-709

Camero-Varo A, Perez-Paredes M, Ruiz-Ros A, Gimenez-Cervantes D, Martinez-Corbalan FR, Cuberto-Lopez T. "Reel syndrome"-a new form of Twiddlers syndrome? Circulation 1990; e45-6

Pereira PL, Trubenbach J, Farnsworth CT, Huppert PE, Claussen CD. Pacemaker and defibrillator Twiddler's syndrome. Eur J Radiol 1999; 30:67-69

Greene TO, Portnow AS, Huang SK. Acute pericarditis resulting from an endocardial active fixation screw-in atrial leads. PACE 1994; 17:21-25

Sivakumaran S, Irwin ME, Gulamhusein SS, and Senaratne PJ. Postpacemaker Implant Pericarditis: Incidence and Outcome with Active-Fixation Leads. PACE 2002; 25:833-837

Goldstein DJ, Losquadro W, Spotnitz HM. Outpatient pacemaker procedures in orally anticoagulated patients. Pacing Clin Electrophysiol 1998; 21:1730-1734

Belott P, Reynolds D. Permanent pacemaker and implantable cardioverter defibrillator implantation. In Ellenbogen K, Kay G, Wilkoff B(Eds): Clinical cardiac pacing and defibrillation, WB Saunders. Philadelphia: Saunders; 2000, 573-644

Pavia S, and Wilkoff B. The management of surgical complications of pacemaker and implantable cardioverter-defibrillators. Current Opinion in Cardiol 2001; 16:66-71

Kiviniemi MS, Pirnes MA, Eranen HJ, Kettunen RV, Hartikainen JE. Complications related to permanent pacemaker therapy. Pacing Clin Electrophysiol 1999; 22:711-720

Harcombe AA, Newel SA, Ludman PF, Wistow TE, Sharples LD, Shofield PM, et al. Late complications following permanent pacemaker implantation or elective unit replacement. Heart 1998; 80:240-244

Griffith MJ, Mounsey JP, Bexton RS, Holden MP. Mechanical, but not infective, pacemaker erosion may be successfully managed by re-implantation of pacemakers. Br Heart J 1994; 71:202-205

Shapiro M, Hanon S, Schweitzer P. A Rare, Late Complication after Automated Implantable Cardioverter-Defibrillator Placement. Indian Pacing Electrophysiol J 2004; 4:213-216

Guiseppe S, Sarubbi B, D'Alto M, Romeo E and Calabro R. Extrusion of the device: a rare complication of the pacemaker implantation. J Cardiovasc Med 2009; 10:330-332

Hayes DL and Loesl K. Pacemaker Component Allergy: Case Report and Review of the Literature. J of Intervent Cardiac Electrophysiol 2002; 6:277-278

Peters MS, Schroeter AL, van Hale HM, Broadbent JC. Pacemaker contact sensitivity. Contact Dermatitis 1984; 11:214-218

Yamauchi R, Morita A, Tsuji T. Pacemaker dermatitis from titanium. Contact Dermatitis 2000; 42:52-53

Iguchi N, Kasanuki H, Matsuda N, Shoda M, Ohnishi S, Hosoda S. Contact sensitivity to polychloroparaxylene-coated cardiac pacemaker. Pacing Clin Electrophysiol 1997; 20:372-373

Landwehr AJ, van Ketel WG. Pompholyx after implantation of a nickel-containing pacemaker in a nickel-allergic patient. Contact Dermatitis 1983; 9:147

Abdallah HI, Balsara RK, O'Riordan AC. Pacemaker contact sensitivity, clinical recognition and management. Ann Thorac Surg 1994; 57:1017-1018

Andersen KE. Cutaneous reaction to an epoxy-coated pacemaker. Arch Dermatol 1979; 115:97-98

Brun R, Hunziker N. Pacemaker dermatitis. Contact Dermatitis 1980; 6:212-213

Laugier P, Hunziker N, Orusco M, Brun R, Reiffers J, Posternak F. Dermite de contact par pace-maker (French). Dermatologie 1975; 150:219-226

Raque C, Goldschmidt H. Dermatitis associated with an implanted cardiac pacemaker. Arch Dermatol 1970; 102:646-649

Tilsey DA, Rotstein H. Sensitivity caused by internal exposure to nickel, chrome, and cobalt. Contact Dermatitis 1980; 6:175-178

Viraben R, Boulinguez S, Alba C. Granulomatous dermatitis after implantation of a titanium-containing pacemaker. Contact Dermatitis 1995; 33:437

Déry JP, Gilbert M, O'Hara G, Champagne J, Desaulniers D, Cartier P, and Philippon F. Pacemaker Contact Sensitivity: Case Report and Review of the Literature. PACE 2002; 25:863-865

Hill PE. Complications of permanent transvenous cardiac pacing: A 14-year review of all transvenous pacemaker inserted at one community hospital. Pacing Clin Electrophysiol 1987; 10:564-570

Kearney R, Eisen HJ, Wolf JE. Nonvalvular infections of the cardiovascular system. Ann Intern Med 1994; 121:219-230

Uslan D, Sohail M, St. Sauver J, Friedman PA, Haye DL, Stoner SM, Wilson WR, Steckelberg JM, Baddour LM. Permanent pacemaker and implantable cardioverter defibrillator infection. A population-based study. Arch Intern Med 2007; 167:669-675

Aggarwal RK, Connelly DT, Ray SG, Ball J, Charles RG. Early complications of permanent pacemaker implantation: no difference between dual and single chamber systems. Br Heart J 1995; 73:571-575

Chauan A, Grace AA, Newell SA, Stone DL, Shapiro LM, Schofield PM, Petch MC. Early complications after dual-chamber versus single-chamber pacemaker implantation. Pacing Clin Electrophysiol 1994; 17:2012-2015

Sohail MR, Uslan DZ, Khan AH, et al. Management and outcome of permanent pacemaker and implantable cardioverter-defibrillator infections. J Am Coll Cardiol 2007; 49:1851-9

Eggimann P, Waldovogel FA. Pacemaker and defibrillator infections. In: Waldvogel FA, Bisno AL, eds. Infections associated with indwelling medical devices. Washington, DC: American Society for Microbiology Press, 2000:247

Bortolotti U, Tursi V, Fasoli G, Milano A, Frigato N, Casarotto D. Tricuspid valve endocarditis: repair with the use of tricuspid chordae. J Heart Valve Dis 1993; 2:567-70

Klug D, Lacroix D, Savoye C, Goullard L. Systemic infection related to endocarditis on pacemaker leads: clinical presentation and management. Circulation 1997; 95:2098-2107

Howarth DM, Curteis PG, Gibson S. Infected cardiac pacemaker wires demonstrated by Tc-99m labeled white blood cell scintigraphy. Clin Nucl Med 1998; 23:74-76

Ellenbogen KA, Kay GN, Lau CP, Wilkoff BL eds. Clinical cardiac pacing, defibrillation, and resynchronization therapy. Saunders Elsevier, Philadelphia 2007; 912-930

Anguera I, Del-Rio A, Miro JM. Staphylococcus lugudensis infective endocarditis: description of 10 cases and analysis of native valve, prosthetic valve and pacemaker lead endocarditis-clinical profiles. Heart 2005; 91:e10

Laguno M, Miro O, Font C, de-la-Sierra A. Pacemaker-related endocarditis. Report of 7 cases and review of literature. Cardiology 1998; 90:244-8

Sharma S, Tieyjeh IM, Espinosa RE, Costello BA, Baddour LM. Pacemaker infection due to Mycobacterium fortuitum. Scand J Infect Dis 2005; 37:66-7

de Oliveira JC, Martinelli M, D'Orio Nishioka SA, Varejao T, Uipe D, Pedrosa AAA, Costa R, Danik SB. Efficacy of Antibiotic Prophylaxis Before the Implantation of Pacemakers and Cardioverter-Defibrillators. Results of a Large, Prospective, Randomized, Double-Blinded, Placebo-Controlled Trial. Circ Arrhythmia Electrophysiol 2009; 2:29-34

Tascini C, Bongiorni MG, Gemignani G, Soldati E. Management of cardiac device infection: A retrospective survey of a non surgical approach combining antibiotic therapy with transvenous removal. J Chemother 2006; 18:157-163

Ruttman E, Hangler HB, Kilo J, Hofer D. Transvenous pacemaker lead removal is safe and effective even in large vegetations: an anlysis of 53 cases of pacemaker lead endocarditis. Pacing Clin Electrophysiol 2006; 29:231-6,

Kaul P, Adluri K, Javangula K and Baig W. Successful management of multiple permanent pacemaker complications-infection, 13 year old silent lead perforation and exteriorisation following failed percutaneous extraction, superior vena cava obstruction, tricuspid valve endocariditis, pulmonary embolism and prosthetic tricuspid valve thrombosis. J of Cardithorac Surg 2009; 4:12

Chua JD, Wilkoff BL, Lee I, Juratli N, Longworth DL, Gordon SM. Diagnosis and management of infections involving implantable electrophysiologic cardiac devices. Ann Intern Med 2000; 133:604-8

17

Conduction Disturbances after the Superior Septal Approach for Mitral Valve Repair

Yoshio Misawa, Shin-ichi Ohki, Yuichiro Kaminishi, Yasuhito Sakano, Kei Aizawa, Tsutomu Saito, Hiroaki Konishi and Arata Muraoka
Division of Cardiovascular Surgery,
Jichi Medical University,
Japan

1. Introduction

The better the operative field, the safer the procedure. In mitral valve surgery, the approach to the left atrium influences the quality of the operation, especially in difficult anatomical situations such as a small left atrium, or technically difficult operations including mitral valvuloplasty. However, it is not always easy to get a good operative field for mitral valve surgery, particularly in cases with a small left atrium.

The conventional approach includes the left atriotomy from the right side and the so-called septal approach. These do not sacrifice the sinus node artery. In contrast, the superior septal approach sacrifices the sinus node artery, and it requires a more invasive incision into the right and left atria. Therefore, postoperative rhythm disturbances, such as supraventricular arrhythmia and atrio-ventricular conduction changes, could arise in patients who had mitral valve surgery via the superior septal approach. However, the superior septal approach provides surgeons with a large operative field even when the left atrium is small. With the superior septal approach, the surgeon and assistants can clearly observe the operative field, whereas with the conventional approach the operative field is not always fully visualzed.

Some studies of rhythm disturbances accompanying the superior septal approach have been published previously, but they covered mainly perioperative events, such as premature contraction and bradycardia. We evaluated perioperative events and postoperative cardiac conduction disturbances in patients who had mitral valve operations by the superior septal approach and compared them with patients who had the conventional surgical approach.

2. Patients and methods

a. Patients profiles:

Between October in 1996 and October in 1998, 52 patients (25 male, 27 female) had mitral valve operations by the superior septal approach, and cardiac rhythm status was assessed (Misawa et al., 1999). The average age of the 52 patients was 55 +/- 14 years (range, 15-76 years). Preoperative mean pulmonary artery pressure was 29 +/- 11 mmHg, and the mean left atrial diameter was 63 +/- 10 mm.

Twelve patients (7 male, 5 female) who underwent mitral surgery by the conventional left atriotomy from the right side served as the control group. The average age of the group was

59 +/- 10 years (range, 36-72 years). Preoperative mean pulmonary artery pressure was 33 +/- 8 mmHg, and the mean left atrial diameter was 68 +/- 19 mm.

b. Our superior septal approach:

To establish cardiopulmonary bypass, bicaval venous drainage is essential for the superior septal approach, and direct caval cannulation is used for the drainage from the superior vena cava. The myocardium was protected during operation with moderate hypothermia (28-32 degree Celsius) and intermittent ante-grade infusion of blood cardioplegic solution. In the case of bradycardia below 70 beats/min, right atrial or ventricular pacing between 70 and 90 beats/min was initiated to obtain a stable postoperative hemodynamic condition.

Our procedure includes a right atriotomy not going beyond the crista terminalis, an atrial septotomy beginning at the fossa ovalis, and a subsequent left atrial incision parallel to the superior vena cava (Figure 1). We did not extend the incision onto the superior portion of the left atrium behind the aorta, but made it parallel to the superior vena cava. The incision length is limited up to a maximum of 2 cm.

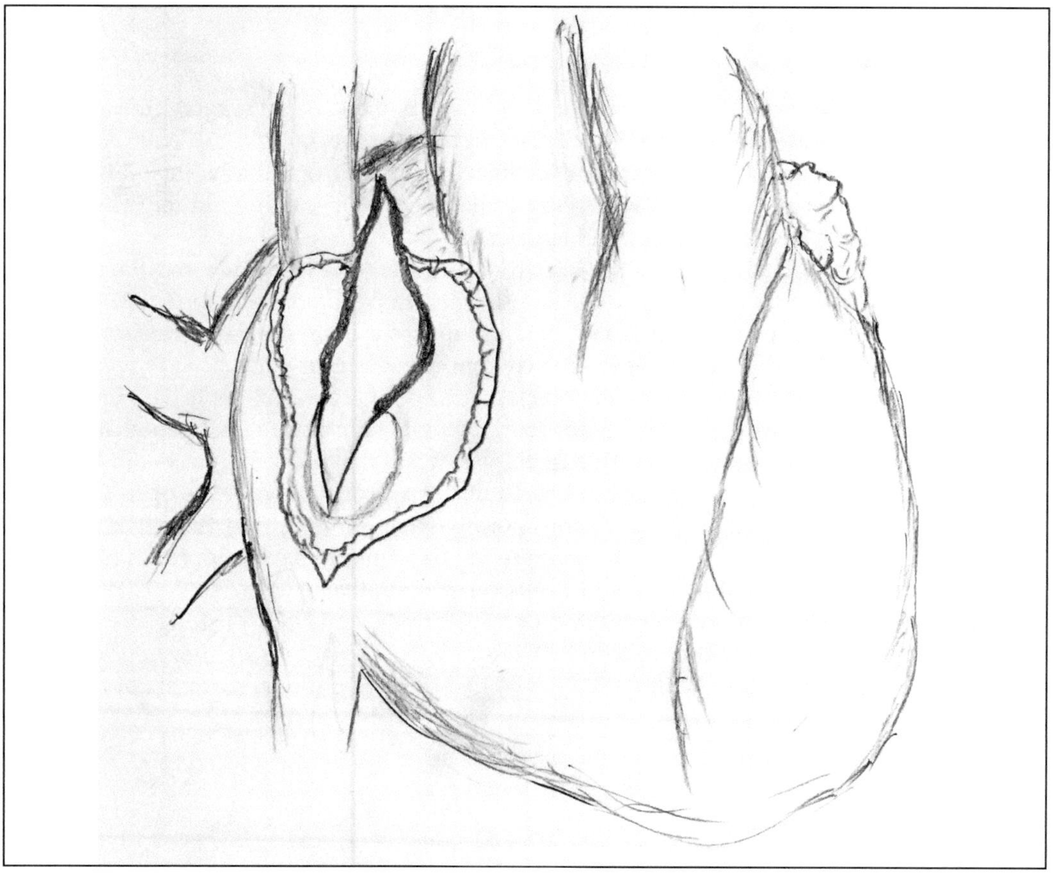

Our procedure includes a right atriotomy not going beyond the crista terminalis, an atrial septotomy beginning at the fossa ovalis, and a subsequent left atrial incision parallel to the superior vena cava. We did not extend the incision onto the superior portion of the left atrium behind the aorta, but made it parallel to the superior vena cava. The incision length is limited up to a maximum of 2 cm.

Fig. 1. Our procedure of the superior septal approach

c. Operations:

Forty-two patients of the superior septal approach group underwent mitral valve replacement, and 10 had mitral valvuloplasty. Twenty-two patients had concomitant operations, including aortic valve replacement in nine, tricuspid annuloplasty in 12, coronary arter bypass grafting in one, atrial septal defect repair in one, atrial septal defect repair plus tricuspid annuloplasty in one, and patch plasty for abscess cavity in the mitral annulus in one. Five patients had previous mitral or aortic valve operations. Cardiopulmonary bypass time was 158 +/- 22 minutes, and ischemic time was 106 +/- 18 minutes.

Eleven patients of the conventional approach group underwent mitral valve replacement, and one had mitral valvuloplasty combined with mitral valve annuloplasty. Three patients had tricuspid annuloplasty, three had the aortic valve replaced, and four had coronary artery bypass grafting. Cardiopulmonary bypass time was 172 +/- 45 minutes, and myocardial ischemic time was 111 +/- 31 minutes.

d. Postoperative follow-ups and complications:

The mean follow-up period of the superior septal approach group was 30 +/- 7 months (range, 23-45 months). The mean follow-up period of the conventional approach group was 15 +/- 8 months (range, 2-25 months).

Postoperative complications were compared in the two groups, and pre- and postoperative electrocardiograms were analyzed in patients with normal sinus rhythms. Serial changes in PR intervals were assessed to study the conduction disturbances that occurred with the two approaches. Holter electrocardiograms were used 6 to 12 months after surgery to assess cardiac rhythm status in the superior septal approach group.

Postoperative mortality and morbidity was analyzed upon the revised guideline (Edmunds et al., 1996). Statistical analysis was based on computer software "STAX '98" produced by Nakayama-shoten, Tokyo, 1998. Data are presented as mean +/- standard deviation, and p-values less than 0.05 were considered significant.

e. Additional studies

Results from a further 61 superior septal approach patients were also included giving a total of 113 patients (Misawa & Kaminishi, 2004). The superior septal approach is also suitable for a left atrial tumor. Recently, the tumor is incidentally diagnosed by echocardiography or chest computed tomography (Misawa et al, 2002).

3. Results

a. Postoperative complications:

In the 52 patients with the superior septal approach, there was no operative death. No intractable arrhythmias occurred in the early postoperative phase. There was one late death from cerebral hemorrhage 4 months postoperatively. Paravalvular leakage was found in one patient 2 months postoperatively, and this patient had a second operation 14 months after the initial surgery because of advancing heart failure. One cirrhotic patient with both aortic and mitral valve replacement underwent reexploration because of mediastinal bleeding 4 hours postoperatively. There were no other valve-related or treatment-related complications.

In the control group of the 12 patients, no intractable arrhythmias occurred in the early postoperative phase. Low cardiac output syndrome developed in the patient who had mitral valvuloplasty 3 hours after the initial operation, and the patient subsequently underwent mitral valve replacement. No other complications were observed in the control group.

b. Changes of postoperative electrocardiograms:

Twenty-six patients had normal sinus rhythms preoperatively. Eleven had transient atrial fibrillation or junctional rhythms for approximately 2 weeks. Twenty-five patients maintained sinus rhythm, and there was atrial fibrillation in one patient at the final follow-up. Five of 26 patients with preoperative atrial fibrillation showed sinus rhythm in the early postoperative phase. In one patient atrial fibrillation recurred within 6 months postoperatively, and another died from cerebral bleeding 4 months postoperatively. Another 10 patients with atrial fibrillation showed transient junctional rhythms postoperatively.

Serial changes in PR intervals were assessed in the 25 patients who maintained their sinus rhythms (Figure 2). The mean preoperative PR interval was 155 +/- 20 milliseconds, indicating no conduction delay. However, postoperative PR intervals were significantly prolonged for 1 week ($p = 0.02$), decreased within 2 weeks postoperatively, and returned to normal by 6 months postoperatively. Five patients developed transient first degree atrioventricular blocks, and one developed a permanent first degree atrioventricular block. No other conduction abnormalities were observed.

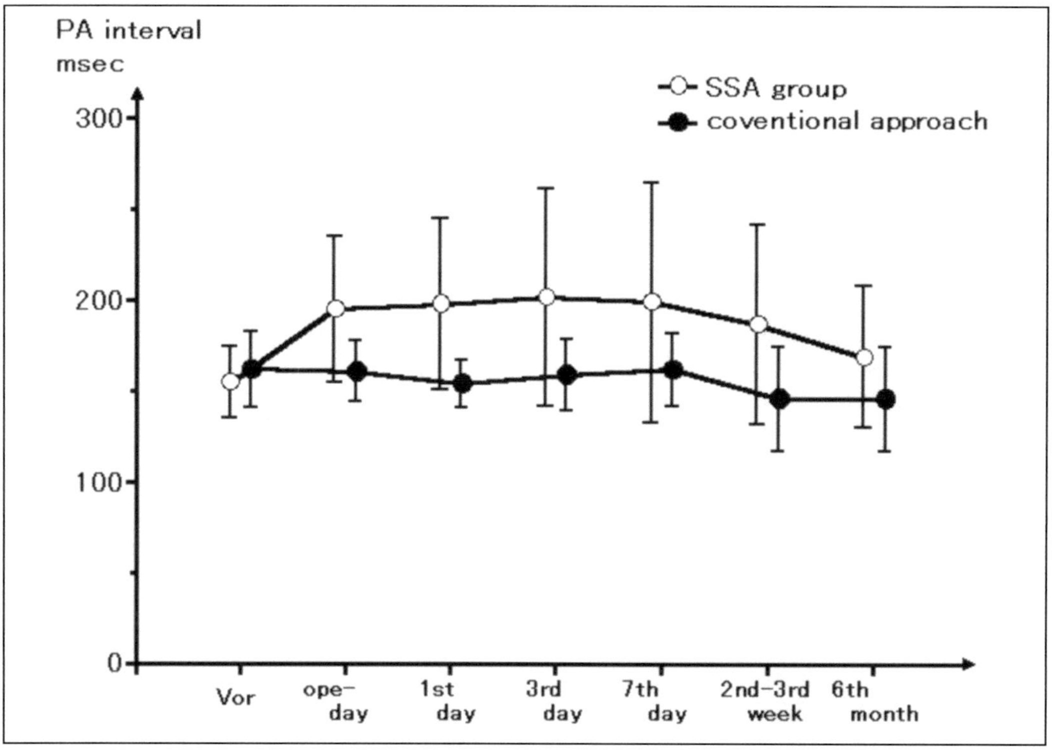

PR intervals of patients undergoing the superior septal approach become longer postoperatively and decreased gradually. Those of patients undergoing the conventional approach show no significant change significantly (p-values between any PR intervals > 0.10). Between the two groups, there is a significant difference in serial PR interval changes (p= 0.05 by the generalized Wilcoxon test).
Abbreviations: SSA; superior septal approach, ope-day; operation day,
msec; milliseconds

Fig. 2. Postoperative serial PR interval changes

Twenty-seven superior septal approach patients underwent Holter electrocardiograms more than 6 months postoperatively. No patient showed bradycardia below 50 /min. Supraventricular arrhythmias such as premature atrial contractions were limited within 3 % of the total beats. Cardiac rhythms responded to the patients' activity levels. None of the 52 superior septal approach patients required pacemaker implantation.

Postoperative echocardiography 1-2 months after operation revealed no case of atrial septal defect.

Five patients maintained normal sinus rhythms perioperatively in the control group. The other patients remained atrial fibrillation throughout the follow-up periods. Mean PR interval of the five patients with sinus rhythm was 162 +/- 21 milliseconds preoperatively, with no significant change postoperatively (p-values of any PR intervals are more than 0.10 , Figure 1). No patient developed atrioventricular blocks. There was a significant serial change between the two groups ($p = 0.05$). None of the 12 patients in the control group also required pacemaker.

c. **Additional studies:**

Including patients from the additional study, 64 of 66 patients with sinus rhythm preoperatively maintained sinus rhythm postoperatively, and seven of 47 with preoperative atrial fibrillation regained sinus rhythm at final follow-up. No patient needed pacemaker implantation, but two had a pacemaker implanted preoperatively.

A left atrial tumor is also a candidate for the superior septal approach (Misawa et al, 2002). We encountered a cardiac myxoma which located on the superior wall of the left atrium. The endoscope-assisted superior septal approach gave an excellent operative view and provided for a safe tumor resection. A 74 year-old man who had been experiencing paroxysmal atrial fibrillation for a few months was admitted to our hospital. Echocardiographic and computer tomographic studies showed a round, homogeneous mass at the free wall of the left atrium. The left atrium was echocardiographically measured at 39 mm in depth beneath the ascending aorta. The patient consented to resection of the tumor. Extracorporeal circulation was established through conventional median sternotomy, and moderate hypothermia and blood cardioplegic solution was used for myocardial protection. The right atrium and atrial septum were incised. A thoracoscope, which is used for routine endoscopic thoracic surgery in our institute, inserted through the atrial septotomy revealed that the stalk of the tumor was located on the superior wall of the left atrium. The incision was extended from the atrial septum to the superior aspect of the left atrium, without incising the stalk (Figure 3). Under thoracoscopic observation, the incision was completed along the superior wall of the left atrium. The stalk was excised together with an adjacent 5 mm of left atrial intima. The intimal defect was closed by direct suture without a patch. Myocardial ischemia time was 55 minutes. Pathological examination showed a completely resected 28x25x17 mm mass compatible with cardiac myxoma. He was discharged with no complications.

4. Comment

a. **Cardiac surgery and postoperative conduction disturbances:**

The risk of developing conduction disturbances after cardiac surgery has been well established. Goldman and associates retrospectively reviewed 5,942 patients who underwent open-heart surgery for acquired heart disease, and they revealed that 123 patients (2.1%) required permanent cardiac pacing postoperatively; 4.6% of these underwent

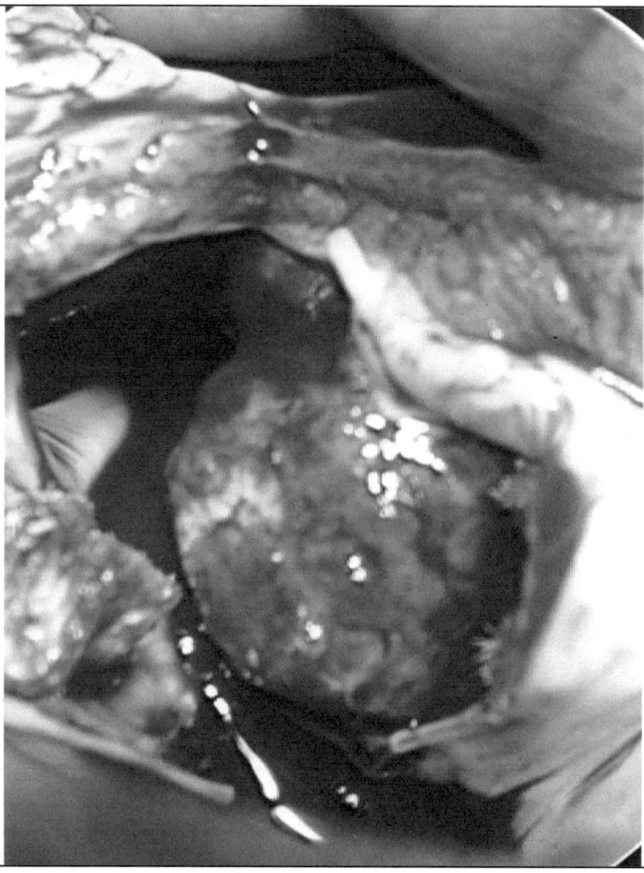

Myxoma of the left atrium was removed via the superior septal approach. The tumor originated from the free wall of the left atrium.

Fig. 3. An operative view in a case of a left atrial tumor

predominantly valvular surgery and 0.6% had coronary bypass (Goldman et al., 1984). They also showed that risk factors of postoperative pacemaker implantation appeared to be: 1) preoperative evidence of a conduction disorder; 2) advanced patient age; 3) dense calcium in the aortic annulus; 4) valvular surgery and, especially, tricuspid valve surgery; and 5) poor myocardial protection.

Another interesting article was published, referring to permanent pace maker implantation following cardiac surgery (Merin et al., 2009). They reviewed 4,999 patients undergoing surgery between 1993 and 2005. The average patient age was 64 +/- 12 years, and 71% were males. Coronary bypass was performed in 4,071, aortic valve replacement in 675, and mitral valve replacement in 968 patients. Seventy-two patients (1.4%) required pacemaker implantation after surgery. Indications for pacemaker implantation included complete atrioventricular block in 59, symptomatic bradycardia/slow atrial fibrillation in nine, second-degree atrioventricular block in two, and other conduction disturbances in two patients. Left bundle branch block and aortic valve replacement were predictors for pacemaker implantation. Of those receiving a pacemaker, about one-third will recover at late follow-up. They did not analyze the differernces in approach in mitral valve surgery, but their study implied that any cardiac surgery has a potential risk of postoperative pacemaker implantation.

Emkanjoo and associates revealed any types of conduction disturbances after open heart surgery (Emkanjoo, et al., 2008). This prospective study included coronary artery bypass (n=128), valve surgery (n=95), coronary artery and valvular surgery (n=6), repair of ventricular septal defect (n=51), repair of tetralogy of Fallot (n=57), and others (n=37). Among 374 patients, 192 developed new conduction disorders including symptomatic sinus bradycardia, atrial fibrillation, first to third atrioventricular block, and new right or left bundle branch block. In 5.6% patients, a permanent pacemaker was implanted, 47.6% of them underwent valvular surgery. In the coronary artery bypass group, 29.7% of patients developed new conduction disturbances; the most common of them was symptomatic sinus bradycardia. After valvular surgery 44.2% of patients developed conduction disturbances, the most common being atrial fibrillation with a slow ventricular response. After ventricular septal defect and tetralogy of Fallot repair, the most common conduction disturbance was new right bundle branch block. In 44.1% of patients the conduction defects occurred in the first 48 hours after surgery. The study showed that valvular surgery has a high potential risk of conduction disturbances during the early postoperative phase.

b. Approaches to the mitral valve and a small left atrium:

Conventionally, a left atriotomy made posterior to the interatrial groove or a transseptal approach was chosen for the mitral valve surgery. However, these approaches often resulted in a limited operative field in the case of a small left atrium or reoperation. Poor observation in the limited field might compromise surgical accuracy. Mitral valvuloplasty, which is more favored than valve replacement because of a better quality of life postoperatively, requires optimal exposure of the valve and the subvalvular apparatus. In such a case, precision and a secure reliable technique are necessary for successful results. Therefore, good exposure of the mitral apparatus is essential for the principal procedure. In addition, a young surgeon would also be able to perform the surgery successfully under a wide operative field where the instructor could also closely observe his procedure. The superior septal approach can provide a wider operative field than conventional approaches.

A tumor can sometimes be found incidentally in the left atrium. In such a case, the left atrium is often small and the superior septal approach is suitable (Misawa et al., 2002). Our patient's small atrium and tumor site prevented us from observing the tumor stalk by the conventional transseptal view. With endoscopic examination, the anatomy of the tumor was clarified, and subsequent operative procedures were easily performed. Our thoracoscope was not flexible because it was designed for use in thoracic surgery. Use of a flexible endoscope in intracardiac procedures would be even more desiable in cases such as ours. With further innovation in endoscopic instruments, complex surgical procedures requiring subtle maneuvers will be possible under endoscopic assistance. Our case exemplifies the increasing usefulness of endoscope-assisted cardiac surgery.

c. Mitral vlave surgery and postoperative conduction disturbances:

Takeshita and associates reviewed the electrocardiograms of 76 patients who underwent mitral valve operations either via the transseptal superior approach or via the right lateral atriotomy (Takeshita et al., 1997). Nine patients who maintained the sinus rhythm for more than one year after surgery via the transseptal superior approach were selected for electrophysiological study to evaluate the sinus node function. They concluded that postoperative electrocardiographic and electrophysiological studies revealed that the sinus node function after the transseptal superior approach was relatively well maintained for more than one year after the operation. The influence of the transseptal superior approach on the sinus node function in the mid-term postoperative period was apparently mild and did not cause a serious problem, and that some of the patients did show abnormal data in terms of sino-atrial conduction time and intrinsic heart rate. Therefore, they recommennded that further follow-up of the sinus node function is necessary in patients who underwent mitral surgery through the transseptal superior approach.

Some investigators mentioned a high risk of loss of sinus rhythm with the superior septal approach, but others showed that the superior septal approach was not associated with a greater incidence of rhythm disturbances. Masuda and assiociates found a higher incidence of dyshythmias with the superior septal approach in the early postoperative period than that with the conventional right lateral left atriotomy and a similar incidence of them in the late period (Masuda et al., 1996). The authors analyzed 152 consecutive patients who underwent mitral valve procedures between 1992 and 1995. Follow-up ranged from 2 to 38 months, and the mean follow-up was 13.8 months in the superior septal group of 83 patients and 16.1 months in the conventional group of 69 patients. They showed that the mortality rate was similar in the two groups, and the causes of death were not related to the left atriotomy. At discharge, 78% of those in the superior septal group remained in sinus rhythm and 96% of the patients in the conventional group who were in sinus rhythm preoperatively. At the last follow-up, 83% of these patients in the former and 88% in the latter remained in sinus rhythm. They concluded that although the incidence of dysrhythmias was higher with the superior septal approach in the early postoperative period, the approach provides an excellent operative view of the mitral valve and similar results in terms of late postoperative cardiac rhythms in comparison with the right lateral left atriotomy.

Lukac and associates retrospectively analyzed consecutive 577 patients after mitral valve surgery with the superior septal approach or the left atrial approach (Lukac et al., 2007). They used the superior septal approach in 150 patients and the left atrial approach in 427. Forty-four patients had a pacemaker implanted after the surgery; 17 in the superior septal group and 27 in the left atrial group (p = 0.010). Nineteen patients had a pacemaker implanted because of sinus node dysfunction; 9 in the former and 10 in the latter (p = 0.017). They concluded that the superior septal approach has a higher risk of clinically significant sinus node dysfunction than the left atrial approach, and that the risk of pacemaker implantation because of atrioventricular conduction disturbances was not different between the two groups.

Utley and Leyland compared the preoperative status, operative factors, and postoperative outcomes among patients having mitral valve operations with three atrial incisions (Utley & Leyland, 1995). The incisions were right lateral (n = 66), superior septal (n = 46), and transseptal (n = 37). Patients in the superior septal group more commonly required permanent pacemakers than those in the right lateral group. In patients with sinus rhythm before operation, sinus rhythm had returned before hospital discharge more commonly in those in the right lateral group (35 of 44, 80%) than in those in the superior septal group (18 of 28, 46%) or in the transseptal group (9 of 13, 69%). With multiple regression analysis the type of atrial incision was not a predictor of postoperative pulmonary failure or need for permanent pacemaker implantation. Right lateral and transseptal atrial incisions were predictors of retention of sinus rhythm after operation. They concluded that the results of the superior septal incision were comparable with those of other incisions except for a slightly greater risk of loss of sinus rhythm, and that one must weigh the technical advantages of the superior septal incision against the risk of loss of sinus rhythm.

Kon and associates used the extended transseptal approach to the mitral valve for 71 consecutive procedures (Kon et al., 1993). Four patients died; none had complications directly attributable to the exposure. Twenty underwent a primary reparative procedure; 30, a primary replacement procedure; and 21, a repeat procedure. Despite division of the sinus node artery, 26 of 32 patients with sinus rhythm preoperatively had sinus rhythm postoperatively; 4 had atrial fibrillation postoperatively. Twenty-seven of 37 patients with atrial fibrillation preoperatively had atrial fibrillation postoperatively; 8 had sinus rhythm postoperatively. They use the extended transseptal approach routinely for mitral valve operations because the exposure provided by the extended transseptal approach is superior to that of standard approaches.

Gaudino and associates evaluated the safety and effectiveness of the superior septal approach for routine mitral valve replacement (Gaudino et al., 1997). One hundred forty-six consecutive patients undergoing mitral valve replacement at their institution were randomly assigned to undergo the procedure using either the conventional left atriotomy or the superior septal approach. Postoperatively and during the follow-up, 12-lead electrocardiography, 24-hour Holter monitoring, and transthoracic and transesophageal echocardiography were performed in all patients. They showed that the cardiopulmonary bypass and cross-clamp times were significantly higher in the superior septal group. No significant difference in blood loss was found between the two groups, and no residual atrial septal defect was found in the superior septal patients. The maintainance of sinus rhythm at late follow-up and the incidences of postoperative arrhythmias and newly developed atrioventricular block were not significantly different between the two groups. They concluded that the use of the superior septal approach to the mitral valve was not associated with a greater incidence of rhythm disturbances or other complications.

In addition, Smith showed an interesting change of P wave axis and morphology in patients who had the superior septal approach (Smith, 1992). The author used the superior septal approach for an excellent exposure in seven patients in whom there were a variety of obstacles to a conventional approach. Four had complex reoperations. There were no bleeding complications. At late follow-up there was no change in rhythm or conduction in four patients with atrial fibrillation preoperatively. A change in P wave axis and morphology was seen at late follow-up in 2 patients with normal sinus rhythm preoperatively, possibly related to division of the sinus node artery. A third patients with normal sinus rhythm preoperatively remained in normal sinus rhythm at late follow-up. The author also confirmed that the superior septal approach could be useful in complex reoperations, in procedures requiring right atriotomy for other reasons, and in patients with a small or inaccessible left atrium.

Yamada and associates reported postoperative premature ventricular contractions arising from the mitral annulus (Yamada et al, 2009). They showed that electroanatomic mapping during the premature ventricular contractions revealed a centrifugal activation pattern arising from the mitral annulus, and the premature ventricular contractions were likely to be idiopathic. They successfully achieved radiofrequency ablation at the site close to the antero-paraseptal end of the mitral annuloplasty ring, which was located adjacent to the fibrous trigone. Their experience indicated that premature ventricular contractions after mitral valve surgery could occur in any approaches to the left atrium.

d. Sinus node function after mitral valve surgery:

Silva Junior and associates studied the interatrial conduction times and atrial node performance in patients submitted to mitral valve surgery with the aid of temporary atrial epicardic electrodes (Silvia et al, 2008). Their approach to the mitral valve was a conventional left atriotmy The atriograms were carried out in the first postoperative day and before the hospital discharge of ten consecutive patients. Sixty percent of the patients could complete the post-operative study protocol. The main results were: a) Post-operative arrhythmias were detected in 50% of the patients; b) There were no statistical differences between the pre and post-operative 12 lead electrocardiograms;. c) The interatrial conduction time ranged from 90 to 140 milliseconds in the first post-operative day, and from 110 to 130 milliseconds at hospital discharge; d) The sinus node recovery time ranged from 250 to 560 milliseconds in the first post-operative day and from 180 to 360 milliseconds at hospital discharge; e) The sinus atrial conduction time remained between 70 and 140 milliseconds, both in the first post-operative day and at hospital discharge, and; f) The interatrial conduction time was normal in patients whose left atrium was less than 50mm in diameter but supranormal in the remaining cases. They concluded that sinus node function and interatrial conduction are not altered by mitral valve operation via the conventional left-sided approach. Their data indicated that the conventional approach to the mitral valve may be more preferable than the superior septal approach from the point of conduction disturbences.

e. Causes of postoperative rhythm disturbances after the superior septal approach:

The sinus node artery arises from the right coronary artery in about 55% of hearts and from the left circumflex or main coronary artery in the remainder. When it originates from the right coronary artery, it runs superiorly over the wall of the right atrium beneath the right appendage to the base of the superior vena cava (Kirklin & Barratt-Boyes, 1993). The sinus node artery must be frequently sacrificed for the superior septal approach, causing potential risks for postoperative arrhythmias such as supraventricular arrhythmias and atrioventricular conduction disturbances. There will be collateral blood flows in the postoperative recovery phase, but blood supply will be reduced in the early postoperatrive phase. Moreover, an atrial incision required for the superior septal approach is longer than that for conventional approaches, which might interfere with the cardiac conduction system, resulting in conduction disturbances and arrhythmias.

Berdajs and associates analyzed 50 human hearts from cadavers without previous pathological alterations (Berdajs et al., 2003). They described the topographic relation between the sinus node artery and the superior posterior border of the interatrial septum with regard to the sinus node dysfunction that follows the superior septal approach to the mitral valve. The position of the sinus node and the course of the sinus node artery were investigated. For identification of the origin of the artery, selective coronary angiograms were performed. The course of the sinus node artery and its topographic relation to the interatrial septum was identified by the dry dissections of the hearts. Based on histologic and dry dissected specimens the exact position of the sinus node was determined. They found that the sinus node artery originates from the right coronary artery in 66% of examined cases and from the left coronary artery in 34% of cases, and that the sinus node artery crosses the superior posterior border of the interatrial septum in 54% of cases. On the basis of morphological and clinical results, they concluded that the risk of intraoperative damage to the sinus node artery during the superior septal approach to the mitral valve is high.

Shin and associates assessed sinus node function after the superior septal approach in 46 patients (Sin et al., 2001). Twelve of 20 patients with preoperative sinus rhythm experienced early postoperative supraventricular arrhythmias, but all spontaneously recovered sinus rhythm. Electrophysiological studies revealed a lack of sinus node dysfunction. During the postoperative period (34 +/- 24 months), 2 of the 20 patients with preoperative sinus rhythm developed persistent atrial fibrillation, and 3 of the 25 patients with preoperative atrial fibrillation achieved normal sinus srhythm. They concluded that the superior septal approach does not appear to cause longterm adverse effects on sinus node function, although temporary effects may occur.

f. Electrical remodeling after mitral valve surgery:

Berdais and associates retrospectively evaluated the causative mechanisms underlying postoperative atrioventricular block following mitral valve replacement and mitral valve annuloplasty (Berdajs et al., 2008). They analyzed 391 patients undergoing mitral valve replacement or ring annuloplasty and quadrangular resection between 1990 and 2003. Their exclusion criteria were preoperative atrioventricular block, two or three valvular procedures, reoperations and procedures combined with coronary artery bypass grafting. The presence of the postoperative atrioventricular block was compared with preoperative and intraoperative variables. On 55 post-mortem specimens the relationship between the atrioventricular node, atrioventricular node artery and mitral valve annulus was investigated. Patients' mean age was 59+/-14 years and 44% of patients were female. Postoperatively atrioventricular block occurred in 92 (23.5%) patients. Third degree atrioventricular block was found in 17 (4%) patents, in whom a pacemaker was implanted within median interval of 4 days. Second degree atrioventricular block occurred and first degree atrioventricular block in five (1.3%) and in 70 (18%) patients respectively. In dry dissected human hearts in 23% of investigated cases the atrioventricular node artery was discovered to run close to the annulus of the mitral valve. Their morphological investigation showed that the atrioventricular node artery runs in close proximity to the annulus in 23% of cases. They speculated that damage of the atrioventricular node artery might play a role in development of atrioventricular block.

The PR intervals on electrocardiogram in our patients who had the superior septal approach were prolonged in the early postoperative phase but returned to normal range in the late phase. We introduce a new concept of electrical remodeling after cardiac surgery, which needs atrial or ventricular iincisions. Coronary artery revascularization can cause such a electrical remodeling because of postischemic reperfusion injuries.

g. Newly developed collateral arteries and electrical remodeling:

We hypothesize that newly developed collateral blood flow to the sinus node or an altered cardiac conduction system caused by the superior septal approach might contribute to transient conduction disturbances (Misawa, 2005). The numerous anastomoses between the surrounding atrial arteries and the arteriolar network of the sinus node, which were mentioned by Kovács (Kovács, 2003), would help lead to preferable clinical outcomes. Cardiac surgeons need to take into consideration the potential risk after the superior septal approach, as implied by Berdajs and colleagues. However, most arrhythmias are transient and can be controlled by ordinary perioperative measures.

The possible causes of the postoperative dysrhythmias with the superior septal approach are mentioned above. The prolongation of the PR interval in the superior septal approach patients in the early postoperative phase and return to normal in the late phase might be caused by newly developed collateral blood flows to the sinus node or cardiac conduction systems. Further studies are required to confirm these hypotheses. The superior septal approach group had the potential risk of an atrial septal defect, but postoperative echocardiography found no cases of such a defect.

Conventional left atrial incision in the control group was longitudinal of approximately 5~6 cm. The sinus node artery is not sacrificed. Even in cases requiring tricuspid surgery, right atrial incision was shorter than the that in the superior septal approach group. This might result in the stable PR intervals after surgery.

h. Postoperative rhythm management:

In our study, patients with bradycardia below 70 beats/min were routinely paced during the early postoperative phase, and no patients developed medically intractable bradycardia more than 2 weeks postoperatively. In addition, no patient required implantation of a permanent pacemaker because of symptomatic or latent bradycardia as detected by Holter electrocardiograms at the median follow-up time of 15 months. As the extended superior septal approach, right atrial and septal incisions are joined at the superior end of the interatrial septum and extended across the dome of the left atrium to the base of the left atrial appendage. Our procedure includes a right atriotomy not going beyond the crista terminalis, an atrial septotomy beginning at the fossa ovalis, and a subsequent left atrial incision 2 cm long parallel to the superior vena cava. The limited incision may contribute to these minimization of postoperative conduction disturbances after the superior septal approach.

i. A modified superior septal approach:

Nguyen showed a modified version of the superior septal approach, which was made without cutting the right atrial appendage and the dome of the right atrium Nguyen, 2009). The modified approach includes three incisions. The first incision is made vertically on the anterolateral aspect of the right atrium, parallel to the atrioventricular groove, from the base of the inferior vena caval cannula to the root of the right atrial appendage. The second incision is made vertically on the transatrial septum, from the base of the inferior vena cava to the middle of the right atrial roof. The third incision extends the second incision 2-3 cm to the left atrial roof, and forward to the root of the left atrial appendage. The author evaluated this shorter procedure in 30 patients aged 4–61 years undergoing complex mitral valve operations including mitral repair (33.3%), reoperation (30%), and small left atrium (30%). The myocardial ischemic time was 117 +/- 29.9 minutes (range, 53–173). Cardiac rhythm resumed spontaneously after release of the aortic clamp in 93.3% of patients, including 36.7% who regained sinus rhythm from arrhythmia preoperatively. There was no heart block, bleeding, or mortality. The author insisted that the modified approach does not cut through the right atrial appendage and part of the right atrium, therefore, it can better nourish the sinus region from the collateral system around the sinus node, and increase the number of atrial muscle fibers that connect the sinus node with the atrioventricular node, thus reinforcing sinoatrial conduction.

5. Conclusions

Excellent visibility of the mitral valve is important for surgical treatment. It yields successful clinical results and educational advantages for surgical residents. Some clinical problems, including postoperative rhythm disturbances, can occur with the superior septal approach, but they can be controlled medically or with transient electrical pacemaking in the early postoperative phase. Conventional approaches for mitral surgery can also produce postoperative rhythm disturbances. We conclude that the superior septal approach is an excellent approach for mitral operations or left atrial tumor resection that overcomes postoperative transient dysrhythmias.

6. References

Berdajs, D. Patonay,l. & Turina, MI. (2003). The clinical anatomy of the sinus node artery. *Ann Thorac Surg* 76,3, (2003, September), 732-5, 0003-4975

Berdajs, D. Schurr, UP. Wagner, A. Seifert, B. Turina, MI. & Genoni, M. (2008). Incidence and pathophysiology of atrioventricular block following mitral valve replacement and ring annuloplasty. *Eur J Cardiothorac Surg* 34,1, (2008, July), 55-61, 1010-7940

Edmunds, LH. Clark, RE. Cohn, LH. Grunkemeier, GL. Miller, DC. & Weisel, RD. (1996). Guideline for reporting morbidity and mortality aftercardiac valvular operations. *Ann Thorac Surg* 62,3,(1996, September)932-935, 0003-4975

Emkanjoo, Z. Mirza-Ali, M. Alizadeh, A. Hosseini,S. Jorat, MV. Nikoo, MH. & Sadr-Ameli, MA. (2008). Predictors and frequency of conduction disturbances after open-heart surgery. *Indian Pacing Electrophysiol J* 8,1, (2008, February), 14-21, 0972-6292

Gaudino, M. Alessandrini, F. Glieca, F. Martinelli, L. Santarelli, P. Bruno, P. & Possati, G. (1997). Conventional left atrial versus superior septal approach for mitral valve replacement. *Ann Thorac Surg* 63,4,(1997, April),1123-7, 0003-4975

Goldman, BS. Hill, TJ. Weisel, RD. Scully, HE. Mickleborough, LL. Pym, J. & Baird, RJ. Permanent cardiac pacing after open-heart surgery: acquired heart disease. *Pacing Clin Electrophysio* 7,3, (1984, May), 367-71, 0147-8389

Kirklin, JW. & Barratt-Boyes, BG. (1993). *Cardiac Surgery. 2nd ed.* Churchill Livingstone, 0-443-07526-3, New York

Kon, ND. Tucker, WY. Mills, SA. Lavender, SW. & Cordell, AR. (1993). Mitral valve operation via an extended transseptal approach. *Ann Thorac Surg* 55,6,(1993, June), 1413-7, 0003-4975

Kovács, GS. (2003). The clinical anatomy of the sinus node artery, *Ann Thorac Surg* 76,3, (2003, September), 735–736, 0003-4975

Lukac, P. Hjortda, VE. Pedersen, AK. Mortensen, PT. Jensen, HK. & Hansen, PS. (2007). Superior transseptal approach to mitral valve is associated with a higher need for pacemaker implantation than the left atrial approach. *Ann Thorac Surg* 83,1,(2007, January), 77-82, 0003-4975

Masuda, M. Tominaga, R. Kawachi, Y. Fukumura, F. Morita, S. Imoto, Y. Toshima, Y. Tomita, Y. & Yasui, H. (1996). Postoperative cardiac rhythms with superior septal approach and lateral approach to the mitral valve. *Ann Thorac Surg* 62,4, (1996, October), 1118-22, 0003-4975

Merin, O. Ilan, M. Oren, A. Fink, D. Deeb, M. Bitran, D. & Silberman, S. (2009). Permanent pacemaker implantation following cardiac surgery: indications and long-term follow-up. *Pacing Clin Electrophysiol* 32,1, (2009, January), 7-12, 0147-8389

Misawa, Y. Fuse, K. Kawahito, K. Saito, T. & Konishi, H. (1999). Conduction disturbances after superior septal approach for mitral valve repair. *Ann Thorac Surg* 68, 4, (1999, October), 1262-5, 0003-4975

Misawa, Y. Saito, T. Fuse, K. Sohara, Y. (2002). Endoscope-assisted superior septal approach for resection of left atrial myxoma. *J Thorac Cardiovasc Surg* 123, 2, (2002, February), 357-358, 0022-5223

Misawa, Y. & Kaminishi, Y.(2004). Early and late arrhythmias in patients in preoperative sinus rhythm after superior septal approach. *Ann Thorac Surg* 77, 6, (2004, June), 2259-9, 0003-4975

Misawa, Y. Kaminishi, Y. Sakano, Y. (2005). Conduction disturbance after shutdown of the sinus node artery. *Ann Thorac Surg* 79, 1, (2005, January), 388-9, 0003-4975

Nguyan, HU (2009). Improved combied superior-transseptal approach to the mitral valve. *Asian Cardiovasc Thorac Ann* 17,2(2009, April), 171-4, 0218-4923

Silva Junior, JR. Ferreira, CA. Rodrigues, AJ. Vicente, WV. & Evora PR. (2008). Sinus node function in patients operated for mitral valve disease; Indirect evaluation with epimyocardial electrodes. *Acta Cir Bras* 23, Suppl 1, (2008), 126-32, 0102-8650

Shin, H. Yozu, R. Higashi, S.Kawada, S. (2001). Sinus node function after mitral valve surgery using the suoerior septal approach. *Ann Thorac Surg* 71, 2, (2001, February), 587-90, 0003-4975

Smith, CR. (1992). Septal-superior exposure of the mitral valve. The transplant approach. *J Thorac Cardiovasc Surg* 103, 4, (1992, April), 623-8, 0022-5223

Takeshita, M. Furuse, A. Kotsuka, Y. & Kubota, H. (1997). Sinus node function after mitral valve surgery via the transseptal superior approach. *Eur J Cardiothorac Surg* 12, 3, (1997, September), 341-4, 1010-7940

Utley, JR. Leyland, SA. & Nguyenduy T. (1995). Comparison of outcomes with three atrial incision for mitral valve operations. *J Thorac Cardiovasc Surg* 109,3, (1995, March), 582-7, 0022-5223

Yamada, T. McElderry, HAT. Doppalapudi, H. Epstein, AE. Plumb, VJ. & Kay. GN. (2009). Catheter ablation of premature ventricular contractions arising from the mitral annulus after mitral valvoplasty. *Pacing Clin Electrophysiol* 32,6, (2009, June), 825-7, 0147-8389

18

Complication of Pacemaker Implantation: An Atrial Lead Perforation

Kenji Sadamatsu
Saga Prefectural Hopital Koseikan
Japan

1. Introduction

The implantation of permanent pacemakers is increasing year by year, and these devices are constantly being improved. Atrial lead perforation is an infrequent but a critical complication of pacemaker implantation. Recently, there have been increasing reports on the complication with the advances made in imaging modalities, and moreover, computed tomography scans can reveal delayed atrial lead perforation even in asymptomatic patients. However, the details of this complication remain unclear, and it is difficult to decide an appropriate strategy for the patients. This chapter thus focuses on this rare but increasing complication of atrial lead following pacemaker implantation.

2. Overview of cardiac perforation following pacemaker implantation

Acute and late complications from pacemaker implantation occur in a variable percentage of patients, ranging 3.2% to 7.5% (Ellenbogen et al., 2003; Healey et al., 2006; Lamas et al., 2002). Cardiac perforation, which can lead to pericarditis, tamponade, or even death, is one of the important complications. The incidence of perforation after permanent pacemaker is reportedly between 0.3% and 1.2% (Aizawa et al., 2001; Ellenbogen et al., 2003; Mahapatra et al., 2005). Most patients with a perforation complain of chest pain, dyspnea, and hypotension, thus making such symptoms important clues to an accurate diagnosis. Abnormal sensing or pacing parameters, and abnormal signs in chest radiography or echocardiography also indicate cardiac perforation. Almost all such instances tend to occur within 1 month after surgery, and the extraction of the lead is recommended when it is identified (Khan et al., 2005). However, some reports have also described successfully managed cases without extraction (Henrikson et al., 2006; Mahapatra et al., 2005).

3. Predictors of cardiac perforation following pacemaker implantation

There are several independent predictors of cardiac perforation following permanent pacemaker implantation. Multivariate analysis of 4280 permanent pacemaker implantations at the Mayo Clinic revealed that the use of a temporary pacemaker, helical screw leads, and steroids are the independent predictors of a perforation, and elevated right ventricular systolic pressure is protective against perforation (Mahapatra et al., 2005). The risk of using screw-in leads has also been demonstrated in other case reports (Akyol et al., 2005; Dilling-

Boer et al., 2003; Ho et al., 1999). A recent review article proposed several candidates in addition to the risk factors of perforation; the type and the location of the leads, the heart muscle characteristics, anticoagulation therapy, patient age, gender, and body mass (Rydlewska et al., 2010). However, the Mode Selection in Sinus Node Dysfunction trial, which was a prospective randomized trial included 2010 patients with sinus node dysfunction, and a report by Laborderie et al., which was a retrospective study from a French institution, could not demonstrate any predictors for cardiac perforation after pacemaker implantation (Ellenbogen et al., 2003; Laborderie et al., 2008), and therefore the early prediction or identification of such conditions continues to be a challenge.

4. Active-fixation atrial leads

An atrial lead is essential for dual chamber pacing, but dislodgement of this lead is not infrequent (Ellenbogen et al., 2003; Lamas et al., 2002). In order to reduce the dislodgement rate, active fixation (screw-in) leads have been developed and have grown in popularity because of their reliability and the relative ease of placement at sites with the optimal pacing and sensing thresholds, adding to lower dislodgement rates. However, active fixation leads are associated with rare complications, including pericarditis, atrial lead perforation, pericardial effusion with or without cardiac tamponade, and death. The leads increase the chance of perforating the thin-walled right atrium, which averages 2mm in wall thickness (Hirschl et al., 2007), compared to passive fixation. Several risk factors may be responsible for the increased complication rate of screw-in leads (Srivathsan et al. 2003). Variations in the anatomy of the right atrium, such as an extremely thin-walled or multi-lobed atrial appendage may therefore play a role in the perforation. Previous reports have suggested that the implantation of active-fixation leads in the right atrial free wall is one of the risk factors responsible for increasing pericardial complications compared to the right atrial appendage, however a study that included 1021 consecutive patients demonstrated that the atrial lead tip in 3 of 4 cases of pericarditis after pacemaker implantation were directed anteromedially to the area of the right atrial appendage (Sivakumaran et al., 2002). A prospective randomized study showed a similar frequency of lead tip positioning in the right atrial appendage and lateral atrial wall among patients with pericardial complications (Luria et al., 2007). In addition, lead factors, such as the design and stiffness of the helix may differ between manufactures and could be important. The experience of the operator regarding pacemaker implantation is equally important. Over-screwing during atrial lead fixation, abrupt lead withdrawal without unscrewing, and distal positioning of the stylet while screwing should be avoided.

5. Differences among atrial lead types

Several types of atrial leads have been available, and active-fixation leads have advantages and disadvantages. However, there is limited data to compare the atrial leads for the choice of fixation (passive or active) or lead shape (J-shape or straight) (Van Herendael & Willems, 2009). A randomized comparison between 2 active-fixation, steroid-eluting, polyurethane-insulated, bipolar atrial lead models that differed only in shape (J-shape or straight) showed equally favorable performance profiles for 1 year of follow-up. Dislodgments were only reported in the straight lead group in 5.9% of cases, while no dislodgments occurred in the J-shaped lead group. The rates of exit block and lead malfunction tended to be higher in the J-shaped group. Pericardial complications occurred in both groups in 1% of cases (Glikson et al., 2000). Moreover, those groups were followed over a 5-year period. Lead macrodislodgment occurred in the straight lead group in another 1.9% of cases during the additional follow-up, and lead malfunction and excessive pacing thresholds without dislodgment occurred in the J-shaped lead group in 10.7% of cases and in the straight lead group in 3.8% of cases (Luria et al., 2005). A prospective randomized comparison of the performance of J-shaped atrial leads with or without active-fixation revealed significantly lower pacing thresholds in the passive-fixation group at implantation, and this difference persisted at 1-year follow-up. The duration of fluoroscopy during the implantation procedure was significantly shorter in the passive-fixation group. Dislodgments were only reported in the passive-fixation group in 2% of cases, while pericardial complications occurred only in the active-fixation group in 6% of cases (Luria et al., 2007). Another report also showed early dislodgment requiring subsequent lead repositioning to occur in 2.4% of passive-fixation leads, but in none of the active-fixation leads. The incidence of pericarditis following implantation of J-shaped active-fixation leads was 5% (Sivakumaran et al., 2002). Passive-fixation leads are reported to have an excellent reliability and a very low incidence of atrial lead perforation (Glikson et al., 1999), while no difference in the J-shaped leads and straight leads in passive-fixation was demonstrated (Krupienicz et al., 2000).

6. Late lead perforation following pacemaker implantation

Late complications of pacemaker implantation that are well recognized include infection, failure of the atiral or ventricular lead to pace or sense appropriately, erosion of the pulse generator, and subclavian vein thrombosis. Delayed lead perforation has been defined as migration and perforation after one month of implantation. This complication has been reported to occur in 0.1-0.8% of pacemaker and 0.6-5.2% of implantable cardioverter defibrillator implantations (Khan et al., 2005; Polin et al., 2006), while recent progress in diagnostic imaging has increased the number of case reports on late lead perforation. Computed tomography is becoming a gold standard used for the diagnosis of a perforation, and asymptomatic perforation cases identified on the scans have been described extensively in the literature. A retrospective investigation of 100 consecutive patients with permanent pacemakers or implantable cardiac defibrillators who underwent multidetector computed tomography revealed that 15% of patients had a lead perforation, and the perforation rate of active- and passive-fixation atrial leads were 12% and 25%, respectively (Hirschl et al., 2007). This common phenomenon was confirmed by an autopsy study. Myocardial perforation or penetration by an electrode was recognized in 5.3% of 111 autopsy cases of patients 60 years of age or over with an implanted pacemaker. The perforation rate was 27.3% in active-fixation atrial leads, and 0% in 10 passive leads. All the atrial leads perforated through the right atrial appendage but did not reach the outside of the pericardium (Ishikawa et al., 1999). In the diagnosis of delayed lead perforation, failure of pacing or sensing of the lead is an important clue. A recent report revealed that detection of lead dysfunction by an automatic home-monitoring system had fast and possibly life-saving capabilities for severe lead perforation (Spencker et al., 2007). Usually, the lead parameters, in particular the pacing threshold, will show a significant change following lead perforation, while many reports have demonstrated normal electrophysiological parameters. Hirschl et al. showed that perforated leads did not show significant difference from nonperforated leads in the impedance, and the pacing threshold of all the perforated leads except for one was categorized as low (Hirschl et al., 2007). A larger part of the electrode may have been in contact with the atrial myocardium, resulting in a lack of change in the lead parameters. Therefore, we should be aware that pacemaker malfunction may indicate perforation, but normal parameters do not exclude a perforation. Risk factors for late perforation have not yet been fully defined, although Polin et al suggested that active fixation leads and anticoagulation therapy may represent predictors for the long-term development of a perforation (Polin et al., 2006). Freedom from symptoms also does not exclude the possibility of there being a perforation, as almost all of the patients were asymptomatic. Therefore, an important question remains how we follow these patients with pacemakers and track down such delayed perforation cases. Interestingly, late lead perforation is characterized by a low rate of tamponade or death (Khan et al.; 2005), although the mechanism underlying subclinical late perforation has not been elucidated.

7. Management of a late lead perforation

A proper management strategy for a late lead perforation remains controversial and should vary among individuals. Altered pacemaker parameters and pericardial complications are the main factors that should be used to decide the strategy. Pacing or sensing failure requires lead repositioning or a new lead insertion for appropriate functioning of the pacemaker. Cardiac tamponade caused by lead perforation requires emergency percutaneous pericardiocenthesis with placement of a drainage catheter. After the stabilization, percutaneous extraction in the operating room with echocardiographic monitoring during and/or after the procedure with the cardiosurgical team backup is one of recommended strategies that can be used instead of conventional open heart lead removal (Geyfman et al., 2007; Laborderie et al., 2008), although this management is classified as a class III indication in the Heart Rhythm Society expert consensus (Wilkoff et al., 2009). Khan et al. reported successful removal of atrial leads in 2 cases of delayed lead perforation with cardiac surgery backup (Khan et al.; 2005). On the other hand, Polin et al. reported that 4 of 5 patients with cardiac tamponade that occurred over 30 days after pacemaker implantation were successfully managed conservatively without lead manipulation at a mean follow-up of 31 months (Polin et al., 2006). Henrikson et al. also demonstrated that a patient with an asymptomatic atrial lead perforation 2 weeks after the implantation was doing well at 1-year follow-up without lead extraction (Henrikson et al., 2006). Although the conservative strategy seems to be reasonable for patients without need of lead repositioning, one case report showed chronic severe pericarditis following acute pericarditis after pacemaker implantation resulted in the lead extraction (Ellenbogen et al., 2002), and another reported an asymptomatic patient with a perforated atrial lead that had to have the lead removed 2 years after the pacemaker implantation (Trigano & Caus, 1996). In addition, a recent report demonstrated that a successful surgical repair in a patient with a perforated right atrial lead migration into the right lung 1 year after the replacement of atrial lead (O'Neill et al., 2010). Although there was no imaging evidence of perforation just after the implantation in these cases, the perforation might have occurred either during or soon after the operation, and thereafter develop progressively over a longer period. A lack of long-term follow-up data remains an important concern that may influence the use of conservative management without lead extraction.

8. Our experience

We have recently reported an asymptomatic case of atrial lead perforation which developed 5 years after pacemaker implantation (Sadamatsu et al., 2009). The patient underwent a pacemaker implantation for sick sinus syndrome via the right subclavian vein (Fig.1A). Because of right breast cancer, the pacemaker and the leads were removed, and new ones were implanted via the left subclavian vein (Fig.1B). Although computed tomography scans, which we examined retrospectively, had already clearly demonstrated a perforation 9 months after the replacement (Fig.2B), another 3 years had passed until we actually noticed the complication because she remained asymptomatic and the lead parameters did not change. Transient pacing failure and the imaging findings (Fig.1EF) made us the diagnosis of perforation, but the patient was asymptomatic and the rhythm became atrial fibrillation.
We therefore managed her condition conservatively by switching the mode from DDD to VVI at first. However, the lead perforation progressed (Fig.1GH, Fig.2CD) and, as a result, open surgery was performed to remove the lead. The lead penetrated the pericardium enclosed in fibrous adhesions. This case suggests that computed tomography for evaluating lead perforation is useful and may be the most effective modality for detection, especially at the earliest possible stage of this complication. Moreover, this case throws some doubt on the safety of conservative management without extraction, and also supports the use of a management algorithm (Ellenbogen et al., 2002; Geyfman et al., 2007), for either the extraction or repositioning of the perforated lead under either fluoroscopic or echocardiographic guidance.

9. Mechanism underlying the delayed pericardial complications

The precise mechanism responsible for such late progression remains unclear, and the mechanism(s) for delayed pericardial effusion and tamponade also have not been elucidated. Surgical and autopsy findings of late atrial lead complications did not reveal any perforation in the atrial wall, which had been observed in the imaging findings (Aizawa et al., 2001; Ishikawa et al., 1999; Kono et al., 2008). These observations seem consistent with the low rate of tamponade or death in late perforation and the successful management with repositioning of the perforated atrial lead. Several recent reports have led to some speculation about the mechanism of pericardial complications. One of the proposed causes is that atrial perforation with partial protrusion of the distal aspect of the fixation screw into the pericardial cavity causes pericardial irritation (Sivakumaran et al., 2002). Another possibility is torsion by the perforated helix on the visceral pericardium during cardiac contraction, which opens a perforation gap allowing for intermittent oozing of blood into the pericardial space out of the right atrium (Geyfman et al., 2007). In addition, a perforation might be sealed by a combination of the lead itself, muscle contraction, and fibrosis, because of the small cross-sectional area of the perforation and the low pressure of the right atrium (Hirschl et al., 2007). On the other hand, the atrial leads in some cases perforate the pericardium completely, and further perforation of the leads would harm other organs, such as the lungs. It is also possible that constant mechanical pressure from the screw could also ultimately culminate in the occurrence of a sudden late myocardial perforation (Ellenbogen et al., 2002).

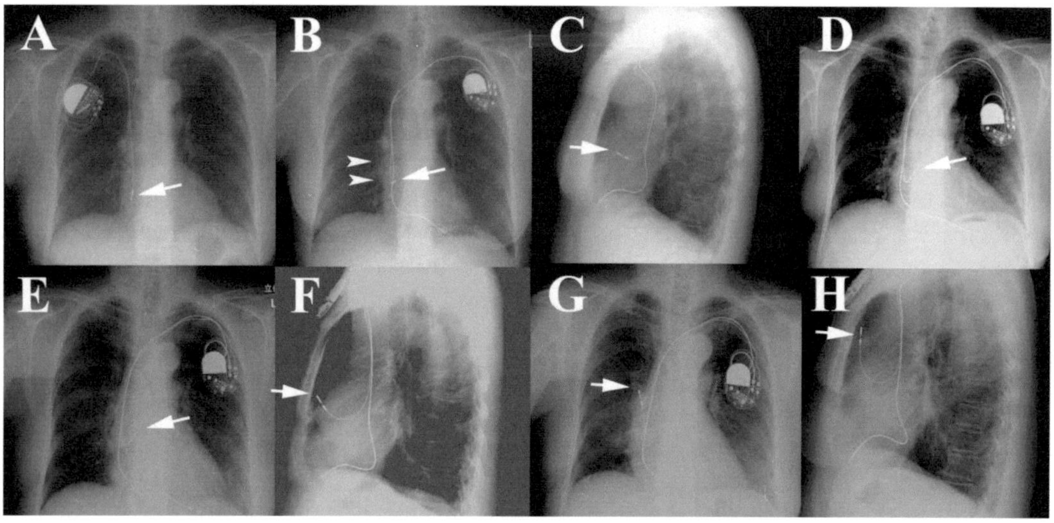

Fig. 1. Chest X-rays. Compared to the image before the replacement of the pacemaker (A), the image taken 1 week after the replacement (B) showed only a focal protrusion from the right side of cardiac silhouette (arrowheads) and the lateral image (C) did not show any abnormalities. The image taken 2 years later had no serial change (D), however the image from 3 years and 9 months later (a lateral view; F) clearly showed atrial lead protrusion, while the lead changed to tip-tilted on the frontal view (E). One year later, both of frontal (G) and lateral views (H) demonstrated the progression of atrial lead protrusion. The arrows indicate the distal tip of the atrial lead. (From Sadamatsu K, et al. (2009). Progressive atrial lead perforation developed 5 years after pacemaker replacement. *J Cardiol*, 53,150-153)

10. Conclusion and future research

Atrial lead perforation, especially late onset perforation, is an infrequent phenomenon. However, recent imaging modalities have revealed that the complication is not as rare as has been previously reported, and the available data and knowledge are limited. The use of active-fixation atrial leads is an independent predictor for cardiac perforation following pacemaker implantation, even though the dislodgment rate is low. In addition, active-fixation leads may also be a risk factor for late lead perforation. In the diagnosis of the perforation, patients are often asymptomatic, and the lead parameters are also normal in many cases. Computed tomography can reveal the perforated lead, however the imaging examination is not appropriate for the routine follow-up. Therefore an important question remains how we follow these patients with pacemakers and track down such perforation cases. Although the proper management strategy remains controversial, percutaneous

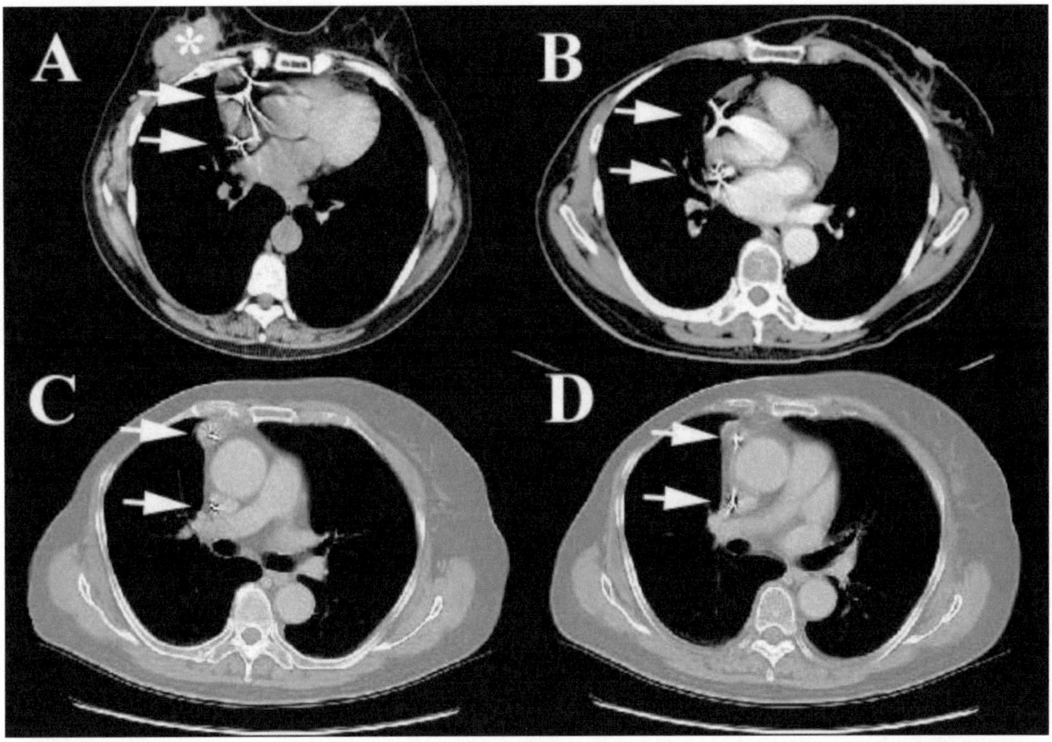

Fig. 2. Computed tomography. (A) Before the replacement of the pacemaker, the scan showed right breast cancer (asterisk) and an atrial lead (arrows). (B) Nine months after the replacement, the new atrial lead (arrows) was screwed in almost the same position as the previous one, and had perforated the right atrial appendage. (C, D) Four years later, consecutive scans clearly showed the progression of the perforated atrial lead (arrows). (From Sadamatsu K, et al. (2009). Progressive atrial lead perforation developed 5 years after pacemaker replacement. *J Cardiol*, 53,150-153)

extraction of the perforated lead in the operating room with a cardiosurgical team backup may be appropriate. Conservative management without extraction is also one of the proposed strategies, however, the long-term safety of this strategy is unknown. Therefore, we should be aware of the potential occurrence of late atrial lead perforation in daily practice for pacemaker follow-up, and large multicenter investigations with long-term follow-up are needed to clarify the details and outcome of this complication.

11. References

Aizawa K, Kaneko Y, Yamagishi T, Utsugi T, Suzuki T, Ishikawa S, Otaki A, Morishita Y, Hasegawa A, Kurabayashi M, Nagai R. (2001). Oozing from the pericardium as an etiology of cardiac tamponade associated with screw-in atrial leads. *Pacing Clin Electrophysiol*, 24, 381-383

Akyol A, Aydin A, Erdinler I, Oguz E. (2005). Late perforation of the heart, pericardium, and diaphragm by an active-fixation ventricular lead. *Pacing Clin Electrophysiol*, 28, 350-351

Dilling-Boer D, Ector H, Willems R, Heidbüchel H. (2003). Pericardial effusion and right-sided pneumothorax resulting from an atrial active-fixation lead. *Europace,* 5, 419-423

Ellenbogen KA, Wood MA, Shepard RK. (2002). Delayed complications following pacemaker implantation. *Pacing Clin Electrophysiol,* 25, 1155-1158

Ellenbogen KA, Hellkamp AS, Wilkoff BL, Camunãs JL, Love JC, Hadjis TA, Lee KL, Lamas G. (2003). Complications arising after implantation of DDD pacemakers: the MOST experience. *Am J Cardiol,* 92, 740-741

Geyfman V, Storm RH, Lico SC, Oren JW 4th. (2007). Cardiac tamponade as complication of active-fixation atrial lead perforations: proposed mechanism and management algorithm. *Pacing Clin Electrophysiol,* 30, 498-501

Glikson M, Hyberger LK, Hitzke MK, Kincaid DK, Hayes DL. (1999). Clinical surveillance of a tined, bipolar, J-shaped, steroid-eluting, silicone-insulated atrial pacing lead. *Pacing Clin Electrophysiol,* 22, 1079-1081

Glikson M, Yaacoby E, Feldman S, Bar-Lev DS, Yaroslavtzev S, Granit C, Rotstein Z, Kaplinsky E, Eldar M. (2000). Randomized comparison of J-shaped and straight atrial screw-in pacing leads. *Mayo Clin Proc,* 75, 1269-1273

Healey JS, Toff WD, Lamas GA, Andersen HR, Thorpe KE, Ellenbogen KA, Lee KL, Skene AM, Schron EB, Skehan JD, Goldman L, Roberts RS, Camm AJ, Yusuf S, Connolly SJ. (2006). Cardiovascular outcomes with atrial-based pacing compared with ventricular pacing: meta-analysis of randomized trials, using individual patient data. *Circulation,* 114, 11-17

Henrikson CA, Leng CT, Yuh DD, Brinker JA. (2006). Computed tomography to assess possible cardiac lead perforation. *Pacing Clin Electrophysiol,* 29, 509-511

Hirschl DA, Jain VR, Spindola-Franco H, Gross JN, Haramati LB. (2007). Prevalence and characterization of asymptomatic pacemaker and ICD lead perforation on CT. *Pacing Clin Electrophysiol,* 30, 28-32

Ho WJ, Kuo CT, Lin KH. (1999). Right pneumothorax resulting from an endocardial screw-in atrial lead. *Chest,* 116, 1133-1134

Ishikawa K, Chida K, Taniguchi T, Watanabe C, Ohkawa S. (1999). Myocardial perforation and/or penetration by a permanent endocardial electrode of the pacemaker in autopsy cases. *J Arrhythmia,* 15, 39-44 [in Japanese]

Khan MN, Joseph G, Khaykin Y, Ziada KM, Wilkoff BL. (2005). Delayed lead perforation: a disturbing trend. *Pacing Clin Electrophysiol,* 28, 251-253

Kono K, Todoroki M, Karasawa T, Ito I, Tadokoro K, Shinbo G, Horinaka S, Matsuoka H, Mochizuki Y. (2008). Delayed pericarditis associated with an implantable cardioverter defibrillator implantation using an active-fixation atrial lead. *Pacing Clin Electrophysiol,* 31, 621-623

Krupienicz A, Karczmarewicz S, Marciniak W, Gniłka A, Kułakowski P, Adamus J. (2000). Passive-fixation J-shaped versus straight leads in atrial position: comparison of efficacy and safety. *Pacing Clin Electrophysiol,* 23, 2068-2072

Laborderie J, Barandon L, Ploux S, Deplagne A, Mokrani B, Reuter S, Le Gal F, Jais P, Haissaguerre M, Clementy J, Bordachar P. (2008). Management of subacute and delayed right ventricular perforation with a pacing or an implantable cardioverter-defibrillator lead. *Am J Cardiol,* 102, 1352-1355

Lamas GA, Lee KL, Sweeney MO, Silverman R, Leon A, Yee R, Marinchak RA, Flaker G, Schron E, Orav EJ, Hellkamp AS, Greer S, McAnulty J, Ellenbogen K, Ehlert F, Freedman RA, Estes NA 3rd, Greenspon A, Goldman L; Mode Selection Trial in Sinus-Node Dysfunction. (2002). Ventricular pacing or dual-chamber pacing for sinus-node dysfunction. *New Engl J Med,* 346, 1854-1862

Luria D, Bar-Lev D, Gurevitz O, Granit H, Rotstein Z, Eldar M, Glikson M. (2005). Long-term performance of screw-in atrial pacing leads: a randomized comparison of J-shaped and straight leads. *Pacing Clin Electrophysiol,* 28, 898-902

Luria DM, Feinberg MS, Gurevitz OT, Bar-Lev DS, Granit C, Tanami N, Eldar M, Glikson M. (2007). Randomized comparison of J-shaped atrial leads with and without active fixation mechanism. *Pacing Clin Electrophysiol,* 30, 412-417

Mahapatra S, Bybee KA, Bunch TJ, Espinosa RE, Sinak LJ, McGoon MD, Hayes DL. (2005). Incidence and predictors of cardiac perforation after permanent pacemaker placement. *Heart Rhythm,* 2, 907-911

O'Neill R, Silver M, Khorfan F. (2010). Pneumopericardium with cardiac tamponade as a complication of cardiac pacemaker insertion one year after procedure. *J Emerg Med,* [Epub ahead of print]

Polin GM, Zado E, Nayak H, Cooper JM, Russo AM, Dixit S, Lin D, Marchlinski FE, Verdino RJ. (2006). Proper management of pericardial tamponade as a late complication of implantable cardiac device placement. *Am J Cardiol,* 98, 223-225

Rydlewska A, Małecka B, Zabek A, Klimeczek P, Lelakowski J, Pasowicz M, Czajkowski M, Kutarski A. (2010). Delayed perforation of the right ventricle as a complication of permanent cardiac pacing - is following the guidelines always the right choice? Non-standard treatment - a case report and literature review. *Kardiol Pol,* 68, 357-361

Sadamatsu K, Enomoto N, Tsuji M, Tashiro H. (2009). Progressive atrial lead perforation developed 5 years after pacemaker replacement. *J Cardiol,* 53, 150-153

Sivakumaran S, Irwin ME, Gulamhusein SS, Senaratne MP. (2002). Postpacemaker implant pericarditis: incidence and outcomes with active-fixation leads. *Pacing Clin Electrophysiol,* 25, 833-837

Spencker S, Mueller D, Marek A, Zabel M. (2007). Severe pacemaker lead perforation detected by an automatic home-monitoring system. *Eur Heart J,* 28, 1432

Srivathsan K, Byrne RA, Appleton CP, Scott LR. (2003). Pneumopericardium and pneumothorax contralateral to venous access site after permanent pacemaker implantation. *Europace,* 5, 361-363

Trigano AJ, Caus T. (1996). Lead explantation late after atrial perforation. *Pacing Clin Electrophysiol,* 19, 1268-1269

Wilkoff BL, Love CJ, Byrd CL, Bongiorni MG, Carrillo RG, Crossley GH 3rd, Epstein LM, Friedman RA, Kennergren CE, Mitkowski P, Schaerf RH, Wazni OM; Heart Rhythm Society; American Heart Association. (2009). Transvenous lead extraction: Heart Rhythm Society expert consensus on facilities, training, indications, and patient management: this document was endorsed by the American Heart Association (AHA). *Heart Rhythm,* 6, 1085-1104

Van Herendael H, Willems R. (2009). Contralateral pneumothorax after endocardial dual-chamber pacemaker implantation resulting from atrial lead perforation. *Acta Cardiol,* 64, 271-273

19

Cardiac Perforation Associated with a Pacemaker or ICD Lead

Seil Oh, MD, PhD, FHRS
Seoul National University Hospital, Seoul, Korea

1. Introduction

Cardiac perforation after pacemaker or implantable cardioverter-defibrillator (ICD) implantation is an infrequent complication. The reported rates of perforation are 0.1-0.8% after pacemaker implantation and 0.6-5.2% after ICD implantation (Khan et al., 2005; Mahapatra et al., 2005). From 1994 to 2009, total 1026 permanent pacemakers and ICDs were implanted in my lab, and two cases (0.2%) developed cardiac perforation without pericardial effusion. However, the incidence rate may be underestimated because some type of perforation does not produce any symptom. Asymptomatic perforation is known to be relatively common (up to 15%) and this can be found incidentally by chest computed tomography (CT) scan (Hirschl et al., 2007).
Although acute presentation is common, delayed presentation can be possible (Khan et al., 2005). The clinical importance is that perforation can lead to longer hospital stays, pacing failure, cardiac tamponade, cardiogenic shock and death (Aizawa et al., 2001; Ellenbogen et al., 2002; Garcia-Bolao et al., 2001; Gershon et al., 2000). In this chapter, information on the overview and management strategy for cardiac perforation will be provided.

2. Cases

2.1 Pacemaker lead perforation

A 64-year-old woman presented to the emergency room with left chest pain which was aggravated with left lateral decubitus position. Four days ago, she underwent implantation of a single chamber permanent pacemaker due to sick sinus syndrome. A passive fixation lead was implanted in the right ventricle. The electrocardiogram and pacemaker analysis revealed sensing and capture failure. Device Interrogation demonstrated unmeasurable capture threshold and normal impedance. Chest X-ray findings indicated lead displacement (Fig. 1). Transthoracic echocardiography excluded pericardial effusion but could not confirm the ventricular lead tip position.
Cardiac CT scan revealed the abnormal lead tip position in the anterior chest wall and confirmed the diagnosis of pacemaker lead perforation (Fig. 2). The displaced lead was removed by open-chest surgery. Surgical exploration showed that the pacemaker lead had perforated the RV and the parietal pericardium without developing hemopericardium. The perforated myocardium was repaired, and a new epicardial pacemaker lead was successfully implanted.

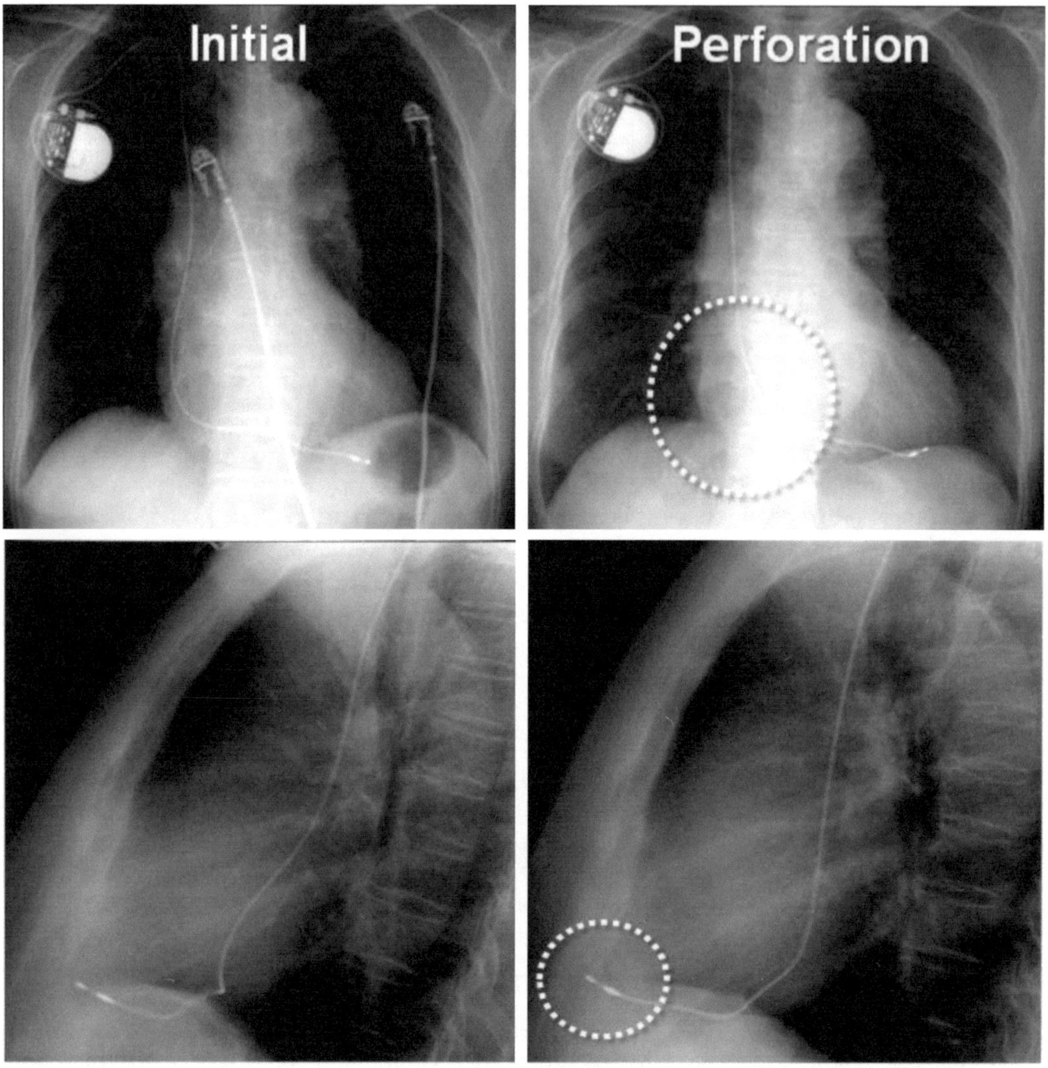

Fig. 1. Initial and perforation chest X-ray. In comparison with the initial images, curvature of the lead in the atrial portion (dotted circle in the posteroanterior view) and the lead tip position (dotted circle in the lateral view) were changed.

2.2 ICD lead perforation

A 32 year-old man with dilated cardiomyopathy underwent ICD implantation due to spontaneous and sustained ventricular tachycardia. Four days after implantation, he experienced one episode of ventricular tachycardia (VT), which was terminated successfully by antitachycardia burst pacing. After the event, he felt left chest pain, which was aggravated by deep inspiration. He visited the device clinic 13 days after the VT event, and device interrogation revealed that the lead parameters were changed as follows: threshold 0.4 volt → capture failure despite 5-volt pacing (Fig. 3); impedance 1080 ohm → 440 ohm; intrinsic sensing 7.0 mV → 3.2 mV. Chest x-ray indicated lead tip displacement, therefore lead repositioning was performed. The migrated lead was removed from the RV apex safely by simple traction under fluoroscopy and echocardiographic monitoring with surgical backup support. Then the lead was re-implanted in the septal area.

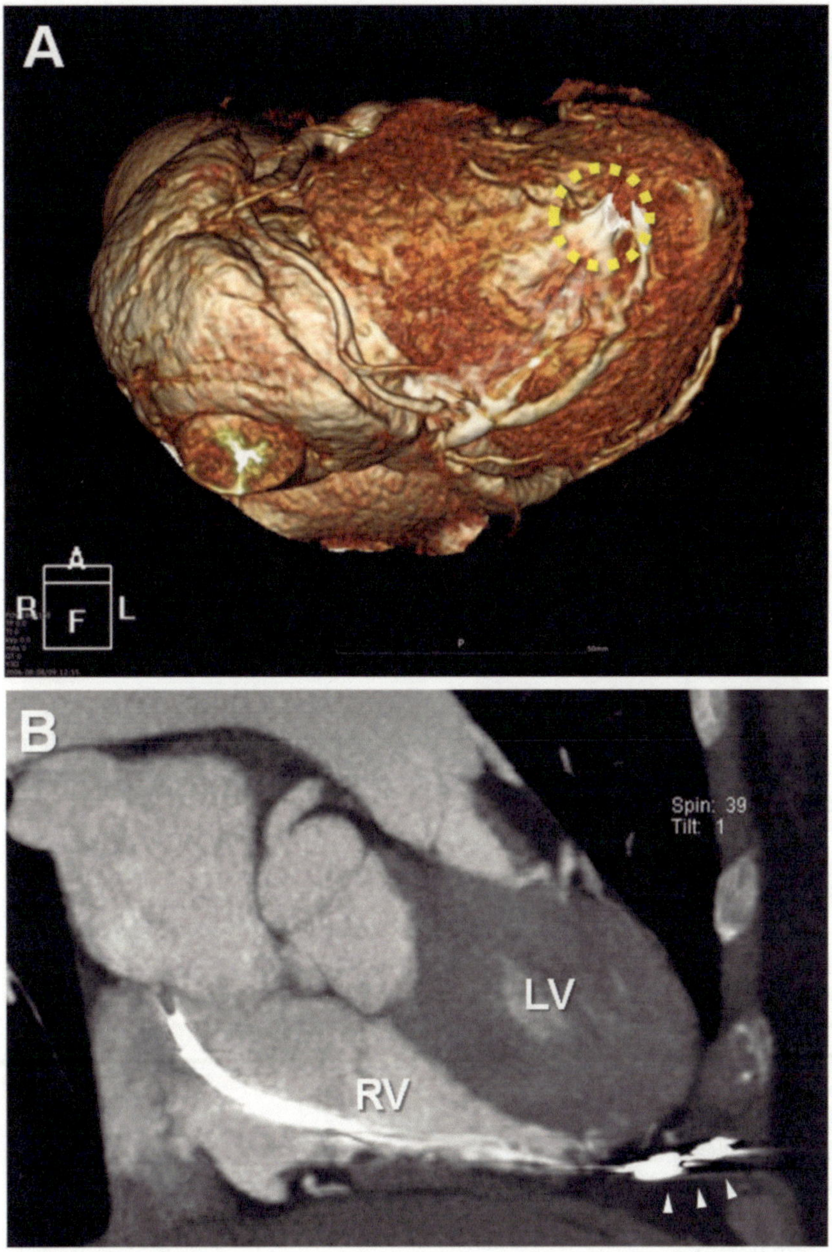

Fig. 2. Multi-detector CT scan images. A, Distal portion of the lead (dotted circle) is observed in the 3D reconstruction image. B, Arrowheads indicate the pacemaker lead penetrating RV apical myocardium and extending to anterior chest wall. LV, left ventricle; RV, right ventricle.

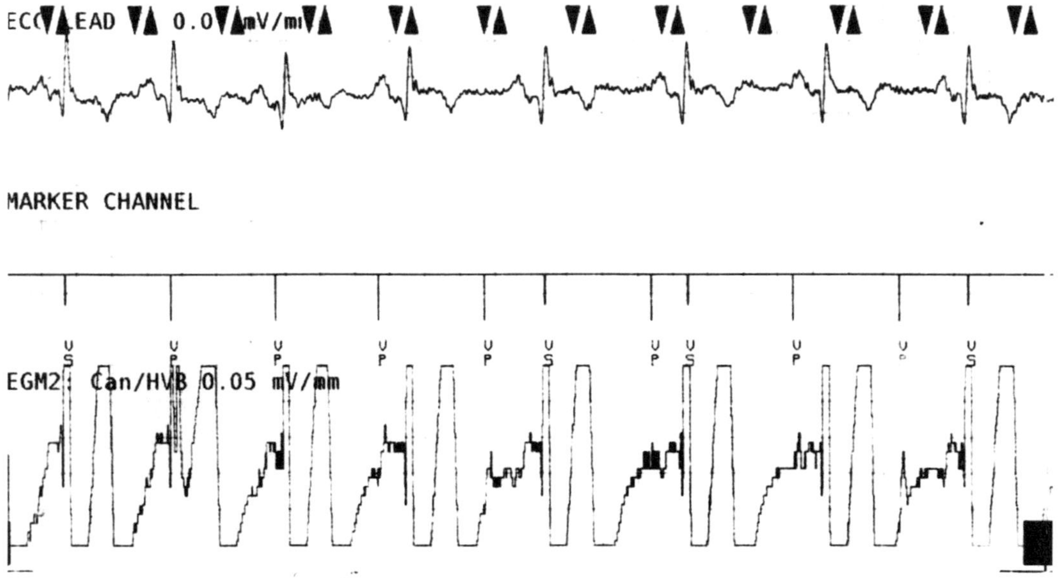

Fig. 3. Capture failure of the ventricular lead. VP, ventricular pacing; VS, ventricular signal sensing.

3. Clinical manifestations

Cardiac perforations are presented with acute, subacute, or delayed manifestations. In general, acute perforation is defined as event within 24 hours after implantation. Delayed perforation is defined by the event which presents at least one month after pacemaker/ICD implantation (Ellenbogen et al., 2002; Rydlewska et al., 2010). Acute perforations usually present with more severe clinical conditions. Delayed perforations seem to have more benign courses because they may be sealed spontaneously.

Symptom, signs and pacing parameter changes would be dependent on the location of the lead tip. A perforated lead tip can be located in pericardial space, extracardiac free space, mediastinum, lung, and chest wall muscles. Therefore, the presenting symptom and signs are variable:

1. Chest pain
2. Dyspnea
3. Hypotension
4. Syncope
5. Capture failure
6. Inappropriate ICD shocks
7. Muscle or diaphragm stimulation
8. Abdominal pain
9. Pericardial effusion
10. Cardiac tamponade
11. Hiccup has been also reported as a result of phrenic nerve stimulation due to cardiac perforation (Celik et al., 2009).

The most common symptom described in the previous reports is pacing or sensing failure. If a lead perforates myocardium, capture threshold will be increased and sensing threshold will be reduced in general. However, impedance will be variable because it depends on the tissue components such as muscle, blood, and air. In some asymptomatic patients with delayed perforation, pacemaker function and electrophysiological parameters appear normal (Hirschl et al., 2007). Therefore, normal pacemaker function cannot exclude cardiac perforation.

Hemodynamic stability is mainly determined by the development of hemopericardium. Hemopericardium and cardiac tamponade needs emergent management and usually requires open-chest surgical correction.

4. Predictors

Cardiac perforation could be associated with any factors that induce myocardial injury or weakening. The predictors of lead perforation have been evaluated by several investigators. They are as follows:

1. Temporary pacemaker implantation
2. Corticosteroid use
3. Active-fixation leads
4. Low body-mass index
5. Older age
6. Longer fluoroscopy times

Mahapatra et al investigated these predictors and found that steroid use was the most powerful predictor by using a multivariate analysis : use of temporary pacemaker (HR 2.7, 95% CI 1.4-3.9, $p = 0.01$), helical screw leads (HR 2.5; 95% CI 1.4-3.8, $p = 0.04$), and steroids (HR 3.2, 95% CI 1.1-5.4, $p = 0.04$) (Mahapatra et al., 2005).

Long-term use of corticosteroid may induce not only skeletal muscle atrophy, but also myocardial atrophy. The effect of chronic steroid use on myocardium may be mediated by some molecules such as muscle ring finger-1, a muscle specific protein (Willis et al., 2009).

Placement of temporary pacemaker before permanent device implantation can affect perforation by several mechanisms. Usually temporary pacing leads are stiffer than permanent leads, thus it could result in more myocardial damage. Situation of temporary pacing such as myocardial infarction might be associated with the risk of cardiac perforation.

A lead type may also increase the risk of cardiac perforation. It may occur more frequently with the following lead types (Rydlewska et al., 2010):

1. Atrial lead
2. Active fixation system
3. ICD lead
4. When excessive length is left.
5. Small diameter
6. High-resistance lead (small tip surface)

However, these have not been evaluated in large clinical trials. An active-fixation lead has a helical screw in its tip to attach the lead tip on the endocardial surface. Mahapatra et al found that ventricular screw leads were associated with cardiac perforation, but Sivakumaran et al reported atrial screw leads were associated with perforation after pacemaker implantation (Sivakumaran et al., 2002). The difference is unclear, which still remains to be elucidated in the further investigations.

Lead location is also a contributing factor. Perforations occur more frequently in the RV apex. This may be associated with the thinner wall thickness of the apex than that of the septum or RV outflow tract (Haq et al., 2008; Khan et al., 2005; Laborderie et al., 2008).
Incidence of cardiac perforations of ICD leads is associated with the number of shocks delivered. Chest trauma may affect perforation, especially during the early period of implantation (Lau et al., 2008; Sassone et al., 2009).
Interestingly, right ventricular systolic pressure >35 mmHg was the only protective factor (HR 0.70, 95% CI 0.50-0.92, P = .02) in Mahapatra et al's study. It may be associated with right ventricular hypertrophy that can be resulted from increased right ventricular pressure. Muscle hypertrophy might be able to reduce cardiac perforation.

5. Diagnosis

A patient with pacemaker and symptom such as chest pain, dyspnea, hypotension, syncope, inappropriate ICD shock, and diaphragm stimulation should be investigated to evaluate the existence of pacemaker-related complications including cardiac perforation. Pacemaker system interrogation, chest radiography and echocardiography can be helpful to evaluate possible extracardiac migration of leads.
Capture and sensing threshold should be compared with the previous values. Usually capture threshold is increased and capture failure is frequently developed as a result. Therefore a highly pacemaker-dependent patient experiences bradycardia-related symptom such as syncope, dizziness and exertional dyspnea. In addition it is easy to develop decrease of sensing threshold. It produces sensing failure and results in inappropriate pacing or ICD shock. Impedance change is variable because it depends on the tissue components such as muscle, blood, and air. If the location of the migrated tip is mainly filled with air (e.g. lung, pericardial space), impedance will be increased. However, if the tip is placed in spaces filled with fluid or blood (e.g. hemothorax, hemopericardium), impedance will not be increased significantly because blood has lower impedance than air. Although inappropriate pacemaker/ICD function may indicate possible perforation, normal function cannot exclude the diagnosis.
Key component of perforation diagnosis is visualization of the lead tip. Therefore, chest radiography, echocardiography (transthoracic or transesophageal), and CT scan are important tests. Chest radiography is useful to compare the lead tip position and lead curvature with those of the initial or previous follow-up data. Lead tip migration may be too subtle to get definite diagnosis in some cases. Diagnosis would be easier if lead migration outside the cardiac silhouette was observed. In addition, it is helpful to evaluate complications associated with perforation: pleural effusion, pericardial effusion, pneumothorax, etc.
Echocardiography is one of the first-line tools to assess the lead location in most cases (Mahapatra et al., 2005). It may show lead tip in the pericardial space and/or pericardial effusion. However, it occasionally fails to demonstrate such findings.
CT scan, especially with multi-detector scanners using cardiac protocols, can be useful when other modalities are nondiagnostic (Henrikson et al., 2006). Thus CT scan is becoming the gold standard in diagnosis of cardiac perforation and lead tip visualization. According to the report on the cases of asymptomatic cardiac perforation in patients who underwent chest CT due to other medical reasons, perforation rates were 15% in atrial leads and 6% in ventricular leads (Hirschl et al., 2007). Sensitivity and specificity of each test modality are still not available due to paucity of systematized studies.

6. Management

Most reports showed that most migrated leads could be removed safely by simple traction under fluoroscopy and/or echocardiographic monitoring in the operating room, with surgical backup support. However, Heart Rhythm Society Expert Consensus classifies this approach as class III for following conditions: *Lead removal is not indicated in patients with known anomalous placement of leads through structures other than normal venous and cardiac structures, (e.g. subclavian artery, aorta, pleura, atrial or ventricular wall or mediastinum) or through a systemic venous atrium or systemic ventricle. Additional techniques including surgical backup may be used if the clinical scenario is compelling* (Wilkoff et al., 2009).

Surgery is generally recommended when cardiac tamponade is expected strongly during extraction, the initial presentation is cardiac tamponade, or the location of the migrated lead is atypical. Therefore management strategy would be dependent on the existence of pericardial effusion. If a case is presented with pericardial effusion, surgical management will be the optimal treatment. If a patient has no pericardial effusion, simple traction can be considered under the guidance of careful monitoring including echocardiography and surgical backups. In asymptomatic cases with normal pacemaker function and no adjacent organ damage, necessity of lead extraction is controversial (Hirschl et al., 2007).

After lead extraction, a new pacemaker lead should be placed at a different location. That is, if the lead was initially placed in the RV apex, RV outflow tract or the septum would be the optimal site. In cases of open-chest surgical correction, epicardial leads would be another option. During the postoperative period, close observation with echocardiography should be performed because delayed cardiac tamponade could develop (Laborderie et al., 2008).

7. Conclusion

Cardiac perforation after pacemaker or ICD implantation is an infrequent complication. The clinical manifestations are variable. The predictors of lead perforation are temporary pacemaker implantation, corticosteroid use, active-fixation leads, low body-mass index, older age, and longer fluoroscopy times. Pacemaker system interrogation, chest radiography and echocardiography can be helpful to evaluate possible extracardiac migration of leads. Computed tomography, especially with multi-detector scanners using cardiac protocols, may be the gold standard. Most migrated leads can be removed safely by simple traction under fluoroscopy and/or echocardiographic monitoring in the operating room, with surgical backup support. Surgery is required when the initial presentation is cardiac tamponade or adjacent structures should be repaired.

8. References

Aizawa K, Kaneko Y, Yamagishi T, Utsugi T, Suzuki T, Ishikawa S, Otaki A, Morishita Y, Hasegawa A, Kurabayashi M and others. (2001). Oozing from the pericardium as an etiology of cardiac tamponade associated with screw-in atrial leads. *Pacing Clin Electrophysiol* 24:381-3.

Celik T, Kose S, Bugan B, Iyisoy A, Akgun V, Cingoz F. (2009). Hiccup as a result of late lead perforation: report of two cases and review of the literature. *Europace* 11:963-5.

Ellenbogen KA, Wood MA, Shepard RK. (2002). Delayed complications following pacemaker implantation. *Pacing Clin Electrophysiol* 25:1155-8.

Garcia-Bolao I, Teijeira R, Diaz-Dorronsoro I. (2001). Late fatal right ventricular perforation as complication of permanent pacing leads. *Pacing Clin Electrophysiol* 24:1036-7.

Gershon T, Kuruppu J, Olshaker J. (2000). Delayed cardiac tamponade after pacemaker insertion. *J Emerg Med* 18:355-9.

Haq SA, Heitner JF, Lee L, Kassotis JT. (2008). Late presentation of a lead perforation as a complication of permanent pacemaker insertion. *Angiology* 59:619-21.

Henrikson CA, Leng CT, Yuh DD, Brinker JA. (2006). Computed tomography to assess possible cardiac lead perforation. *Pacing Clin Electrophysiol* 29:509-11.

Hirschl DA, Jain VR, Spindola-Franco H, Gross JN, Haramati LB. (2007). Prevalence and characterization of asymptomatic pacemaker and ICD lead perforation on CT. *Pacing Clin Electrophysiol* 30:28-32.

Khan MN, Joseph G, Khaykin Y, Ziada KM, Wilkoff BL. (2005). Delayed lead perforation: a disturbing trend. *Pacing Clin Electrophysiol* 28:251-3.

Laborderie J, Barandon L, Ploux S, Deplagne A, Mokrani B, Reuter S, Le Gal F, Jais P, Haissaguerre M, Clementy J and others. (2008). Management of subacute and delayed right ventricular perforation with a pacing or an implantable cardioverter-defibrillator lead. *Am J Cardiol* 102:1352-5.

Lau EW, Shannon HJ, McKavanagh P. (2008). Delayed cardiac perforation by defibrillator lead placed in the right ventricular outflow tract resulting in massive pericardial effusion. *Pacing Clin Electrophysiol* 31:1646-9.

Mahapatra S, Bybee KA, Bunch TJ, Espinosa RE, Sinak LJ, McGoon MD, Hayes DL. (2005). Incidence and predictors of cardiac perforation after permanent pacemaker placement. *Heart Rhythm* 2:907-11.

Rydlewska A, Malecka B, Zabek A, Klimeczek P, Lelakowski J, Pasowicz M, Czajkowski M, Kutarski A. (2010). Delayed perforation of the right ventricle as a complication of permanent cardiac pacing - is following the guidelines always the right choice? Non-standard treatment - a case report and literature review. *Kardiol Pol* 68:357-61.

Sassone B, Gabrieli L, Boggian G, Pilato E. (2009). Management of traumatic implantable cardioverter defibrillator lead perforation of the right ventricle after car accident: a case report. *Europace* 11:961-2.

Sivakumaran S, Irwin ME, Gulamhusein SS, Senaratne MP. (2002). Postpacemaker implant pericarditis: incidence and outcomes with active-fixation leads. *Pacing Clin Electrophysiol* 25:833-7.

Wilkoff BL, Love CJ, Byrd CL, Bongiorni MG, Carrillo RG, Crossley GH, 3rd, Epstein LM, Friedman RA, Kennergren CE, Mitkowski P and others. (2009). Transvenous lead extraction: Heart Rhythm Society expert consensus on facilities, training, indications, and patient management: this document was endorsed by the American Heart Association (AHA). *Heart Rhythm* 6:1085-104.

Willis MS, Rojas M, Li L, Selzman CH, Tang RH, Stansfield WE, Rodriguez JE, Glass DJ, Patterson C. (2009). Muscle ring finger 1 mediates cardiac atrophy in vivo. *Am J Physiol Heart Circ Physiol* 296:H997-H1006.

20

Long-Term Consequences of Endocardial Leads Present in Cardiovascular System

Barbara Małecka
Department of Electrocardiology, Institute of Cardiology, Jagiellonian University Collegium Medicum, John Paul II Hospital in Krakow, Krakow Poland

Acknowledgements to Andrzej Ząbek for his authorship of Figures Section as well as Multimedia Section.

1. Introduction

Endocardial leads for permanent heart stimulation and cardioverter/defibrillator ones have been implanted for 52 and 20 years, respectively. From the very beginning of the age of heart stimulation with the use of endocardial leads, there have been considered reactions of coagulation and immunological systems as well as the changes to the endocardium and the blood vessels in response to the leads in them. In the technological process the leads are covered by external insulation made by polymer materials with bio-compatible properties, that is ones not inducing side effects. Mass implantation of systems for permanent stimulation and implantable cardioverter/defibrillator (ICD) could take place only at the age of developed electronics. Recently we have celebrated the 50th anniversary of permanent heart stimulation. Since that time the number of patients with cardio implants in the right heart have proliferated and also their life expectancy have become substantially prolonged. Over a 50 year-old history of permanent heart stimulation presents a number of arguments to show that ideas of full bio-compatibility of polymer covered leads (usually silicone and polyurethane) were only a wishful thinking. Patients with pacemaker (PM) and ICD systems tend to live longer and possess more, sometimes up to 20 or 30 years old leads in their hearts, which causes a variety of complications.

2. Cardiovascular system response to the leads

2.1 Vegetations and a need for broadening indications for anticoagulant treatment in patients with endocardial leads

Nowadays, an easy access to the echocardiography and especially transesophageal echocardiography (TEE), allows to reveal in the hearts of some patients (5-14%) masses of various consistency, shape and diameter, associated with the leads or the surrounding endocardium, called vegetations (Lo et al., 2006). The term 'vegetation' is a histological term

and means *"a shapeless mass of platelets or fibre, which can contain microorganisms and inflammatory cells"*.
In the echocardiography there can be observed vegetations in shape of loose, moving whips or spherical, compact ones. The former occur in connection with the leads coming across the cavity lumen and follow the flow of blood filling or emptying the heart. The latter, spherical, compact vegetations are sometimes connected with the endocardium surrounding the leads like the stalk. It follows the Byrd division (Byrd, 2007), according to which the right heart vegetations divide into:

1. less compact, long, greatly movable (clot) and
2. more compact, spherical, sometimes having a stalk and less movable (thrombus).

TEE examinations repeated several times in the same patients revealed that vegetations in the right heart are not permanent phenomena, but tend to appear and disappear in the same place; some of them undergo lysis, and other move to the pulmonary bed. According to the above, the existence of vegetations and accounting from it danger of pulmonary embolism needs further detailed studies. Nowadays, there are only case reports of a pulmonary embolism on removal of an infected stimulation system, or an embolism caused by a missing part of a broken lead.
Theoretically there is a number of reasons for pulmonary embolism after an implantation of a PM/ICD system. They are as follows:

1. Stimulation system is a foreign body and stimulates clotting.
2. Anti-thrombotic drugs are stopped for the time of the procedure.
3. In the lead dependent infective endocarditis (LDIE) infected vegetations move to the pulmonary bed.

Yet, the guidelines for the prophylactic anticoagulant drug administration do not list endocardial leads as one of the threats. That suggests the need for broadening the indications for anticoagulant treatment in patients with multi-lead PM/ICD systems, especially in patients with incidentally diagnosed asymptomatic vegetations. Until now, the existence of a vegetation in the left heart could be revealed only after the diagnosis or the suspection of endocarditis.
A vegetation in the right heart with multiple leads constitutes an element of the diagnosis of the endocarditis only in presence of other infective clinical or laboratory symptoms. Finally, the importance of an isolated vegetation with no inflammatory symptoms, is still an unknown. Does the vegetation lead to the infection or result from it?
A conception of the thrombotic endocarditis casts some light on the above doubt. The damage of the endothelium leads to the creation of the microscopic thrombus composed of platelets and fiber and much more exposed to bacterial colonization than healthy endothelium. Two mechanisms take part in the primary creation of the thrombus: damaged endothelium and hyper-coagulability. Hemodynamic situations increasing the turbulence of the blood flow lead to endothelium lesions. A logical conclusion, thus, is that the leads, moving in the blood that continuously flows, can stimulate clotting along their surface, and the thrombi, created in that way, can become infected. An additional stimulus for clotting can be rubbing of the endocardium with the leads moving around or abrasion of the external lead insulation with exposure of its internal metal wire.

2.2 Endothelialization processes

Observations made by cardio-surgeons during the lead removal procedures with the use of cardio-pulmonary bypass present the effects of the productive changes connected with the existence of the leads in the heart cavities. One of those changes is the endothelialization, that is process of covering the leads with smooth endothelium and attaching them firmly to the walls of the cardiovascular system. Thus, the lead, which is a foreign body, becomes separated from the blood flow which makes contact with the bacteria during periods of bacteremia impossible. Endothialization takes place in the regions where the lead is relatively stable regarding the walls of the blood vessel or the heart and adheres well to their endothelium (Esposito et al., 2002).

Can we assume that the process of endothalialization has been already well known, altogether with all its consequences during removal procedures? It is well known though, that it doesn't cover the whole length of the lead. The extent of the lead closed in the tunnel created by the endothelium depends most probably on the polymer used for the lead's insulation, as well as on the spatial localization of the leads in regards to the walls of the blood vessels and the heart cavities. The most privileged places of in growing of the leads to the walls of the blood vessels and the heart, observed during percutaneous and cardio-surgical procedures of lead extraction, constitute a marked map of technical difficulties during these procedures. The strongest, most durable and therefore most difficult to cut off adhesions occur at the junction of the vena innomina and vena cava superior, in the upper part of the right atrium, in the vicinity of the tricuspid valve as well as in the very right auricle (Byrd, 2007). In these places there is an increased risk of perforation and bleeding during lead removal procedures.

3. Lead dependent infective endocarditis

Infective endocarditis (IE) was first described over a 100 years ago. Since late 20th century New Duke's criteria, broadened by echocardiographic examination results, have been introduced. Textbook descriptions of this disease mention, insufficiently though, the difference in the course of IE regarding the left and the right heart. There are significant differences in etio-pathogenetic factor, clinical course of disease and prophylactic indications. The descriptions of the disease and the experience gained after observing the course of IE were obtained on the basis of observation of infected left heart valves and their prostheses. Such observations were possible due to the development of cardio-surgical methods of valve defect corrections since mid 20th century and because of an increasing popularity of left heart implants. IE proceeds with bacteremia of the systemic circulation and severe infection symptoms such as fever (80%), weakness (25-40%), joint and muscle pain (15-30%), appetite and weight loss (30%) accompanied by characteristic skin color (café au lait). The object examination revealed symptoms of heart failure, valve damage, and the effects of complications caused by embolism in the systemic circulation (spleen, skin, kidneys, brain, extremities). There were also noted spectacular but rare vascular symptoms (5-15%): skin extravasations, the effect of a splinter driven into the nail, Ossler's nodules, Roth's retinal spots and a Janeway symptom (Habib et al., 2009). The second part of the 20th century brought the news about the bacterial endocarditis of the right heart. The problem was noticed in drug addicts, and as a iatrogenic complication in patients with catheters in their right heart cavities as well as in patients under long-term hospitalization (Baddour et al., 2003). In the recent years infective complication of long term existence of endocardial leads in the blood vessels and heart cavities have been increasingly observed. Possibility of the right heart infective endocarditis was implicated in patients with permanent PM/ICD systems (Klug et al., 1997). A certain delay in appreciation of the right heart IE in patients

with PM/ICD can be well understood in the face of a later development of the contemporary electrotherapy compared to the cardio-surgical corrections of heart valve defects.
Risk factors of infections connected with PM/ICD systems are as follows: fever prior to the implantation procedure, temporary stimulation, repeated procedure e.i. exchange /revision of a system, early repairs and lack of antibiotic prophylaxis (Klug et al., 2007).
The etiology of the LDIE is predominantly bacterial (90%) and the pathogens responsible are mainly Staphylococci (Aureus and Epidermidis), Streptococci, Enterococci, Pneumococci, Gonococci, group HACEK gram- bacteria, mycobacterium and sporadically fungi (Candida albicans, Aspergillus sp., Histoplasma capsulatum) and other (chlamydia, rickettsias, mycoplasmus).
From the pathomorphologic point of view LDIE is characterized by vegetations visible in the echocardiography, especially in TEE. Vegetations can, in a natural way, migrate to the pulmonary circulation and consequently, lead to pulmonary embolism.
Classic symptoms of LDIE are:

1. Local PM/ICD pocket infection (of different frequency).
2. Pulmonary symptoms: cough and pleural chest pain, dyspnoea, advanced symptoms of pneumonia, atypical lung changes in the x-ray chest scan suggesting pulmonary embolism by infected vegetations (26-41%).
3. Severe inflammatory state of the whole organism: persistent fever (80%), shivers (75%), weakness, feeling tired (75%), loss of appetite (36%), sweats (32%), café au lait skin color (relatively late).
4. Laboratory IE indicators such as blood culture tests results (about 70%), anaemia (66%), leukocytosis (59), increased ESR, CRP (59%), erythrocyturia and albuminuria are rare symptoms of the disease (Greenspon et al., 2008; Massour et al., 2007; Sohail et al., 2008).

This disease entity lacks the symptoms typical for infected vegetations in the left heart (small Duke's symptoms). Vegetations and embolisms do exist but in the pulmonary circulation. For the fact that several symptoms may not reveal, the disease is usually diagnosed very late, and sometimes left undiagnosed until patient's death. Patients with LDIE happen to be referred for pulmonary, medical or even oncologic diagnostic investigations due to atypical and ambiguous changes seen in their chest x-ray scans. Those changes usually subside after antibiotic treatment, with no permanent recovery, though. The disappearance of a vegetation from the echocardiography picture is not synonymous with recovery if the leads are left in heart cavities. In case of repetitive infections it is crucial to consider LDIE in a patient with a cardio-implant in the form of a lead in the right heart, with possible vegetations on it [Figure 1].

4. Multiple endocardial leads, abandoned, migrated – a growing problem in electrotherapy

4.1 Multiple leads

It was assumed that the implanted lead is inexchangable and should be sufficient for the patient's whole life. Thanks to the extended life expectancy of patients with PM/ICDs there has appeared an opportunity to observe endocardial leads staying long in the human body. However, time has verified the above assumption negatively. A logical conclusion seems to be, that the risk of breakage, abrasion or migration ('dropping in') of the inactive lead

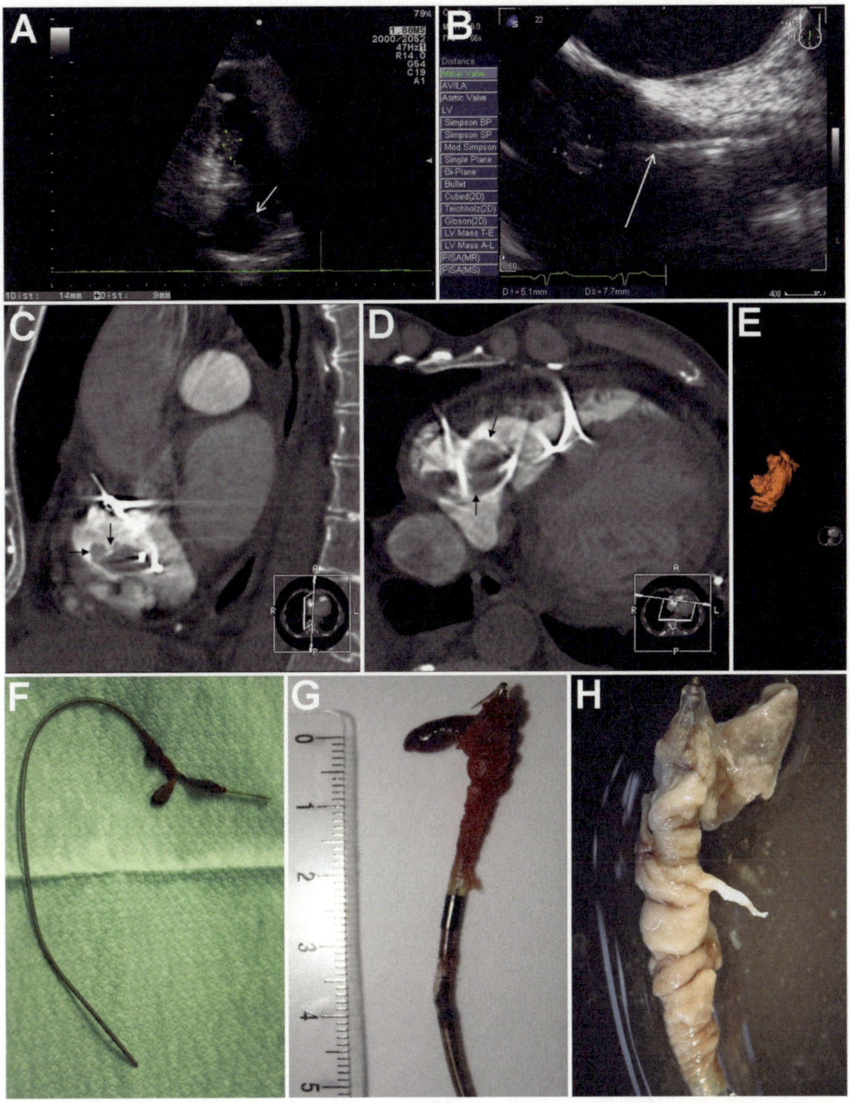

Fig. 1. Vegetations in the course of LDIE visualized by different techniques.

A. TTE: modified 4 - cavity projection. The vegetation connected with the lead in the right ventricle (crosses); the lead (arrow).
B. TEE: 2 - cavity projection. The vegetation connected with the lead in the right atrium (crosses); the lead (arrow).
C. C,D,E. Figures presented thanks to courtesy of dr E. Czekajska - Chehab; Lublin Medical University.
D. C,D. MSCT (Multi Sliced Computer Tomography) of the thorax. MIP (maximum intensity projection) reconstructions. The vegetation connected with the lead in the right atrium (arrow).
E. 3D reconstruction of the vegetation in the patient from figure C&D.
F. Intraoperative picture of the endocardial lead removal procedure with cardio - pulmonary bypass. Visible vegetation connected with the lead.
G. Magnified vegetation from fig. F.
H. Vegetation connected with the lead under the optic microscope.

increases every year further from the implantation. All inactive leads need to be substituted with new ones, older systems can be upgraded and PM systems changed into ICD systems, which results in multiple lead existence in cardiovascular system [Figure 2].

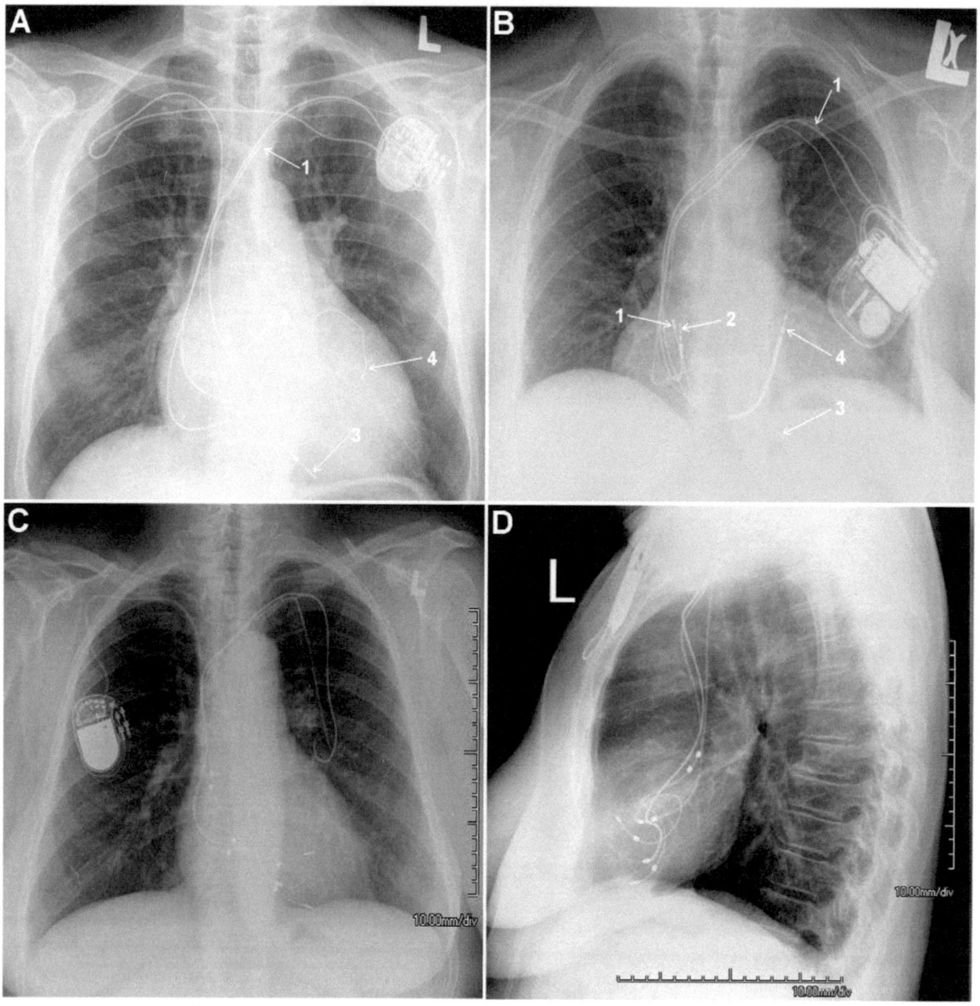

Fig. 2. Multiple leads in chest x-ray scan.

A. Postero-anterior projection in a patient with PM - CRT (Cardiac Resynchronization Therapy).Visible 4 leads: One of the atrial leads broken and migrated to the left subclavian vein (arrow 1); Second atrial lead implanted from the right subclavian vein and lead to the left PM pocket due to the obstruction of the left subclavian vein (arrow 2); Remaining leads: right ventricular (arrow 3) and left ventricular (arrow 4).

B. Postero - anterior projection in the patient with ICD. Visible 4 leads: one of the atrial leads broken and migrated to the left subclavian vein (arrows 1), the other atrial lead is active (arrow 2), abandoned PM lead for right ventricle apical stimulation (arrow 3), ICD lead implanted to the right ventricle outlet track (arrow 4).

C. Postero - anterior projection in the patient with a single lead atrio - ventricular PM system on the right side. Additionally visible two abandoned leads implanted from the left side.

D. Lateral projection in the patient with from fig. C.

4.2 Vascular obstruction

The existence of leads in the veins causes thrombosis and vascular obstruction in high percentage of patients (Rozmus et al., 2005) [Figure 3]. This lead dependent complication of a permanent stimulation can sometimes significantly lower the quality of life of a patient

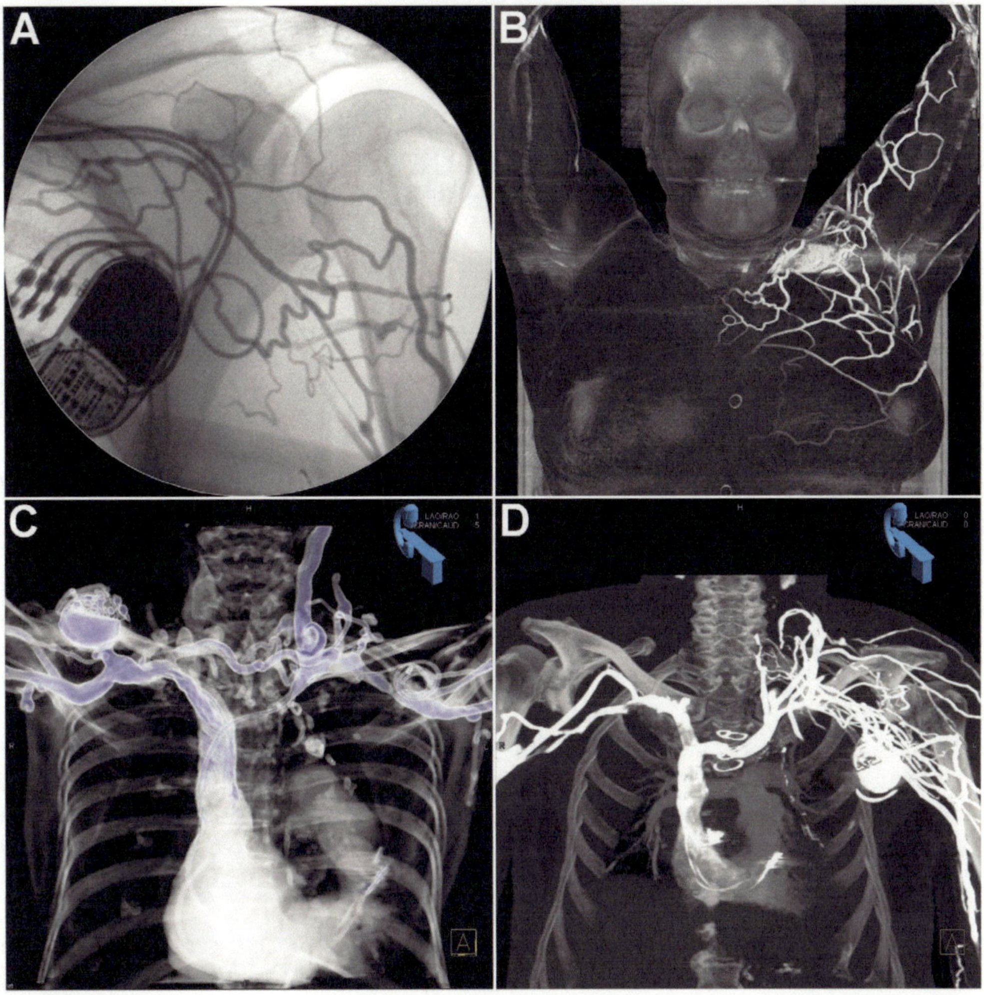

Fig. 3. Vascular obstruction in the presence of the endocardial leads visualized by different techniques

A. Chest X-ray scan: postero-anterior projection. Intraoperative venography of the left vein flow in a patient with PM - CRT. Visible lateral circulation as a result of the obstruction of the left subclavian vein.
B. MSCT in a patient with PM. Visible lateral circulation as a result of obstruction of the left subclavian vein.
C. MSCT in the patient with PM on the right side and abandoned leads on the left side. Visible obstruction of the innominate vein and current lateral circulation as well as narrowing of the right subclavian vein lumen.
D. MSCT in the patient with PM. Visible lateral circulation as a result of obstruction of the left subclavian vein.

(edema of an upper limb, face, in extreme cases a typical vena cava syndrome) but, what is even more important, it makes an implantation of the lead for the planned system upgrade impossible. In such situations it is possible to regain vein lumen by removal of one of the leads, since the lead in the obstructed vein constitutes "the access door" to the heart. There is also a possibility to treat the vascular obstruction by plastic surgery (with the use of the stent or without). The analysis of long-term efficiency of plastic surgery of great veins with endocardial leads present in them has not been made so far.

4.3 Abandoned leads resulting in multiple lead existence in cardio-vascular system

What do we know about the potential risk of abandoning inactive leads in the heart cavities? From the clinical practice it is known that increased number of the leads in the cardio-vascular system causes negative effects to the veins, to the function of the tricuspid valve and PM/ICD pocket. Multiple leads in the heart increase the risk of lead external insulation abrasions, for the fact that the leads continuously rub against one another with frequency of the heart rhythm. External insulations of the leads can, for that reason, undergo mechanical abrasion, exposing their metal wire, and generate thrombosis and secondary pulmonary embolism in those places. In this way a place for 'anchorage' of the dangerous LDIE is created. Coils of the leads' proximal part lying in the pocket enlarge its volume and so increase the risk of the decubitus of the skin which covers the PM/ICD pocket. Apart from that there is a high risk of migration of the proximal end of the abandoned lead inside the vascular system, which can trigger a number of further complications (Bohm et al., 2001). Even though Heart Rhythm Society (HRS) 2009 guidelines present indications for lead removal in particular cases, we should focus not on asking whether to remove an inactive lead but whether if and when we are allowed to leave it in the cardiovascular system (Wilkoff et al., 2009).

4.4 Migrating leads

An abandoned, cut short and not sufficiently fixed lead creates the risk of migration to the cardiovascular system. Active endocardial leads may also migrate to the cardiovascular system after being damaged up to the total break-up. This may occur as a result of the crush syndrome in case of unfavorable position of the lead and the clavicle (Magney et al., 1993). There is also a risk of lead's break-up at the site of ligature tightening on the lead in the pacemaker pocket.

The migration of the lead's proximal end to the subclavian, brachio-cephalic vein or vena cava superior creates loops, which in turn move through the tricuspid valve to the right ventricle provoking valve dysfunction and ventricular arrhythmias [Figure 4].

Sometimes the free end of the lead drops in the right heart cavities or pulmonary artery causing pulmonary embolism.

Practically, every lead, the free end of which is dropped in the cardiovascular system becomes a potential source of the consequences mentioned above and is class 1 (*lead with ending in CVS, which may pose an immediate threat to the patient if left in place, life threatening arrhythmias secondary to retained lead or lead fragment*) or class 2b (*lead which may pose a potential future threat to the patient if left in place*) according to the latest guidelines of the HRS (Wilkoff et al., 2009).

There are no descriptions of percutaneous lead removal procedures with free ends migrated to the cardiovascular system, based on a larger population of patients with such a problem, except single or a few patients case reports.

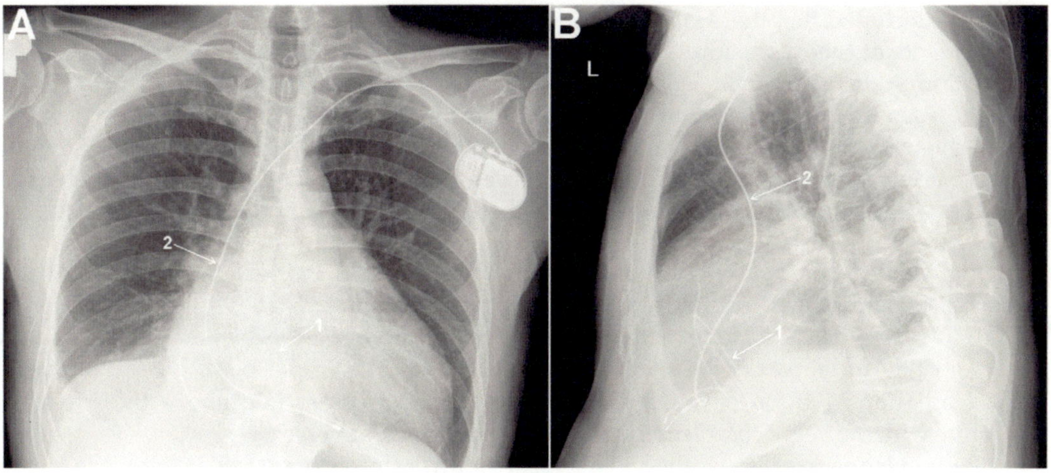

Fig. 4. The lead dropped in and coiled in the heart in the X-ray chest scan in a patient with PM.

A. Postero-anterior projection. Dropped in lead (arrow 1); Active lead (arrow 2)
B. Lateral projection. Labeling leads in A.

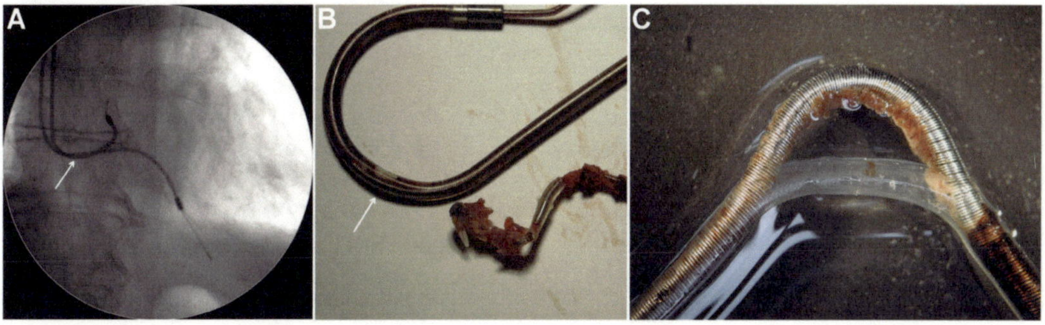

Fig. 5. Inside-heart abrasions of leads in a patient with PM.

A. Chest X-ray scan: postero-anterior projection. Atrio-ventricular PM system with 2 leads. Visible mutual contact of two leads at the bottom of the right atrium (arrow).
B. Intraoperative picture with the removed atrial lead in a patient from figure A: visible abrasion of the lead's silicone insulation (arrow).
C. Optic microscope picture: visible abrasion of the silicone external insulation.

4.5 Mechanical damage of the leads

Studies on the subject have given a number of information about mechanical damage to the endocardial leads resulting from their construction imperfections, implantation procedures as well as human anatomy. A phenomenon of lead abrasion between the clavicle and the first rib in the 'crush syndrome' mechanism as well as external insulation abrasions of the leads coiled in the PM/ICD pocket caused by rubbing against the system can are well known phenomena.

Inside-heart abrasions of silicone lead insulations have also been discovered (Kutarski et al., 2009; Kołodzińska et al., 2010) [Figure 5]. This phenomenon is probably a significant factor in creation and/or generation of vegetations, thrombi and LDIE. It has been proved, that in the group of patients with abraded leads, patients with several leads are predominant. Thus, it can be concluded that there is a certain relation between the number of leads in the heart and incidents of their abrasion. The abrasions have been observed more often in the older stimulation systems: after at least 2 years in the CRT systems and four years in DDD systems. Such findings mean that probability of leads' abrasions is similar in every multi-lead system. A condition under which an abrasion occurs is a specific spacial localization of multiple leads in the right heart. It predisposes bumping or/and rubbing of the leads against one another, with the frequency of the heart beat. The phenomenon of lead abrasion occurs only in the right heart cavities, especially in the atrium and sporadically in the ventricle. Leads' abrasions are possible to occur only when the leads move in opposite directions to one another, with different spatial configurations:

a. a too long atrial lead loop with its distal end in the auricle, which continously rubs against the atrial part of the ventricular lead,
b. a lead running through the coronary sinus outlet crosses right above the tricuspid valve with the ventricular lead running towards the right ventricle,
c. two lead loops cross each other in the right ventricle.

The discovery of endocardial lead abrasions puts the durability of leads for permanent heart stimulation as well as current techniques of their implantation in a new light. Abrasions in the atrio-ventricular systems in which the atrial lead was implanted in the sites where it couldn't move was not observed. This applies to Bachman's bunch (roof of the right atrium), as well as to the anterior part of the atrial septum.

Prospective, randomized research of lead abrasions in people are not possible for ethic reasons. They would have to assume planned lead removals for solely cognitive reasons, with no therapeutic indications for the procedure carrying nearly 1% risk of death. The process of abrasion takes too long to observe it in studies on animals. Endocardial lead external insulation abrasions have been discovered in the leads covered with silicone, which does not exclude the possibility of abrasions in the leads covered with polyurethane or other polymer materials.

4.6 Choice of the lead model

Considering to use a lead for heart stimulation we often tend to forget about possible late, even very far away complications. A lead which is too long for the patient's heart needs to be looped in the pocket several times. In this way a skin decubitus or abrasion of the lead's insulation inside the stimulator pocket is created. We pay too much attention to stimulation conditions ('low-treshold) and leads' dislocation percentage (non-dislocating leads) and much too little to the ways of removing the leads years later. Deffibrillation leads cause most technical problems. Most adhesions (bridges) of the connective tissue are formed in the vena innomina and vena cava superior, and the strongest ones (often obstructing the vein's lumen) are formed on the proximal coil. However, removability constitutes one of the most crucial features of the lead.

5. Lead removal procedures

Percutaneous removal of endocardial leads is the most difficult electrotherapy procedure carrying 1% risk of intraoperative death. It is still an alternative for cardio-surgical procedures, which are more strenuous for the patients and carry 10 times as high percentage of death (Camboni et al., 2008). The later from the implantation procedure the more technical difficulties are encounted during removal with significant increase of its risk. The

growth of the connective tissue around the leads is a well known factor which makes the procedures of percutaneous lead removal more difficult. It increases the risk of great vein and the right heart ruptures with fatal bleeding.
Technical details of every lead removal can contain elements going beyond a stereotypical procedure. Individual anatomical conditions or specific leads' configuration force the operators to create unique, original modifications.
A percutaneous lead removal in presence of large (over 2cm in diameter) vegetations with protection of the pulmonary bed against the pulmonary embolism becomes the challenge of the oncoming times (Małecka el al., 2010). The literature describing lead removal with no laser or radiofrequency back up presents Bongiorni's technique, which uses rotation-cutting forces with/and change of the leads into free floating ones (Bongiorni et al. 2008).

5.1 Removal of leads with proximal ends accessible in the PM/ICD pockets with the use of rotation-cutting forces

Extraction of the leads is initiated by removing the stimulator from the pocket. In presence of an infection, a smear of the pocket discharge and/or blood culture test of the tissue is required. Next, the leads are let off the ligatures in the pocket and the tunnel leading to the large vessel (usually the subclavian vein). Inside the leads 'anchoring' or ' non-anchoring' leaders are introduced. The choice of the type of the leader mostly depends on the condition of the lead's lumen. Our own experience shows that it is usually impossible to use the 'anchoring' leader, which is supposed to carry the pulling forces onto the distal end (of the lead) or the whole lead. It is connected with the advanced age of the removed leads and resulting from it destruction of their structure, a common phenomenon of a 'crush syndrome" in Polish patients (having leads implanted from the unfavourable peristernal puncture of the subclavian vein or working physically hard despite implantation of the endocardial leads).
Not infrequently it is associated with failed attempts to remove the stimulation system in patients' home centers. In the situation when the lead's lumen is distorted and the leader cannot reach the very end of the lead, it seems to be the best solution to stiffen as long section of the lead as possible with a 'non-anchoring' metal leader.
At a later stage of the procedure the proximal lead ends are secured with long, strong, ligatures, which, at the same time, tighten the lead during the process of its being freed from the connective tissue bridges. Those strong ligatures are tied to the leads in such a way to crush and connect all layers of the lead, together with the metal leader inside. The ligatures are tied around the lead in a way to prevent leads' diameter from considerable growth , as well as from cutting it. In case of an 'anchoring' leader being used, the ligatures are additional elements of the traction system.
Steel preparation sheaths of possibly smallest diameter are used to overcome the resistance of tissues in the subclavian region. Having gained the access to the subclavian vein the steel sheaths are substituted with a pair of teflon or polypropylene sheaths, so called Byrd dilators, which act in a telescopic way. The experience shows that the operator should have all dilator sizes (according to colors) and two standard lengths 33/38 and 41/46 cm at hand. In case of encountering a significant resistance (usually in vena cava superior) polypropylene dilators are exchanged for the other ones, usually of a bigger diameter (blue, yellow, green, white, and orange). Recommendations of the company can be confirmed that unipolar leads can usually be removed with the use of blue and yellow dilators, bipolar ones

with yellow or green sheaths, and ICD leads with green or white and sporadically orange dilators.

The lead removal procedure builds upon slow (millimeter after millimeter!) freeing the lead from connective tissue bridges, vegetations, endothelialization tunnels with the use of rotation of a catheter cut diagonally, that is with the use of rotation-cutting forces. At this stage of the procedure and maneuvers associated with it, it is essential for the other operator to keep a proper tension of the lead. The first operator is at the same time highly occupied with proper position (i.e. lengthwise to the wall the blood vessel and later to the heart cavities) of the dilators during maneuvers, which are mainly rotation movements exerting delicate pressure on the lead. A single catheter meets the increased friction resistance the deeper it goes into the vascular system, whereas the technique of a 'catheter in a catheter' allows to move (rotate) dilators with much less resistance from the tissues and a lower risk of breaking or wrenching the dilator off.

From the moment of reaching the ingrown distal end of the lead with the dilators, the phenomenon of a counter traction is put into use, i.e. supporting the tissue around the lead's end and preventing it from moving along with the lead which is being freed and pulled outside.

At all stages of the procedure a careful observation of patient's heart rhythm and vital signs is necessary.

5.2 Removal of dropped-in leads

Such procedures usually do not proceed in a typical way. Most frequently they are a demonstration of operators skills in using various types of anchoring and pulling catheters, and *ad hoc* modifications of techniques offered by the companies.

In order to remove a lead without its end accessible in the pocket, a Byrd workstation is introduced into one of the femoral veins. The catheters to catch the lead are introduced via the workstation. The choice of the catheter depends on the experience and liking of an operator and also on the spatial situation. The 'pigtail' catheter is considered to be the one of the first choice.

The next popular catheter is the Dotter's basket.' Needle snare eye', though, has proved to be of little use in many of the procedures performed so far. It is probably connected with presence of multiple leads in the heart and with the situation when the coiled lead being removed is only one of the leads in the heart. Having grasped the floating end of the lead, it is moved outside the femoral vein. Then the traction used in the sheath that creates counter traction should be sufficient, according to the equipment producers, for pulling the lead from the adhesion in the heart. Own experience shows that the situation is much more complicated. Usually, the lead being removed has some more adhesions to the heart or to another lead. In such cases cutting properties of polypropylene Byrd dilators or other diagonally cut, sharpened catheters can be successfully used.

5.3 Potential complications and safety precautions during percutaneous lead removal procedures

Contrary to the general opinion, the possibility to damage the wall of the right ventricle does not constitute the greatest danger caused by releasing the leads from the connective tissue bridges or the endothelialization tunnels. During percutaneous removals of the old and strongly ingrown and immobilized leads we are mostly concerned with the following:

- Damage of the subclavian vein / vena innomina / vena cava superior: the surgical intervention is most difficult due to the difficult access,
- Damage of the subclavian artery, creation of V –A fistula to a lesser extent,
- Massive pulmonary embolism by the torn off large vegetation,
- Damage of the coronary sinus: applies to removals of left - atrial leads and left - ventricular leads.

During the procedures we are much less concerned with their consequences in the form of damage of the right atrium, right ventricle or tricuspid valve. In such situations the cardio-surgical intervention is not always necessary, and technically easier due to the easy access in case the intervention is indispensable. Massive bleeding to the mediastinum or pleural cavity or massive pulmonary embolism are the most dangerous complications and can lead to death before the delayed cardio-surgical intervention. Thus, the back up of the cardio-surgical and anaesthesiological team ready to act at any moment is essential.

In the presented technique of percutaneous lead removal the key role is the experience of the main operator. Independently from the degree of their training and having in mind the risk of potential complications, it is necessary to backup every procedure of percutaneous lead removal by an experienced cardio-surgeon, prepared for a quick joining of the great vessels or removing of the embolic material from the pulmonary trunk. Safety of such procedures is also increased by the angio-surgeon being available and, if possible, an experienced operative radiologist. It is also desirable to perform the procedure in a cardio-surgical operation room with a high class X-ray apparatus.

6. Spontaneous delayed heart perforation caused by endocardial lead

Incidence of the delayed heart perforation is proved to be low (at 0,1-0,8% for pacemakers implantation and 0,6-5,2% in ICDs) (Khan et al., 2005), probably due to "self-sealing" properties of the ventricle wall: fibrosis, muscle contraction or by the lead itself.

Suspected risk factors for heart perforation are as follows:

- temporary stimulation,
- atrial stimulation,
- stimulation with active fixation system,
- defibrillator leads, with double spirals (more wires, stiffer),
- when excessive length during implantation is left,
- small diameter (increased force per unit area),
- the so-called high resistance (small tip surface).

The literature presents reports about higher perforation rate in case of a certain lead types (eg. Riata ST Jude Medical leads), which might indicate that some constructive elements of the leads may predispose heart perforation. It is known that this condition occurs more often in localizations of the distal end of the lead such as right ventricular apex.

Apart from the two above conditions the state of the heart may also favor perforation.

Anticoagulation and steroid therapy, low body mass index, female gender and incidental chest trauma may trigger perforation.

Delayed right ventricle perforation may have several clinical symptoms:

- chest pain,
- dyspnea,
- syncope (due to improper stimulation or its complete failure),

- inadequate ICD shocks,
- muscle or diaphragm stimulation,
- abdominal pain (due to diaphragm stimulation or lead migration to the peritoneal cavity),
- hiccup (as a symptom of the phrenic nerve stimulation),
- mammary hematoma,
- consequences of the diaphragm, lung, chest wall perforation,
- pleural or pericardial effusion, rarely demanding drainage.

The most common symptom is the electric dysfunction: sensing, pacing and impedance. Sometimes perforation occurs also with normal electrophysiological parameters. Thus, it can be concluded, that improper function may indicate perforation but its normal function does not exclude it.

Perforation diagnosis can be confirmed by visualization techniques:

chest X-ray, transthoracic (TTE) or transoesophageal (TEE) echocardiography and computed tomography [Figure 6]. X-ray is efficient in revealing distal lead end migrations outside the heart and assessing pleural effusion.

Echocardiography can present more discreet changes in lead migration. It is also a good technique for assessing pericardial effusion. The golden mean, however, stays computed tomography (CT).

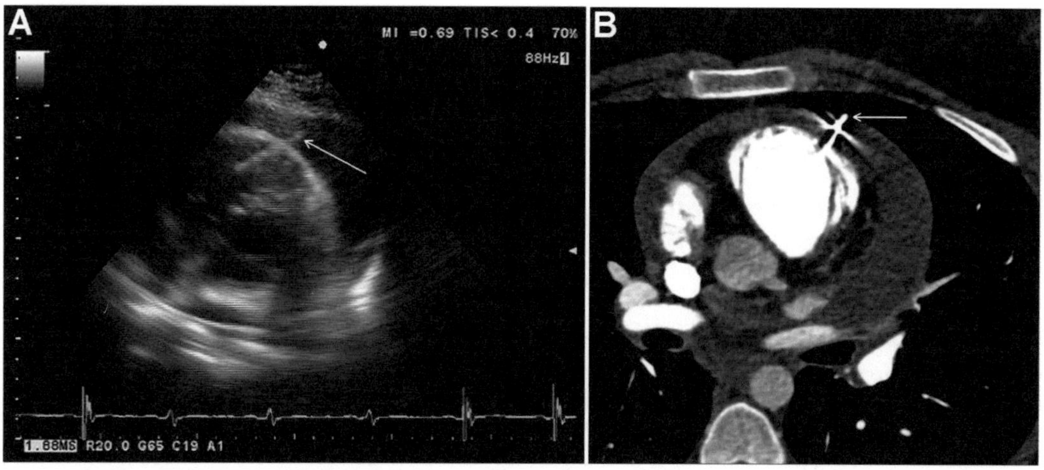

Fig. 6. Delayed heart perforation by endocardial lead visualised by different techniques.

A. Transthoracic echocardiography (TTE).

B. MSCT in the same patient. MIP projection. The lead is perforating the wall of the right ventricle (arrow).

7. References

Baddour L.M., Bettmann M.A., Bolger A.F., Epstein A.E, Ferrieri P., Gerber M.A., Gewitz M.H., Jacobs A.K., Levison M.E., Newburger J.W., Pallasch T.J., Wilson W.R., Baltimore R.S., Falace D.A., Shulman S.T., Tani L.Y., Taubert K.A. (2003). Nonvalvular Cardiovascular Device-Related Infections. *Circulation*, Vol. 108, No. 16 pp. 2015-2031, ISSN 0009-7322

Bohm A., Pinter A., Duray G., Lehoczky D., Dudas G., Tomcsanyi I., Preda I. (2001). Complications due to abandoned noninfected pacemaker leads. *PACE*, Vol. 24, No. 12, pp. 1721-1724, ISSN 0147-8389

Bongiorni M.G., Soldati E., Zucchelli G., Di Cori A., Segreti L., De lucia R., Solarino G., Balbarini A., Marzilli M., Mariani M. (2008). Transvenous removal of pacing and implantable cardiac defibrillating leads using sheath mechanical dilatation and multiple venous approaches: high success rate and safety in more than 2000 leads. *Eur. Heart J.*, Vol. 29, No. 23, pp. 2886-2893, ISSN 0195-668X

Byrd C. L. Managing Device-Related Complications and Transvenous Lead Extraction 855. Ellenbogen K. A., Kay G. N., Lau C.P., Wilkoff B. L. *Clinical Cardiac Pacing, Defibrillation, and Resynchronization Therapy*, Third Edition, Saunders Elsevier 2007. ISBN 978-1-4160-2536-8

Camboni D., Wollmann C. G., Löher A., Gradaus R., Scheld H. H., Schmid C. (2008). Explantation of Implantable Defibrillator Leads Using Open Heart Surgery or Percutaneous Techniques. *Ann Thorac Surg* Vol. 85, No. 1, pp. 50-55, ISSN 0003-4975

Esposito M., Kennergren C., Holmström N., Nilsson S., Eckerdal J., Thomsen P. (2002). Morfologic and Immunohistochemical Observations of Tissues Surrounding Retriver Transvenous Pacemaker Leads. *Biomed Mater Res* Vol. 63, No. 5, pp. 548-558, ISSN 1552-4965

Greenspon A.J., Rhim E.S., Mark G., Desimone J., Ho R.T. (2008). Lead-Associated Endocarditis: The Important Role of Methicillin-Resistant Staphylococcus aureus. *PACE* Vol. 31, No. 5, pp. 548-553, ISSN 0147-8389

Habib G., Hoen B., Tornos P., Thuny F., Prendergast B., Isidre Vilacosta I., Moreillon P., Antunes M., Thilen U., Lekakis J., Maria Lengyel M., Muller L., Naber CK., Nihoyannopoulos P., Moritz A., Zamorano JL., ESC Committee for Practice Guidelines: Guidelines on the prevention, diagnosis, and treatment of infective endocarditis (new version 2009) (2009). Task Force on the prevention, diagnosis, and treatment of infective endocarditis of the European Society of Cardiology; European Society of Clinical Microbiology and Infectious Diseases; International Society of Chemotherapy for Infection and Cancer, *Eur. Heart J.*, Vol. 30, No. 19, pp 2369-2413, ISSN 0195-668X

Khan M., Joseph G., Khaykin Y, Ziada K. M., Wilkoff B. L. (2005). Delayed lead perforation: a disturbing trend. *PACE*, Vol. 28, No. 3, pp. 251-253, ISSN 0147-8389

Klug D., Lacrox D., Savoye C., Goullard L., Grandmougin D., Hennequin J. L., Kacet S., Lekieffre J. (1997). Systemic infection related to endocarditis on pacemaker leads. Clinical presentation and management. *Circulation*, Vol. 95, No. 8, pp. 2098-2107, ISSN 0009-7322

Klug D., Balde M., Pavin D., Hidden_lucet F., Clementy J., Sadoul N., Rey J. L., Lande G., Lazarus A., Victor J., Barnay C., Grandbastien B., Kacet S., for the People Study Group. (2007). Risk Factors Related to Infections of Implanted Pacemakers and Cardioverter-Defibrillators: Results of a Large Prospective Study. *Circulation*, Vol. 116, No. 12, pp. 1349-1355, ISSN 0009-7322

Kołodzińska A., Kutarski A., Grabowski M., Małecka B., Opolski G. (2010). The Late Silicone Leads Abrasions In Their Intracardiac Part. *Heart Rhythm* , Vol. 7, No. 5S, pp. S248-9, ISNN 1547-5271

Kutarski A., Małecka B., Ząbek A. (2009). Mutual abrasions intracardiac leads-important finding among explanted leads. *Europace*, Vol. 11, No. S2, ISNN 1099-5129

Lo R., D'Anca M., Cohen T., Kervin T. (2006). Incidence and prognosis of pacemaker lead-associated masses: a study of 1,569 transesophageal echocardiograms. *J Invasive Cardiol*, Vol.18, No. 12, pp. 599-601, ISSN 1042-3931

Magney J.E., Flynn D.M., Parsons J.A., Staplin D.H., Chin-Purcell M.V., Milstein S., Hunter D.W. (1993). Anatomical mechanisms explaining damage to pacemaker leads, defibrillator leads, and failure of central venous catheters adjacent to the sternoclavicular joint. *PACE*, Vol. 16, No. 3 Pt 1, pp. 445-457, ISSN 0147-8389

Małecka B., Kutarski A., Tomaszewski A., Czekajska - Chehab E., Ząbek A. (2010). Transvenous removal of endocardial leads with coexisting great vegetation (3.5 cm) - case report. *Europace* , Vol. 12, No. 3, pp. 445-446, ISSN 1099-5129

Massoure P-L., Reuter S., Lafitte S., Laborderie J., Bordachard P., Clementy J., Raudaut R. (2007). Pacemaker Endocarditis: Clinical Features and Management of 60 Consecutive Cases. *PACE*, Vol. 30, No. 1, pp. 12-19, ISNN 0147-8389

Rozmus G., Daubert J. P., Huang D. T., Rosero S., Sala B., Francis C. (2005). Venous Thrombosis and Stenosis After Implantation of Pacemakers and Defibrillators. *Journal of Interventional Cardiac Electrophysiology* 2005, Vol. 13, No. 1, pp. 9-19, ISNN 1383-875X

Sohail M. R., Uslan D. Z., Khan A. H., Friedman P.A., Hayes DL, Wilson W.R., Steckelberg JM, Jenkins S.M., Baddour L.M. (2008). Infective Endocarditis Complicating Permanent Pacemaker and Implantable Cardioverter-Defibrillator Infection. *Mayo Clin Proc*. Vol. 83, No. 1, pp. 46-53, ISNN 0025-6196

Wilkoff B.L., Love C.J., Byrd C.L., Bongiorni M.G., Carrillo R.G., Crossley G.H. 3rd, Epstein L.M., Friedman R.A., Kennergren C.E., Mitkowski P., Schaerf R.H., Wazni O.M. (2009). Transvenous lead extraction: Heart Rhythm Society expert consensus on facilities, training, indications, and patient management: this document was endorsed by the American Heart Association (AHA), *Heart Rhythm*, Vol. 6, No. 7, pp. 1085-104, ISNN 1547-5271

21

Pacing System Malfunction: Evaluation and Troubleshooting

Majid Haghjoo, MD, FACC, FESC
Rajaie Cardiovascular Medical and Research Center,
Iran University of Medical Sciences,
Iran

1. Introduction

Currently, most of the time spent caring for the patients with permanent pacemaker will be concerned with evaluating the function of the previously implanted pacing system. Pacing system malfunction can be secondary to pacemaker circuitry failure or to lead dysfunction. Various tools are available to help evaluation of the pacing system malfunction, including physical examination, standard 12-lead ECG, ambulatory ECG monitoring, stored telemetry data, chest x-ray, and fluoroscopy.
This chapter will discuss the differential diagnosis, evaluation, and management of the common malfunctions encountered in the single-chamber, dual-chamber, and biventricular pacing system.

2. Single-chamber pacing system malfunction

Although many pacing system malfunction are common to single-chamber and dual-chamber devices, the latter are more challenging. This section will discuss the common malfunctions associated with single-chamber pacing systems. The subsequent sections will focus on specific abnormalities associated with dual-chamber and biventricular pacing systems.
Depending on the presence or absence of pacing artifact, the potential problems identifiable on an ECG can generally be assigned to three categories: 1) pacing artifact present with failure to capture, 2) pacing artifact absent with failure to pace, 3) pacing artifact present with failure to sense.

2.1 Pacing artifact present with failure to capture

To differentiate between different categories of the pacing system malfunctions, it is essential to identify the pacing artifact. This can be done easily in unipolar system with large pacing artifact. However, it can problematic in dual-chamber devices with diminutive pacing artifact. There are two important issues related to the pacing artifact that can cause great difficulty in differential diagnosis of pacing system malfunction. Some ECG recording systems, such as holter monitoring and in-hospital monitoring units, contain special filter to eliminate baseline noise (Sheffield et al, 1985).These filters can markedly reduce the size of pacing artifact in the unipolar pacing system and effectively erase the pacing stimuli in the bipolar system. In these situations, recording of the multiple simultaneous or sequential ECG leads with older analog ECG machines would be highly helpful. In addition, newer recording systems (e.g. telemetry system and holter recorder) have unique algorithms for pacemaker pulse detection that generate a discrete artifact in response to any high-frequency signal. Therefore, even nonpacemaker signals may be displayed as pacing artifact. Electromagnetic interference, loose ECG electrode connections, and subthreshold pulses (minute ventilation sensors) are examples of nonpacemaker signals.

The causes of failure to capture with pacing artifact present are summarized in Table 1. The onset of malfunction in relation to implantation of pacing system can provide valuable data to identification of the cause. If failure to capture occurred shortly (hours or days) after implant, the most likely diagnosis is lead dislodgment or perforation. Loss of capture weeks to months after implantation is most probably due to lead maturation process. Currently, this problem is rarely seen because of routine use of the steroid-eluting electrodes. This malfunction occurs between 2 to 6 weeks after implantation. If loss of capture of capture occurs several months to years after implantation, structural injury in the lead insulation or conductor should be suspected. Other less common causes in this period are exit block, metabolic abnormalities, pharmacological agents, misprogramming, and battery depletion.

Lead dislodgment is accompanied by a change in the paced QRS morphology and/or the lead position in repeat chest x-rays. A change in the paced QRS morphology is diagnostically useful when fusion with native QRS complexes is absent. Depending on presence or absence of a visible change in the lead position on a repeat chest x-ray, lead dislodgment can classified as "macro-dislodgment" or "micro-dislodgment". Other distinguishing features are normal pacing impedance and elevated thresholds. Incidence of the lead dislodgment has markedly reduced with the introduction of active fixation leads. However, active lead implantation does not guarantee long-term lead stability (Furman et al, 1975). Correction of this malfunction requires surgical intervention. Before reoperation, the cause of dislodgment should be identified. An examination of anchoring sleeve for adequate fixation, looking for adequate amount of current-of-injury in the recorded electrograms at the implant time, and looking for proper lead slack on postimplant chest x-ray would be highly informative. In most cases, lead repositioning is enough but thrombus developed around the lead tip may effectively prevent the lead tip to be fixed at new position. The latter situation, lead dislodgement with no identifiable cause and repeated dislodgment after prior lead repositioning requires new active lead implantation. *Lead perforation* usually occurs at the time of implant or within the first 24 hours (Aggarwal et al, 1995), although this complication has been reported up to 10 months after the device implantation (Haghjoo, 2010). In addition to loss of capture, perforation manifests itself by lead migration to pericardial, pleural, or peritoneal space. Lead perforation can be confirmed by the negative current of injury at implant. *Lead maturation* is an inflammatory reaction that is produced following lead tip contact with endocardium (Furman et al, 1979; Furman et al, 1977). Local tissue swelling displaces the electrode tip from excitable myocardium and, consequently, increases the capture threshold. Although incidence of this problem was significantly reduced in steroid-eluting leads (Mond et al, 1988; Kein et al, 1990), a significant rise in threshold may occur despite the introduction of steroid-eluting leads and other innovation in lead design (Ellenbogen et al, 1999). This process occurs between 2 to 6 weeks after implantation. To minimize the probability of noncapture, a high output setting is recommended during this period. Any threshold rise after this period is considered to be in the chronic phase of lead maturation. If the threshold rise resulted in noncapture, it is referred to as exit block (Sheppard et al, 1991; Davies & Sowton, 1966). Acute and chronic phase of lead maturation are not associated with a change in paced QRS morphology or lead location in chest x-ray. Acute threshold rise occasionally responds to systemic steroids. A regimen of prednisone, 60 mg (1 mg/kg) per day, is found to be effective in one-half of the patients (Levine, 2005). Exit block does not respond to systemic steroids and require lead repositioning or new lead implantation.

Lead dislodgment
Micro-dislodgment
Macro-dislodgment
Perforation
Lead maturation process
Early inflammation
Late fibrosis- exit block
Mechanical lead injury
Insulation failure
Conductor fracture
Iatrogenic malfunctions
Loose setscrew
Misprogramming
Elevated pacing thresholds
Metabolic abnormalities
Electrolyte disturbances
Myocardial infarction
Cardiomyopathy
Pharmacological agents
Pseudomalfunctions

Table 1. Causes of failure to capture with pacing artifact present

Lead insulation failure is mainly due to extrinsic forces exerted to the lead either at or following implantation. Insulation damage has reported both in silicone- and polyurethane-coated leads (Kertes et al, 1983). Excessively tight suture on the anchoring sleeve, lead passage between clavicle and first rib, and abrasion between overlapping coils or between leads and housing of the pulse generator are three common causes of the insulation defect in clinical practice (Dunlap et al, 1983; Magney et al. 1993). ECG with an insulation failure involving a unipolar lead will show a decrease in amplitude of pacing artifact. An insulation damage involving outer insulation of a coaxial bipolar lead will show an increase in the amplitude of the pacing artifact (unipolarization). Failure of the internal insulation of a coaxial bipolar lead will results in a decrease in the amplitude of pacing artifact. This is best identified with an analog ECG recording system. Chest x-ray is normal in the patients with insulation failure because insulation material is radiolucent. Another specific feature of insulation defect is reduced lead impedance.

Lead conductor fracture is the most common cause of an open circuit. Although the clinician might expect that fracture of a lead would result in the absence of any visible pacing artifact, this is frequently not the case. This occurs because the current passes across the gap in the conductor coil though the fluid in the lead with high resistance. In such circumstances, energy reaching the heart is subthreshold with no capture, but a stimulus will be present. The ECG with an intermittent conductor fracture may show a varying amplitude artifact if recorded with an analog machine. Lead fracture is associated with infinitely high lead impedance if the insulation remains intact. However, total lead transsection (concomitant conductor fracture and insulation defect) may show normal or minimally elevated impedance. Chest x-ray may show conductor fracture (figure 1). In contrast to the unipolar lead, diagnosis of the conductor fracture is very difficult in a coaxial bipolar lead unless there is total disruption of both conductors at the same place. Reprogramming to unipolar mode is a temporary measure in partial fracture of bipolar lead. In pacemaker-dependent patients with complete lead transsection, temporary pacemaker implantation is necessary before definitive management. Definitive treatment of conductor fracture is lead replacement.

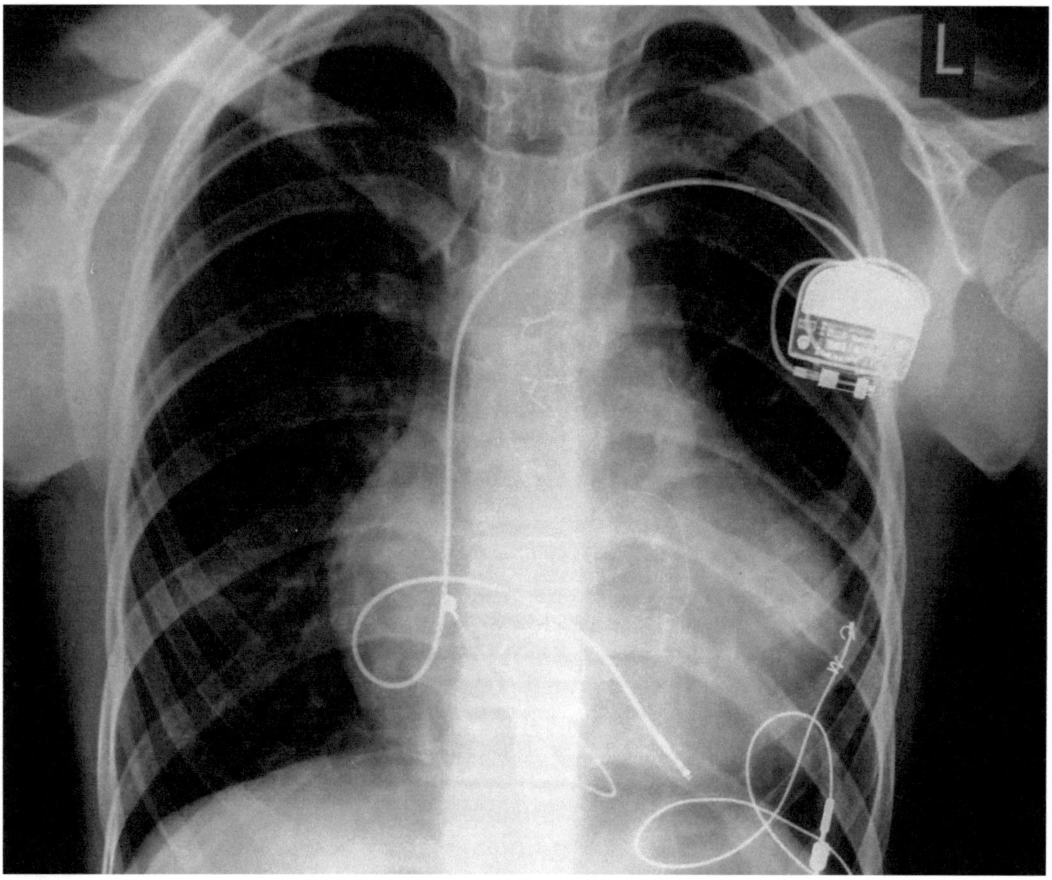

Fig. 1. This chest x-ray illustrates a typical example of conductor fracture with intact insulation. Conductor fracture occurred near to the fixation sleeve.

Loose set screw usually presents with failure to output due to complete disconnection of the lead pin and the connector. Sometimes, minimal contact between the pin and the connector may permit the transmission of the electrical current, but delivered energy is not enough to capture the paced chamber. This problem is produced because of the inadequate tightening of the lead pin within the connector block. The presence of air or fluid within the connector can produce similar clinical picture. ECG usually may show a decrease in the amplitude of the pacing artifact. Chest x-ray clearly shows the displacement of the terminal pin out of the head of pacemaker. Reoperation with pin reconnection is necessary to correct these malfunctions.

Battery depletion manifests several years after device implantation. Pacemaker-dependency is major determinant of the battery longevity. Although modern pacemakers attempt to maintain the programmed values until the battery is depleted, actual output will fall below the capture threshold and resulting in the loss of capture. ECG and chest x-ray show no abnormalities. Pacing threshold is increased as measured via depleted generator but is normal through the pacing system analyzer. Definitive management requires the generator replacement.

Late rise in the pacing threshold may also occur secondary to the *myocardial infarction, cardiomyopathy, metabolic abnormalities, and pharmacologic agents* (Schlesinger et al, 1980; Hughes, et al, 1975; Preston & Judge 1969; Guarnieri et al, 1988). Any severe electrolyte or metabolic abnormalities can increase pacing threshold. These abnormalities include acidosis, alkalosis, hypoxemia, hypercarbia, hyperkalemia, hyperglycemia, and hypothyroidism. In addition, threshold rise and noncapture may be due to some pharmacological agents such as bretylium, class Ic antiarrhythmic drugs, sotalol, and mineralocorticoids. Myocardial infarction and cardiomyopathy can cause noncapture by producing nonexcitable tissue near the lead tip. Increasing the programmed output, correcting the cause, and the lead repositioning are the therapeutic options in these situations.

2.2 Pacing artifact absent with failure to pace

In this category of pacing system malfunction, the clinician must be certain that a malfunction truly exists before taking any corrective measure. Already diminutive pacing artifact of the bipolar pacing may be further obscured by being isoelectric in a given lead. New pacemaker algorithms for minimal ventricular pacing may also present with absence of the pacing artifact. Similarly, hysteresis and sleep function can mimic this malfunction.

Differential diagnosis of pacing artifact present with failure to pace is listed in Table 2. *Oversensing* is the most common cause of intermittent pauses without pacing artifact.

Oversensing
Physiological signals- T-wave, myopotential
Nonphysiologic signals- Electromagnetic interference
Nonphysiologic signals- Make-break signals
Open circuit
Conductor fracture
Loose set screw
Insulation failure
Battery depletion
Pulse generator component malfunction
Pseudomalfunctions
Sleep function
Hysteresis
Algorithms for minimizing ventricular pacing

Table 2. Causes of failure to pace

Oversensing is the sensing of a physiologically inappropriate or nonphysiologic signal. Oversensing is more common in the unipolar pacing. T-waves and myopotentials are major sources of the physiologically inappropriate signals. Myopotential oversensing either inhibits the ventricular output in the ventricular channel or triggers ventricular output when sensed on the atrial channel of a DDD pacemaker. T-wave oversensing can similarly produce long asystole in pacemaker-dependent patients. If the native signal is sufficiently large, reducing the ventricular sensitivity can easily correct this abnormality.

Nonphysiologic electrical signals may also cause oversensing. The potential sources of electromagnetic interference (EMI) are electrocautery, electrolysis, radiofrequency (RF) ablation, cardioversion, defibrillation, lithotripsy, magnetic resonance scanner, positron emission tomographic scanner, high voltage power line, cellular and cordless phone, transcutaneous electrical nerve stimulation, and radiotransmission (AM and FM). Other nonphysiologic source of oversensing is make-break signals. If of sufficient amplitude, these signals can cause significant oversensing and long pauses. The most common sources of make-break signals are loose set-screw, partial conductor fracture, failure of the internal insulation of bipolar lead, loose active fixation screw, and interaction between active and abandoned leads. Diagnosis of the oversensing can be confirmed by applying magnet or programming to asynchronous mode. The oversensing-related pauses are relieved by before-mentioned maneuvers. The definitive treatment differs depending on the sources of oversensing. The lead problems require lead replacement, or repositioning, or correction of the loose connection. Oversensing related to the physiological signals can be treated by reprogramming or lead repositioning. EMI-related oversensing needs avoidance from EMI sources.

Open circuit secondary to conductor fracture or loose set screw are second most common cause of pauses associated with absence of the pacing artifact. As it was mentioned previously, open circuit usually present with loss of capture in the absence of pacing artifact. Measured data telemetry will show infinitely high pacing impedance. Chest x-ray can be diagnostic in unipolar lead but conductor fracture is difficult to detect in case of a bipolar lead. Magnet application has no effect on pauses associated with open circuit. Definitive treatment is the lead replacement or tightening of the pin within the header.

Lead insulation failure can cause failure to capture in the absence of pacing artifact mainly because of oversensing. Again, malfunction persists after magnet application. Reprogramming to unipolar mode can temporarily correct the malfunction until definitive treatment is done.

Pulse generator malfunction is the least common cause of the pacing system malfunction. This malfunction does not respond to magnet application. Pacemaker interrogation shows inconsistent measurements or inaccessible data. Pulse generator replacement is the only effective treatment.

2.3 Pacing artifact present with failure to sense

A proper sensing require good quality signal with adequate amplitude and slew rate. Apparently high amplitude signal may not be appropriately sensed because of the slow slew rate (Furman et al, 1977). Undersensing is characterized by the inappropriate pacing because of underdetection of the intrinsic signals (figure 2). The etiologies of the undersensing are listed in Table 3. As in failure to capture, onset of the undersensing in relation to implantation time may direct the clinician to the correct diagnosis. Early-onset undersensing is most probably due to *lead dislodgment or lead perforation.* Late-onset undersensing is frequently caused by *mechanical lead problems (insulation failure and partial open circuit) or programming errors*. Occasionally, they are attributable to a *change in the morphology of the intrinsic cardiac signal*.

In addition to failure to capture, the *lead dislodgment* is frequently associated with undersensing. In this circumstance, displaced lead will record a signal different from and usually smaller than that recorded at implant. Perforated lead similarly records a smaller signal. Therefore, sensing failure will occur in both situations. Definitive management is the lead replacement.

Lead insulation failure can be associated with sensing failure due to attenuation of the incoming signal. Other corroborating features are increased capture threshold, decreased pacing impedance, increased battery drain, and reduced amplitude of the pacing artifact. Curative treatment will require lead replacement or repair.

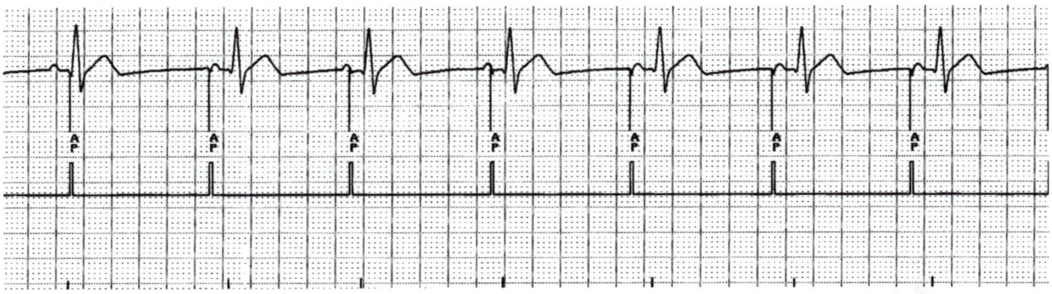

Fig. 2. This tracing shows inappropriate atrial pacing because intrinsic depolarization is not seen by the pacemaker.

Lead dislodgment
Micro-dislodgment
Macro-dislodgment
Perforation
Lead maturation process
Mechanical lead injury
Insulation failure
Partial open circuit
Battery depletion
Elevated pacing thresholds
Metabolic abnormalities
Electrolyte disturbances
Myocardial infarction
Cardiomyopathy
Pharmacological agents
Pseudomalfunctions
Asynchronous mode
Triggered mode
DVI mode
Safety pacing

Table 3. Causes of sensing failure

Partial open circuit is another cause of the undersensing. If the two ends of the conductor are making any contact at all, resistance to incoming signal will reduce the amplitude of the filtered signal and undersensing will occur. Infinitely high impedance is an important diagnostic feature. Chest x-ray is also diagnostic in some cases. Correction of this malfunction requires lead replacement or reconnection of the lead pin within the connector block.

Change in the native signal amplitude occurs secondary to myocardial infarction, cardiomyopathy, metabolic abnormalities, and some pharmacologic agents.

As the *pulse generator begins to become depleted,* intermittent or persistent undersensing may occur. *Stuck reed switch* is another rare cause of the undersensing. Placing *magnet over the pacemaker or triggered mode* are other causes of the failure to sense. In pacemakers using *impedance plethysmography as a rate modulation sensor,* removal of generator out of the pocket will result in the asynchronous pacing in response to a lot of electrical noise. Definitive treatment of the undersensing depends on the underlying cause.

3. Dual-chamber pacing system malfunction

Dual-chamber pacing system malfunctions can be categorized into two groups: 1) general dual-chamber pacing system malfunctions; 2) specific dual-chamber pacing system malfunctions.

3.1 General dual-chamber pacing system malfunctions

All abnormalities previously discussed in the section of the single-chamber pacing system malfunctions can occur with either channel of the dual-chamber pacemakers. However, malfunctions easily detected in single-chamber pacemakers may be very difficult to diagnose in dual-chamber devices. For example, detection of the ventricular loss of capture may be very challenging in the presence of normal atrioventricular (AV) conduction. In this situation, changing the AV interval can be very useful. Occasionally, it is not easy to detect atrial noncapture in the dual-chambers pacing systems. In this situation, programming to AAI mode or increasing AV interval will readily unmask the malfunction. Atrial undersensing may be difficult to recognize in the presence of an intact sinus node function. Oversensing in dual-chamber pacing systems can result in inappropriate inhibition or triggering depending on the channel on which oversensing occurs and the programmed pacing mode. Atrial channel oversensing will result in rapid ventricular pacing whereas oversensing in the ventricular channel will inhibit both atrial and ventricular channels.

3.2 Specific dual-chamber pacing system malfunctions

Crosstalk is the sensing of the far-field signal in the opposite chamber, causing the pacemaker to either inhibit or trigger an output depending on its design. Crosstalk can occur in any dual-chamber mode in which atrium is paced and the ventricle is sensed and paced (DVI, DDI, and DDD). In the presence of complete heart block, inhibition of the ventricular pacing can be life-threatening (Sweesy et al, 1988). Crosstalk is more difficult to detect in the presence of intact AV conduction. Several factors predispose the patients to crosstalk inhibition of the ventricular output: unipolar atrial and ventricular leads, high atrial output, high ventricular sensitivity, and short ventricular blanking and refractory periods. Crosstalk is diagnosed by the ventricular sensing in the absence of a QRS complex in the telemetered marker channels and corrected by the magnet application.

There are several preventive strategies to avoid the crosstalk or its sequel. Use of a bipolar lead with adequate amplitude and pulse width, proper ventricular sensitivity, use of the ventricular blanking period, and safety pacing are the main approaches to prevent the crosstalk (Batey et al, 1985; Barold & Belott, 1987).

Pacemaker-mediated tachycardia (PMT) is characterized by the active participation of the pacemaker in the tachycardia (figure 3). There are several forms of PMT. Typical form of PMT is endless-loop tachycardia (ELT). ELT only occur in patients with P-synchronous dual-chamber pacing (DDD, VDD) and intact retrograde ventriculoatrial conduction. ELT is classically initiated by a PVC. If the PVARP has expired and retrograde P-wave is sensed, the sensed atrial event triggers the ventricular output. This setups a repetitive sequence of the sensed retrograde P-wave, triggering a ventricular output at the end of maximum tracking rate interval (Den Dulk et al, 1982). In addition to PVC, atrial undersensing, atrial oversensing, and atrial noncapture may initiate ELT. PVARP extension after a sensed ventricular event is the main defense against the ELT. If ELT is initiated, PVARP extension and withholding the ventricular output for one cycle are the major modalities to terminate ELT. Second form of PMT is secondary to tracking of atrial signals (atrial tachycardia/flutter/fibrillation) (figure 4) or oversensing on the atrial channel (Greenspan et al, 1984). This is not a pacemaker malfunction and terminated by applying magnet. Third form of PMT is called repetitive nonreentrant ventriculoatrial synchronous rhythm (Love, 2007). Several factors predispose the patient to this kind of PMT. First, intact ventriculoatrial conduction is needed. Second, a sufficiently long PVARP should be programmed to avoid ELT induction. Third, a relatively rapid baseline rate is also required to render the atrial tissue refractory. In this condition, retrograde P-wave is not sensed (functional undersensing) allowing atrial escape interval to be completed and atrial pulse is delivered with no capture (functional noncapture). Then, the ventricular output is delivered at the end of the programmed AV interval. Therefore, this rhythm is characterized by ventricular pacing, atrial undersensing, and atrial noncapture in the presence of normally functioning dual-chamber DDDR or DDIR pacemakers (figure 5). To prevent this rhythm, a new algorithm called noncompetitive atrial pacing (NCAP) has been introduced. Other preventive strategies are providing short AV intervals at high rates or AAI pacing.

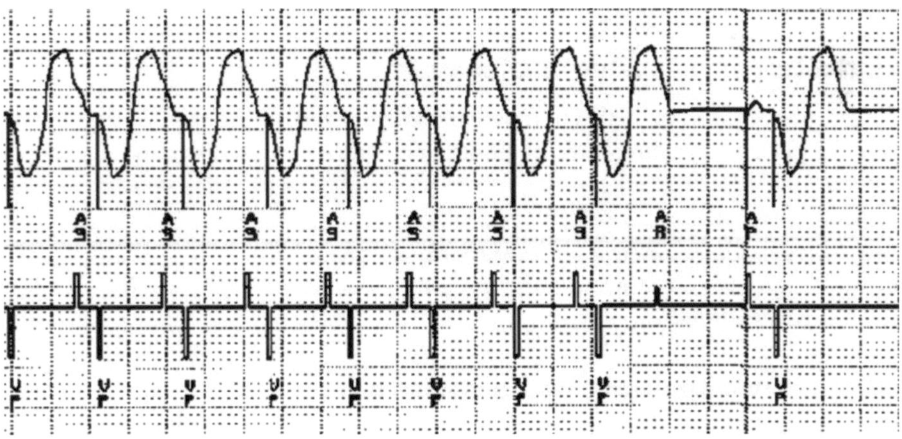

Fig. 3. This tracing was recorded from a patient with dual-chamber pacemakers who presented with frequent palpitations. Pacemaker interrogation showed frequent episodes of pacemaker-mediated tachycardia initiated by a PVC and terminated by a P-wave falling within the PVARP.

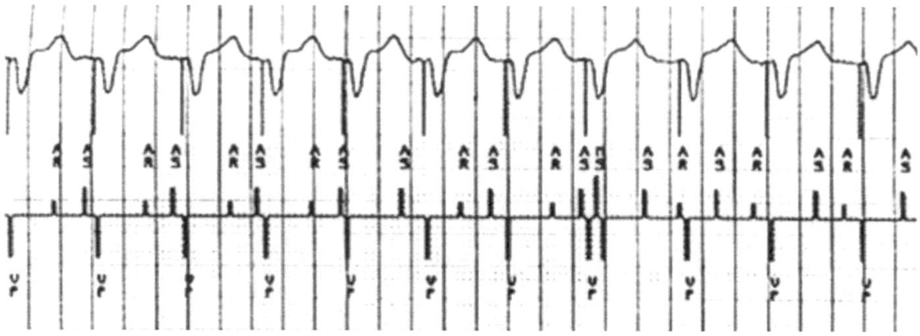

Fig. 4. This figure is recorded from a patient with dual-chamber pacemaker and paroxysmal palpitations. Device interrogation showed tracking of the atrial signals during paroxysmal atrial tachycardias.

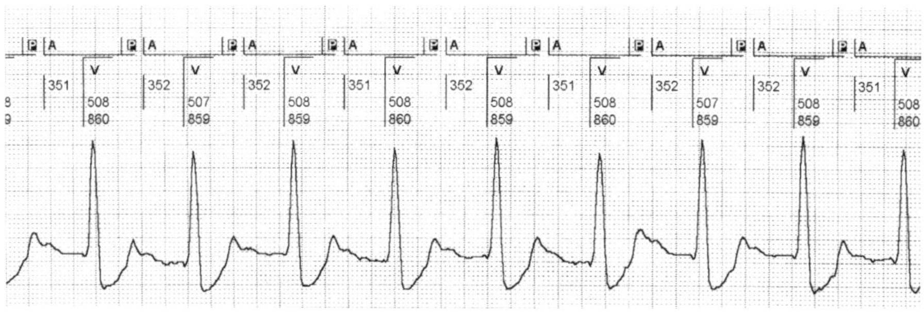

Fig. 5. This figure shows a classical example of repetitive nonreentrant ventriculoatrial synchronous rhythm. This rhythm is characterized by ventricular pacing, atrial undersensing, and atrial noncapture in the presence of normally functioning dual-chamber pacemakers.

4. Biventricular pacing system malfunction

Biventricular pacing system malfunctions can be categorized into two groups: 1) general biventricular pacing system malfunctions; 2) specific biventricular pacing system malfunctions.

4.1 General biventricular pacing system malfunction

This category includes all abnormalities previously discussed in the section of single- and dual-chamber pacemakers.

4.2 Specific biventricular pacing system malfunction

As the left ventricular (LV) lead is not as secure as the right ventricular (RV) lead, LV lead dislodgment is more common than RV lead. However detection of noncapture in the LV lead is very difficult because of the intact RV pacing. Baseline ECG recording after implant would be highly useful in this regard. Therefore, LV lead noncapture mainly present with heart failure decompensation.

5. Pseudomalfunctions

Pseudomalfunctions are defined as unexpected ECG findings that appear to result from pacemaker malfunction but that represent normal pacemaker function. Pseudomalfunctions should be ruled out as the cause(s) of an anomalous ECG strip before corrective measures are taken.

Pseudomalfunctions may be classified into three categories: 1) rate change, 2) anomalous AV interval or refractory period, and 3) mode change.

5.1 Rate change

Rate changes in the presence of normal pacemaker function may occur secondary to magnet operation, timing variations (A-A vs. V-V), upper rate behavior (wenckebach or 2:1 block), electrical reset, PMT intervention, and rate response. Furthermore, hysteresis, rate drop response, mode switching, and sleep function have varying degrees of impact on the rate. *Magnet operation* varies within different products and from manufacturer to manufacturer, but will usually involve a rate change (increase or decrease depending on manufacturer) when the magnet is applied. *Wenckebach block* has the characteristic Wenckebach pattern of the PR interval gradually extending beat-to-beat until a ventricular beat is dropped. Wenckebach block occurs when the intrinsic atrial rate begins to exceed the upper rate limit. The ventricular response to the intrinsic atrial event cannot exceed the upper rate limit, so the AV interval is lengthened until the upper rate expires and a ventricular pace can be delivered. An atrial sensed event eventually falls into the refractory period and is not seen, and therefore not followed, by a ventricular pace. *Two to one block* is characterized by atrial rates that occur at intervals less than the total atrial refractory period (TARP). Every other P-wave falls into the refractory period and is therefore not preceded by a paced ventricular event. Patients who experience 2:1 block, particularly those who are active at the time the event occurs, will feel the precipitous drop in rate, which is cut in half. *Electrical reset* may occur secondary to exposure to EMI such as electrocautery, defibrillation, etc. These EMI sources can cause both rate and mode changes (back-up mode). As it was mentioned previously, *PMT intervention* is designed to terminate PMT. In Medtronic pacemakers, when PMT intervention is turned ON, the PVARP will be forced to 400 msec after the ninth paced ventricular event. By extending the PVARP, the intent is to interrupt atrial tracking for one cycle and break the PMT. After an intervention, PMT Intervention is automatically suspended for 90 seconds before the pacemaker can monitor for a PMT again. In *rate responsive pacemakers*, physical activity will cause an increase in the pacing rate. However, some patients may experience "false positive" increases in rate from their sensors. In the case of a piezoelectric crystal, the pacemaker may begin pacing at a faster rate if, for example, the patient is either lying on the side that the pacemaker is implanted on or experiencing a bumpy car ride. Similarly, minute ventilation sensors measure the change in respiration rate and tidal volume. If a patient experiences rapid respiration resulting from a cause other than exercise (e.g., hyperventilation), the pacemaker may begin pacing at a faster rate. *Hysteresis* provides the capability to maintain the patient's intrinsic heart rhythm as long as possible, while providing back-up pacing if the intrinsic rhythm falls below the hysteresis rate. Because hysteresis exhibits longer intervals after sensed events, it may be perceived as oversensing. *Rate drop response* will exhibit pacing at high rates if the detection criteria are met. Rate drop response therapy prevents a precipitous decrease in the rate in patients experiencing cardioinhibitory neurally-mediated syncope. *Mode switching* is used to prevent the tracking of the atrial signals in paroxysmal atrial tachycardia, atrial flutter, or atrial fibrillation in the DDD(R) and VDD(R) modes. Mode switching is associated both with rate slowing and mode change to DDI(R) or VVI(R). Sleep function is designed to provide a slower rate while patient sleeping.

5.2 Anomalous AV interval and refractory period

AV interval or refractory periods may appear anomalous due to safety pacing, blanking, rate-adaptive AV delay, sensor-varied PVARP, PVC response, and NCAP. *Safety pacing* is designed to prevent inhibition due to crosstalk. This algorithm delivers a ventricular output 110 ms after an atrial paced event. Therefore, safety pacing is manifested as abbreviated AV interval. *Blanking* is the first portion of the refractory period during which the pacemaker is "blind" to any activity. Blanking is designed to prevent multiple detection of a single paced or sensed event by the sense amplifier. However, if the blanking period is too long, it may not sense an event and cause inappropriate pacing. *Rate-adaptive AV delay* is designed to mimic the intrinsic response to increasing heart rate. In a normal heart, PR intervals decrease as the heart rate increases. Conversely, as the heart rate decreases, PR intervals increase. The rate-adaptive AV delay can be programmed to mimic the normal physiologic response of the PR interval to increasing heart rates. When *sensor-varied PVARP* is enabled, the duration of the PVARP will shorten as the rate increases. *PVC response* designates a PVC as a ventricular sensed event following a ventricular event with no intervening atrial event. When a PVC is detected, and PVC response is programmed ON, the PVARP is extended in order to avoid sensing the retrograde P-wave that could occur as a result of the PVC. Pacemaker-defined PVC will initiate a V-A interval. This extended PVARP (if PVC response is ON) and subsequent resetting of the timing interval may appear anomalous on an ECG. *NCAP* can be used in an effort to prevent atrial pacing from occurring too close to a refractory sensed event. If NCAP is programmed ON, the scheduled atrial output will be delayed until at least 300 msec has elapsed since the refractory sensed P wave occurred. PAV interval may then be shortened to maintain a stable ventricular rate.

5.3 Mode change

Change in pacing mode may occur secondary to electrical reset, mode switching, and noise revision. Electrical reset and mode switching have been described in the section of mode change. The portion of the refractory period after the blanking period ends is commonly called the "noise sampling period." A sensed event in the noise sampling period will initiate a new refractory period and blanking period. Continuous refractory sensing is called *noise reversion* and will cause pacing to occur at the sensor-indicated rate for rate-responsive modes and cause pacing to occur at the lower rate for non-rate responsive modes.

6. Conclusions

Pacing system malfunctions can be secondary to the pacemaker circuitry failure or to the lead dysfunction. Although primary malfunctions of the pulse generators do occur, they are least common cause of the malfunctions related to the pacing system. More commonly, problems are related to the damaged leads or primary abnormality at electrode-myocardial interface. Not uncommonly what appears to be pacemaker malfunction may actually represent normal functioning of the pacemaker.

7. References

Aggarwal, R.; Connelly, D.; Ray, S.; Ball, J. & Charles, R. (1995). Early complications of permanent pacemaker implantation: no difference between dual and single chamber systems. *Br Heart J*, 73, 6, (June 1995), 571-575, 1355-6037.

Barold, S. & Belott, P. (1987). Behavior of the ventricular triggering period of DDD pacemakers. *Pacing Clin Electrophysiol*, 10, 6, (November 1987), 1237-1252, 0147-8389.

Combs, W.; Reynolds, D.; Sharma, A. & Bennett, T. (1989). Crosstalk in bipolar pacemakers. *Pacing Clin Electrophysiol*, 12, 10, (October 1989), 1613-1621, 0147-8389.

Davies, J. & Sowton, E. (1966). Electrical threshold of the human heart. *Br Heart J*, 28, 2, (March 1966), 231-239, 1355-6037.

Dulk, K.; Lindemans, F.; Bar, F. & Wellens, H. (1982). Pacemaker-related tachycardias. *Pacing Clin Electrophysiol*, 5, 4, (July 1982), 476-485, 0147-8389.

Dunlap, T.; Popak, K. & Sorkin, R. (1983). Radiographic pseudofracture of the Medtronic bipolar polyurethane pacing lead. *Am Heart J*, 106, 1, (July 1983), 167-168, 0002-8703.

Ellenbogen, K.; Wood, M.; Gilligan, D.; Zmijewski, M. & Mans, D. (1999). Steroid eluting high impedance pacing leads decrease short- and long-term current drain: results from a multicenter clinical trial. CapZure Z investigators. *Pacing Clin Electrophysiol*, 22, 1, (January 199), 39-48, 0147-8389.

Furman, S.; Hurzeler, P. & De Caprio, V. (1977). Cardiac pacing and pacemakers III: Sensing the cardiac electrogram. *Am Heart J*, 93, 6, (June 1977), 794-801, 0002-8703.

Furman, S.; Hurzeler, P. & Mehra, R. (1977). Cardiac pacing and pacemakers IV. The threshold of cardiac stimulation. *Am Heart J*, 94, 1, (July 1977), 115-124, 0002-8703.

Furman, S.; Pannizzo, F. & Campo, I. (1979). Comparison of active and passive adhering leads for endocardial pacing. *Pacing Clin Electrophysiol*, 2, 4, (July 1979), 417-427, 0147-8389.

Greenspan, A.; Greenberg, R. & Frank, W. (1984). Tracking of atrial flutter by DDD pacing, another form of pacemaker-mediated tachycardia. *Pacing Clin Electrophysiol*, 7, 6, (November 1984), 955-960, 0147-8389.

Guarnieri, T.; Datorre, S.; Bondke, H.; Brinker, J.; Myers, S. & Levine, J. (1988). Increased pacing threshold after an automatic defibrillatory shock in dogs: effects of class I and class II antiarrhythmic agents. *Pacing Clin Electrophysiol*, 11, 9, (September 1988), 1324-1330, 0147-8389.

Haghjoo, M.; Alizadeh, A.; Fazelifar, A.; Hajahmadi, M. & Sadr-Ameli M. (2010). Delayed cardiac perforation by one small body diameter defibrillator lead. *J Electrocardiol*, 43, 1o, (January-February 2010), 71-73, 0022-0736.

Hughes, J.; Tyers, G. & Torman, H. (1975). Effects of acid-base imbalance on myocardial pacing thresholds. *J Thorac Cardiovasc Surg*, 69, 5, (May 1975), 743-746, 0022-5223.

Kein, H.; Steinberger, J. & Knack, W. (1990). Stimulation characteristics of a steroid-eluting electrode compared with three conventional electrodes. *Pacing Clin Electrophysiol*, 13, 2, (February 1990), 134-137, 0147-8389.

Kertes, P.; Mond, H.; Sloman, G.; Vohra, J. & Hunt, D. (1983).Comparison of lead complications with polyurethane tined, silicone rubber tined, and wedge tip leads: clinical experience with 822 ventricular endocardial lads. *Pacing Clin Electrophysiol*, 6, 5, (September 1983), 957-962, 0147-8389.

Levine, P. (2005). Evaluation and management of pacing system malfunctions, In: *Cardiac pacing and ICDs*, Ellenbogen, K. & Wood, M. (4th Ed.), p.329, Blackwell publishing, 978-1-4051-0447-0, Massachusetts.

Preston, T. & Judge, R. (1969). Alteration of pacemaker threshold by drug and physiologic factors. *Ann N Y Acad Sci*, 167, No, (October 1969), 686-692, 0077-8923.

Love, C. (2007). Pacemaker troubleshooting and follow-up, In: *Clinical cardiac pacing, defibrillation, and resynchronization therapy*, Ellenbogen, K.; Kay, G.; Lau, C. & Wilkoff, B. (3rd Ed.), pp.1054-1055, WB Saunders, 978-1-4160-2536-8, Philadelphia.

Mond, H.; Strokes, K.; Helland, J.; Grigg, L.; Kertes, P; Pate, B. & Hunt D. (1988). The porous titanium steroid-eluting electrode: a double-blind study assessing the stimulation threshold effects of steroid. *Pacing Clin Electrophysiol*, 11, 2, (February 1988), 214-219, 0147-8389.

Magney, J.; Flynn, D.; Parsons, J.; Staplin, D; Chin-Purcel, M.; Milstein, S. & Hunter, D. (1993). Anatomical mechanisms explaining damage to pacing leads, defibrillator leads and failure of central venous catheters adjacent to the sternoclavicular joint. *Pacing Clin Electrophysiol*, 16, 3, (March 1993), 445-457, 0147-8389.

Schlesinger, Z.; Rosenberg, T.; Stryjer, D. & Gilboa, Y. (1980). Exit block in myxedema, treated effectively with thyroid hormone therapy. *Pacing Clin Electrophysiol*, 3, 6, (November 1980), 737-739, 0147-8389.

Sheffield, L.; Berson, A.; Bragg-Remschel, D.; Gillette, P.; Hermes, R.; Hinkle, L.; Kennedy, H.; Mirvis, D. & Oliver, C. (1985). AHA special report: recommendation for standards of instrumentation and practice in the use of ambulatory electrocardiography. *Circulation*, 71, 3, (March 1985), 626A-636A, 0009-7322.

Shepard, R.; Kim, J.; Colvin, E.; Slabaugh, J.; Epstein, A. & Bargeron Jr, L. (1991). Pacing threshold spikes months and years after implant. *Pacing Clin Electrophysiol*, 14, 11, (November 1991), 1835-1841, 0147-8389.

Sweesy, M.; Batey, R. & Forney, RC. (1988). Crosstalk during bipolar pacing. *Pacing Clin Electrophysiol*, 11, 11, (November 1988), 1512-1516, 0147-8389.

22

Infections of Permanent Pacemakers and Implantable Cardioverter- Defibrillators

Metallidis Symeon – Pilalas Dimitris
Aristotle University of Thessaloniki
Greece

1. Introduction

The rapid evolution of technology in recent decades has led to the development of several new implantable devices that help to improve or sustain life. Both cardiovascular and orthopedic medicines are among the specialties most affected by these advances. New and improved versions of early devices are being introduced routinely.

Cardiac prosthetic devices have become an integral part of modern cardiovascular medicine. Since the initial use of prosthetic heart valves in 1953 as a treatment for aortic regurgitation, other permanent indwelling devices, including permanent pacemakers (PPMs) and implantable cardioverter defibrillators (ICDs), have been shown to improve survival rates, reduce symptoms, or both. The growing number of evidenced-based indications for cardiac devices coupled with an aging population ensures a continued increase in the implantation of cardiac devices for the foreseeable future.

Worldwide, there are approximately 3.25 million functioning pacemakers and 180000 functioning implantable cardioverter defibrillators (Chua, Wilkoff et al. 2000). Although cardiac devices have prolonged the lives of countless patients, they also paradoxically place these same patients at risk for a number of complications, including infection. Infection rates for these devices range from 1% to 7%, and the optimal method for management of such infection has yet to be defined.

In 2003, the American Heart Association published a scientific statement that reviewed a variety of nonvalvular cardiovascular device infections (Baddour, Bettmann et al. 2003). The 7 years after the publication of the 2003 document have witnessed exceptional advances of several clinical aspects of cardiovascular device infections. In particular, CIED infections have received the bulk of the attention, with sentinel observations regarding the epidemiology, associated risk factors, and management and prevention of permanent pacemaker (PPM) and implantable cardioverter-defibrillator (ICD) infections.

In an analysis of CIED implantation in the United States between 1997 and 2004, implantation rates for PPMs and ICDs increased by 19% and 60%, respectively (Zhan, Baine et al. 2008). Approximately 70% of device recipients were 65 years of age or older and more than 75% of them had 1 or more coexisting illnesses. Similarly, the frequency of ICD implantation increased in the elderly (70 to 79 years of age) and very elderly (80 years of age or older) (Uslan, Tleyjeh et al. 2008). The 2001 World Survey found that in developed countries, between 20% and 35% of CIED recipients were more than 80 years old. The

National Hospital Discharge Survey found a 49% increase in the number of new CIED implantations, including both PPMs and ICDs, in the United States between 1999 and 2003 (Voigt, Shalaby et al. 2006).

2. Incidence and epidemiology

PPM endocarditis has been recognized since the early 1970s. In earlier years, the rates of PPM infection ranged widely between 0.13% and 19.9% (Bluhm 1985). Although most infections have been limited to the pocket, PPM endocarditis accounts for approximately 10% of PPM infections (Arber, Pras et al. 1994).

The first ICD was implanted in 1980 (Mirowski, Reid et al. 1980). Subsequent decreases in the size of ICDs permitted implantation without thoracotomy, although initially, abdominal implantation with tunneling was required. Subsequently, the entire device could be implanted prepectorally. The infection rate with these less extensive operations was lower (7%) (Mela, McGovern et al. 2001).

Cabell et al reported that among Medicare beneficiaries, the rate of cardiac device infections (PPMs, ICDs, valves, and ventricular assist devices) increased from 0.94 to 2.11 per 1000 beneficiaries between 1990 and 1999, a 124% increase during the study period. The rate of endocarditis was relatively unchanged (0.26 and 0.39 cases/ 1000 beneficiaries, respectively) (Cabell, Heidenreich et al. 2004).

The National Hospital Discharge Survey similarly showed that between 1996 and 2003, the number of hospitalizations for CIED infections increased 3.1-fold (2.8-fold for PPMs and 6.0-fold for ICDs). The numbers of CIED infection–related hospitalizations increased out of proportion to rates of new device implantation. Moreover, CIED infection increased the risk of in-hospital death by more than 2-fold (Voigt, Shalaby et al. 2006). The number of CIED implantations continued to increase after 2003 from 199516 in 2004 to 222940 in 2006, representing a 12% increment. In the same period the number of CIED infections increased from 8273 in 2004 to 12979 in 2006, representing a 57% increment as seen in figure 1. From 1996 to 2006, co morbid illnesses in recipients of new CIED devises became more prevalent with an increasing percentage of patients with end-organ failures (6.5% in 1996 vs 8% in 2006) and diabetes mellitus (14.5% in 1996 vs 16.5% in 2006) (Voigt, Shalaby et al. 2006) (Voigt, Shalaby et al. 2010).

It also results in significant financial costs, including prolonged hospitalization, prolonged antimicrobial therapy, management of systemic complications of sepsis, and the costs involved in device extraction and potential re-implantation. According to one US study, the mean hospital cost for treating a single PPM or ICD infection is $24 459 or $57 213, respectively.

3. Risk factors

In a prospective cohort of 6319 patients receiving CIED implantation in 44 medical centers, Klug et al identified 42 patients who developed CIED infection during 1 year of follow-up. The factors associated with an increased risk of infection included fever within 24 hours before implantation (OR 5.83), use of preprocedural temporary pacing (OR 2.46), and early reintervention (OR_15.04). Implantation of a new system (OR_0.46 compared with partial or complete system replacement) and use of periprocedural antimicrobial prophylaxis (OR 0.40) were both associated with a lower risk of infection (Klug, Balde et al. 2007).

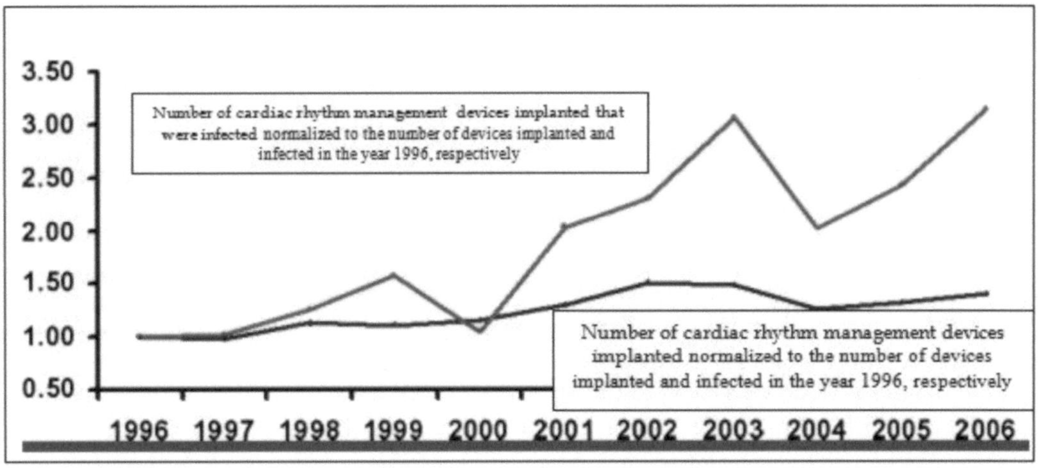

Fig. 1. Trends in Cardiovascular Implantable Devises and Infection in the United States (Adapted from Voigt, A., A. Shalaby, et al. (2010). "Continued rise in rates of cardiovascular implantable electronic device infections in the United States: temporal trends and causative insights." Pacing Clin Electrophysiol 33(4): 414-9.)

Johansen et al followed up 36 076 patients in the Danish Pacemaker Register. The incidence of explantation due to infection was significantly higher after replacement procedures than after first implantation (2.06% versus 0.75%). Device revision was associated with CIED infection in another investigation described recently. Although the incidence of infection decreased in the past 3 years of the study, the shorter follow-up of patients was thought to be a possible explanation. Whether multiple device revisions increasethe risk of CIED infection exponentially is undefined (Johansen, Feychting et al. 2002).

Another retrospective study was contacted in Minnesota (Sohail, Uslan et al. 2007). From 1 January 1991 to 31 December 2003, 12,799 PPMs were implanted at the Mayo Clinic-Rochester. Potential study subjects among the patients who received these devices were identified by searching the aforementioned databases. Twenty-nine case patients and 58 control subjects met the inclusion criteria. On univariate analysis, previous PPM infection, malignancy, long-term corticosteroid use, multiple device revisions, a permanent central venous catheter, the presence of 12 pacing leads, and a lack of antibiotic prophylaxis at the time of PPM placement were associated with an increased risk of PPM infection. A multivariable logistic regression model identified long-term corticosteroid use (odds ratio [OR], 13.90; 95% confidence interval [CI], 1.27–151.7) and the presence of 12 pacing leads versus 2 leads (OR, 5.41; 95% CI, 1.44–20.29) as independent risk factors for PPM infection. In contrast, use of antibiotic prophylaxis prior to PPM implantation had a protective effect (OR, 0.087; 95% CI, 0.016–0.48).

Among patients with bloodstream infection, the organism involved is strongly associated with the likelihood of serving as a manifestation of CIED infection, even in patients with no other evidence of CIED infection. In a cohort of 33 patients with implanted devices and subsequent *Staphylococcus aureus* bacteremia, 26 nearly one half (45.4%) had confirmed CIED infection, and only a minority had local signs or symptoms that suggested generator-pocket infection (Chamis, Peterson et al. 2001).

Physician experience in CIED implantation may also play a role in the rate of subsequent CIED infection. In a study of Medicare administrative data, Al-Khatib et al found a significantly higher risk of ICD infection within 90 days of device implantation in patients whose device was placed by physicians in the lowest quartile of implantation volume (OR 2.47 compared with physicians in the highest-volume quartile). Rates of mechanical complications at 90 days were also higher for lower-volume physicians (Al-Khatib, Lucas et al. 2005).

Finally Baman et al. evaluated risk factors for mortality in patients with cardiac-device related infection. Two hundred ten patients with cardiac-device related infection were identified at the University of Michigan between 1995 and 2006. Mean age for our study population was 63 ±17 years, and 72 (44%) were women. All-cause 6-month mortality was 18% (n=37). Independent variables associated with death were systemic embolization (hazard ratio 7.11; 95% CI 2.74 to 18.48), moderate or severe tricuspid regurgitation (hazard ratio 4.24; 95% CI 1.84 to 9.75), abnormal right ventricular function (hazard ratio 3.59; 95% CI 1.57 to 8.24), and abnormal renal function (hazard ratio 2.98; 95% CI 1.17 to 7.59). Size and mobility of cardiac device vegetations were not independently associated with mortality (Baman, Gupta et al. 2009).

In summary, several factors associated with a greater risk of CIED infection have been described in this section, including the following:

1. Fever within 24 hours of implantation
2. Lack of antibiotic prophylaxis before device implantation
3. Temporary pacing before permanent device placement
4. Presence of tunneled central venous catheter (such as hemodialysis catheter)
5. Operator inexperience
6. History of cardiac rhythm management device infection
7. History of multiple device-related procedures
8. Recent device manipulation (i.e., generator exchange or lead revision)
9. Presence of more than two electrode leads
10. Long-term corticosteroid therapy
11. Anticoagulation
12. Comorbid conditions (diabetes mellitus, heart failure, renal failure, malignancy)

4. Microbiology

Staphylococcal species cause the bulk of CIED infections and account for 60% to 80% of cases in most reported series. In a recent investigation, coagulase-negative staphylococci (42%), followed by S. aureus (29%) were responsible for more than two thirds of cases of device infection (2) (Sohail, Uslan et al. 2007). Early device infections (within 2 weeks of implantation) are primarily caused by S. aureus. Prevalence of oxacillin-resistant S. aureus is variable depending on the geographic location of reporting institutions. In one study, gram-negative bacteria, other gram-positive cocci (including enterococci, streptococci, and micrococci), and fungi (Candida spp. and Aspergillus fumigatus) were isolated in 9%, 4%, and 2% of cases, respectively. A variety of coagulase-negative *Staphylococcus* (CoNS) species have been described to cause CIED infections. CoNS is well recognized as a common cause of microbiological specimen contamination, and thus, repeated isolation of the same species of CoNS with an identical antibiotic susceptibility pattern is desired to support its role as an etiologic agent in CIED infections. Distinguishing skin flora, particularly coagulase-negative staphylococci, as either pathogen or culture contaminant is a frequent diagnostic dilemma. Multiple sets of blood cultures should yield the pathogen if endovascular infection is present. Skin flora that grow in culture from percutaneous aspirates of fluid or abscess collection should be considered as pathogens. Recovery of skin flora at driveline transcutaneous exit sites or in open wounds in proximity to a device is more difficult to define as pathogen versus contaminant; a Gram's stain may be helpful.

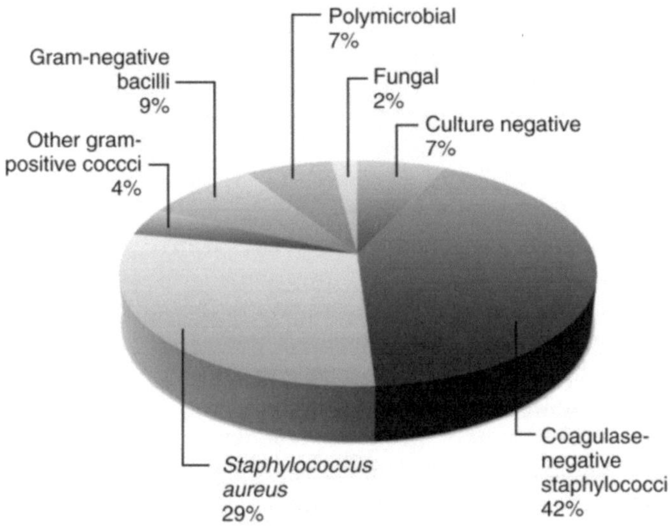

Fig. 2. Microbiology of cardiac rhythm management device infections. (Adapted from Sohail MR, Uslan DZ, Khan AH, et al. Management and outcome of permanent pacemaker and implantable cardioverter defibrillator infections. J Am Coll Cardiol 2008;49;1851-1859.)

Polymicrobial infection sometimes involves more than 1 species of CoNS (Cacoub, Leprince et al. 1998). The prevalence of oxacillin resistance among staphylococcal strains has varied among studies, but it is prevalent and should influence initial empirical therapy decisions in CIED infections. *Corynebacterium* species, *Propionibacterium acnes*, Gram-negative bacilli including *Pseudomonas aeruginosa*, and *Candida* species account for a minority of CIED infections. Fungi other than *Candida (Metallidis, Chrysanthidis et al. 2008)* and nontuberculosis mycobacteria are rarely identified as pathogens in CIED infection. We have recently described a rare case of lead endocarditis caused by mucor sp.

The microorganisms that cause CIED infections may be acquired either endogenously from the skin of patients or exogenously from the hospital inanimate environment or from the hands of hospital workers. In support of endogenous acquisition, an association has been noted between the presence of pre-axillary skin flora and the pathogens isolated from pacemaker infection.

In a study by Da Costa et al specimens were collected at the site of implantation for culture from the skin and the pocket before and after insertion in a consecutive series of patients who underwent elective permanent pacemaker implantation. There were 103 patients (67 men and 36 women) whose age ranged from 16 to 93 years. At the time of pacemaker implantation, a total of 267 isolates were identified. The majority (85%) were staphylococci. During a mean follow-up of 16.5 months (range, 1 to 24), infection occurred in four patients (3.9%). In two of them, an isolate of *Staphylococcus schleiferi* was recognized by molecular method as identical to the one previously found in the pacemaker pocket. In one patient, *Staphylococcus aureus*, an organism that was absent at the time of pacemaker insertion, was isolated. In another patient, a *Staphylococcus epidermidis* was identified both at the time of pacemaker insertion and when erosion occurred; however, their antibiotic resistance profiles were different (Da Costa, Lelievre et al. 1998).

Although low concentrations of methicillin-resistant CoNS have been detected in individuals with no healthcare contact and no recent antibiotic exposure, a disproportionate frequency of CIED infections due to multidrug-resistant staphylococci suggests that a healthcare environment is the site of infection acquisition.

5. Pathogenesis

Microbial contamination of a device generator or leads with skin flora at the time of implantation is the most likely mechanism of infection in the large majority of cases. This likely explains the preponderance of staphylococci as causative pathogens. Colonization and subsequent infection of CIEDs are facilitated by an ability of these organisms to adhere to device surfaces and produce biofilm. This causes an inability of the host's immune system to eliminate infection due to neutrophil dysfunction, poor penetration of antibiotics into the biofilm, and down regulation of metabolic activity in infecting organisms that makes them less susceptible to some antimicrobials, necessitating device removal for the best chance of infection cure. Once a generator or pocket is colonized, bacteria can migrate along the electrode leads and manifest as tunnel infection, bacteremia, or infected vegetations on electrode leads or cardiac valves. Incorporation of lead segments in the vascular endothelium or endocardial tissue may provide some protection from hematogenous seeding of microorganisms. Nevertheless, hematogenous seeding of leads is a major concern, particularly when Staphylococcus aureus is the pathogen

The pocket may become infected at the time of implantation, during subsequent surgical manipulation of the pocket, or if the generator or subcutaneous electrodes erode through the skin. In the latter case, erosion can also occur as a secondary event due to underlying infection. Pocket infection may track along the intravascular portion of the electrode to involve the intracardiac portion of the pacemaker or ICD. Alternatively, the pocket or intracardiac portion of the electrode may become infected as a result of hematogenous seeding during about of bacteremia or fungemia secondary to a distant infected focus. Hematogenous seeding of a CIED is unlikely to occur in cases of Gram-negative bacillary bacteremia, as discussed below. Bacteremia due to *S aureus* can result in device infection, but the prevalence of this occurrence and the differentiation of this mechanism of device infection from intraoperative contamination at the time of device placement or manipulation are difficult to determine. There are no data that examine the likelihood of hematogenous seeding of a device due to other Gram-positive cocci that are more common causes of bloodstream infection or due to fungi, in particular *Candida* species. Device-related infection is the result of the interaction between the device, the microbe, and the host. Initial attachment of bacteria to the device is mediated by physicalchemical properties, such as hydrophobicity, surface tension, and electrostatic charge, of the plastic surface of the device and the bacterial surface (Vuong and Otto 2002). Bacteria, particularly Gram positive cocci, can also adhere to and be engulfed by endothelial cells that can cover an endothelialized lead over a period of time, which is thought to be an important mechanism of device infection by the hematogenous route.

Pathogen Virulence Factors: Two major areas of investigation of microbial virulence factors are (1) tissue and foreign body adherence molecules and (2) foreign body surface biofilm formation.

There are several *S aureus* adhesins that are operative in the binding of microorganisms to extracellular and host plasma proteins that coat the surface of indwelling medical devices. These host proteins are exposed in areas where endothelium has been denuded by contact with or attachment to indwelling devices. The adhesins, known as extracellular matrix-binding proteins or microbial surface components recognizing adhesive matrix molecules (MSCRAMM), have been studied in a number of in vitro adherence assays and in animal models of infection and have demonstrated their importance in microbial virulence. Much of the work has examined *S aureus* surface proteins, including fibronectin-binding protein A or B, clumping factor A or B, and collagen-binding protein (Veenstra, Cremers et al. 1996). The only experimental model of cardiovascular infection that has been used to examine these putative virulence factors is the animal endocarditis model. Findings derived from experimental endocarditis investigations may be applicable to cardiovascular device–related infections in humans.

The layers of bacteria on the surface of an implanted device are encased in this extracellular slime and constitute a biofilm. Biofilm is defined as a surface-associated community of 1 or more microbial species that are firmly attached to each other and the solid surface and are encased in an extracellular polymeric matrix that holds the biofilm together. Microbes in a biofilm are more resistant to antibiotics and host defenses, perhaps as a result of the dense extracellular matrix that protects the microbes secluded in the interior of the community. When a bacterial cell switches modes from free-floating (planktonic) organisms to biofilm, it undergoes a phenotypic shift in behavior in which large groups of genes are regulated (Francois, Vaudaux et al. 1998).

Device Factors: Device-related factors, such as the type of plastic polymer, irregularity of its surface, and its shape, can affect bacterial adherence to the device. Plastic polymers that encase medical devices, as well as the pathogens that adhere to them, are hydrophobic. The greater the degree of hydrophobicity, the greater is the adherence. Polyvinyl chloride favors more adherence than Teflon (duPont, Wilmington, Del), polyethylene more than polyurethane, silicone more than polytetrafluoroethylene, and latex more than silicone; some metals (eg, stainless steel) favor adherence more than others (eg, titanium). An irregular surface of the device favors microbial adherence more than a smooth surface.

6. Clinical manifestations

CRMD infection has three important presentations (Sohail, Uslan et al. 2007). The most common presentation is pocket site infection (>60%). Patients generally present with localized inflammatory changes at the generator pocket site including erythema, pain, swelling, warmth, drainage, or dehiscence of overlying skin. Systemic signs of sepsis or positive blood cultures are present in less than one half of these cases. The second presentation is occult bacteremia or fungemia and no local changes at the pocket site. The third presentation is CRMD-related endocarditis (lead and/or valvular vegetations) in 10% to 23% of cases. Patients with device-related endocarditis are defined by modified Duke criteria (Arber, Pras et al. 1994). When vegetations are visualized on cardiac structures, the tricuspid valve is the most common site of infection (as many as 25% of cases with CRMD-related endocarditis). However, vegetations can develop on the pulmonic or left-sided valves, especially in the setting of *S. aureus* bacteremia (SAB). Patients who are bacteremic with *S. aureus* have radiographic or computed tomography (CT) findings of multiple focal pulmonary infiltrates or abscesses due to septic emboli in as many as 40% (Klug, Lacroix et al. 1997). Patients with CRMD-related endocarditis have a higher mortality (14% to 21%) compared with those without it (<5%), even with percutaneous device extraction. A small proportion (<5%) of patients can present with erosion of a device lead or generator only in the absence of inflammatory signs at the pocket and positive blood cultures. Whether erosion is caused by low-grade infection or purely by mechanical factors may not be entirely clear in all patients. Median time from device implantation to infection was much shorter for ICD recipients (125 days) compared with those with PPM implantation (414 days) in a recent investigation. Early onset of infection in patients with ICDs may be, in part, due to higher prevalence of comorbid conditions and an increased rate of *S. aureus* infection in this group of patients (Uslan, Tleyjeh et al. 2008).

7. Diagnosis

A diagnosis of CRMD infection is apparent when pocket site inflammatory changes are present. For some patients, a diagnosis is more difficult to confirm. Blood cultures should be obtained in all cases before starting empirical antibiotics. If drainage is present, swab specimens should be submitted for cultures. Abnormal laboratory findings (leukocytosis, anemia, high erythrocyte sedimentation rate or C-reactive protein) are present in 50% or less of cases, and the absence of these findings should not dissuade clinicians from considering a possibility of CIED infection in the appropriate setting. At least 2 sets of blood cultures should be obtained before the initiation of antimicrobial therapy in all patients with suspected CIED infection; some patients with bloodstream infection may not manifest systemic toxicity or peripheral leukocytosis. Positive blood cultures, particularly due to staphylococcal species, provide a strong clue that the clinical syndrome is due to CIED infection.

Laboratory, radiological, and echocardiographic procedures are helpful in making a diagnosis of cardiovascular device-related infection. Occult bacteremia or fungemia with no other evidence of infection should prompt serious concerns of device infection. In patients with SAB, concomitant CIED infection is present in as many as 50% of the patients (Klug, Balde et al. 2007). Risk is especially high within the first year after device implantation. Local signs or symptoms of pocket or tunnel infection may be absent in more than 50% of cases. A thorough evaluation for focal infection, including echocardiography and possibly an ultrasound scan of the generator pocket (to evaluate for fluid collection) in patients with SAB and the presence of CIED is recommended. Although fluid can be present early after surgical implantation of the device generator, its accumulation months to years after device placement would be unusual. Ultrasonography-directed diagnostic aspiration could be considered. However, it carries a risk of introducing infection in an otherwise sterile collection during this procedure. Indium-labeled leukocyte or gallium scanning may be helpful in differentiating an inflammatory fluid collection from a noninfected pocket site fluid collection. A technetium-labeled white blood cell scan may aid in the differentiation of noninfected versus septic thrombi attached to pacing leads. CIED removal may also be considered in patients who have no identified focus of SAB. Failure to remove an infected device is associated with an increased risk of treatment failure with relapsing bacteremia. In patients with no evidence of CIED infection (after a thorough evaluation) at the time of SAB and for whom a decision is made to treat conservatively, there should be close follow-up over the next 12 weeks to monitor for relapsing bacteremia. In untreated patients with bacteremia, blood cultures are usually positive. Culture of purulent drainage from a percutaneous driveline exit site or from a subcutaneous pocket or other site identifies a specific pathogen. Gram's stain of the drainage material is useful in demonstrating neutrophils and infecting bacteria. Despite collection of clinical specimens for microbiological examination, stains and cultures fail to demonstrate a pathogen in some patients with nonvalvular cardiovascular device–related infections. These culture-negative cases, much like those seen with infective endocarditis, are often due to recent antibiotic administration, which may diminish the sensitivity of subsequent microbiological studies. Unlike infective endocarditis, fastidious and uncommon microorganisms that do not grow or stain positive by routinely used laboratory methods have not been identified as pathogens in nonvalvular device-related infections. These groups of rare pathogens that are now being identified as causes of culture-negative endocarditis by technical advances in the laboratory have not accounted for culture-negative nonvalvular infections.

Lead tip cultures are frequently used to confirm the diagnosis of CRMD-related infective endocarditis. However, most transvenous leads are extracted percutaneously in current practice, and lead tips may be contaminated during removal through the incision of an infected pocket (Sohail 2007). Lead tip cultures are more reliable if they are extracted using a sterile technique (via protected sleeve) or if removed from a different incision than that used at the generator pocket site.

Transesophageal echocardiography (TEE) may be useful in demonstrating CIED-related endocarditis in adults. Because of its poor sensitivity, transthoracic echocardiography is frequently not helpful in ruling out a diagnosis of lead-related endocarditis, particularly in adults. Moreover, patients can develop both right-sided (lead-related) and left-sided endocarditis; the sensitivity of TEE for left-sided involvement and for perivalvular extension of infection is superior to that of transthoracic echocardiography. Additionally, visualization of the lead in the proximal superior vena cava from TEE views may identify tissue along that region that is difficult to visualize by other methods. TEE examination is critical among patients with S aureus bacteremia, because the rate of endocarditis is significant (Fowler, Li et al. 1997). Several prognostic features may be better defined on transthoracic echocardiography than on TEE, such as pericardial effusion, ventricular dysfunction and dyssynchrony, and pulmonary vascular pressure estimations.

A mass adherent to the lead that is seen on echocardiography is usually a thrombus or infected vegetation. Because it is impossible to distinguish between the 2 with echocardiography and recognizing that 5% of adherent masses were deemed thrombus in 1 retrospective survey, there will be some patients who are labeled as manifesting CIED-related endocarditis who may not have a lead infection (Vilacosta, Sarria et al. 1994; Victor, De Place et al. 1999). Masses that are detected in patients without positive blood cultures or other suggestive features for infection are likely to represent thrombus and by themselves do not require lead removal or antibiotic treatment. In addition, the failure to visualize a mass adherent to a lead with TEE does not exclude lead infection. Cultures of generator-pocket–site tissue and lead tips at the time of device removal are useful in identifying the causative organism and to support a diagnosis of CIED infection. The sensitivity of pocket-site tissue culture is higher than that of swab culture of the pocket. In a study by Chua et al seventy-one patients with implantable pacemaker (n = 49, 69%), implantable defibrillator (n

= 18, 25%), or both devices (n = 4, 6%) requiring lead extraction had pocket swab and tissue cultures for analysis. Infection was evident clinically in 35 (49%) of the patients and absent in the remainder. Patients with clinical infection had positive cultures more frequently (P = 0.002) by pocket tissue culture (n = 24, 69%) than by swab culture (n = 11, 31%). However, patients without clinical infections had positive cultures at similar rates by pocket tissue culture (n = 10, 28%) and by swab culture (n = 8, 22%). Gram staining, in addition to both anaerobic and aerobic bacterial cultures, should be done (Chua, Wilkoff et al. 2000).

Both tissue and the lead tip should be cultured for fungi and mycobacteria if the initial Gram stain is negative; mycobacteria and fungal stains also should be obtained on resected pocket tissue. Percutaneous aspiration of the device pocket should not be done, in general, because of the lack of adequate diagnostic yield and the theoretical risk of introducing microorganisms into the pocket site and causing device infection. Because leads are extracted through an open generator pocket in most cases, lead contamination can occur if a pocket is infected. This likely explains the lack of systemic manifestations and negative blood cultures in many cases in which a positive lead-tip culture is demonstrated.

8. Management

The primary focus of treatment should be complete removal of the PPM or ICD system. Although no prospective, randomized trials have been conducted to evaluate the role of medical (antimicrobial) therapy alone versus a combined medical-surgical treatment approach, data from several retrospective analyses show a clear and clinically important advantage of complete device removal. For example, the reported mortality rate of CRMD-related endocarditis ranges from 31% to 66% if the infected device is retained compared with 18% or less in patients managed with a combined approach of complete device removal and parenteral antibiotics. Patients with partial device removal (generator only) or those treated conservatively with antibiotics alone have a higher risk of treatment failure or relapse.

CIED removal is not required for superficial or incisional infection at the pocket site if there is no involvement of the device. Seven to 10 days of antibiotic therapy with an oral agent with activity against staphylococci is reasonable.

Complete removal of all hardware, regardless of location (subcutaneous, transvenous, or epicardial), is the recommended treatment for patients with established CIED infection (Love, Wilkoff et al. 2000). This includes cases in which a localized pocket infection occurs in the absence of signs of systemic infection. Complete removal of hardware is needed because infection relapse rates due to retained hardware are high (Gaynor, Zierer et al. 2006; Field, Jones et al. 2007). Erosion of any part of the CIED should imply contamination of the entire system, including the intravascular portion of leads, and complete device removal should be performed.

In a study by Anna del Rio a total of 31 patients, 25 men and 6 women aged 61 ±15 years (mean ±SD), with pacemaker or ICD endocarditis were identified among 669 consecutive patients (4.6%) with IE. Medical treatment without removal of the pacing system was initially performed on seven patients; all of them (100%) had relapses of endocarditis, and one patient died. The remaining 24 patients underwent surgical removal of the pacing system; 1 patient had one relapse, 3 patients died after surgical treatment, and the others were successfully cured with no relapses after a mean follow-up of 38 ±9 months. The only prognostic factor for failure of treatment or mortality was the absence of surgical treatment (del Rio, Anguera et al. 2003).

Complete CIED removal should be performed when patients undergo valve replacement or repair for infective endocarditis, because the CIED could serve as a nidus for relapsing infection and subsequent seeding of the surgically treated heart valve. An epicardial system should be considered if a new CIED is required after valve surgery with initial CIED removal.

The first issue to address in the treatment of CIED infections is the approach to hardware removal. As newer technologies have emerged and the experience has grown, percutaneous lead extraction has become the preferred method for removal of CIED hardware. However, these procedures involve significant risks, including cardiac tamponade, hemothorax, pulmonary embolism, lead migration, and death, even in experienced hands. Thus, the performance of these procedures should be limited to centers with the appropriate facilities and training, which includes the presence and imminent availability of cardiothoracic surgery on site to provide backup in the event of complications. In high-volume centers, percutaneous lead removal can be accomplished relatively safely with a high rate of success (Jones, Eckart et al. 2008).

In a study by Grammes et al a total of 984 patients underwent extraction of 1,838 leads; local or systemic infection occurred in 480 patients. One hundred patients had intracardiac vegetations identified by transesophageal echocardiogram, and all underwent percutaneous lead extraction (215 leads). Mean age was 67 years. Median extraction time was 3 min per lead; median implant duration was 34 months. During the index hospitalization, a new device was implanted in 54 patients at a median of 7 days after extraction. Post-operative 30-day mortality was 10%; no deaths were related directly to the extraction procedure (Grammes, Schulze et al. 2010).

A primary surgical approach to lead removal in patients with CIED infection should be limited to patients who have significant retained hardware after attempts at percutaneous removal. Another scenario in which a preference for surgical lead removal has been advocated is in patients with lead vegetations >2 cm in diameter, because of concerns about the risk of pulmonary embolism with percutaneous lead extraction (Smith and Love 2008). Experience suggests, however, that percutaneous removal in patients with large vegetations can be done without precipitating a clinically apparent pulmonary embolism. Until additional data are available, decisions regarding percutaneous versus surgical removal of leads with vegetations larger than 2 cm in diameter should be individualized and based on a patient's clinical parameters and the extractor's evaluation.

Antimicrobial therapy is adjunctive in patients with CIED infection, and complete device removal should not be delayed, regardless of timing of initiation of antimicrobial therapy. Selection of the appropriate antimicrobial agent should be based on identification and in vitro susceptibility testing results. Because the bulk of infections are due to staphylococcal species, and some of them will be oxacillin resistant, vancomycin should be administered initially as empirical antibiotic coverage until microbiological results are known. Patients with infections due to oxacillin-susceptible staphylococcal strains can be given cefazolin or nafcillin alone with discontinuation of vancomycin. Vancomycin should be continued in patients who are not candidates for b-lactam antibiotic therapy and those with infections due to oxacillin-resistant staphylococci. Pathogen identification and in vitro susceptibility testing can be used to direct treatment in the minority of patients with nonstaphylococcal CIED infections.

There are no clinical trial data to define the optimal duration of antimicrobial therapy for CIED infections, regardless of the extent of infection, or to determine when conversion to an oral agent is appropriate once complete device removal has been achieved. Factors that influence medical decision making include the extent of device infection, the causative organism, the presence and duration of bloodstream infection, and associated complications such as valvular involvement, septic thrombophlebitis, or osteomyelitis. Blood cultures should be obtained from all patients after device removal. When CIED infection is limited to the pocket site, 7 to 10 days of therapy after device removal is reasonable if the presentation is device erosion without inflammatory changes; otherwise, 10 to 14 days of antimicrobial treatment is recommended. Therapy can be switched to an oral regimen once susceptibility results are known if there is an oral agent available that is active against the pathogen and the infected CIED has been removed.

At least 2 weeks of parenteral therapy is recommended after extraction of an infected device for patients with bloodstream infection. Patients with sustained (>24 hours) positive blood cultures despite CIED removal and appropriate antimicrobial therapy should receive parenteral therapy for at least 4 weeks, even if TEE is negative for valvular vegetations (Sohail, Uslan et al. 2007).

It is intuitive that adequate debridement and control of infection at all sites, both at the generator site and metastatic, if present, be achieved before new device placement. The contralateral side is preferred for new device placement, if required. There are several aspects of CIED removal for which data are needed so that management recommendations can be provided. These include whether the infected pocket site should be closed before new device placement, whether generator-capsule debridement is appropriate, and how to manage patients who have undergone device removal but have a remaining lead remnant. A practical approach to CIED infections is provided in figure 3.

Patients with bloodstream infection and no localizing evidence of either generator-site infection or lead or endocardial involvement represent a difficult management group. Although bloodstream infection can be a manifestation of CIED infection, it can occur without CIED infection. There are several clinical parameters that may better characterize patients who have CIED infection and *S aureus* bacteremia but no localizing evidence of infection. These include the following: (1) Relapsing bacteremia after a course of appropriate antibiotic therapy; (2) if there is no other identified source for bacteremia; (3) if bacteremia persists more than 24 hours; (4) if the CIED is an ICD; (5) presence of a prosthetic cardiac valve; and (6) bacteremia within3 months of device placement.

As reported by Uslan et al from forty-nine patients with gram-negative bacteremia who had PPM/ICD only 3 (6%) had either definite (2 patients) or possible (1 patient) PPM/ICD infection. Both patients with definite PPM/ICD infection had clear infection of the generator pocket. None of the other patients with alternate sources of bacteremia developed PPM/ICD infection. Thirty four patients with retained PPM/ICD were observed for 112 weeks (median time, 759 days), and 2 (6%) developed relapsing bacteremia, although they each had alternative sources of relapse. In sharp contrast to *S. aureus* infection, PPM/ICD infection in patients with gram-negative bacteremia was rare, and no patients appeared to have secondary PPM/ICD infection due to hematogenous seeding of the system. Despite infrequent system removal in these patients, relapsing bacteremia among patients who survived initial bacteremia was rarely seen. If secondary PPM/ICD infection occurs in patients with gram-negative bacteremia, it is either uncommon or it is cured with antimicrobial therapy despite device retention (Uslan, Sohail et al. 2006).

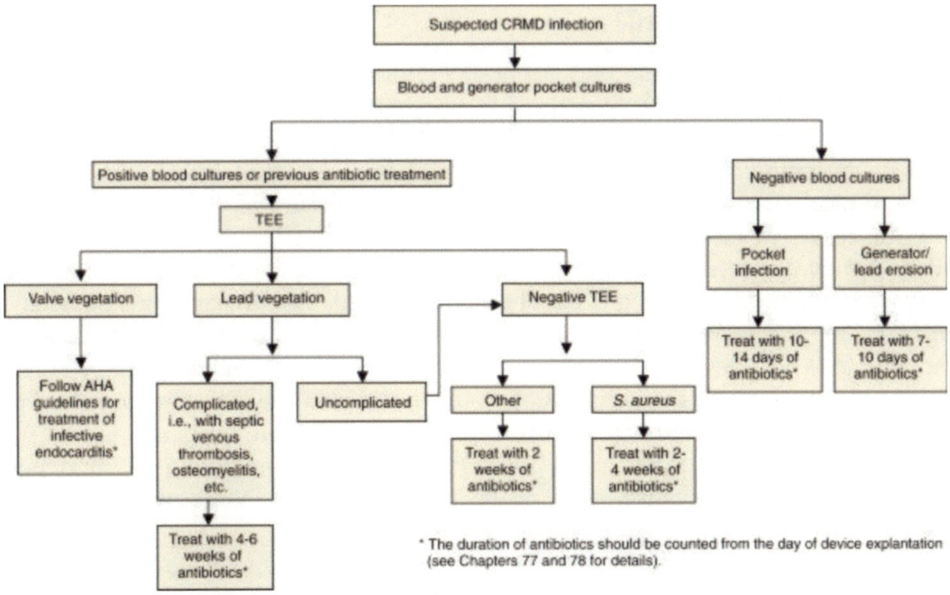

Fig. 3. Approach to the management of adults with cardiac rhythm management device infection. This algorithm applies only to the patients who are managed with complete device removal. AHA, American Heart Association; CRMD, cardiac rhythm management device; TEE, transesophageal echocardiogram.(Adapted from Sohail MR, Uslan DZ, Khan AH, et al. Management and outcome of permanent pacemaker and implantable cardioverter defibrillator infections. J Am Coll Cardiol. 2008;49;1851-1859.)

Chamis et al evaluated prospectively in a cohort all adult patients with SAB and permanent pacemakers or implantable cardioverterdefibrillators over a 6-year period. The overall incidence of confirmed CDI was 15 of 33 (45.4%). Confirmed CDI occurred in 9 of the 12 patients (75%) with early SAB (1 year after device placement). Fifteen of 21 patients (71.5%) with late SAB (1 year after device placement) had either confirmed (6 of 21, 28.5%) or possible (9 of 21, 43%) CDI. In 60% of the patients (9 of 15) with confirmed CDI, no local signs or symptoms suggesting generator pocket infection were noted (Chamis, Peterson et al. 2001). The incidence of CDI among patients with SAB and cardiac devices is high. Neither physical examination nor echocardiography can exclude the possibility of CDI. In patients with early SAB, the device is usually involved, and '40% of these patients have obvious clinical signs of cardiac device involvement. Conversely, in patients with late SAB, the cardiac device is rarely the initial source of bacteremia, and there is a paucity of local signs of device involvement. The cardiac device is involved, however, in 28% of these patients.

The likelihood of CIED infection in patients with bacteremia or fungemia due to organisms other than *S aureus* or Gram-negative bacilli that more commonly cause bloodstream infection (coagulase-negative staphylococci, streptococci, enterococci, and *Candida* species) and no other evidence of CIED infection has received limited attention. Results of 2 relatively small case series suggest that the risk of CIED infection in these patients is low; however, more data are clearly needed in this clinical setting to permit recommendations on whether device removal is warranted (Camus, Leport et al. 1993; Sopena, Crespo et al. 2010).

9. New device implantation

It is imperative that there be an assessment of the need for new device placement in each patient with an infected CIED. One third to one half of patients in some series will not require new CIED placement (Sohail, Uslan et al. 2007). There are several factors, including reversal of the pathological processes that precipitated the need for CIED implantation, changing clinical circumstances, and lack of appropriate clinical indication initially, that obviate the need for new CIED placement and thus result in avoidance of new device infection. Removal of infected hardware should not be attempted until a careful assessment of a new implantation strategy has been performed, particularly in patients with pacemakers for complete heart block and resynchronization therapy devices. When implantation of a new device is necessary, it should be performed on the contralateral side if possible to avoid relapsing device infection. If this is not possible, a transvenous lead can be tunneled to a device placed subcutaneously in the abdomen. Implantation is usually postponed to allow for resolution of infection, but patients who are PPM dependent represent a challenge, because they cannot be discharged home with a temporary pacemaker.

Because of complications with passive-fixation leads that have been used in the past for temporary pacing in CIED infection cases, active-fixation leads attached to pacing generators or defibrillators are now being used as a "bridge" until PPM implantation is deemed appropriate. Use of active fixation leads connected to external devices in stimulation dependent patients with infection permits earlier mobilization of the patient and has been associated with a reduced risk of pacing-related adverse events, including lead dislocation, resuscitation due to severe bradycardia, and local infection (Braun, Rauwolf et al. 2006).

The optimal timing of device replacement is unknown (Mansour, Kauten et al. 1985). Some have advocated proceeding 24 hours after removal. Sohail et al demonstrated a difference in timing of replacement based on (1) blood culture results (median time of 13 days for bacteremic patients versus 7 days for nonbacteremic patients) and (2) type of pathogen identified (median 7 days for CoNS versus 12 days for *S aureus*) (Sohail, Uslan et al. 2007).

There have been no prospective trial data that examined timing of new device replacement and risk of relapsing infection; however, several investigators recommend waiting for blood cultures to be negative before a new device is placed (Figure 4).

Only 1 medical center has described simultaneous contralateral (side-to-side) replacement of an infected CIED. A 1-stage exchange was performed in 68 consecutive patients over almost a 14-year period by 1 cardiologist, and two thirds of patients had dual-chamber devices. Clinical presentations included device erosion (41%), cellulitis or abscess (35%), and endocarditis (24%). Fifty-nine patients (87%) were followed up for more than 1 year, and 9 patients were lost to follow-up after 1 to 10 months after 1-stage contralateral device exchange, with no new identified CIED infections (Nandyala and Parsonnet 2006). Additional experience with 1-stage contralateral device exchange is needed, however, before it can be recommended for routine use. There are reports of successful implantations of previously implanted devices from either deceased patients or from the same patient with a prior PPM infection (Panja, Sarkar et al. 1996). Mansour and coworkers described 17 patients with a previously infected PPM who underwent successful implantation (at a new site and after resterilization) without relapsing infection. The practice of reusing CIEDs after sterilization is not advocated, however (Mansour, Kauten et al. 1985).

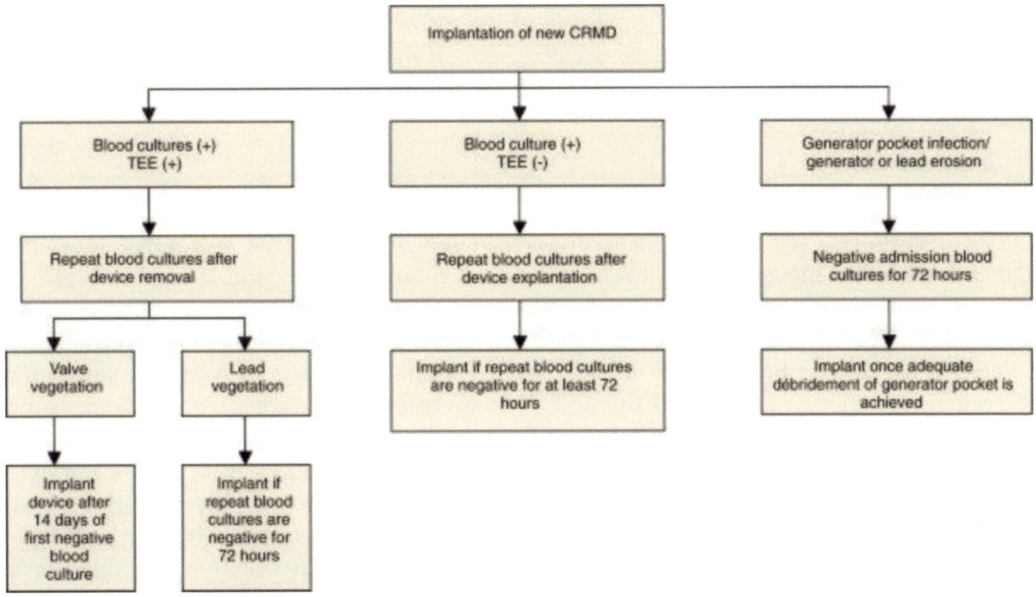

Fig. 4. Guidelines for implantation of a new device in patients with cardiac rhythm management device infection. CRMD, cardiac rhythm management device; TEE, transesophageal echocardiogram.(Adapted from Sohail MR, Uslan DZ, Khan AH, et al. Management and outcome of permanent pacemaker and implantable cardioverter defibrillator infections. J Am Coll Cardiol. 2008;49;1851-1859.)

10. Long-term suppressive antimicrobial therapy

Long-term antimicrobial suppressive therapy is used in selected patients with CIED infections who, for a variety of reasons, are not candidates for device removal either by percutaneous or surgical methods (Baddour 2001). Often, these patients have a limited life expectancy or refuse device removal. Long-term suppressive therapy can be attempted in these cases if they meet several criteria, which include a stable cardiovascular status, clinical improvement with initial antimicrobial therapy, and clearance of bloodstream infection. Because there are no comparative trials, the optimal choice of antimicrobial therapy and its dosing are undefined. Moreover, treatment options are frequently limited, because many CIED infections are caused by multidrug-resistant pathogens that are acquired in the healthcare or nosocomial environment. Thus, prolonged suppression of infection can be difficult to achieve with oral antimicrobial therapy. Little is known about CIED infection relapse rates despite use of long-term suppressive therapy. Other factors that are relevant to the use of long-term suppressive therapy include the likelihood for selection of resistant organisms, both for the identified pathogen being suppressed and for normal colonizing strains; safety profile; patient compliance; and financial expense.

11. Complications of device infection

Complications of CRMD infection may include valvular endocarditis (mostly right sided), septic arthritis, vertebral osteomyelitis, sternal wound infection, metastatic abscesses (lung, liver, spleen, brain, renal), and thrombosis of a subclavian vein or superior vena cava. In patients with metastatic abscesses or osteomyelitis, it may be difficult to decipher whether an ectopic site is the source of bacteremia with hematogenous seeding of a cardiac device or vice versa.

12. Outcomes

CIED infection is a serious complication associated with substantial morbidity, mortality, and cost. Reported mortality rates for these infections range widely and tend to be higher in patients with confirmed device-related endocarditis and in those treated without device removal (Molina 1997; Bracke, Meijer et al. 2002; Rundstrom, Kennergren et al. 2004; Sohail, Uslan et al. 2008). Because of a lack of adequate comparison groups, substantial heterogeneity among studies and marked differences in populations who do and do not receive device removal, precise estimates of the benefits of device removal are not available. A risk factor analysis was conducted that examined clinical and echocardiographic variables that identified patients with CIED infections who were at increased risk of mortality. All-cause mortality at 6 months among 210 patients with CIED infections was 18% (Baman, Gupta et al. 2009). Variables associated with increased mortality risk among this cohort included systemic embolization, moderate to severe tricuspid regurgitation, abnormal right ventricular function, and abnormal renal function. Size and mobility of lead vegetations were not independently associated with mortality.

13. Prophylaxis at CIED implantation

Prevention of CIED infection can be addressed before, during, and after device implantation. Before device implantation, it is important to ensure that patients do not have clinical signs of infection. A parenterally administered antibiotic is recommended 1 hour before the procedure. Data from a meta-analysis (Da Costa, Kirkorian et al. 1998), 2 case-control studies (Klug, Balde et al. 2007; Sohail, Uslan et al. 2007) that examined purported risk factors of CIED infection, and a large, prospective, randomized, double-blinded, placebo-controlled trial (de Oliveira, Martinelli et al. 2009) strongly support the administration of antibiotic prophylaxis for CIED implantation. Most experts continue to advocate a first-generation cephalosporin, such as cefazolin, for use as prophylaxis. Although not generally recommended, some advocate the use of vancomycin instead of cefazolin, particularly in centers where oxacillin resistance among staphylococci is high. If vancomycin is used, then it should be administered 90 to 120 minutes before the procedure. Vancomycin also represents an alternative to a first-generation cephalosporin in patients who are allergic to cephalosporins. In patients who are allergic to both cephalosporins and vancomycin, daptomycin and linezolid represent prophylaxis options. Antibiotic prophylaxis is also recommended if subsequent invasive manipulation of the CIED is required.

Preoperative antiseptic preparation of the skin of the surgical site should be done. Intraprocedurally, compulsive attention to sterile technique is mandatory. If a patient has limited subcutaneous tissue and/or poor nutrition and is at increased risk for erosion, a retropectoral pocket should be considered. In a survey of pediatric patients, 9 (13.8%) of 65 with subcutaneously placed device-pocket transvenous systems developed infection compared with none of the 82 who underwent retropectorally placed systems. Hematoma within the pocket that complicates CIED placement or invasive manipulation has been identified as a risk factor associated with device placement (Cohen, Bush et al. 2002). Therefore, prevention of hematoma during the procedure is desirable, and several interventions have been used, although there are no data to support their use. This can be achieved by meticulous cautery of bleeding sites and consideration of packing the pocket with antibiotic-soaked sponges to provide tamponade while leads are being placed. The application of topical thrombin may be helpful, particularly in anticoagulated patients. Irrigation of the pocket is useful to remove debris and may reveal persistent bleeding that could lead to a pocket hematoma. In addition, irrigation with an antimicrobial-containing solution for pocket cleansing has been used. Use of monofilament suture for closure of the subcuticular layer may avoid superficial postoperative cellulitis. A pressure dressing applied for 12 to 24 hours after skin closure and dressing may further decrease the risk of hematoma formation.

In the immediate postoperative period, recent data indicate that low-molecular-weight heparin predisposes to hematoma formation and should be avoided (Robinson, Healey et al. 2009). A hematoma should be evacuated only when there is increased tension on the skin. Needle aspiration should otherwise be avoided because of the risk of introducing skin flora into the pocket and subsequent development of infection.

Routine ambulatory care follow-up after CIED placement to detect early infectious complications has been performed in many centers. Recent data from 1 investigation (Deuling, Smit et al. 2009) failed to demonstrate the utility of early follow-up and advocated that instead, patients should be instructed to call their implanting physician for development of fever or incision findings of inflammation.

Currently, there are no data to support the administration of postoperative antibiotic therapy, and it is not recommended because of the risk of drug adverse events, selection of drug-resistant organisms, and cost.

14. Antibiotic prophylaxis for invasive procedures

Since the original American Heart Association recommendations were made more than 50 years ago, there has been a proliferation of purported indications for the use of prophylactic antibiotics for patients thought to be at risk for distant site infection from invasive procedures. There is little, if any, scientific justification for administration of antibiotic prophylaxis for invasive procedures, although there is a wide range of opinions.96 A review of the literature from 1950 to 2007 for publications on cardiac electrophysiological device infections reveals more than 140 articles, none of which report hematologic infection from dental, gastrointestinal, genitourinary, dermatologic, or other procedures (Tong and Rothwell 2000; Lockhart, Brennan et al. 2002; Wilson, Taubert et al. 2008).

The predominance of staphylococci as pathogens in CIED infections rather than oral flora suggests that antibiotic prophylaxis for dental procedures is of little or no value (Aas, Paster et al. 2005). In the rare event of a device infection due to an oral pathogen, it is most likely to have arisen from a bacteremia from a common daily event such as toothbrushing or chewing food. Therefore, there is currently no scientific basis for the use of prophylactic antibiotics before routine invasive dental, gastrointestinal, or genitourinary procedures to prevent CIED infection.

15. Conclusion

As the number of CIED implantations continued to increases, the numbers of CIED infections are following the increment (57% increment from 2004 to 2006). All physicians must be aware of the potential role of implantable cardiovascular devices in infection. Diagnosis and management might be difficult, so guidelines must be followed. As conclusion we will provide the recommendations made by the American Heart Association (Baddour, Epstein et al. 2010).

Diagnosis:

1. All patients should have at least 2 sets of blood cultures drawn at the initial evaluation before prompt initiation of antimicrobial therapy for CIED infection.
2. Generator-pocket tissue Gram's stain and culture and lead-tip culture should be obtained when the CIED is explanted.
3. Patients with suspected CIED infection who either have positive blood cultures or who have negative blood cultures but have had recent antimicrobial therapy before blood cultures were obtained should undergo TEE for CIED infection or valvular endocarditis.
4. All adults suspected of having CIED-related endocarditis should undergo TEE to evaluate the left-sided heart valves, even if transthoracic views have demonstrated lead-adherent masses. In pediatric patients with good views, transthoracic echocardiography may be sufficient.

Management:

5. Choice of antimicrobial therapy should be based on the identification and in vitro susceptibility results of the infecting pathogen.
6. Duration of antimicrobial therapy should be 10 to 14 days after CIED removal for pocket-site infection.
7. Duration of antimicrobial therapy should be at least 14 days after CIED removal for bloodstream infection.
8. Duration of antimicrobial therapy should be at least 4 to 6 weeks for complicated infection (ie, endocarditis, septic thrombophlebitis, or osteomyelitis or if bloodstream infection persists despite device removal and appropriate initial antimicrobial therapy.
9. Complete device and lead removal is recommended for all patients with definite CIED infection, as evidenced by valvular and/or lead endocarditis or sepsis.
10. Complete device and lead removal is recommended for all patients with CIED pocket infection as evidenced by abscess formation, device erosion, skin adherence, or chronic draining sinus without clinically evident involvement of the transvenous portion of the lead system.
11. Complete device and lead removal is recommended for all patients with valvular endocarditis without definite involvement of the lead(s) and/or device.
12. Complete device and lead removal is recommended for patients with occult staphylococcal bacteremia.

New device implantation:

1. Each patient should be evaluated carefully to determine whether there is a continued need for a new CIED.
2. The replacement device implantation should not be ipsilateral to the extraction site. Preferred alternative locations include the contralateral side, the iliac vein, and epicardial implantation.

Prevention:

1. A parenterally administrated antibiotic is recommended 1 hour before the implantation of the device
2. Cefazolin is the preferred regimen
3. Vancomycin must be use particularly in centers where oxacillin resistance among staphylococci is high
4. Preoperative antiseptic preparation of the skin and sterile technique is mandatory.
5. Antimicrobial prophylaxis is not recommended for dental or other invasive procedures not directly related to device manipulation to prevent CIED infection.
6. Clinical trials and large nationals registries must be done in order to increase the knowledge of handling such infections.

16. References

Aas, J. A., B. J. Paster, et al. (2005). "Defining the normal bacterial flora of the oral cavity." J Clin Microbiol 43(16272510): 5721-5732.

Al-Khatib, S. M., F. L. Lucas, et al. (2005). "The relation between patients' outcomes and the volume of cardioverter-defibrillator implantation procedures performed by physicians treating Medicare beneficiaries." J Am Coll Cardiol 46(8): 1536-40.

Arber, N., E. Pras, et al. (1994). "Pacemaker endocarditis. Report of 44 cases and review of the literature." Medicine (Baltimore) 73(6): 299-305.

Baddour, L. M. (2001). "Long-term suppressive antimicrobial therapy for intravascular device-related infections." Am J Med Sci 322(4): 209-12.

Baddour, L. M., M. A. Bettmann, et al. (2003). "Nonvalvular cardiovascular device-related infections." Circulation 108(16): 2015-31.

Baddour, L. M., A. E. Epstein, et al. (2010). "Update on cardiovascular implantable electronic device infections and their management: a scientific statement from the American Heart Association." Circulation 121(3): 458-77.

Baman, T. S., S. K. Gupta, et al. (2009). "Risk factors for mortality in patients with cardiac device-related infection." Circ Arrhythm Electrophysiol 2(2): 129-34.

Bluhm, G. (1985). "Pacemaker infections. A clinical study with special reference to prophylactic use of some isoxazolyl penicillins." Acta Med Scand Suppl 699: 1-62.

Bracke, F., A. Meijer, et al. (2002). "Extraction of pacemaker and implantable cardioverter defibrillator leads: patient and lead characteristics in relation to the requirement of extraction tools." Pacing Clin Electrophysiol 25(7): 1037-40.

Braun, M. U., T. Rauwolf, et al. (2006). "Percutaneous lead implantation connected to an external device in stimulation-dependent patients with systemic infection--a prospective and controlled study." Pacing Clin Electrophysiol 29(16923004): 875-879.

Cabell, C. H., P. A. Heidenreich, et al. (2004). "Increasing rates of cardiac device infections among Medicare beneficiaries: 1990-1999." Am Heart J 147(4): 582-6.

Cacoub, P., P. Leprince, et al. (1998). "Pacemaker infective endocarditis." Am J Cardiol 82(4): 480-4.

Camus, C., C. Leport, et al. (1993). "Sustained bacteremia in 26 patients with a permanent endocardial pacemaker: assessment of wire removal." Clin Infect Dis 17(8353245): 46-55.

Chamis, A. L., G. E. Peterson, et al. (2001). "Staphylococcus aureus bacteremia in patients with permanent pacemakers or implantable cardioverter-defibrillators." Circulation 104(9): 1029-33.

Chua, J. D., B. L. Wilkoff, et al. (2000). "Diagnosis and management of infections involving implantable electrophysiologic cardiac devices." Ann Intern Med 133(8): 604-8.

Cohen, M. I., D. M. Bush, et al. (2002). "Pediatric pacemaker infections: twenty years of experience." J Thorac Cardiovasc Surg 124(12324742): 821-827.

Da Costa, A., G. Kirkorian, et al. (1998). "Antibiotic prophylaxis for permanent pacemaker implantation: a meta-analysis." Circulation 97(18): 1796-801.

Da Costa, A., H. Lelievre, et al. (1998). "Role of the preaxillary flora in pacemaker infections: a prospective study." Circulation 97(18): 1791-5.

de Oliveira, J. C., M. Martinelli, et al. (2009). "Efficacy of antibiotic prophylaxis before the implantation of pacemakers and cardioverter-defibrillators: results of a large, prospective, randomized, double-blinded, placebo-controlled trial." Circ Arrhythm Electrophysiol 2(1): 29-34.

del Rio, A., I. Anguera, et al. (2003). "Surgical treatment of pacemaker and defibrillator lead endocarditis: the impact of electrode lead extraction on outcome." Chest 124(4): 1451-9.

Deuling, J. H. H., M. D. Smit, et al. (2009). "The value and limitations of a wound inspection clinic after cardiac device implantation." Eur J Cardiovasc Nurs 8(19299201): 288-292.

Field, M. E., S. O. Jones, et al. (2007). "How to select patients for lead extraction." Heart Rhythm 4(17599690): 978-985.

Fowler, V. G., J. Li, et al. (1997). "Role of echocardiography in evaluation of patients with Staphylococcus aureus bacteremia: experience in 103 patients." J Am Coll Cardiol 30(9316542): 1072-1078.

Francois, P., P. Vaudaux, et al. (1998). "Role of plasma and extracellular matrix proteins in the physiopathology of foreign body infections." Ann Vasc Surg 12(9451994): 34-40.

Gaynor, S. L., A. Zierer, et al. (2006). "Laser assistance for extraction of chronically implanted endocardial leads: infectious versus noninfectious indications." Pacing Clin Electrophysiol 29(17201842): 1352-1358.

Grammes, J. A., C. M. Schulze, et al. (2010). "Percutaneous pacemaker and implantable cardioverter-defibrillator lead extraction in 100 patients with intracardiac vegetations defined by transesophageal echocardiogram." J Am Coll Cardiol 55(9): 886-94.

Johansen, C., M. Feychting, et al. (2002). "Risk of severe cardiac arrhythmia in male utility workers: a nationwide danish cohort study." Am J Epidemiol 156(9): 857-61.

Jones, S. O., R. E. Eckart, et al. (2008). "Large, single-center, single-operator experience with transvenous lead extraction: outcomes and changing indications." Heart Rhythm 5(18325849): 520-525.

Klug, D., M. Balde, et al. (2007). "Risk factors related to infections of implanted pacemakers and cardioverter-defibrillators: results of a large prospective study." Circulation 116(12): 1349-55.

Klug, D., D. Lacroix, et al. (1997). "Systemic infection related to endocarditis on pacemaker leads: clinical presentation and management." Circulation 95(8): 2098-107.

Lockhart, P. B., M. T. Brennan, et al. (2002). "Decision-making on the use of antimicrobial prophylaxis for dental procedures: a survey of infectious disease consultants and review." Clin Infect Dis 34(12032898): 1621-1626.

Love, C. J., B. L. Wilkoff, et al. (2000). "Recommendations for extraction of chronically implanted transvenous pacing and defibrillator leads: indications, facilities, training. North American Society of Pacing and Electrophysiology Lead Extraction Conference Faculty." Pacing Clin Electrophysiol 23(4 Pt 1): 544-51.

Mansour, K. A., J. R. Kauten, et al. (1985). "Management of the infected pacemaker: explantation, sterilization, and reimplantation." Ann Thorac Surg 40(6): 617-9.

Mela, T., B. A. McGovern, et al. (2001). "Long-term infection rates associated with the pectoral versus abdominal approach to cardioverter- defibrillator implants." Am J Cardiol 88(7): 750-3.

Metallidis, S., T. Chrysanthidis, et al. (2008). "A fatal case of pacemaker lead endocarditis caused by Mucor spp." Int J Infect Dis 12(6): e151-2.

Mirowski, M., P. R. Reid, et al. (1980). "Termination of malignant ventricular arrhythmias with an implanted automatic defibrillator in human beings." N Engl J Med 303(6991948): 322-324.

Molina, J. E. (1997). "Undertreatment and overtreatment of patients with infected antiarrhythmic implantable devices." Ann Thorac Surg 63(9033328): 504-509.

Nandyala, R. and V. Parsonnet (2006). "One stage side-to-side replacement of infected pulse generators and leads." Pacing Clin Electrophysiol 29(16650268): 393-396.

Panja, M., C. N. Sarkar, et al. (1996). "Reuse of pacemaker." Indian Heart J 48(9062017): 677-680.

Robinson, M., J. S. Healey, et al. (2009). "Postoperative low-molecular-weight heparin bridging is associated with an increase in wound hematoma following surgery for pacemakers and implantable defibrillators." Pacing Clin Electrophysiol 32(19272069): 378-382.

Rundstrom, H., C. Kennergren, et al. (2004). "Pacemaker endocarditis during 18 years in Goteborg." Scand J Infect Dis 36(9): 674-9.

Smith, M. C. and C. J. Love (2008). "Extraction of transvenous pacing and ICD leads." Pacing Clin Electrophysiol 31(18507548): 736-752.

Sohail, M. R. (2007). "Concerning diagnosis and management of pacemaker endocarditis." Pacing Clin Electrophysiol 30(6): 829; author reply 830.

Sohail, M. R., D. Z. Uslan, et al. (2008). "Infective endocarditis complicating permanent pacemaker and implantable cardioverter-defibrillator infection." Mayo Clin Proc 83(1): 46-53.

Sohail, M. R., D. Z. Uslan, et al. (2007). "Management and outcome of permanent pacemaker and implantable cardioverter-defibrillator infections." J Am Coll Cardiol 49(18): 1851-9.

Sohail, M. R., D. Z. Uslan, et al. (2007). "Risk factor analysis of permanent pacemaker infection." Clin Infect Dis 45(2): 166-73.

Sopena, B., M. Crespo, et al. (2010). "Individualized management of bacteraemia in patients with a permanent endocardial pacemaker." Clin Microbiol Infect 16(19456825): 274-280.

Tong, D. C. and B. R. Rothwell (2000). "Antibiotic prophylaxis in dentistry: a review and practice recommendations." J Am Dent Assoc 131(10715929): 366-374.

Uslan, D. Z., M. R. Sohail, et al. (2006). "Frequency of permanent pacemaker or implantable cardioverter-defibrillator infection in patients with gram-negative bacteremia." Clin Infect Dis 43(6): 731-6.

Uslan, D. Z., I. M. Tleyjeh, et al. (2008). "Temporal trends in permanent pacemaker implantation: a population-based study." Am Heart J 155(5): 896-903.

Veenstra, G. J., F. F. Cremers, et al. (1996). "Ultrastructural organization and regulation of a biomaterial adhesin of Staphylococcus epidermidis." J Bacteriol 178(8550477): 537-541.

Victor, F., C. De Place, et al. (1999). "Pacemaker lead infection: echocardiographic features, management, and outcome." Heart 81(1): 82-7.

Vilacosta, I., C. Sarria, et al. (1994). "Usefulness of transesophageal echocardiography for diagnosis of infected transvenous permanent pacemakers." Circulation 89(6): 2684-7.

Voigt, A., A. Shalaby, et al. (2006). "Rising rates of cardiac rhythm management device infections in the United States: 1996 through 2003." J Am Coll Cardiol 48(3): 590-1.

Voigt, A., A. Shalaby, et al. (2010). "Continued rise in rates of cardiovascular implantable electronic device infections in the United States: temporal trends and causative insights." Pacing Clin Electrophysiol 33(4): 414-9.

Vuong, C. and M. Otto (2002). "Staphylococcus epidermidis infections." Microbes Infect 4(11932199): 481-489.

Wilson, W., K. A. Taubert, et al. (2008). "Prevention of infective endocarditis: guidelines from the American Heart Association: a guideline from the American Heart Association Rheumatic Fever, Endocarditis and Kawasaki Disease Committee, Council on Cardiovascular Disease in the Young, and the Council on Clinical Cardiology, Council on Cardiovascular Surgery and Anesthesia, and the Quality of Care and Outcomes Research Interdisciplinary Working Group." J Am Dent Assoc 139 Suppl(18167394): 24.

Zhan, C., W. B. Baine, et al. (2008). "Cardiac device implantation in the United States from 1997 through 2004: a population-based analysis." J Gen Intern Med 23 Suppl 1: 13-9.

Part 5

Non-cardiac Pacemakers

23

Pacemaker and Network Mechanisms of Neural Rhythm Generation

Thomas Nowotny[1] and Mikhail I. Rabinovich[2]
[1]*University of Sussex*
[2]*University of California, San Diego*
[1]*UK*
[2]*USA*

1. Introduction

The origin of flexible rhythmic activity in brain circuits, or even in smaller neural networks, like central pattern generator (CPG) motor networks, is still not fully understood. The main unresolved questions are (i) what are the respective roles of intrinsic neuronal rhythms and network based dynamics in systems of coupled, heterogeneous, intrinsically complex, even chaotic, neurons? and (ii) what mechanisms are underlying the coexistence of robustness and flexibility in the observed rhythmic spatio-temporal patterns?

One common view is that particular neurons provide the rhythmogenic component while the connections between different neurons are responsible for the regularization and synchronization of groups of neurons and for specific phase relationships in multi-phasic bursting patterns. The opposing view is that constituent neurons are by themselves non-rhythmogenic and the emergence of rhythmic bursting behaviors is entirely due to the network interactions. The reality is more interesting and challenging, especially, when we are concerned about the brain. Usually, different mechanisms of rhythm generation coexist in the brain and rhythms from different sources and different levels of integration interact closely. It is important to emphasize that fast rhythms and slow rhythms need different levels of abstraction for describing and understanding them. It is reasonable to consider three such levels: (i) the neuronal level, (ii) the neuronal module or neuronal mass level, and (iii) the mental mode level. The analysis of low frequency (< 0.1 Hz) oscillations, for example, needs coarse-grained models of the interaction of mental modes, i.e., perceptional, cognitive and emotional modes.

The chapter is organized in the following way. In the first part (neuronal level) we describe the results of computer simulations examining how spatio-temporal rhythmic patterns emerge in motif networks of Hodgkin-Huxley (H-H) neurons connected by slow inhibitory synapses with a non-symmetric pattern of coupling strengths. We demonstrate that the interplay between intrinsic and network dynamics can lead to either cooperation or competition, depending on three basic control parameters identified in the models: (i) the shape of intrinsic bursts, (ii) the strength of the coupling between neurons and (iii) the degree of asymmetry in the connectivity matrix.

The cooperation of intrinsic dynamics and network mechanisms is shown to correlate with bistability, i.e., the coexistence of two different attractors in the phase space of the system

corresponding to different rhythmic spatio-temporal patterns. In contrast, if the network mechanism of rhythmogenesis dominates, monostability is observed with a typical pattern of winnerless competition between neurons. The analysis of bifurcations between the two regimes reveals how they provide robustness and flexibility to the network performance.
In the second part of the chapter (neuronal module level) we discuss the interaction of different motif networks that produce rhythmic activities and analyze their (periodic or chaotic) cooperative dynamics. One of the promising applications of the general analysis is building a mathematical theory for hippocampal theta rhythms known to be crucial for spatial memory. It is interesting that the interaction of two or more core motif networks could generate chaotic rhythms with very specific dynamical features that we discuss in detail here. We also analyze here the interaction of network oscillations with external periodic fields. One aspect that we have investigated in detail is heteroclinic synchronization that can explain the coordination of different rhythms in the brain (see Fig 6).
In the third part of the chapter (mental mode level) we describe rhythmic mental dynamics. In particular, based on an ecological model of cognitive and emotional modes that compete for energy and informational resources, we have discovered a new instability that can be the origin of low frequency oscillations in the brain. It is an envelope or modulation instability that is typical for the brain resting state. Our modeling has demonstrated the emergence of pulsations of brain activity with a time scale of about 25-30 s. The mathematical object that represents this rhythmic activity is a heteroclinic cycle that appears in the phase space of the three clusters of modes which we identify as the cognitive, emotional and resources clusters.

2. Small neuronal motif networks

Oscillatory neural circuits and, in particular, central pattern generators (GPGs) contain both basic rhythmogenic and pattern forming mechanisms. A question fundamental to such networks is how the specific intrinsic activity of individual neurons can be constrained by synaptic dynamics and network organization and, conversely, how the network output emerges from the cooperative activity of the network components.
Over the last three decades, neurophysiologists have proposed two different mechanisms for the generation of neuronal network oscillations: rhythmogenesis by one or more pacemaker neurons and rhythm generation by network mechanisms. Pacemaker mechanisms are based on a single neuron, or a synchronized neural group, that generates bursting activity as a result of intrinsic cellular properties, while the rest of the network orchestrates the phase relationships between different principal cells (or cell groups) to generate a specific spatio-temporal pattern (Rabinovich, Huerta, Varona & Afraimovich, 2006; Selverston & Miller, 1980; Yuste et al., 2005; Buzsaki, 2006; Kopell et al., 2005; Börgers et al., 2005). In network-based rhythm generation the spatio-temporal dynamics result from the excitatory and inhibitory synaptic connections between neurons, which do not have intrinsic rhythmic activity. In this case, networks of tonically spiking neurons are able to generate rhythmic bursts as a result of a cooperative, synapse-mediated, modulational instability (Nowotny & Rabinovich, 2007).
Rhythmogenesis based on inhibition has been studied extensively in the past (see e.g., (Whittington et al., 2000) for a review). However, the existing theoretical work was often focused on networks with symmetric reciprocal inhibition. In this earlier work it has been well established that, depending on synaptic characteristics (e.g synaptic timescale, synaptic depression) and intrinsic neuronal characteristics (e.g. spike frequency adaptation) the

inhibition between two neurons can produce synchronous or anti-phase activity (Calabrese, 1995; Wang & Rinzel, 1993; Skinner et al., 1994). Concurrent gap-junction coupling is, furthermore, known to complement burst generation through inhibition and its synchronization (in-phase or anti-phase) (Skinner et al., 1999; Mancilla et al., 2007). These ideas have shown a vast potential for modeling coordination, memory and decision-making tasks like artificial CPG design (Lewis et al., 2003) or the two-interval discrimination problem (Machens et al., 2005). Generalization to two competing neural populations in the context of explaining binocular rivalry yields essentially similar phenomena (Tong et al., 2006). The emphasis was typically on the case of symmetrical coupling, because asymmetry seemed to add little qualitative change to the dynamics, if any.

Another approach is analyzing symmetry breaking bifurcations and arising stable heteroclinic cycles (the image of alternating neural activity) in networks with ring topology (Buono et al., 2000; Golomb & Ermentrout, 2002). In this case the symmetry of coupling strengths was the key demand for the analytical treatment to be fulfilled. A step towards understanding the principal role of asymmetry in the rhythmogenesis in multi-cell motifs was made in a series of papers by (Rabinovich et al., 2001; Afraimovich et al., 2004; Rabinovich et al., 2008) and (Nowotny & Rabinovich, 2007). They revealed the origin of sequential bursting activity in inhibitory spiking neural ensembles (the minimal motif had three neurons). These oscillations were shown to bifurcate from stable heteroclinic sequences in the phase space of the network. Moreover, it was proved that sequences are uniquely determined by the given asymmetry of the network.

Little is known about the dynamical principles that govern the interplay between intrinsic bursting and network mechanisms when both are found in a single system. There is growing experimental evidence suggesting that in some neural systems, like the respiratory CPG of mammals, the rhythm is generated by a combined pacemaker-network mechanism (Johnson et al., 2007; Rybak et al., 2004; 2007; Calabrese, 1998; Sohal et al., 2006), in this case operating on a distributed population of coupled, bursting pacemaker neurons. It has been suggested that such hybrid mechanisms of rhythmogenesis are potentially more robust, more reliable and more flexible than mechanisms based on pacemakers or network topology alone. They may, therefore, be more frequently at work in neuronal systems than previously assumed, which motivated us to examine their fundamental dynamical properties.

2.1 From tonic-spiking neuronal activity to network bursting

There is a growing body of evidence that slow brain rhythms are generated by simple inhibitory neuronal networks. Sequential switching emerging from a modulation instability of tonic spiking activity is a widespread phenomenon underlying such rhythms. A basic dynamical system demonstrating reproducible switching is a network or motif realizing the Winnerless Competition Principle (WLC) (Rabinovich et al., 2001; Afraimovich et al., 2004). Below we analyze a minimal, reciprocally connected motif of three spiking units and explore observable dynamical regimes and transitions between them. We show that a tonic spiking regime loses its stability due to a Neimark-Sacker bifurcation. As computer modeling suggests, a heteroclinic cycle appears at the moment of bifurcation.

In general, the dynamical image of the bursting dynamics for the network-induced bursting is an attractor (limit cycle or strange attractor) in the vicinity of the heteroclinic manifold, which consists of saddle limit cycles and one-dimensional separatrix manifolds connecting them (see Fig. 1). The saddle limit cycles correspond to spiking in one of the neurons while

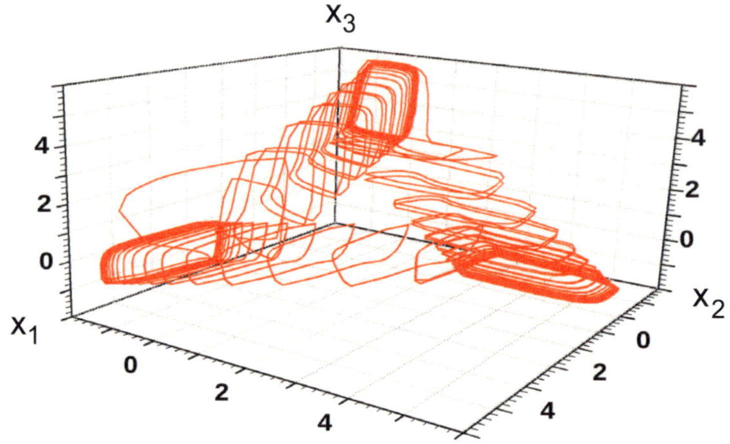

Fig. 1. Heteroclinic cycle (image of rhythmic bursting activity) in a 3D projection of the motif's phase space. Modified from (Rabinovich et al., 2000)

the others are silent. The sequential visits of the system to the neighborhoods of the saddle cycles is the origin of a periodic switching dynamics between silence and spiking in all neurons. The strength of the asymmetric inhibition between neurons determines the proximity of the attractor to the saddle cycles and the frequency of the network dynamics (Rabinovich, Huerta & Varona, 2006). The stronger the inhibition, the closer the attractor is to these saddles. To begin with, let us analyze the motif dynamics with a small network of simple spiking neurons described by the Bonhoeffer-Van der Pol model

$$\tau_1 \frac{dx_i(t)}{dt} = x_i(t) - \frac{1}{3}x_i^3(t) - y_i(t) - z_i(t)(x_i(t) - V) + S_i, \tag{1}$$

$$\frac{dy_i(t)}{dt} = x_i(t) - by_i(t) + a, \quad i = 1,\ldots,3, \tag{2}$$

which are connected by an inhibitory synaptic coupling described by

$$\tau_2 \frac{dz_i(t)}{dt} = \sum_j g_{ij} F(x_j) - z_i(t), \tag{3}$$

where $x_i(t)$ denotes the membrane potential of the ith neuron, $y_i(t)$ the variable corresponding to the action of all ionic currents, S_i the external stimuli to each neuron, V the reversal potential, g_{ij} the coupling coefficients between the ith and jth neuron and $F(x_j) = 1/(1+\exp((0.5-x_j)/20))$. The values of the parameters are fixed in all simulations to a=0.7, b = 0.8, τ_1 = 0.08, τ_2 = 3.1, and V = −1.5, and we chose the parameter S_i > 0.35 which corresponds to the tonic spiking regime of individual uncoupled neurons. Depending on the level of asymmetry of the inhibitory coupling, this simple network demonstrates a variety of dynamical regimes. In particular, regimes in which (i) one of the neurons generates tonic spiking and two other neurons are suppressed, (ii) two neurons are active and one is suppressed, (iii) all three neurons exhibit synchronous in-phase spiking oscillations ($x_1 = x_2 =$

x_3), and (iv) sequential bursting activity emerges. In terms of the dynamical system, a stable limit cycle (of tonic spiking) transforms after bifurcation into a saddle cycle. Local bifurcation analysis and computer modeling of the global network dynamics of the system described by (1)-(3) was performed in (Komarov et al., 2009). The local bifurcation that corresponds to a modulation instability was identified to be a Neimark-Sacker bifurcation. In a dynamical system with discrete time (an iterated map) this bifurcation is characterized by the birth of a closed invariant curve from a fixed point when the fixed point changes stability via a pair of complex eigenvalues with unit modulus. We are interested in a sub-critical Neimark-Sacker bifurcation, which results in an unstable limit cycle (within an invariant two-dimensional manifold). When this happens in the Poincaré map of a limit cycle, the bifurcation generates an invariant two-dimensional torus in the corresponding dynamical continuous time model (Kuznetsov, 1998). The stable two-dimensional torus is a geometrical image of stable rhythmic burst oscillations.

To analyze the emergence of such a regime it is necessary to investigate the dependence of the Floquet multipliers of the limit cycles which correspond to tonic spiking regimes on the control parameters $\alpha_i = g_{ij}/g_{ji}$, i.e., the degree of asymmetry of the inhibitory coupling strengths. In the absence of resonance the modulation appears when two conjugate complex multipliers reach the unit circle. Fig. 2 illustrates how multipliers change with increasing asymmetry of inhibitory connections. For the parameters of the system (1)-(3) a heteroclinic torus appears when the asymmetry of the connections becomes strong enough, i.e., $\alpha_i \gg 7.36 > 1$.

When considering biologically more plausible Hodgkin-Huxley neurons, the analysis of the global bifurcations of the phase portrait of the motif dynamics becomes quickly analytically and numerically intractable. Nowotny & Rabinovich (2007) demonstrated, however, that if no resonance between cooperative bursting and individual neuronal spiking dynamics exists, an elegant direct reduction of the H-H model to an average (rate) description of the activity of individual neurons can be used to analyze the bifurcations of the system. The results of this analysis, comparing the bifurcations of the model at the two different levels of description, are presented in Fig. 3.

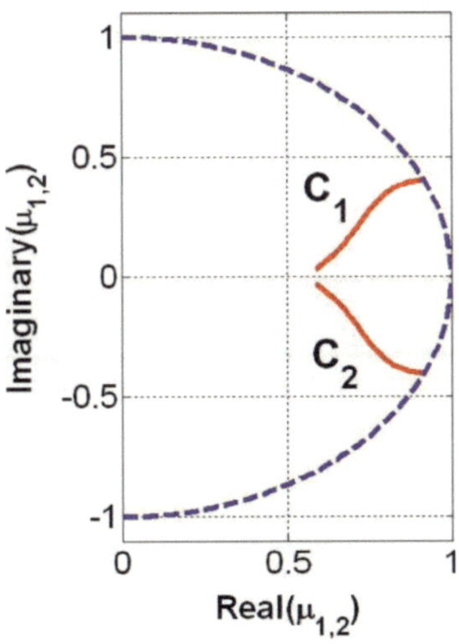

Fig. 2. The trajectories of two complex conjugate Floquet multipliers (red lines) as the system (1)-(3) approaches a Neimark-Sacker bifurcation. The bifurcation occurs when the multipliers reach the unit circle (dashed blue line). Modified from Komarov et al. (2009)

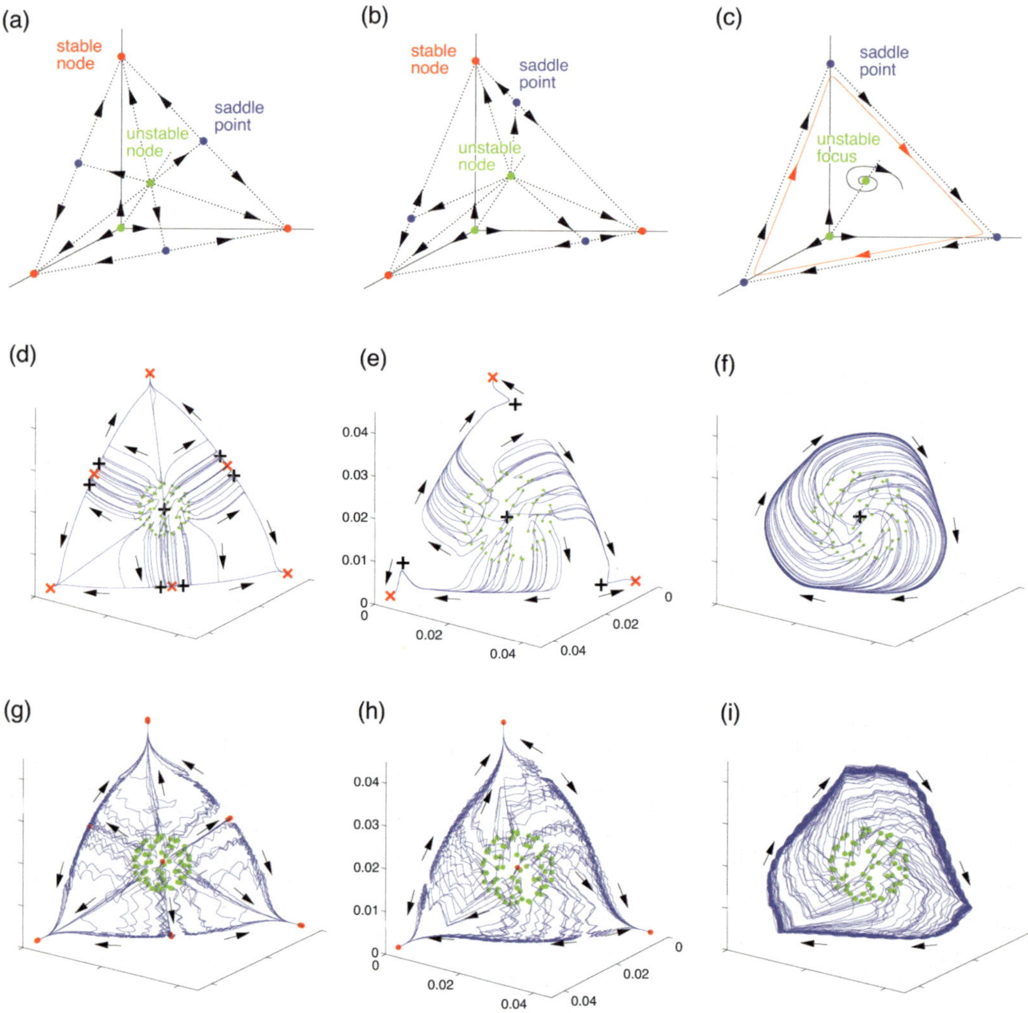

Fig. 3. Bifurcation towards rhythmic bursting in the Lotka-Volterra model, a biologically more plausible H-H type circuit model, and its average rate description. The Lotka-Volterra model with three units (a-c), undergoes a simultaneous saddle-node bifurcation in the three corners of the shown phase space simplex with increasing asymmetry of the connections (red points - stable fixed points (FP), blue points - saddles, green points - unstable FP). Numerical evidence for a similar bifurcation can be found in a system of realistic Hogkin-Huxley neurons (g-i) (Nowotny & Rabinovich, 2007). This is confirmed by a systematic reduction of the biophysical Hodgkin-Huxley model to an equivalent rate model (d-f) and a subsequent numerical bifurcation analysis (red and black crosses in d-f denote the calculated FPs - red crosses are stable FP and black markers are FP with at least one unstable direction (saddles or unstable FP)). Modified from (Nowotny & Rabinovich, 2007)

The modulation instability that is related to a sub-critical Neimark-Sacker bifurcation is a general mechanism of the emergence of Low Frequency Oscillation (LFO) on all levels of neural network complexity (see also below). The necessary condition for such an instability is a non-symmetric competition between agents, i.e., neurons, oscillating neuronal masses, or mental modes.

2.2 Competition-cooperation of bursting neurons in inhibitory networks

Let us now analyze bifurcations between the pacemaker and network regimes and understand how they provide robustness and flexibility to the network performance. Based on a simple model network (a motif, see e.g., (Sporns & Kötter, 2004; Milo et al., 2002; Zhigulin, 2004)) of three conditionally bursting Hodgkin-Huxley (H-H) type neurons with reciprocal inhibitory coupling, we elucidate some of the important properties of pacemaker-network interactions (Ivanchenko et al., 2008). The model network was inspired by the stomatogastric system of lobsters and we use the term conditional to signify that the biological bursting requires the presence of appropriate neuromodulators. In the model this corresponds to the presence of appropriate de- or hyperpolarization of the somatic compartment. The model neurons are similar to the lateral pyloric (LP) neurons in the lobster *Panulirus interruptus*, which normally burst irregularly when isolated. The model neurons also mimic real LP neurons in that being depolarized causes them to burst at higher frequencies and with longer bursts and being hyperpolarized slows the burst frequency down and decreases the burst duration (Nowotny et al., 2008). Furthermore, similar to the graded synapses in the lobster stomatogastric CPG, the model synapses are slow enough to implement an interaction between bursts rather than responding to single spikes. We are interested in the drastic changes (bifurcations) in the network dynamics which occur when the strength of intrinsic pacemaker activity is altered by passage of DC current and/or when the strength of the synaptic connections changes. The two-compartment neuron model used in this study was built based on voltage clamp recordings and extensive fits to data from isolated lobster LP neurons (Nowotny et al., 2008). The LP neuron plays an important role in the dynamics of the pyloric CPG of the lobster and is known to be a conditional burster with a wide range of dynamics from tonic spiking to irregular spiking, chaotic bursting, and regular bursting for polarizations ranging from depolarization to increasing levels of hyperpolarization. The LP neuron model is particularly well suited for our purposes because it replicates this wide range of dynamics. As we have already mentioned, burst generation in the circuit is based on two separate mechanisms.

Intrinsic bursting: In this case the synaptic connections determine the relative phases and detailed timings of the bursting activity of the pacemaker-type neurons. Pacemaker neurons can drive single-phase rhythms, such as heartbeat, by themselves and in synaptically connected clusters they can produce multi-phase rhythms as seen in the pyloric CPG in lobster. It has generally been assumed that pacemaker neurons lend a degree of robustness to rhythmic systems and they have indeed been found in almost all small circuits that have been described.

Network bursting: Here, the mechanism of rhythmogenesis is a modulation instability of the network (also known as winnerless competition). The constituent neurons of the circuit are tonic spiking neurons and the sequential bursting emerges due to synaptic interactions for sufficiently asymmetric connections between the neurons of the motif (Rabinovich et al., 2001; Afraimovich et al., 2004; Rabinovich et al., 2008). The sequence of bursting is uniquely determined by the network structure: in our case the chosen asymmetry of the inhibitory synapses will usually select a clockwise sequence of bursts; a reversal of the asymmetry would produce an opposite temporal sequence by default. This mechanism does not depend on the details of the dynamics of the constituent neurons other than that they are intrinsically active (Nowotny & Rabinovich, 2007). An example of a network bursting system of Hodgkin-Huxley neuron is illustrated in figure 4. In this particular example, the system undergoes a bifurcation with increasing intrinsic excitability of the neurons, in which the heteroclinic orbit underlying network bursting becomes stable and causes an infinite slowdown of the bursting dynamics (Fig. 4c and d).

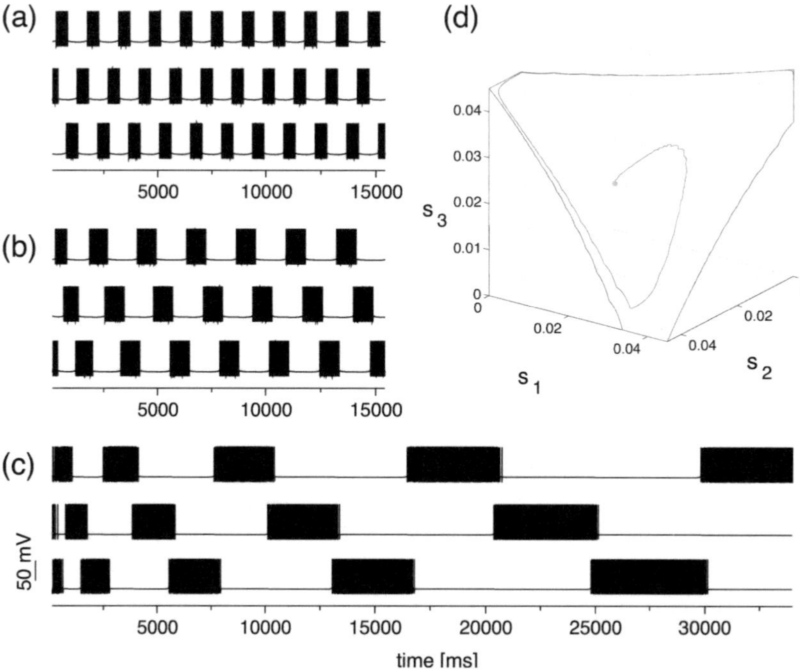

Fig. 4. Example of an entirely network driven rhythm in a model of biophysical Hodgkin-Huxley model neurons. When increasing the intrinsic neuronal excitability of the neurons in the 3-neuron circuit modeled (a to c), the heteroclinic orbit underlying the rhythmic bursting becomes attracting, leading to an infinite slowdown of bursting as the trajectory of the system approaches it (c). The corresponding phase space picture in terms of the synaptic activation (which can be used as a proxy for firing rate) is shown in d). The trajectory starts in the green point and then approaches the stable heteroclinic orbit. Modified from Nowotny & Rabinovich (2007)

If the neurons can exhibit both intrinsic bursting and tonic spiking activity, network-induced bursting and pacemaker-type bursting dynamics may coexist and interact. Numerical experiments reveal at least two types of dynamics resulting from the interaction of intrinsic and network mechanisms.

When the neurons are hyperpolarized, network and intrinsic burst generation interact (cooperate) in forming network oscillations. Bursting is dominantly characterized by post-inhibitory rebound (PIR) and spontaneous burst termination of the neurons. Interestingly, the cooperation of network and intrinsic bursting mechanisms leads to bi-stability: A clockwise bursting sequence and an anti-clockwise bursting sequence coexist and are both stable. This bistability exists for a wide range of coupling strengths. Figure 5 shows an example of this phenomenon. In the clockwise bursting sequence $1 \rightarrow 2 \rightarrow 3$, the less

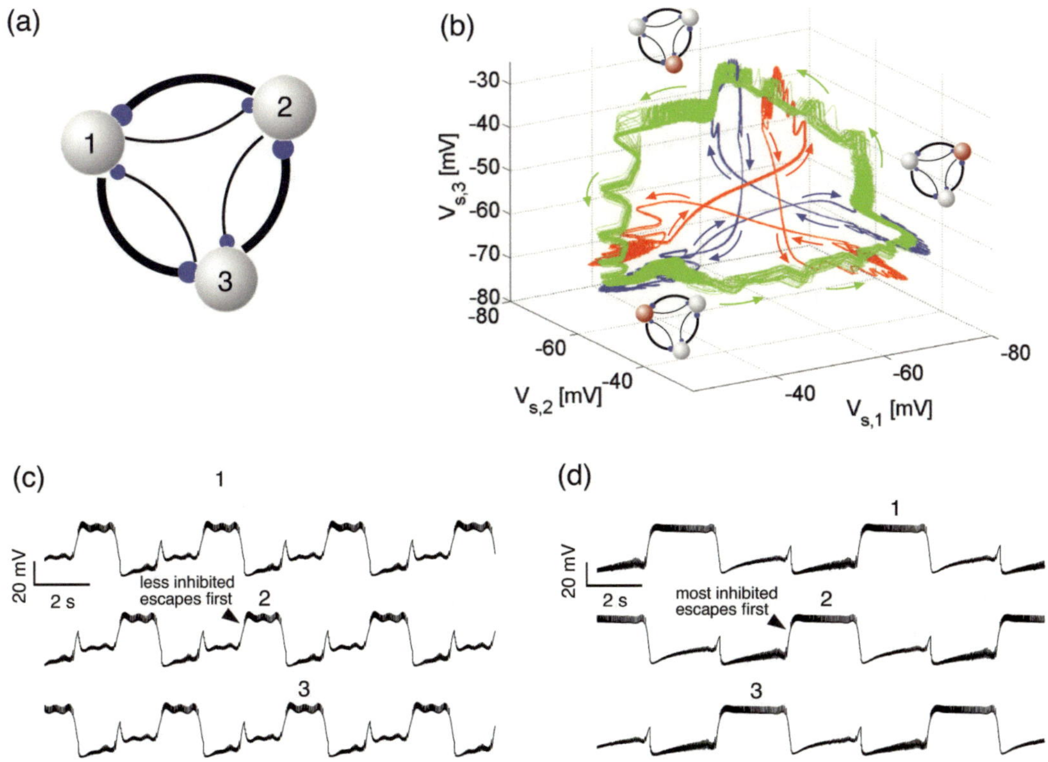

Fig. 5. A bifurcation towards bistability appears as a function of the "strength" of intrinsic bursting. A) face portraits of two co-existing attractors for strong bursting, *i.e.* for short bursts, (I_{DC} = −6 nA): Sequences 1→2→3 (blue) and 3!2!1 (red) are both stable limit cycles. At weaker bursting, *i.e.* for long intrinsic bursts (I_{DC} = −1.0 nA) only a 1→2→3 sequence exists (green). B) Example time series data for the 1 → 2 → 3 (top) and 3 → 2 → 1 sequence (bottom). Note how the less inhibited neuron escapes from inhibition first in the former and the more inhibited neuron escapes first in the latter. Modified from (Ivanchenko et al., 2008)

inhibited neuron escapes first from inhibition and continues the cycle (Fig. 5c). In the other case, the most inhibited neuron escapes first due to PIR and the sequence is counter-clockwise, 3 → 2 → 1 (Fig. 5d).

With decreasing intrinsic hyperpolarization of the neurons, the system undergoes a bifurcation towards mono-stability, where the network mechanism of burst generation persists, leading to a single attractor of clock-wise bursting (green trace in Fig. 5b). Intuitively, we can understand this transition as a transition of the neurons from strong bursters with strong PIR to weak bursters with long bursts and short, comparatively weak, hyperpolarization episodes. Consistently with this interpretation the bifurcation towards mono-stability occurs approximately at the point where the length of the intrinsic bursts of the neurons starts to exceed the duration of bursts in the network. With respect to the network dynamics, the neurons then act essentially like tonically spiking neurons.

With this model we are now also able to address some additional questions: i) What are the characteristics of the hybrid pacemaker-network mechanisms of bursting in the elementary network? ii) What combination of neural circuit parameters, e.g., synaptic strengths or length of bursts, control the qualitative changes of the rhythmic patterns? iii) Do the concurrent mechanisms provide robustness and flexibility to the motif network, i.e., the ability to generate input-specific but reproducible responses under the action of an informational signal?

In the monostable regime of long intrinsic bursts the network activity is based on a competitive interaction of neurons that essentially restructures (shortens) the bursts, when inhibition strengthens. This interaction yields the unique bursting pattern, with characteristics that sensitively depend upon the level of inhibition (as with a pure network mechanism of burst generation).

Short intrinsic bursts on the other hand allow cooperative network oscillations, in which inhibitory interactions promote subsequent activity in inhibited neurons by PIR, in addition to the competition scenario. This leads to explained bistability of bursting patterns. Two parameters control the emergence of bistability: the asymmetry of reciprocal inhibition and the length of intrinsic bursts. Because of the interaction of intrinsic and synaptic dynamics both types of bursting patterns are highly robust, i.e., even if one of the neurons is changed to a tonic spiking regime, the other two neurons make it resume bursting and produce almost the same network patterns as if all neurons are identical (Ivanchenko et al., 2008). The hybrid pacemaker-network bursting does show a well-pronounced flexibility as well. The level of DC-input to the cells (interpreted as their intrinsic excitability) and synaptic plasticity can make the circuit switch between bistability and monostability, and modulating the overall synaptic strength can change the characteristics of bursting on a large scale.

Thus the hybrid pacemaker-network mechanism has modes of cooperation or of competition between the cellular and network dynamics and demonstrates both robustness (stability of the produced patterns) and flexibility (the ability to produce different patterns in response to appropriate stimuli) concurrently. The consequence of cooperation or competition is the bistability or monostability of spatio-temporal bursting patterns, and the decisive factors for either cooperation or competition are the parameters underlying intrinsic bursting. The other basic control parameter to switch between cooperation and competition is the asymmetry of coupling. Surprisingly it has been found that bistability only disappears for strong asymmetry, which suggests that comparatively weak background synaptic interactions could still qualitatively change the overall network dynamics and give rise to new bursting patterns and therefore cannot be neglected *a priori*.

3. Oscillatory motifs interaction

In complex hierarchical neural systems like the brain the oscillatory motifs that we have considered so far can play the role of individual dynamical agents. The cooperation and competition between them are the origin of many phenomena observed in the brain such as synchronization, low frequency oscillations, chaotic modulation of brain rhythms and so on.

3.1 Motifs activity clustering and synchronization.

EEG recordings of brain activity exhibit multiple frequency peaks or rhythms in the range from < 1 Hz, up to > 100 Hz. These rhythms are able to synchronize with each other even when they have very different frequencies (Roopun et al., 2008). The functional roles played by these synchronized neuronal oscillations vary widely – synchronized rhythms can facilitate synaptic plasticity (Buzsaki & Draguhn, 2004), correlate with attention (Womelsdorf et al., 2006), allow perceptual binding (Lachaux et al., 2005), and are involved in many others mechanisms (Palva & Palva, 2007). Recently, (Canolty et al., 2006) have observed robust coupling between the high- and low-frequency bands of ongoing electrical activity in the human brain. In particular, they indicated that the phase of the low-frequency theta (4 to 8 Hz) rhythm modulates the power in the high gamma (80 to 150 Hz) band of the electrocorticogram. The dynamical origin of such an interaction between rhythms with frequency ratios on the order of 15 − 20 is still unclear. We propose that the mechanism underlying this extraordinary phenomenon may be related to the heteroclinic modulation instability that we discussed above. It is well known that interneurons are able to cooperate in distinct local inhibitory networks (motifs) that are well-suited for generating synchronous gamma frequency rhythmic activity in the cortex (Whittington & Traub, 2003; Buzsaki, 2006). Because of the synchronization, such inhibitory motifs form clusters that compete with each other through slow inhibitory interaction. Thus, it is reasonable to hypothesize that the low frequency theta rhythm is a result of cyclic competition of different "theta clusters". As a result of such a competition the power of gamma oscillations has to be strongly modulated by the rhythmic slow switching, i.e., the low frequency theta rhythm.

Another problem that is related to this subject is the synchronization of different low frequency theta-motifs by high frequency global brain rhythms. The existence of this type of synchronization supports the popular explanation of long-range coordination of distinct brain region's activities (see (Fries, 2005) for review).

To illustrate the dynamical origin of such disparate-frequency synchronization we suppose that the theta rhythm is generated by WLC motifs and that different theta-motifs have no other interactions except for a joint external oscillatory field. In this case we can focus the analysis on the entrainment of the oscillations of one motif under the action of an oscillating external field.

The results of modeling the equations

$$\dot{a}_i = a_i\left[1-\left(a_i+\sum_{j\neq i}^{N}\rho_{ij}a_j\right)+\xi(t)\right]+\gamma\varphi_i(\omega_f t, a_i), \tag{4}$$

where $a_i(t) \geq 0$ represents the rate of the neural activity of the ith neural pool in the motif, $0 < \rho_{ij} < 1$, $\rho_{ii} = 1$ is an inhibitory connectivity matrix, $\varphi_i(\omega t, a_i) \geq 0$ is a periodic function with period $T = 2\pi/\omega$, $\xi(t)$ is Gaussian white noise, and $\gamma \ll 1$ is the coupling to the external field, are illustrated in Fig. 6.

Similarly, when considering a motif of spiking H-H type neurons coupled asymmetrically with inhibitory synapses, we observe wide areas of synchronization to an external oscillation continuing to very high frequency ratios (see Fig. 7). Surprisingly, this sub-harmonic synchronization already appears for fairly weak oscillatory drive, and even if only one of the neurons in the network is driven by it.

3.2 Chaotically modulated ordered sequences.

A related, but at first sight seemingly different, phenomenon is the emergence of reproducible but irregularly timed (chaotically modulated) sequences that have been proposed to underlie the chaotic hunting patterns by the marine mollusk *Clione* (Varona et al., 2002). In this work it was suggested, that the statocyst network, a small inhibitory micro-

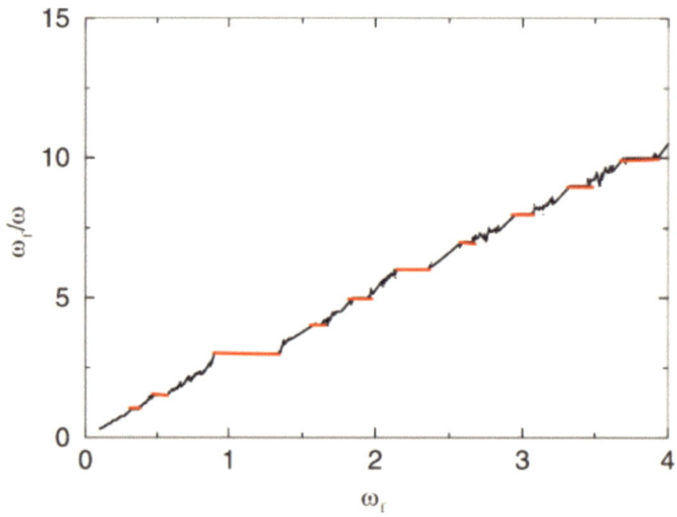

Fig. 6. Devil's Staircase and bands of heteroclinic synchronization between low- and highfrequency oscillations. Modified from (Rabinovich, Huerta & Afraimovich, 2006)

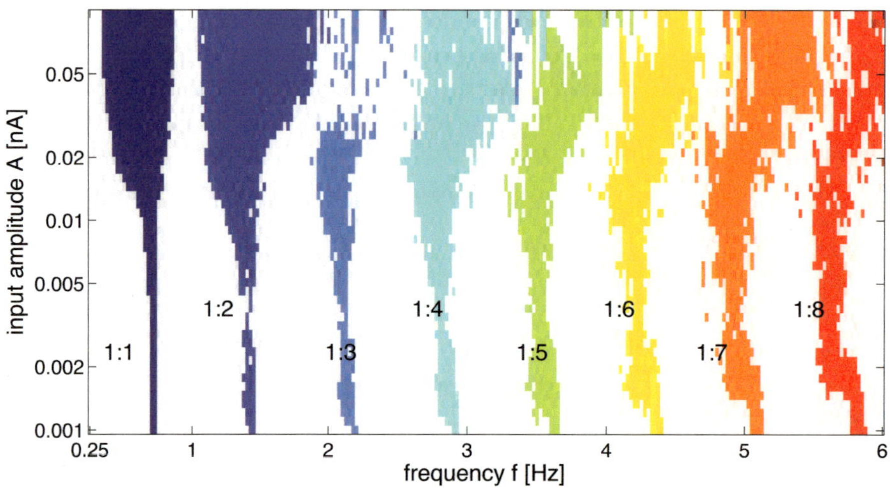

Fig. 7. Arnold tongues for a network of Hodgkin-Huxley model neurons. One of the neurons received the negative part of a sinusoidal external input. The oscillation frequency of the circuit was measured as the inverse of the average burst to burst period of all three neurons.

circuit in the brain of *Clione* that normally is used to balance the mollusk's body position, is driven by a global excitatory drive from the "hunting neuron" whenever the mollusk senses the vicinity of its prey. This global excitation causes the network of the statocyst receptor cells (SRCs) to generate a complex output due to the intrinsic network dynamics (winnerless competition). This output is directed to the cerebral ganglia to participate in forming a search motor program. The theoretical validity of this hypothesis was demonstrated in the model study of Varona et al. (2002). It was found that a simple network formed by neuron-like elements with non-reciprocal inhibitory connections generated a complex switching

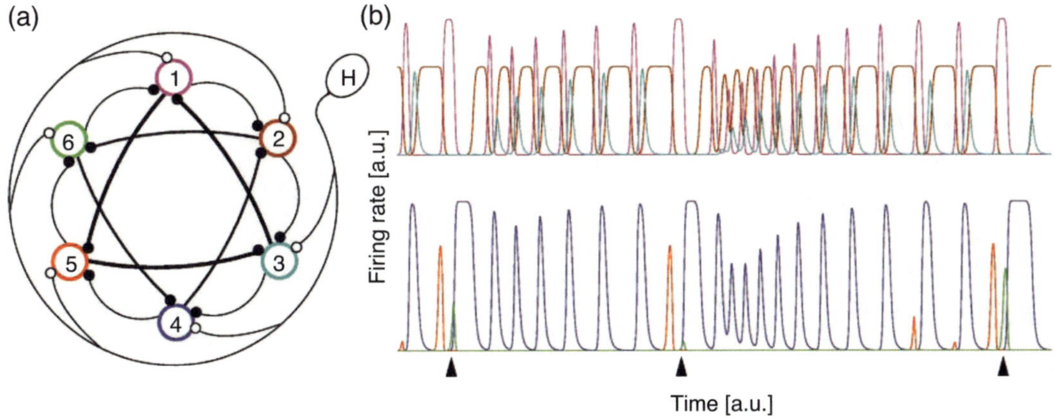

Fig. 8. Model for the statocyst network dynamics. A: architecture of the model network: color circles represent 6 model receptor neurons (MSRCs), and k circles represent inhibitory connections; thicker traces mean stronger connections. CHunINs are represented by H, and excitatory connections to the MSRCs are depicted with small white circles. B: firing rates of the MSRCs induced by activating the model CHunIN (H). Activities of the 1st MSRCs (units 13 in A) are shown in the top panel; the bottom panel corresponds to the activity of units 4 6; the colors used correspond to the colors of MSRCs shown in A. Arrows show an example of the coordinated activation among units even when the neurons are silent for a long period. Firing rates and time scale are arbitrary. Modified from (Levi et al., 2004)

activity in response to the excitatory input (H in Fig. 8), mimicking the effect of the *Clione* hunting interneurons (CHunINs). The excitation from the hunting neuron in the model was only used to trigger the activation of the receptor network dynamics. The model CHunIN activity did not require any temporal structure to produce the switching dynamics. In addition, the model showed that such a network can produce an ordered pattern of activation in otherwise irregular activity. This is a desirable feature to organize a complex but coordinated motion. The known anatomical connections suggest that the statocyst output can be reflected, at least partly, in the activity of tail motoneurons. Therefore, the model results are in correspondence with results obtained in electrophysiological experiments (Levi et al., 2004; 2005).

4. Neuronal mass network oscillations

The execution of cognitive functions and information processing in the brain in general are largely based on dynamic interactions within a complex network of neurons. Neuronal mass modeling is one of the approaches that play an important role in investigating these processes. It can, in contrast to single neuron activity, be supported by non-invasive measurements such as EEG, MEG and fMRI. The analysis of the dynamics of interconnected neural mass networks can help to understand the origin of some brain activity and to find the relationship of it with brain measurements and psychological functions. Below we illustrate the phenomenon of emergent network rhythms in systems with random excitatory-inhibitory synaptic connections based on the Wilson-Cowan model of excitatory and inhibitory neuronal mass interaction. The Wilson-Cowan formalism (Wilson & Cowan, 1972; 1973) can be reduced to the following equations:

$$\mu\frac{\partial E(x,t)}{\partial t}=-E(x,t)+(1-rE(x,t))\mathcal{L}_e\Big(\int E(y,t)w_{ee}(y,x)dy-\int I(y,t)w_{ei}(y,x)dy+S_e(x,t)\Big),\quad(5)$$

$$\mu\frac{\partial I(x,t)}{\partial t}=-I(x,t)+(1-rI(x,t))\mathcal{L}_i\Big(\int E(y,t)w_{ie}(y,x)dy-\int I(y,t)w_{ii}(y,x)dy+S_i(x,t)\Big),\quad(6)$$

where $E(x, t)$ and $I(x, t)$ are the proportions of firing neurons in the excitatory and inhibitory populations, the coordinate x is a continuous variable that represents the position in the cortical surface, w_{ee}, w_{ei}, w_{ie}, and w_{ii} are the connectivity weights, and S_e and S_i are external inputs to the excitatory and inhibitory populations, respectively. The gain functions $\mathcal{L}_e$ and $\mathcal{L}_i$ reflect the expected proportions of excitatory and inhibitory neurons receiving at least threshold excitation per unit of time. One subtle trick used in the derivation of this model is that the membrane integration time is introduced through synaptic connections. The model expressed in this form attempts to eliminate the uncertainty of single neurons by grouping them according to those with reliable common responses. We are still left with the problem of what to expect in a network of neuronal masses connected randomly to each other.

In a random network of excitatory and inhibitory neurons, it is not uncommon to find oscillatory activity (Jin & Seung, 2002; Huerta & Rabinovich, 2004). Huerta & Rabinovich (2004) showed, using the Wilson-Cowan formalism, that periodic sequential activity, i.e., limit cycles, is more likely to be found in regions of the control parameter space where inhibitory and excitatory synapses are slightly out of balance. They have analyzed the Wilson-Cowan model in the form

$$\mu\frac{dx_i(t)}{dt}=\Theta\left(\sum_{j=1}^{N_E}w_{ij}^{EE}x_j(t)-\sum_{j=1}^{N_I}w_{ij}^{EI}y_j(t)+S_i^E\right)-x_i(t),\quad(7)$$

$$\mu\frac{dy_i(t)}{dt}=\Theta\left(\sum_{j=1}^{N_E}w_{ij}^{IE}x_j(t)-\sum_{j=1}^{N_I}w_{ij}^{II}y_j(t)+S_i^I\right)-y_i(t),\quad(8)$$

where $x_i(t)$ and $y_i(t)$ represent the fractions of active neurons in cluster i of the excitatory and inhibitory populations, respectively. The numbers of excitatory and inhibitory clusters are N_E and N_I. The labels E and I are used to denote quantities associated with the excitatory or inhibitory populations, respectively. The external inputs $S_{E,I}$ are instantaneous kicks applied to a fraction of the total population at time zero. The gain function is $\Theta(z) = (\tanh((z-b)/\sigma) + 1)/2$, with a threshold $b = 0.1$ below the excitatory and inhibitory synaptic strength of a single connection. Clusters are taken to have very sharp thresholds of excitability by choosing $\sigma = 0.01$. The time scale is set to $\mu = 10$ ms as originally done by Wilson & Cowan (1972). The connectivity matrices w_{ij}^{XY} have entries drawn from a Bernoulli process (Huerta & Rabinovich, 2004). The main control parameters in this problem are the probability of connections from population to population.

Now we can answer the important question: What kind of activity can a network with many neurons and random connections produce? Intuition suggests that the answer has to be complex multidimensional dynamics. However, this is not the case. The results presented in Fig. 9 tell us that most observable stimulus-dependent dynamics are more simple and reproducible: periodic dynamics, transient dynamics, or low dimensional chaos.

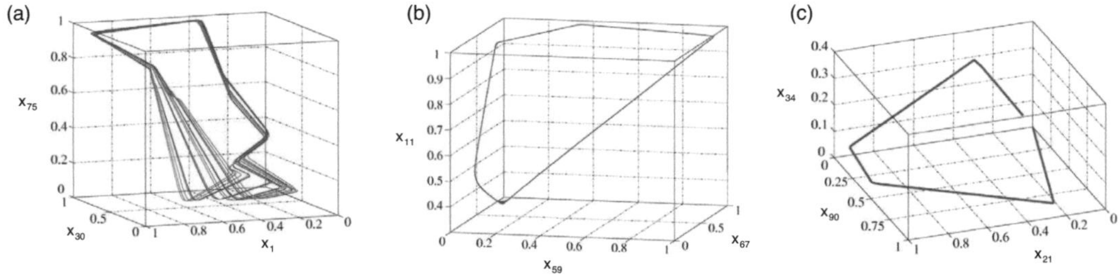

Fig. 9. Three-dimensional projections of simulations of random networks of 200 neurons. For illustrative purposes we show three types of dynamics that can be generated by a random network: a) chaos, b) limit cycle, both regimes in the areas of parameter space that are close to balance and c) transient dynamics far from balance of excitatory-inhibitory connections. Modified from (Rabinovich, Varona, Selverston & Abarbanel, 2006)

5. Mental mode network: Low frequency (< 0.1 Hz) rhythm generation

Now let us consider the spontaneous rhythmic dynamics of mental modes in a stationary environment where the brain is not engaged in a particular cognitive function, i.e., the resting-state brain dynamics. Mental modes have been introduced in (Rabinovich & Muezzinoglu, 2010) in the following way: The cognitive cooperative activity at time t can be represented as $\sum_{i=1}^{N} A_i(t)V(i)$, where $V(i)$ is a fixed distributed neuronal set that forms the i-th cognitive mode, and $A_i(t) \geq 0$ is its level of activity, in particular, the average intensity of all voxels covering the spatial pattern $U(i)$ in an fMRI image at time t. Some of the cognitive modes can be responsible for the interaction with emotion, i.e., valence, arousal and generation of any given coping strategy (see also (Damasio, 1994)). The number N of these cognitive modes depends on the level of detail that is necessary to describe the particular brain state. Emotional activity is represented in the same way, $\sum_{i=1}^{M} B_i(t)U(i)$, where $B_i(t) \geq 0$ are dynamical variables and $U(i)$ is the structure of the ith emotional mode. The ensemble of emotional modes includes both positive and negative emotions in the model. Resources are represented in a similar manner.

Mental modes competition - Describing the interaction between mental modes, specifically cognitive and emotional modes that compete for the mental resources (memory, attention and so on), Rabinovich & Muezzinoglu (2010) have suggested a model of mental mode dynamics. This model is built for the variables, $A_i(t)$, $B_i(t)$, and $R_i(t)$, which characterize mental resources, according to

$$\tau_A^i \frac{d}{dt} A_i(t) = A_i(t)\left(\sigma_i(S,B,R_A) - \sum_{j=1}^{N} \rho_{ij} A_j(t) \right) + A_i(t)\eta_A(t), \quad i = 1,\ldots,N \tag{9}$$

$$\tau_B^i \frac{d}{dt} B_i(t) = B_i(t)\left(\zeta_i(S,A,R_B) - \sum_{j=1}^{M} \xi_{ij} B_j(t) \right) + B_i(t)\eta_B(t), \quad i = 1,\ldots,M \tag{10}$$

$$\theta_A^i \frac{d}{dt} R_A^i(t) = R_A^i(t)\left(\sum_{j=1}^{N} A_j(t) - \sum_{j=1}^{K_A} R_A^j(t) - \phi_A \sum_{j=1}^{K_B} R_B^j(t) + d_A(t)\right), \quad i = 1,\ldots,K_A \tag{11}$$

$$\theta_B^i \frac{d}{dt} R_B^i(t) = R_B^i(t)\left(\sum_{j=1}^{M} B_j(t) - \sum_{j=1}^{K_B} R_B^j(t) - \phi_B \sum_{j=1}^{K_A} R_A^j(t) + d_B(t)\right), \quad i = 1,\ldots,K_B \tag{12}$$

As the authors proposed, this model reflects mutual inhibition and excitation within and among the three sets of modes (cognitive, emotional and resources). These modes depend on the external inputs through parameter S (e.g., stress, cognitive load, physical state of the body). Characteristic times of the cognitive and emotional activities are τ_A and τ_B, respectively. The variables R_A^i and R_B^i characterize the K_A and K_B resource items that are allocated to cognition and emotion, respectively. The vectors R_A and R_B are the collections of these items that gate the increments of the cognitive and emotional modes in competition. The characteristic times θ of the different resources may vary. The coefficients ϕ_A and ϕ_B determine the level of competition between cognition and emotion for these resources. Each process is open to the multiplicative noise denoted by the η and d terms in the equations.
We have chosen the control parameters of the model (9)-(12) in the area of the control parameter space where the basic dynamics of both cognitive and emotional modes

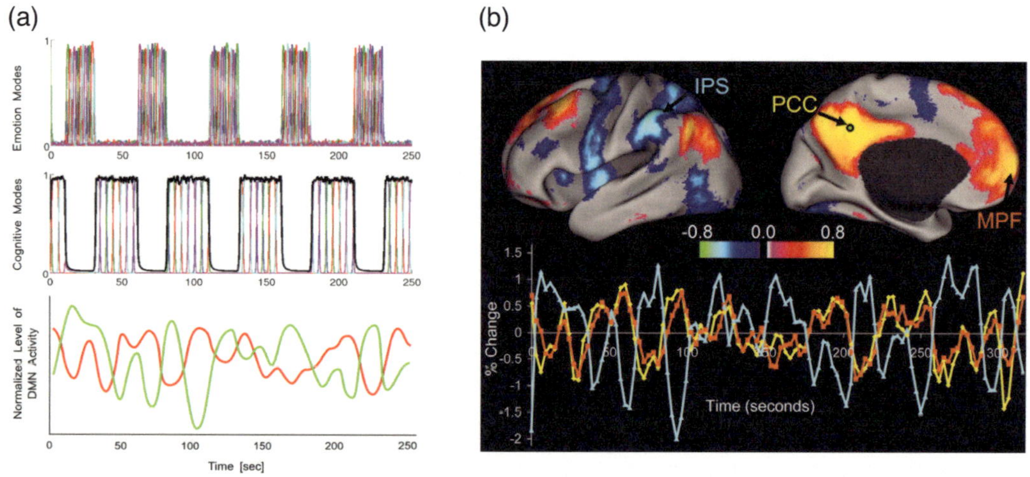

Fig. 10. Anti-phase Low-Frequency Oscillation of mental activity in the resting state (no external stimuli) is a result of two groups of default modes competition – modulation instability (a), modified from Rabinovich et al. (2010). The black envelope on the middle plot (a) is the total cognitive activity as predicted by the model. Its competition with the emotion modes (top row) results in a pulsation as observed in many EEG and fMRI studies. The bottom figure, reconstructed based on the data presented in (b), adapted from Fox et al. (2005), shows one such observation in the brain's resting state. (The resting state is related to the dynamics of the default-mode network (DMN), which is a set of specific brain regions whose activity is predominant during the resting state (Ben-Simon et al., 2008)).

demonstrate simple rhythmic activity (oscillations with the characteristic time of about 2 – 3 s). Such "independent" emotional and cognitive activity has been observed during weak competition. When the competition becomes larger than a critical value, this simple rhythmic activity becomes unstable due to a modulation instability, whereby a stable limit cycle appears on the phase plane of the mean activity $\tilde{A}(t)=\frac{1}{N}\sum_{i=1}^{N}A_i$ and $\tilde{B}(t)=\frac{1}{M}\sum_{i=1}^{M}B_i$. This modulation instability leads to a stable LFO, as shown in Fig. 10 (S is constant and N = M = 5 in the model (9)-(12)). The time-averaged oscillogram indicates that the observed robust modulation process is close to the quasi-periodic LFO. LFOs represent a fundamental component of brain activity. In particular, resting state fMRI measures show stable properties of LFO (see Fig. 10), the nature of which is only beginning to be uncovered and is producing numerous debates. For example, the LFO fluctuations observed with fMRI are not the same as the underlying neuronal fluctuations, because they have been passed through a hemodynamic response function. LFOs observed in fMRI could therefore simply be due to the band-pass filtering effect of this hemodynamic response function. However, some data (Tomasi & Volkow, 2010; Lörincz et al., 2009; Taylor et al., 2009; Buckner, 2010) support the hypothesis that LFOs are correlated with the network activity, i.e., the cooperative dynamics of network modes (e.g. due to their modulation or synchronization). The modulation instability that has been observed in the discussed computer experiments suggests a plausible dynamical origin of low frequency mental mode dynamics in brain resting states.

6. Conclusion

Integrating the results that have been discussed in this chapter, we can formulate some general statement, which sounds trivial enough: interactions between pacemaker and network mechanisms of rhythmic activity in neural systems are very diverse at all levels of the neuronal hierarchy. In complex systems, the role of the pacemaker can be played by neuronal clusters that are able to synchronize complex spatio-temporal patterns. However, what we can say more or less definitely is the following: *Low frequency oscillations* in complex systems, including the brain, are usually the result of cooperative activity of many neurons, brain centers, or modes. And, vice versa, (not necessary rhythmic) *fast switching between different states* is, as a rule, the result of activity of individual neurons. A recent report of Li et al. (2009) supports this point of view. In this study the authors showed that repetitive high-frequency bursts in a single cortical neuron of a rat could trigger a switch between the cortical states resembling slow-wave and rapid-eye-movement sleep.

7. References

Afraimovich, V. S., Zhigulin, V. P. & Rabinovich, M. I. (2004). On the origin of reproducible sequential activity in neural circuits., *Chaos* 14(4): 1123–1129. URL: *http://dx.doi.org/10.1063/1.1819625*

Ben-Simon, E., Podlipsky, I., Arieli, A., Zhdanov, A. & Hendler, T. (2008). Never resting brain: simultaneous representation of two alpha related processes in humans., *PLoS One* 3(12): e3984.

URL: *http://dx.doi.org/10.1371/journal.pone.0003984*

Börgers, C., Epstein, S. & Kopell, N. J. (2005). Background gamma rhythmicity and attention in cortical local circuits: a computational study., *Proc Natl Acad Sci U S A* 102(19): 7002– 7007. URL: *http://dx.doi.org/10.1073/pnas.0502366102*

Buckner, R. L. (2010). Human functional connectivity: new tools, unresolved questions., *Proc Natl Acad Sci U S A* 107(24): 10769–10770. URL: *http://dx.doi.org/10.1073/pnas.1005987107*

Buono, P.-L., Golubitsky,M. & Palacios, A. (2000). Heteroclinic cycles in rings of coupled cells, *Physica D: Nonlinear Phenomena* 143: 74–108.

Buzsaki, G. (2006). *Rhythms of the Brain*, Oxford University Press, New York.

Buzsaki, G. & Draguhn, A. (2004). Neuronal oscillations in cortical networks., *Science* 304(5679): 1926–1929. URL: *http://dx.doi.org/10.1126/science.1099745*

Calabrese, R. L. (1995). Oscillation inmotor pattern-generating networks., *Curr Opin Neurobiol* 5(6): 816–823.

Calabrese, R. L. (1998). Cellular, synaptic, network, and modulatory mechanisms involved in rhythm generation., *Curr Opin Neurobiol* 8(6): 710–717.

Canolty, R. T., Edwards, E., Dalal, S. S., Soltani, M., Nagarajan, S. S., Kirsch, H. E., Berger, M. S., Barbaro, N. M. & Knight, R. T. (2006). High gamma power is phase-locked to theta oscillations in human neocortex., *Science* 313(5793): 1626–1628. URL: *http://dx.doi.org/10.1126/science.1128115*

Damasio, A. (1994). *Descartes' Error: Emotion, Reason and the Human Brain,* Putnam, New York.

Fox, M. D., Snyder, A. Z., Vincent, J. L., Corbetta, M., Essen, D. C. V. & Raichle, M. E. (2005). The human brain is intrinsically organized into dynamic, anticorrelated functional networks., *Proc Natl Acad Sci U S A* 102(27): 9673–9678. URL: *http://dx.doi.org/10.1073/pnas.0504136102*

Fries, P. (2005). A mechanism for cognitive dynamics: neuronal communication through neuronal coherence., *Trends Cogn Sci* 9(10): 474–480. URL: *http://dx.doi.org/10.1016/j.tics.2005.08.011*

Golomb, D. & Ermentrout, G. B. (2002). Slow excitation supports propagation of slow pulses in networks of excitatory and inhibitory populations., *Phys Rev E Stat Nonlin Soft Matter Phys* 65(6 Pt 1): 061911.

Huerta, R. & Rabinovich, M. (2004). Reproducible sequence generation in random neural ensembles., *Phys Rev Lett* 93(23): 238104.

Ivanchenko, M. V., Nowotny, T., Selverston, A. I. & Rabinovich, M. I. (2008). Pacemaker and network mechanisms of rhythm generation: cooperation and competition., *J Theor Biol* 253(3): 452–461. URL: *http://dx.doi.org/10.1016/j.jtbi.2008.04.016*

Jin, D. Z. & Seung, H. S. (2002). Fast computation with spikes in a recurrent neural network, *Phys. Rev. E* 65(5): 051922.

Johnson, S. M., Wiegel, L. M. & Majewski, D. J. (2007). Are pacemaker properties required for respiratory rhythm generation in adult turtle brain stems in vitro?, *Am J Physiol Regul Integr Comp Physiol* 293(2): R901–R910.

URL: *http://dx.doi.org/10.1152/ajpregu.00912.2006*

Komarov, M. A., Osipov, G. V., Suykens, J. A. K. & Rabinovich,M. I. (2009). Numerical studies of slow rhythms emergence in neural microcircuits: bifurcations and stability., *Chaos* 19(1): 015107.
URL: *http://dx.doi.org/10.1063/1.3096412*

Kopell, N., Börgers, C., Pervouchine, D., Malerba, P. & Tort, A. (2005). Gamma and theta rhythms in biophysical models of hippocampal circuits, *in* V. Cutsuridis, S. Cobb,
B. Graham & I. Vida (eds), *Hippocampal Microcircuits: A Computational Modeler's Re- source Book*, Springer, New York, pp. 423–457.

Kuznetsov, Y. (1998). *Elements of Applied Bifurcation Theory, Vol. 112 of Applied Mathematical Sciences,* Springer, New York.

Lachaux, J.-P., George, N., Tallon-Baudry, C., Martinerie, J., Hugueville, L., Minotti, L., Kahane, P. & Renault, B. (2005). The many faces of the gamma band response to complex visual stimuli., *Neuroimage* 25(2): 491–501.
URL: *http://dx.doi.org/10.1016/j.neuroimage.2004.11.052*

Levi, R., Varona, P., Arshavsky, Y. I., Rabinovich,M. I. & Selverston, A. I. (2004). Dual sensory motor function for a molluskan statocyst network., *J Neurophysiol* 91(1): 336–345.
URL: *http://dx.doi.org/10.1152/jn.00753.2003*

Levi, R., Varona, P., Arshavsky, Y. I., Rabinovich, M. I. & Selverston, A. I. (2005). The role of sensory network dynamics in generating a motor program., *J Neurosci* 25(42): 9807–9815.
URL: *http://dx.doi.org/10.1523/JNEUROSCI.2249-05.2005*

Lewis, M. A., Etienne-Cummings, R., Hartmann, M. J., Xu, Z. R. & Cohen, A. H. (2003). An in silico central pattern generator: silicon oscillator, coupling, entrainment, and physical computation., *Biol Cybern* 88(2): 137–151.
URL: *http://dx.doi.org/10.1007/s00422-002-0365-7*

Li, C.-Y. T., Poo, M.-M. & Dan, Y. (2009). Burst spiking of a single cortical neuron modifies global brain state., *Science* 324(5927): 643–646.
URL: *http://dx.doi.org/10.1126/science.1169957*

Lörincz,M. L., Geall, F., Bao, Y., Crunelli, V. & Hughes, S.W. (2009). ATP-dependent infra-slow (<0.1 Hz) oscillations in thalamic networks., *PLoS One* 4(2): e4447.
URL: *http://dx.doi.org/10.1371/journal.pone.0004447*

Machens, C. K., Romo, R. & Brody, C. D. (2005). Flexible control of mutual inhibition: a neural model of two-interval discrimination., *Science* 307(5712): 1121–1124.
URL: *http://dx.doi.org/10.1126/science.1104171*

Mancilla, J. G., Lewis, T. J., Pinto, D. J., Rinzel, J. & Connors, B. W. (2007). Synchronization of electrically coupled pairs of inhibitory interneurons in neocortex., *J Neurosci* 27(8): 2058–2073.
URL: *http://dx.doi.org/10.1523/JNEUROSCI.2715-06.2007*

Milo, R., Shen-Orr, S., Itzkovitz, S., Kashtan, N., Chklovskii, D. & Alon, U. (2002). Network motifs: simple building blocks of complex networks., *Science* 298(5594): 824–827.
URL: *http://dx.doi.org/10.1126/science.298.5594.824*

Nowotny, T., Levi, R. & Selverston, A. I. (2008). Probing the dynamics of identified neurons with a data-driven modeling approach., *PLoS One* 3(7): e2627.
URL: *http://dx.doi.org/10.1371/journal.pone.0002627*

Nowotny, T. & Rabinovich, M. I. (2007). Dynamical origin of independent spiking and bursting activity in neural microcircuits., *Phys Rev Lett* 98(12): 128106.

Palva, S. & Palva, J. M. (2007). New vistas for alpha-frequency band oscillations., *Trends Neurosci* 30(4): 150–158.
URL: *http://dx.doi.org/10.1016/j.tins.2007.02.001*

Rabinovich, M. I., Huerta, R. & Afraimovich, V. (2006). Dynamics of sequential decision making., *Phys Rev Lett* 97(18): 188103.

Rabinovich, M. I., Huerta, R. & Varona, P. (2006). Heteroclinic synchronization: ultrasubharmonic locking., *Phys Rev Lett* 96(1): 014101.

Rabinovich, M. I., Huerta, R., Varona, P. & Afraimovich, V. S. (2006). Generation and reshaping of sequences in neural systems., *Biol Cybern* 95(6): 519–536.
URL: *http://dx.doi.org/10.1007/s00422-006-0121-5*

Rabinovich, M. I., Huerta, R., Varona, P. & Afraimovich, V. S. (2008). Transient cognitive dynamics, metastability, and decision making., *PLoS Comput Biol* 4(5): e1000072.
URL: *http://dx.doi.org/10.1371/journal.pcbi.1000072*

Rabinovich, M. I., Huerta, R., Volkovskii, A., Abarbanel, H. D., Stopfer, M. & Laurent, G. (2000). Dynamical coding of sensory information with competitive networks., *J Physiol Paris* 94(5-6): 465–471.

Rabinovich, M. I., Muezzinoglu, M. K., Strigo, I. & Bystritsky, A. (2010). Dynamical principles of emotion-cognition interaction: Mathematical images of mental disorders, PLoS ONE 5(9): e12547.
URL: *http://dx.doi.org/10.1371/journal.pone.0012547*

Rabinovich, M. I., Varona, P., Selverston, A. I. & Abarbanel, H. D. I. (2006). Dynamical principles in neuroscience, *Rev Mod Phys* 78: 1213–1265.

Rabinovich, M. & Muezzinoglu, M. (2010). Nonlinear dynamics of the brain: emotion and cognition, *Physics-Uspekhi* 53(4): 357–372.

Rabinovich, M., Volkovskii, A., Lecanda, P., Huerta, R., Abarbanel, H. D. & Laurent, G. (2001). Dynamical encoding by networks of competing neuron groups: winnerless competition., *Phys Rev Lett* 87(6): 068102.

Roopun, A. K., Kramer,M. A., Carracedo, L.M., Kaiser,M., Davies, C. H., Traub, R. D., Kopell, N. J. & Whittington, M. A. (2008). Temporal interactions between cortical rhythms., *Front Neurosci* 2(2): 145–154.
URL: *http://dx.doi.org/10.3389/neuro.01.034.2008*

Rybak, I. A., Abdala, A. P. L., Markin, S. N., Paton, J. F. R. & Smith, J. C. (2007). Spatial organization and state-dependent mechanisms for respiratory rhythm and pattern generation., *Prog Brain Res* 165: 201–220.
URL: *http://dx.doi.org/10.1016/S0079-6123(06)65013-9*

Rybak, I. A., Shevtsova, N. A., Paton, J. F. R., Pierrefiche, O., St-John, W. M. & Haji, A. (2004). Modelling respiratory rhythmogenesis: focus on phase switching mechanisms., *Adv Exp Med Biol* 551: 189–194.

Selverston, A. I. & Miller, J. P. (1980). Mechanisms underlying pattern generation in lobster stomatogastric ganglion as determined by selective inactivation of identified neurons. i. pyloric system., *J Neurophysiol* 44(6): 1102–1121.

Skinner, F. K., Kopell, N. & Marder, E. (1994). Mechanisms for oscillation and frequency control in reciprocally inhibitory model neural networks., *J ComputNeurosci* 1(1-2): 69–87.

Skinner, F. K., Zhang, L., Velazquez, J. L. & Carlen, P. L. (1999). Bursting in inhibitory interneuronal networks: A role for gap-junctional coupling., *J Neurophysiol* 81(3): 1274–1283.

Sohal, V. S., Pangratz-Fuehrer, S., Rudolph, U. & Huguenard, J. R. (2006). Intrinsic and synaptic dynamics interact to generate emergent patterns of rhythmic bursting in thalamocortical neurons., *J Neurosci* 26(16): 4247–4255.
URL: *http://dx.doi.org/10.1523/JNEUROSCI.3812-05.2006*

Sporns, O. & Kötter, R. (2004). Motifs in brain networks., *PLoS Biol* 2(11): e369.
URL: *http://dx.doi.org/10.1371/journal.pbio.0020369*

Taylor, K. S., Seminowicz, D. A. & Davis, K. D. (2009). Two systems of resting state connectivity between the insula and cingulate cortex., *Hum Brain Mapp* 30(9): 2731–2745.
URL: *http://dx.doi.org/10.1002/hbm.20705*

Tomasi, D. & Volkow, N. D. (2010). Functional connectivity density mapping., *Proc Natl Acad Sci U S A* 107(21): 9885–9890.
URL: *http://dx.doi.org/10.1073/pnas.1001414107*

Tong, F., Meng, M. & Blake, R. (2006). Neural bases of binocular rivalry., *Trends Cogn Sci* 10(11): 502–511.
URL: *http://dx.doi.org/10.1016/j.tics.2006.09.003*

Varona, P., Rabinovich, M. I., Selverston, A. I. & Arshavsky, Y. I. (2002). Winnerless competition between sensory neurons generates chaos: A possible mechanism for molluscan hunting behavior., *Chaos* 12(3): 672–677.
URL: *http://dx.doi.org/10.1063/1.1498155*

Wang, X. J. & Rinzel, J. (1993). Spindle rhythmicity in the reticularis thalami nucleus: synchronization among mutually inhibitory neurons., *Neuroscience* 53(4): 899–904.

Whittington, M. A. & Traub, R. D. (2003). Interneuron diversity series: inhibitory interneurons and network oscillations in vitro., *Trends Neurosci* 26(12): 676–682.

Whittington, M. A., Traub, R. D., Kopell, N., Ermentrout, B. & Buhl, E. H. (2000). Inhibition-based rhythms: experimental and mathematical observations on network dynamics., *Int J Psychophysiol* 38(3): 315–336.

Wilson, H. R. & Cowan, J. D. (1972). Excitatory and inhibitory interactions in localized populations of model neurons., *Biophys J* 12(1): 1–24.
URL: *http://dx.doi.org/10.1016/S0006-3495(72)86068-5*

Wilson, H. R. & Cowan, J. D. (1973). A mathematical theory of the functional dynamics of cortical and thalamic nervous tissue., *Kybernetik* 13(2): 55–80.

Womelsdorf, T., Fries, P., Mitra, P. P. & Desimone, R. (2006). Gamma-band synchronization in visual cortex predicts speed of change detection., *Nature* 439(7077): 733–736.
URL: *http://dx.doi.org/10.1038/nature04258*

Yuste, R., MacLean, J. N., Smith, J. & Lansner, A. (2005). The cortex as a central pattern generator., *Nat Rev Neurosci* 6(6): 477–483.
URL: *http://dx.doi.org/10.1038/nrn1686*

Zhigulin, V. P. (2004). Dynamical motifs: building blocks of complex dynamics in sparsely connected random networks., *Phys Rev Lett* 92(23): 238701.

24

Network of Gut Pacemaker Cells: Spatio-Temporal Evaluation of Electrical Activity by Use of Microelectrode Array

Shinsuke Nakayama, Mizuki Taniguchi and Hong-Nian Liu
Nagoya University Graduate School of Medicine, Japan

1. Introduction

The word 'pacemaker' prompts us to imagine 'heart beats' and also an 'electric cardiogram'. However, spontaneous electrical activity occurs in numerous tissues and organs in the autonomic nervous system, such as in the gastrointestinal and urinary tracts, trachea, uterus, lymph ducts, etc. (Takaki et al, 2010). Recent studies have revealed that special interstitial cells in these tissues and organs act as pacemaker cells. In particular, in the gastrointestinal tract, pacemaker cells surround the myenteric plexus between the circular and longitudinal muscle layers. Since these cells express abundant tyrosine kinase, Kit receptors, on the surface, Kit-immunoreactivity and *kit* cDNA are used as markers for special pacemaker cells. Moreover, these cells are now referred to as interstitial cells of Cajal (ICC) due to their histological features of the network (Maeda et al. 1992; Faussone-Pellegrini and Thuneberg, 1999; Sanders et al. 1999; Rumessen and Vandervinden, 2003; Takaki, 2003).

It is widely accepted that peristaltic movement of the gastrointestinal tract is organized by a network of enteric neurons in the myenteric plexus: Ascending contraction and descending relaxation simultaneously occur to forward luminal contents. It is hypothesized that ICC may also make an essential contribution to the co-ordinated actions of gastrointestinal motility through their network (Nakayama et al. 2006; 2009, see also Fig. 7).

There are an increasing number of papers that report the impairment of ICC in GI motility disorders, for example, in inflammatory bowel diseases (IBD) (Suzuki et al. 2004; Wang et al. 2002; 2007; Kinoshita et al. 2007), diabetic gastroparesis (Camilleri, 2002; Ordög et al. 2000; Vittal et al. 2007), slow transit constipation (He et al. 2000; Lyford et al. 2002; Wedel et al. 2002), Hirschsprung's disease (Vanderwinden et al. 1996), etc. In these studies, the impairment of ICC has been evaluated in histological terms, such as apoptotic changes and reduction of ICC number. However, in some stage of these diseases, GI motility disorders may be caused by functional impairment of ICC preceded by or not linked with histological changes. Therefore, tools for evaluating ICC spatio-temporal activity are now anticipated.

We have thus employed a microelectrode array (MEA) in order to study ICC pacemaker activity. In this chapter, we describe our methods of MEA measurements and provide evidence showing that ICC play crucial roles in propagating electrical activity as well as in pacemaking. In some experiments, we compare ileal muscle preparations of wild-type (WT) and W/W^v mice as a model to evaluate the impairment of ICC, because it is well known that the latter has a largely reduced population of ICC in the myenteric region due to partial loss-of-function mutation of Kit receptors (Reith, 1990; Ward et al. 2004; Iino et al. 2007).

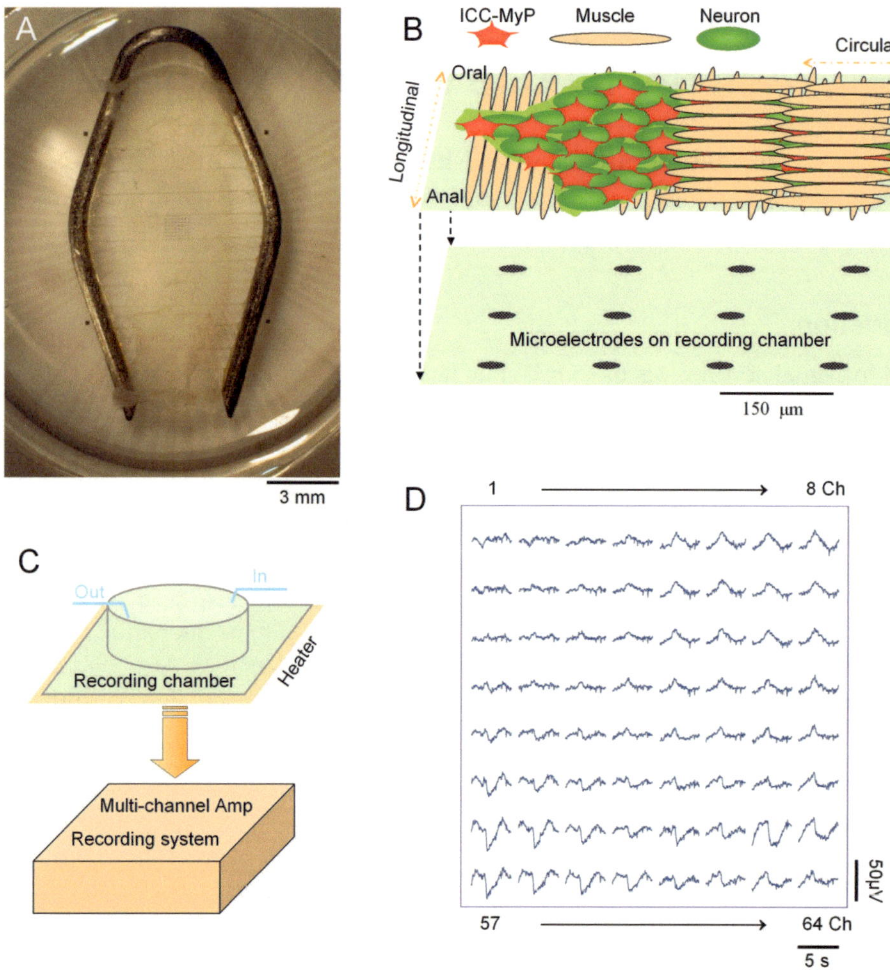

Fig. 1. MEA system to measure gut pacemaker electrical activity (modified from Fig. 1, Nakayama et al. 2009). As an example, an MEA recording from ileal musculature is shown. It is known that network-forming ICC in the myenteric plexus (ICC-MyP) generate pacemaker potentials in the ileum.

2. Microelectrode array measurements

In order to analyze spatio-temporal properties of gut pacemaker cells, we employed an MEA system (Nakayama et al. 2006; 2009), which was previously used for brain slice and explant preparations (Shimono *et al.* 2000; Nakamura *et al.* 2002). Musculature preparations isolated from animals were mounted in a recording chamber with an 8 x 8 planar MEA (Fig. 1). The chamber was kept warm and continuously perfused with physiological solutions. Gut pacemaker electrical activity was recorded at 64 channels simultaneously.

2.1 Animals

The animals used were treated in accordance with the Animal Experimental Guides of Nagoya University Graduate School of Medicine. Guinea-pigs, and WT (BALB/c) and *W/W^v^* mice were used. The gastrointestinal tract was quickly excised. The mucosa was removed with fine scissors in the stomach, and with fine forceps in the ileum. Small segments of the whole-muscle layer containing the myenteric plexus were dissected and mounted in a recording chamber. The musculature preparations were held down under the strings of a slice anchor (SDH series, Harvard Apparatus Japan, Tokyo, Japan), and were superfused with modified Krebs solution (normal extracellular solution) at a constant rate of 2 ml/min, and placed on a heater kept at 35°C.

2.2 Electrical recordings

In this MEA system 8 x 8 planar electrodes (150 or 300 μm in polar distance) were connected to a 64-channel amplifier (MED 64 System, Alpha Med Science, Osaka, Japan). Electrical potentials at 64 channels were recorded simultaneously at a sampling rate of 20 kHz, after low-pass filtering at 10 kHz. Also, a high-pass filter (HPF) of 0.1 Hz was applied to stabilise the baseline drift of the DC potential (Brock & Cunnane, 1987). The low impedance of microelectrodes (<10 kΩ, at 1 kHz) and a HPF of 0.1 Hz enabled us to follow slow electrical oscillations of gut pacemaker activity (Nakayama et al. 2006; 2009).

2.3 Solutions and drugs

The composition of the "normal" extracellular solution, a modified Krebs solution, was (in mmol/L): NaCl, 125; KCl, 5.9; $MgCl_2$ 1.2; $CaCl_2$ 2.4; glucose 11; Tris-HEPES, 11.8 (pH 7.4). Nifedipine and tetrodotoxin (TTX) were purchased from Sigma (St Louis, MO, USA).

Gut musculature preparations contain three major cell types which generate electrical activity: smooth muscle cells, neurons and ICC. It is well known that TTX suppresses neural activity by blocking voltage-gated Na^+ channels. In gut smooth muscle, contractility and excitability largely depend on Ca^{2+}-influx via L-type voltage-gated Ca^{2+} channels. Dihydropyridine (DHP) Ca^{2+} antagonists e.g. nifedipine and nicardipine, which selectively block L-type Ca^{2+} channels, nearly completely suppress spontaneous contractile and electrical activities in gut smooth muscle (Nakayama et al. 2007). On the other hand, ICC pacemaking also requires extracellular Ca^{2+} , but DHP Ca^{2+} antagonists have little effect on ICC electrical activity (Dickens et al. 1999; Huang et al. 1999), probably because L-type Ca^{2+} channels are not major Ca^{2+} influx pathways in ICC.

In MEA measurements of gut pacemaker activity, the extracellular solution contained nifedipine (1 μmol/L) in order to suppress smooth muscle electrical activity, and to reduce electrical artefacts due to muscle contractions. In addition, the extracellular solution always contained TTX (500 nmol/L) in order to rule out electrical signals from enteric neurons and neural modulation of ICC activity (linked with neurotransmitter release by action potentials in neurons). MEA measurements started ~30 min after superfusing with the extracellular solution containing nifedipine and TTX.

2.4 Data analysis

Arrayed data of field potentials were normally thinned by a 1000-fold time domain, thereby the sampling interval was increased to 50 ms. This sampling frequency was enough to follow gut pacemaking electrical activity. Cross-correlation, power spectrum, and digital filtering of spontaneous electrical potentials were performed using commercial add-in software (Kyowa Electronic Instruments, Tokyo, Japan). Two-dimensional field potential images were constructed by calculating values at the desired location via spline interpolation, using the MATLAB software package (Mathworks: Natick, MA, USA)(Shimono et al. 2000; Nakayama et al. 2009).

Numerical data are expressed as means±S.D. Significant differences were evaluated by unpaired t-tests.

3. Gut pacemaker activity

3.1 Stomach ICC activity

The stomach is divided into the fundus, corpus, antrum and pylorus. Typical pacemaker potentials are relatively easily observed in the gastric antrum of guinea-pigs, therefore we used musculature preparations in this part of the stomach. It is known that network-forming ICC in the myenteric plexus (ICC-MyP) of the antral muscle act as primary pacemaker cells, while intramuscular ICC (ICC-IM) in the circular muscle amplify the pacemaker electrical activity (Dickens et al. 1999; Hirst & Ward, 2003).

Musculature preparations were placed with the circular muscle layer down, and fixed in a recording chamber with an array of 8 x 8 MEA with 300 μm in interpolar distance. The recording area was ~4mm^2. Figure 2 shows an example of field potential recordings in the guinea-pig stomach, by use of the MEA. In Aa, a muscle preparation was under superfusion with a "normal" (modified Krebs) extracellular solution. The upper and lower ends correspond to the anal and oral ends of the gastric antrum, respectively, while the left and right correspond to the lesser and greater curvature ends. This set of MEA recordings is plotted with the same scale of amplitude, indicating the existence of a gradient in the field potential amplitude.

In Fig. 2B, the amplitude (y-axis) of MEA recording was expanded to more clearly display spontaneous electrical activity recorded in each planar electrode, indicating that the occurrence of spontaneous electrical activity was well synchronised over the electrode array area. Essentially, the synchoronicity of electrical activities was similar in all antral muscle preparations tested.

As described in Section 2.3, DHP Ca^{2+} channel antagonists can be used to isolate ICC pacemaker electrical activity by suppressing smooth muscle contractility and excitability. As shown in Fig. 2Ab, nifedipine, a DHP Ca^{2+} antagonist had little effect on the frequency of spontaneous electrical activity, and also did not significantly alter the shape of the field potential in the majority of recording channels. Also, additional application of TTX had little or no further effect on these field potential recordings (Fig. 2Ac). These results indicated that ICC make a predominant contribution to the generation of spontaneous electric activity in the stomach musculature.

The shape of the spontaneous electrical activity (≈ ICC pacemaker activity) in the stomach musculature varied greatly, but usually consisted of an initial, fast negative potential (red arrow in Fig. 2D) followed by a slowly decaying component (green double arrow).

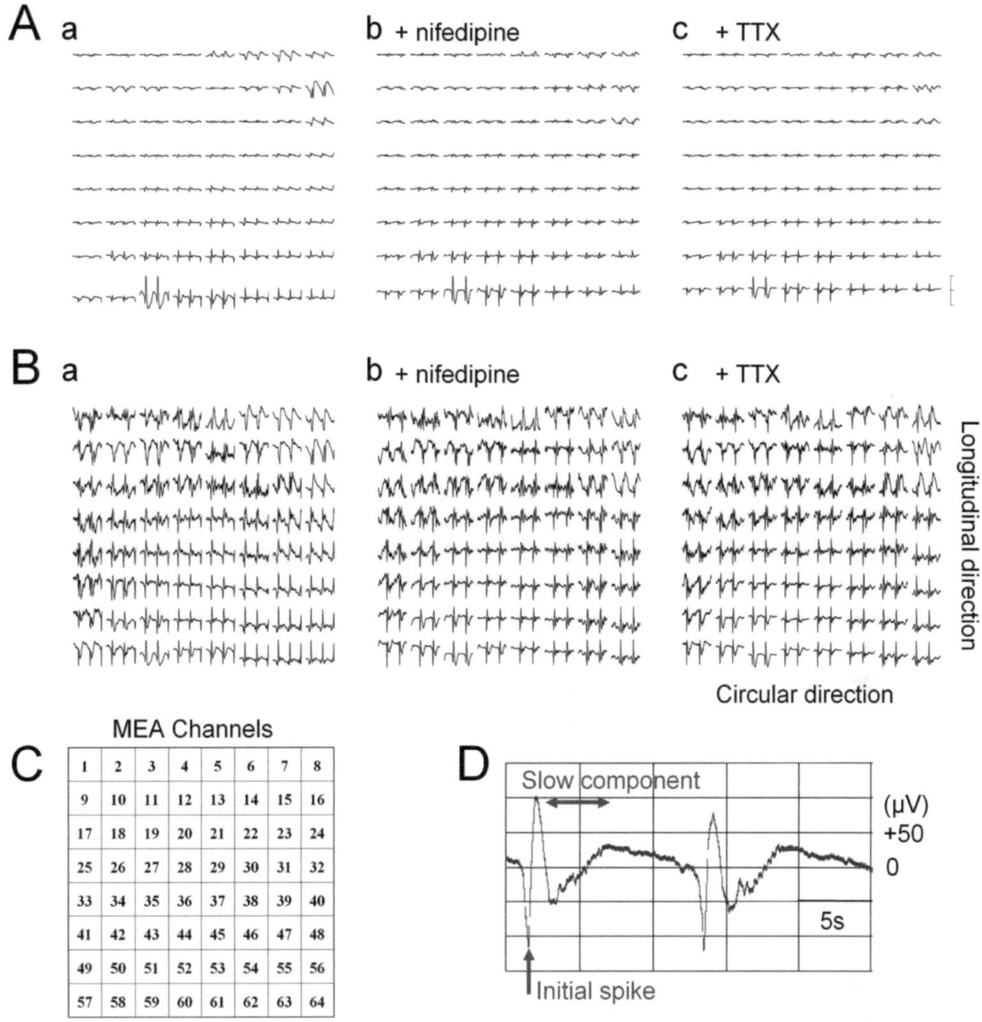

Fig. 2. An example of the distribution of spontaneous electrical activities in a stomach muscle preparation recorded using an 8 x 8 MEA with a polar distance of 300 μm (Modified from Figs. 1 and 3, Nakayama et al. 2006). Each trace in A shows the normalised field potential with a y-range of ±150 μV (scale bar). In B, the y-range was adjusted to more clearly show the shape of spontaneous electrical activity at each recording channel. The channel number of the arrayed electrodes is shown in C. Panel D shows an expanded typical pacemaker activity with initial spike followed by a slow component.

3.2 Reversible propagation

ICC pacemaking field potentials were well synchronized over the recording area; however, phase differences were clearly observed between some of the recording channels. Figure 3A shows an example in which the pacemaker potentials propagate from the oral to anal end. The field potential traces (a-c) were recorded in Ch. 25, 27, and 29, respectively. The initial spike (down-stroke) in trace (a) was followed by those in (b) and (c). The field potential images (d) show excitation (yellow area) running from the right to the left, indicating the oral to anal propagation.

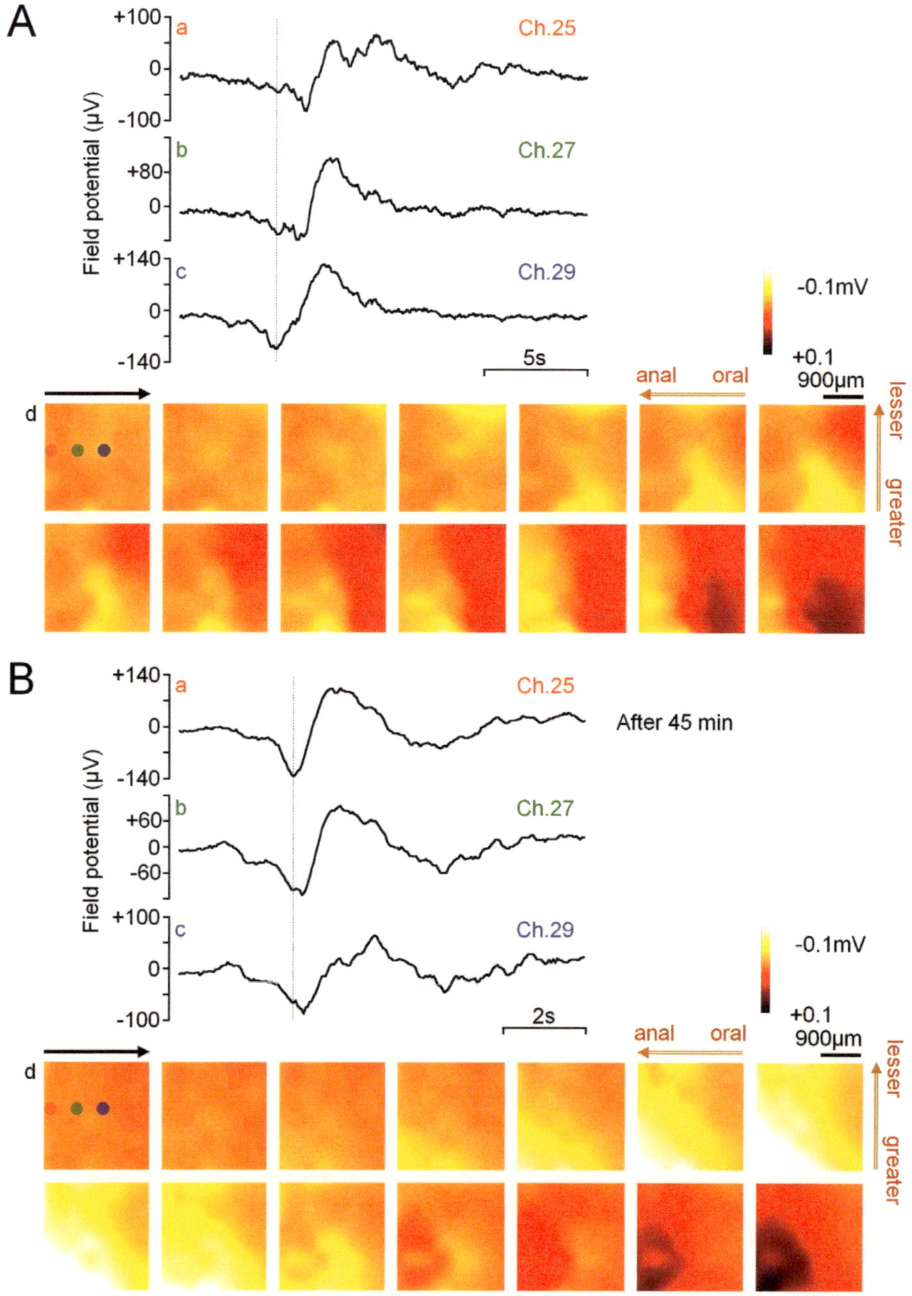

Fig. 3. An example of reversed ICC pacemaker activity (Modified from Fig. 8, Nakayama et al. 2006).

The field potential traces and images in Fig. 3B were obtained from the same gastric antrum preparation used in A, after approximately 45 min. This preparation was continuously superfused with the same extracellular solution (containing nifedipine). The field potential traces and images clearly show reversed electrical excitation, running from the anal to the oral end.

A phase shift proceeding from the oral end was observed in the majority (15 out of 18) of the stomach preparations. The propagation velocity of the spontaneous electrical activity along the longitudinal muscle ranged from –14.25 to +13.27 mm s^{-1}, but it was around ~1 (or –1) mm s^{-1} in the majority (13 out of 18) of preparations (plus indicates the oral to anal propagation). In 10 antral muscle preparations with the pacemaker phase shift proceeding from the oral end in the initial observation, field potentials were continuously recorded for ~30 min. The direction of propagation was reversed in four out of 10 preparations (Nakayama et al. 2006). Altogether, these results indicate that coupling of ICC pacemaker activity has plasticity and that that an ICC network can even produce reversible propagation of pacemaker potentials in the stomach.

3.3 Ileal ICC activity in wild-type and *W/W^v* mice

Musculature preparations isolated from the mouse ileum were placed with the longitudinal muscle layer down on an 8 x 8 MEA with a polar distance of 150 μm. The recording area was ~1 mm^2. Ileal musculature preparations contained both circular and longitudinal muscle layers and the myenteric plexus between these muscle layers. In order to suppress smooth muscle and neural activities, the extracellular solution contained nifedipine and TTX, respectively.

In the WT mouse ileum, network-forming ICC-MyP predominantly contribute to the generation of pacemaker potentials. W/W^v mice are known to lack or largely reduce pacemaking ICC-MY in the ileum (Reith, 1990; Ward et al. 1994; Iino et al. 2007). Therefore in the presence of nifedipine and TTX, only little spontaneous electrical activity was anticipated in ileal preparations from W/W^v mice. Figure 4 shows such the difference between WT and W/W^v mice. In WT mice spontaneous electrical potentials occurred regularly, while in W/W^v mice electrical activity was significantly smaller in amplitude and irregular in occurrence.

Power spectra over the recording area (Fig. 5A and B) were constructed from field potentials of all 64 channels for approximately 40 s recorded from the same preparations shown in Fig. 4. The power spectrum of WT mice had a prominent peak corresponding to the frequency of ileal ICC electrical activity, but that of W/W^v mice did not, reflecting an irregular occurrence of small electrical activities. Essentially the same tendencies were observed in other WT (n=28) and in W/W^v (n=27) ileal musculature preparations. In all preparations of WT mice, the spectral peak was normally observed between 9.4-27.0 cpm, thereby, the ratio of spectral power in this frequency range ($Pw_{9.4\text{-}27.0cpm}$) was significantly greater in WT mice (74.8±15.9%, n=29) than in W/W^v mice (38.0±15.6%, n=28) ($P<0.0001$, Fig. 5C).

3.4 Spatio-temporal analysis

Pacemaker potential images were constructed from field potentials measured by MEA. Panels in Fig. 6A show a sequence of field potential images obtained from the same WT mouse ileum preparation in Fig. 4. The top and bottom of each image correspond to the oral and anal ends of the MEA recording region, respectively. In this preparation, initial

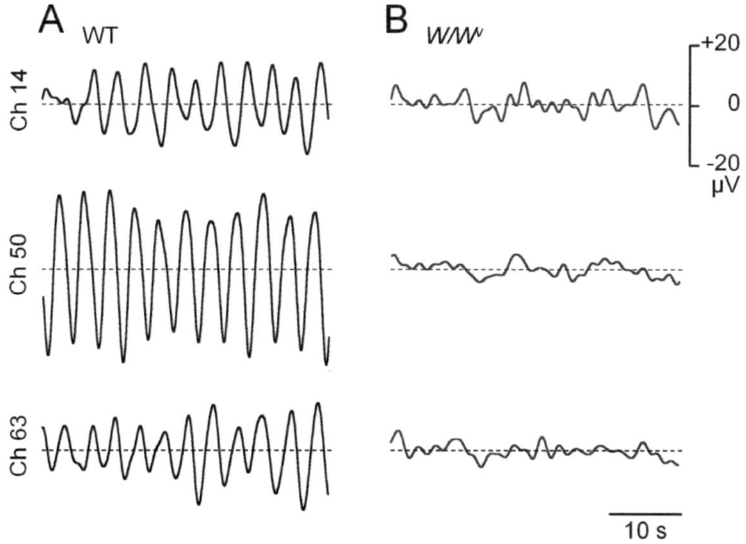

Fig. 4. Examples of field potentials recorded from ileal muscle preparations of WT (A) and W/W^v mice (B) (Reproduced from Fig. 2, Nakayama et al. 2009). Field potentials were plotted after digital band-pass filtering at 0.05-0.5 Hz.

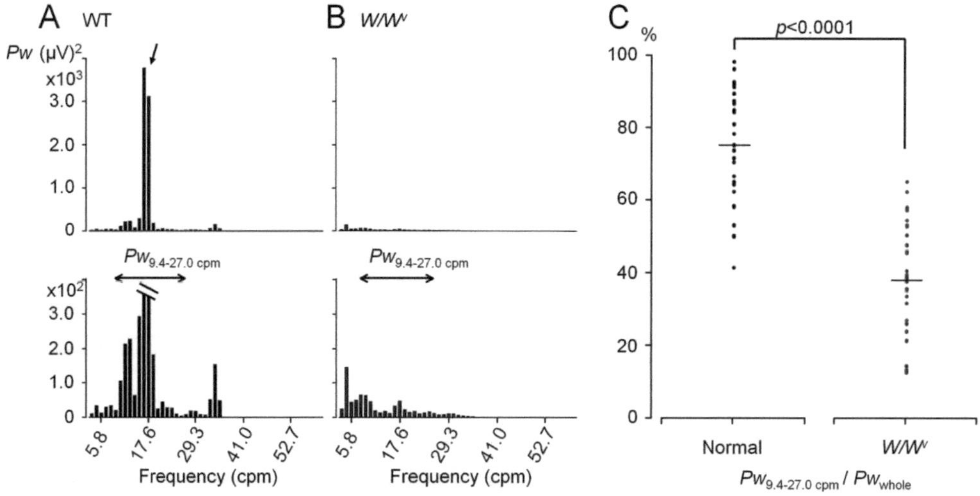

Fig. 5. Power spectrum analysis (Reproduced from Fig. 3, Nakayama et al. 2009). A-B: Field potential recordings from the same preparations shown in Fig. 4 were used. C: Summary of power spectra in WT (n=29) and W/W^v mice (n=28). The ratio of the spectral power (*Pw*) between 9.4-27.0 cpm to the whole *Pw* is plotted. Horizontal lines represent mean values.

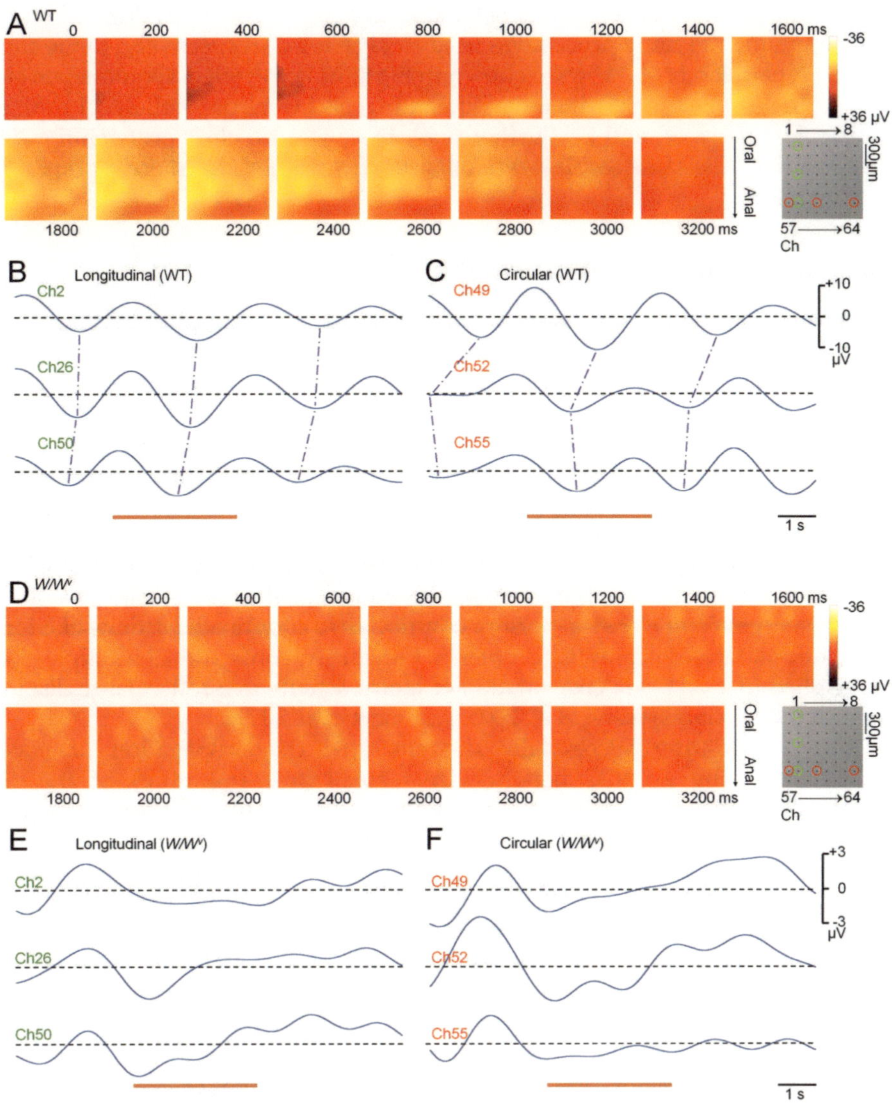

Fig. 6. Spatio-temporal analysis of pacemaker electrical activity in the ileum isolated from WT wild-type (A-C) and *W/W^v* mice (D-F) (Reproduced from Fig. 4, Nakayama et al. 2009). The peaks of electric excitation (down-stroke corresponding to depolarization) are connected by blue dotted lines. The red horizontal lines indicate the period of the potential images acquired.

excitation occurred in the right bottom of MEA near Ch62. Next, the excitation propagated along the circular muscle toward both ends, and then propagated along the longitudinal muscle toward the oral end. Field potential traces in Figs 6B and C show three cycles of spontaneous electrical oscillations recorded in Ch2, 26, and 50 (lined along longitudinal muscle), and Ch49, 52, and 55 (lined along circular muscle), respectively. As shown in Fig. 6A-C, in 29 preparations in WT mice, electrical activities were synchronised, and the propagation velocity of the excitation was ~1.4 mm s^{-1} in both directions. The propagating velocity was, however, changeable.

The sequence of potential images in Fig. 6D and field potential traces in Figs. 6E and F were obtained by applying the same procedures used in Figs. 6A-C, respectively, to the same ileal musculature preparation of *W/W^v* mice shown in Fig 4. In *W/W^v* mice, spontaneous electrical activities were smaller in amplitude, were fluctuating, and were not well-synchronized over the recording area (Figs. 6E and F). Furthermore, there was no clear propagating direction observed. Essentially the same results were obtained from other ileal muscle preparations of WT and *W/W^v* mice.

4. Applications of MEA in gut pacemakers

The mechanisms underling gut spontaneous electrical activity are becoming clearer. Conventional microelectrodes have elucidated that Kit-reactive interstitial cells in the myenteric plexus, i.e. ICC-MyP generate basal pacemaking electrical potentials (Dickens et al. 1999; Kito et al. 2005). Further, there is a growing body of evidence that Ca^{2+} mechanisms provide these cells with fundamental rhythmicity (Nakayama et al. 2007). Namely, intracellular Ca^{2+} release channels and Ca^{2+}-permeable channels in the plasmalemma co-ordinately produce ICC Ca^{2+} oscillations underlying the generation of pacemaker electrical activity (Aoyama et al. 2004; Liu et al. 2005a; b).

Since ICC-MyP are network-forming cells, the next step in the understanding of GI motility and in the treatment of GI dismotility is how these interstitial cells communicate with each other, and how pacemaking electrical activity contributes to coordinated actions of GI motility, i.e. to digest, mix and transport luminal contents. Previously, conventional multiple electrodes have been applied to investigate coordination of motor activity in a rather large distance, e.g. antroduodenal coordination (Wang et al. 2005; Lammers et al. 2005).

Recently, our MEA study successfully demonstrated the propagation of pacemaker potentials generated by an ICC network in a small area (~4 mm^2) of the stomach musculature (Nakayama et al. 2006). It is likely that such a phase shift (propagation delay) of pacemaker activity even in a few hundred micrometers enables smooth GI motility. Namely, the contractions of small segments of the gut linked with a linear phase shift in distance would elaborately squeeze luminal contents in a certain direction.

Coupling of pacemaker activity is changeable (plasticity) in the gut. Further, the propagation direction of pacemaker activity is reversible (Fig. 3), in contrast to the enteric neural network. Using this network system, luminal contents stimulate primary afferent neurons, and subsequently co-activate ascending excitatory and descending inhibitory neurons of the myenteric plexus via interneurons, causing ascending contraction and descending relaxation simultaneously (Furness, 2006; Wood, 2006). It is hypothesized that chained reactions of this reflex (i.e. peristaltic reflex) transport luminal contents throughout the gastrointestinal tract. Presumably the ICC network which can produce reversible activity, cooperates with the neural network, resulting in complex gut motility to efficiently digest luminal contents.

MEA has also been applied to investigate spontaneous electrical activity between ileal musculature preparations from WT and W/W^v mice. This comparison provides a model to evaluate impairment of the ICC network, because it is well known that the latter has a largely reduced population of ICC-MyP due to a partial loss-of-function mutation of Kit receptors (Reith, 1990; Ward et al. 2004; Iino et al. 2007). Analyses with power spectrum and potential mapping successfully distinguished electrical properties of these musculature preparations, indicating that network-forming ICC-MyP not only generates pacemaker potentials but also co-ordinates basal electrical activities. Disorders of gut motility based on morphological and/or functional impairments of the ICC network with a range of several hundred micrometers could be uncovered in future extensive studies, including model animals. As described earlier, there is a considerable body of evidence for the impairment of the ICC network in GI motility disorders. Furthermore, there is also a growing body of evidence that ICC-like interstitial cells are widely distributed outside the GI tract, for example in small vessels, the lymph duct, urinary tract, uterus, and also accessory organs of the GI tract (Huizinga, and Faussone-Pellegrini, 2005; Brading, and McCloskey, 2005; McCloskey et al. 2002; Harhun et al. 2005; Ciontea et al. 2005; Sun et al. 2006). MEA could also be a useful tool to evaluate a wide range of spontaneous rhythmicities and related dismotilities, e.g. unstable urinary bladder in geriatrics.

5. Conclusions

MEA has enabled spatio-temporal analysis of gut pacemaker activity in a small area. Network-forming ICC not only generates pacemaker potentials but also co-ordinates basal electrical activities. The propagation velocity of pacemaker potential (i.e. phase shift of ICC electrical activity) is changeable, and even reversible under certain conditions. It is likey that co-contribution of the ICC network and neural network organizes complex gut motility.

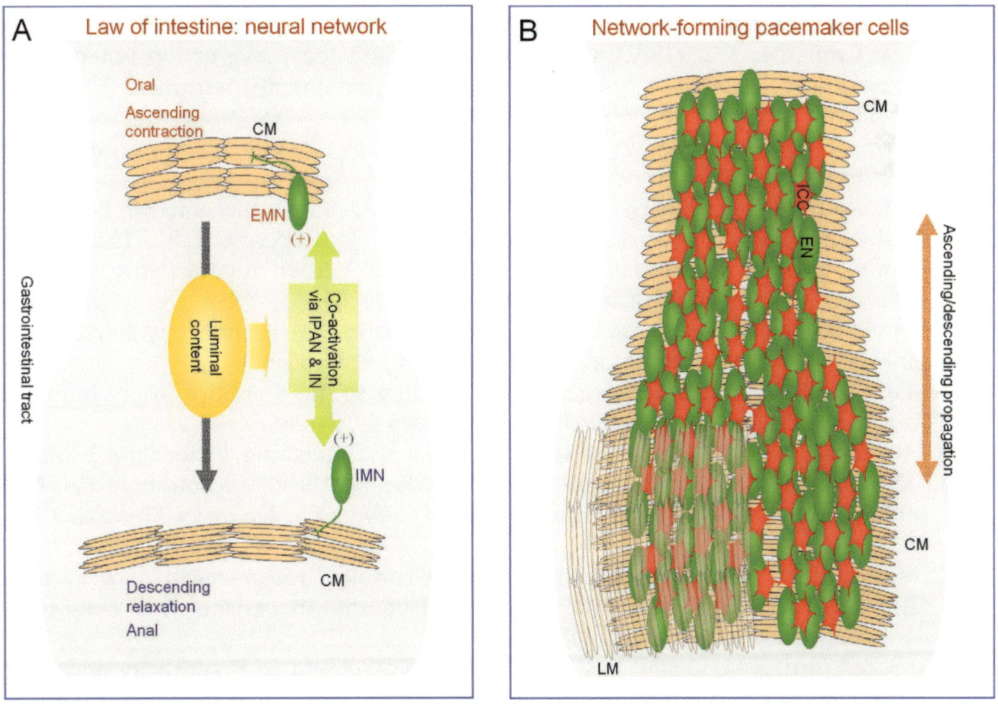

Fig. 7. Schematic diagrams of mechanisms underlying gut motility. A: Generally accepted 'law of intestine' is controlled by neural network. Luminal contents co-activate oral excitatory and anal inhibitory neurons (EMN and IMN) via intrinsic primary afferent neurons (IPAN) and interneurons (IN), thereby produce ascending contraction and descending relaxation simultaneously. B: A new contributor, 'network-forming pacemaker cells'. ICC-MyP surrounding the myenteric plexus between circular and longitudinal muscle layers (CM and LM), propagate as well as generate pacemaker activity. Propagation of pacemaker activity is changeable (plasticity), even reversed under some conditions. ICC network along with intrinsic neural network appears to elaborately control gut motility.

Future extensive studies using MEA will uncover disorders of gut motility based on morphological and/or functional impairments of the ICC network with the range of several hundred micrometers.

6. Acknowledgements

This work was partially supported by the Japan Society for the Promotion of Science and Takeda Science Foundation.

7. References

Aoyama, M.; Yamada, A.; Wang, J.; Ohya, S.; Furuzono, S.; Goto, T.; Hotta, S.; Ito, Y.; Matsubara, T.; Shimokata, K.; Chen, S.R.W.; Imaizumi, Y. & Nakayama, S. (2004). Requirement of ryanodine receptors for pacemaker Ca^{2+} activity in ICC and HEK293 cells. *Journal of Cell Science* 117, 2813-2825

Brading, A.F. & McCloskey, K.D. (2005). Mechanisms of disease: specialized interstitial cells of the urinary tract—an assessment of current knowledge. *Nature Clinical Practice Urology* 2, 546-554.

Brock, J.A. & Cunnane, T.C. (1987). Relationship between the nerve action potential and transmitter release from sympathetic postganglionic nerve terminals. *Nature* 326, 605-607.

Camilleri, M. (2002). Advances in diabetic gastroparesis. *Reviews in Gastroenterological Disorders* 2, 47-56.

Ciontea, S.M.; Radu, E.; Regalia, T.; Ceafalan. L.; Cretoiu, D.; Gherghiceanu, M.; Braga., R.I.; Malincenco, M.; Zagrean, L.; Hinescu, M.E. & Popescu, L.M. (2005). C-kit immunopositive interstitial cells (Cajal-type) in human myometrium. *Journal of Cellular and Molecular Medicine* 9, 407-420.

Dickens, E.J.; Hirst, G.D.S. & Tomita, T. (1999). Identification of rhythmically active cells in guinea-pig stomach. *Journal of Physiology (Lond.)* 514, 515-531.

Faussone-Pellegrini, M.S. & Thuneberg, L. (1999). Guide to the identification of interstitial cells of Cajal. *Microscopy Research and Technology* 47, 248-66.

Furness, J.B. (2006). The enteric nervous system. Blackwell Publishing, Oxford, pp.1-274.

Harhun, M.I.; Pucovsky, V.; Povstyan, O.V.; Gordienko, D.V. & Bolton, T.B. (2005). Interstitial cells in the vasculature. *Journal of Cellular and Molecular Medicine* 9, 232-243.

He, C.L.; Burgart, L.; Wang, L.; Pemberton, J.; Young-Fadok, T.; Szurszewski, J. & Farrugia, G. (2000). Decreased interstitial cell of cajal volume in patients with slow-transit constipation. *Gastroenterology* 118, 14-21.

Hirst, G.D.S. & Ward, S.M. (2003). Interstitial cells: involvement in rhythmicity and neural control of gut smooth muscle. *Journal of Physiology (Lond.)* 550, 337-346.

Huizinga, J.D. & Faussome-Pellegrini, M.S. (2005). About the presence of interstitial cells of Cajal outside the musculature of the gastrointestinal tract. *Journal of Cellular and Molecular Medicine* 9, 468-73.

Huang, S.-M.; Nakayama, S.; Iino, S. & Tomita, T. (1999). Voltage sensitivity of Slow wave frequency in isolated circular muscle strips from guinea pig gastric antrum. *American Journal of Physiology Gastrointeststinal and Liver Physiology* 276, G518-528.

Iino, S.; Horiguchi, S.; Horiguchi, K. & Nojyo, Y. (2007). Interstitial cells of Cajal in the gastrointestinal musculature of W mutant mice. *Archives of Histology and Cytology* 70, 163-173.

Kinoshita, K.; Horiguchi, K.; Fujisawa, M.; Kobirumaki, F.; Yamato, S.; Hori, M. & Ozaki, H. (2007). Possible involvement of muscularis resident macrophages in impairment of interstitial cells of Cajal and myenteric nerve systems in rat models of TNBS-induced colitis. *Histochemistry and Cell Biology* 127, 41-53.

Kito, Y.; Ward, S.M. & Sanders, K.M. (2005). Pacemaker potentials generated by interstitial cells of Cajal in the murine intestine. *American Journal of Physiology Cell Physiology* 288, C710-720.

Lammers, W.J.; Ver Donck, L.; Schuurkes, J.A. & Stephen, B. (2005). Peripheral pacemakers and patterns of slow wave propagation in the canine small intestine in vivo. *Canadian Journal of Physiology and Pharmacology* 83, 1031-1043.

Liu, H.-N.; Ohya, S.; Furuzono, S.; Wang, J.; Imaizumi, Y. & Nakayama, S. (2005a). Co-contribution of IP_3R and Ca^{2+} influx pathways to pacemaker Ca^{2+} activity in stomach ICC. *Journal of Biological Rhythms* 20, 15-26.

Liu, H.-N.; Ohya, S.; Wang, J.; Imaizumi, Y. & Nakayama, S. (2005b). Involvement of ryanodine receptors in pacemaker Ca^{2+} oscillation in murine gastric ICC. *Biochemica et Biophysica Research Communications* 328, 640-646.

Lyford. G.L.; He, C.L.; Soffer, E.; Hull, T.L.; Strong, S.A.; Senagore, A.J.; Burgart, L.J.; Young-Fadok, T.; Szurszewski, J.H. & Farrugia, G. (2002). Pan-colonic decrease in interstitial cells of Cajal in patients with slow transit constipation. *Gut* 51, 496-501.

Maeda, H.; Yamagata, A.; Nishikawa, S.; Yoshinaga, K.; Kobayashi, S.; Nishi, K. & Nishikawa, S.-I. (1992). Requirement of c-kit for development of intestinal pacemaker system. *Development* 116, 369-375.

McCloskey, K.D.; Hollywood, M.A.; Thornbury, K.D.; Ward, S.M. & McHale, N.G. (2002). Kit-like immunopositive cells in sheep mesenteric lymphatic vessels. *Cell and Tissue Research* 310, 77-84.

Nakamura, W.; Honma, S.; Shirakawa, T. & Honma K. (2002). Clock mutation lengthens the circadian period without damping rhythms in individual SCN neurons. *Nature Neuroscience* 5, 399-400.

Nakayama, S; Ohishi, R.; Sawamura, K.; Watanabe, K. & Hirose K. (2009). Microelectrode array evaluation of gut pacemaker activity in wild-type and W/W^v mice. *Biosensors and Bioelectronics* 25, 61-67.

Nakayama, S.; Shimono, K.; Liu, H.-N.; Jiko, H; Katayama, N; Tomita, T. & Goto K. (2006). Pacemaker phase shift in the absence of neural activity in guinea-pig stomach: a microelectrode array study. *Journal of Physiology (Lond.)* 576, 727-738.

Nakayama, S.; Kajioka, S.; Goto, K.; Takaki, M. & Liu, H.N. (2007). Calcium-associated mechanisms in gut pacemaker activity. *Journal of Cellular and Molecular Medicine* 11, 958-968.

Ordög, T.; Takayama, I.; Cheung, W.K.; Ward, S.M. & Sanders, K.M. (2000). Remodeling of networks of interstitial cells of Cajal in a murine model of diabetic gastroparesis. *Diabetes* 49, 1731-1739.

Reith, A.D.; Rottapel, R.; Giddens, E.; Brady, C.; Forrester, L. & Bernstein, A. (1990). W mutant mice with mild or severe developmental defects contain distinct point mutations in the kinase domain of the c-kit receptor. *Genes & Development* 4, 390-400.

Rumessen, J.J. & Vandervinden, J.-M. (2003). Interstitial cells in the musculature of the gastrointestinal tract: Cajal and beyond. *International Review of Cytology* 229, 115-208.

Sanders, K.M.; Ordög, T.; Koh, S.D.; Torihashi, S. & Ward, S.M. (1999). Development and plasticity of interstitial cells of Cajal. *Neurogastroenterology and Motility* 11, 311-338.

Sun, X.; Yu, B.; Xu, L.; Dong, W. & Luo, H. (2006). Interstitial cells of Cajal in the murine gallbladder. *Scandinavian Journal of Gastroenterology* 2006; 41: 1218-26.

Suzuki, T.; Won, K.J.; Horiguchi, K.; Kinoshita, K.; Hori, M.; Torihashi, S.; Momotani, E.; Itoh, K.; Hirayama, K.; Ward, S.M.; Sanders, K.M. & Ozaki, H. (2004). Muscularis inflammation and the loss of interstitial cells of Cajal in the endothelin ETB receptor null rat. *American Journal of Physiology Gastrointeststinal and Liver Physiology* 287, G638-646.

Takaki, M. (2003). Gut pacemaker cells: The interstitial cells of Cajal. *Journal of Smooth Muscle Research* 39, 137-161.

Takaki, M.; Suzuki, H. & Nakayama, S. (2010). Recent advances in studies of spontaneous activity in smooth muscle: ubiquitous pacemaker cells. *Progress in Biophysics and Molecular Biology* 102, 129-135.

Torihashi, S.; Fujimoto, T.; Trost, C. & Nakayama, S. (2002). Calcium oscillation linked to pacemaking of interstitial cells of Cajal. *Journal of Biological Chemistry* 277, 19191-19197.

Yamazawa, T. & Iino, M. (2002). Simultaneous imaging of Ca^{2+} signals in interstitial cells of Cajal and longitudinal smooth muscle cells during rhythmic activity in mouse ileum. *Journal of Physiology (Lond.)* 538, 823-835.

Vanderwinden, J.M.; Rumessen, J.J.; Liu, H.; Descamps, D.; De Laet, M.H. & Vanderhaeghen, J.J. (1996). Interstitial cells of Cajal in human colon and in Hirschsprung's disease. *Gastroenterology* 111, 901-910.

Vittal, H.; Farrugia, G.; Gomez, G. & Pasricha, P.J. (2007). Mechanisms of disease: the pathological basis of gastroparesis--a review of experimental and clinical studies. *Nature Clinical Practice Gastroenterology and Hepatology* 4, 336-346.

Wang, X.Y.; Berezin, I.; Mikkelsen, H.B.; Der, T.; Bercik, P.; Collins, S.M. & Huizinga, J.D. (2002). Pathology of interstitial cells of Cajal in relation to inflammation revealed by ultrastructure but not immunohistochemistry. *American Journal of Pathology* 160, 1529-1540.

Wang, X.Y., Lammers, W.J., Bercik, P., Huizinga, J.D. (2005). Lack of pyloric interstitial cells of Cajal explains distinct peristaltic motor patterns in stomach and small intestine *American Journal of Physiology Gastrointeststinal and Liver Physiology* 289, G539-549.

Wang, X.Y.; Zarate, N.; Soderholm, J.D.; Bourgeois, J.M.; Liu, L.W. & Huizinga, J.D. (2007). Ultrastructural injury to interstitial cells of Cajal and communication with mast cells in Crohn's disease. *Neurogastroenterology and Motility* 19, 349-364.

Ward, S.M.; Burns, A.J.; Torihashi, S. & Sanders, K.M. (1994). Mutation of the proto-oncogene c-kit blocks development of interstitial cells and electrical rhythmicity in murine intestine. *Journal of Physiology (Lond.)* 480, 91-97.

Wedel, T.; Spiegler, J.; Soellner, S.; Roblick, U.J.; Schiedeck, T.H.; Bruch, H.P. & Krammer, H.J. (2002). Enteric nerves and interstitial cells of Cajal are altered in patients with slow-transit constipation and megacolon. *Gastroenterology* 123, 1459-1467.

Wood, J.D. 2006. Integrative function of enteric nervous system. in: Barrett, K.E., Ghishan, F.K., Merchant, J.L., Said, H.M., Wood, J.D., Johnson, L.R. (eds.) Physiology of the Gastrointestinal Tract. Volume 2. fourth ed. Academic Press, New York, pp.665-684.

25

Possible Role of Respiratory Pacemaker Neurons in the Generation of Different Breathing Patterns

Peña-Ortega F
Instituto de Neurobiología, UNAM.
México

1. Introduction

Rhythmic output is a common feature of several neuronal networks throughout the brain (Arshavsky 2003; Llinas 1988; Buzsaki & Draguhn 2004; Ramirez et al., 2004; Selverston 1999; Harris-Warrick & Marder 1991). Despite the fact that rhythmogenic networks were initially described for simple motor behaviors produced by invertebrates (Selverston 1999; Harris-Warrick & Marder 1991), there is increasing evidence suggesting that basic mechanisms revealed in these simple networks are conserved in mammalian circuits in the neocortex or other subcortical networks involved in more complex behaviors (Ramirez et al. 2004; Yuste et al., 2005). Recent findings indicate that network oscillations determine synaptic input selection, neuronal assemblies formation as well as synaptic plasticity (for a review see Buzsaki & Draguhn 2004). Rhythmic network activity emerges from the combination of synaptic network interactions and intrinsic cellular properties (Vergara et al., 2005; Peña et al., 2004; Cunningham et al., 2004; Yuste et al. 2005; Peña & Ramirez 2005; Peña et al., 2006; Mellen & Mishra, 2010). However the relative contribution of those mechanisms may be state dependent (Llinas 1988; Yuste et al. 2005; Peña & Ramirez 2005; Doi & Ramirez, 2010). Examples of state-dependency in neuronal network activity can be observed during sleep/wake states in the cortex or normoxia/hypoxia in the respiratory network (Llinas 1988; Yuste et al. 2005; Peña & Ramirez 2005; Peña & Aguileta, 2007). Moreover, neuronal network properties may be altered by several intracellular and extracellular environmental conditions (i.e. the action of neuromodulatory systems; Steriade 2004; Traub et al., 2003; Peña & Ramirez 2002; 2004; Johnson et al., 2003; van den Top et al., 2004; Doi & Ramirez, 2008). Regardless of the old dilemma on the relative contribution of intrinsic and synaptic properties to circuit activity (Vergara et al. 2003; Egorov et al., 2002; Shu et al., 2003; 2006; Cunningham et al. 2004; Cardin et al., 2005), there is increasing evidence supporting the participation of intrinsic pacemaker neurons in the generation of network rhythmic activity (Llinas & Sugimori 1980; Schwindt & Crill 1982; Freund & Antal 1988; King et al., 1998; Stewart & Fox 1989; 1990; Leresche et al., 1991; Tresch & Kiehn 2000; Wang 2002; Sotty et al., 2003; Cunningham et al. 2004; Peña et al. 2004; Ramirez et al. 2004; Sipilä et al., 2005).

2. Pacemaker neurons

Pacemaker neurons can be considered as neurons with the intrinsic ability to generate bursts of action potentials at regular intervals (in the absence of synaptic interactions; Ramirez & Peña, 2005; Peña, 2008). Pacemaker neurons posses a particular combination of ion currents, that allows them to amplify synaptic inputs, as well as to promote general network excitation and synchrony (Llinas & Sugimori 1980; Llinas 1988; Del Negro et al. 2002; Arshavsky 2003; Ramirez et al. 2004; Schwindt & Crill 1982; Tresch & Kiehn 2000; Harris-Warrick 2002; Shu et al. 2006). The well stablished role of pacemaker neurons commanding rhythmic neuronal networks in invertebrates (Selverston 1999; Harris-Warrick & Marder 1991; Ramirez et al. 2004), is now been suggested for mammalian neuronal networks as well. For instance, GABAergic pacemaker neurons from the medial septum seem to be essential for theta rhythm generation (Freund & Antal 1988; Stewart & Fox, 1989; 1990; King et al. 1998; Sotty et al. 2003; Wang 2002); bursting CA3 pyramidal neurons seem to be responsible for spontaneous rhythmic activity observed in the newborn hippocampus (Sipilä et al. 2005), bursting reticular thalamic neurons might be responsible for generation of several thalamocortical rhythms (Leresche et al. 1991) and fast rhythmic bursting neurons seem to be essential for gamma rhythm generation in the cortex (Cunningham et al. 2004). Pacemaker neurons may also be involved in generation of different breathing patterns.

3. Respiratory rhythms generation

Ventilation of the lungs as consequence of rhythmic contractions of the respiratory muscles constitutes a complex neuromuscular function that involves several brainstem and spinal cord circuits, several muscles such as the diaphragm, intercostal, laryngeal and pharyngeal muscles, as well as the lungs and the vasculature (Richter, 1982; Bianchi et al., 1995; Feldman, 1995) A reduction in such function can cause hypoxia, that evokes a response of the respiratory network that leads to the generation of gasping, which is considered to be the 'last-resort' respiratory effort to autoresuscitate and sustain life (Poets et al., 1999; Sridhar et al., 2003; Peña, 2009). Indeed, failure to respond to severe hypoxia via gasping and autoresuscitation can result in death. Thus, dysregulation of the generation of gasping rhythm and/or autoresuscitation has been hypothesised to contribute to Sudden Infant Death Syndrome (SIDS; Poets et al., 1999; Sridhar et al., 2003; Peña, 2009).

Breathing is commanded and regulated by the respiratory centres of the brainstem (Richter, 1982; Bianchi et al., 1995; Feldman, 1995). The central respiratory pattern generator consists of two interacting oscillators, one controlling inspiration (the pre-Bötzinger complex; PreBötC) and other, located in the parafacial respiratory group (pFRG), possibly controlling active expiration (Smith et al., 1991; Onimaru & Homma, 2006; Janczewski & Feldman, 2006; Peña, 2009). In contrast with the pFRG, the vital role of the PreBötC in the generation of respiratory rhythms is supported by a variety of experimental data. First, during embryonic development there is a coincidence between the appearance of the PreBötC and initial respiratory rhythmic activity *in vitro* (Pagliardini et al., 2003; Thoby-Brisson et al., 2005; Greer et al., 2006). Second, brain stem rhythmic respiratory output is eliminated when the PreBötC is ablated (Smith et al., 1991; Ramirez et al., 1998; Wenninger et al., 2004). Finally, perturbations of neuronal function in and around the PreBötC severely disrupt breathing in mammals (Ramirez et al., 1998; Gray et al., 2001; Wenninger et al., 2004).

We have been characterizing pacemaker activity in the PreBötC in a slice preparation, which is able to produce, in normoxic conditions, the neural correlate of two respiratory rhythms observed *in vivo*: fictive eupneic activity and fictive sighs. If this preparation is challenged with hypoxia, fictive eupnea and sighs are supplanted by another rhythm called fictive gasping (Lieske et al. 2000; Ramirez & Lieske 2003). It has been proposed that the PreBötC is a multifunctional neural network, able to produce multiple rhythmic activities by the reconfiguration of network interactions (Lieske et al. 2000; Peña et al., 2004).

4. Respiratory pacemaker neurons

The PreBötC contains several types of neurons, including expiratory, inspiratory and postinspiratory neurons (Peña & Ramirez, 2002; Peña et al., 2004; Ramirez et al., 1997). Based just on their intrinsic properties and their ability to burst in synaptic isolation, we can distinguish two major types of neurons: pacemaker and non-pacemaker neurons (Thoby-Brisson & Ramirez 2001; Del Negro et al. 2002; Peña et al. 2004). Regardless of the evidence that there is a *continuum* between the intrinsic properties of pacemaker and non pacemaker neurons (Ramirez et al. 2004); most respiratory neurons in the PreBötC have been considered non-pacemakers (Ramirez et al. 1997; Peña et al. 2004). On the other hand, PreBötC pacemaker neurons reported so far, express a quite variable range of interburst and intraburst frequencies; amplitude of the plateau potential underlying bursting firing; as well as the voltage trajectory of such plateau (Thoby-Brisson & Ramirez 2001; Del Negro et al. 2002; 2005; Peña et al. 2004; Viemari & Ramirez 2006; Tryba et al. 2006, Mellen & Mishra, 2010, Table 1).

An initial pharmacological characterization has shown that there are at least two types of respiratory pacemakers neurons in the PreBötC (Thoby-Brisson & Ramirez 2001; Peña et al. 2004; Del Negro et al. 2005; Table 1). Despite the fact that all of them are sensitive to tetrodotoxin (TTX) (Thoby-Brisson & Ramirez 2001), two groups have been identified based on their sensitivity to the general calcium channel blocker Cd^{2+} (Elsen & Ramirez 1998): One group of pacemakers stop bursting in the presence of Cd^{2+}, whereas another group continued bursting in the same conditions. Such pacemaker neurons were originally identified as Type II (or Cd^{2+}-sensitive) and Type I (or Cd^{2+}-insensitive) pacemaker neurons, respectively (Thoby-Brisson & Ramirez 2001, Table 1). In the last two decades, some other differences have also been identified: In general, type I pacemaker neurons produce bursts of shorter duration than type II pacemaker neurons (Thoby-Brisson & Ramirez 2001; Peña & Ramirez 2002; 2004; Peña et al. 2004). Whereas type I pacemaker neurons are present during all postnatal development, it seems like type II pacemakers are scarce at early postnatal age (P0-P5) and increase their presence afterwards (Peña et al. 2004, Table 1).

The identification of the ion channels involved in bursting properties of these groups of respiratory pacemaker neurons, has provided us with some pharmacological tools that have helped to test the role of these neurons in the generation of the different respiratory rhythms (Del Negro et al. 2002; 2005; Peña et al. 2004; Paton et al., 2006; Tryba et al. 2006). The sensitivity of PreBötC pacemaker neurons to either Cd^{2+} or TTX (Thoby-Brisson & Ramirez 2001), does not help much for this purpose, since both channel blockers produce a generalized disturbance of neuronal firing and neurotransmitter release (Onimaru et al. 1989; Peña & Tapia 2000; Peña et al., 2002). Further pharmacological characterization revealed that most type I (or Cd^{2+}-insensitive) pacemaker neurons rely on the activity of a persistent Na^+ current and that bursting activity of most of them might be abolished by persistent Na^+ current blockers, including riluzole (Del Negro et al. 2002; 2005; Peña et al. 2004; Tryba et al. 2006). It is important to mention that around 25 % of type I (or Cd^{2+}-insensitive) pacemaker neurons were not sensitive neither to riluzole nor to Cd^{2+} (Peña et al. 2004).

	Type I Pacemaker	**Type II Pacemaker**	**References**
Blocked by tetrodotoxin	Yes	Yes	Thoby-Brisson & Ramirez, 2001 Peña et al. 2004
Blocked by Cd^{2+}	No	Yes	Thoby-Brisson & Ramirez, 2001 Peña et al. 2004 Tryba et al. 2006
Presence at: P0-P5	Scarce	Yes	Peña et al. 2004 Del Negro et al. 2002; 2005
Presence at: >P5	Yes	Yes	Peña et al. 2004 Del Negro et al. 2002; 2005
Blocked by riluzole	Yes (around 75 % of them*)	No	Peña et al. 2004 Del Negro et al. 2002; 2005 Paton et al. 2006 Tryba et al. 2006
Blocked by FFA	No	Yes (around 90 % of them*)	Peña et al. 2004 Del Negro et al. 2005 Tryba et al. 2006
$5\text{-}HT_{2A}R$-dependent	Yes	No	Peña et al. 2004 Tryba et al. 2006
Substance P-potentiated	No	Yes	Peña et al. 2004 Ben-Mabrouk & Tryba, 2008
Noradrenaline-potentiated	No	Yes	Viemari & Ramirez, 2006
Necessary for eupnea generation	Yes[a]	Yes[a]	Peña et al. 2004 Tryba et al., 2006 Peña and Aguileta, 2007
Bursting in hypoxia	Yes	No	Thoby-Brisson & Ramirez, 2000 Peña et al. 2004 Paton et al. 2006 Tryba et al. 2006
Necessary for gasping generation	Yes	No	Peña et al. 2004 Paton et al. 2006 Tryba et al. 2006 Peña and Aguileta, 2007

Abbreviations: FFA: flufenamic acid; $5\text{-}HT_{2A}R$: $5\text{-}HT_{2A}$ receptors. *From data reported in Peña et al. 2004.[a]Both populations have to be blocked to abolish eupnea.

Table 1. Properties of pacemaker neurons localized in the preBötC.

On the other hand, type II pacemaker neurons, which are both TTX and Cd^{2+}-sensitive, seem to rely on a Ca^{2+}-activated unspecific cationic current (ICAN) (Peña et al. 2004; Del Negro et al. 2005; Tryba et al. 2006; Ben-Mabrouk & Tryba, 2010), which may arise from TRP channels (Ben-Mabrouk & Tryba, 2010). This is supported by the fact that around 90% of these pacemakers were blocked by the ICAN blocker flufenamic acid (FFA) (Peña et al. 2004; Ben-Mabrouk & Tryba, 2010). Remarkably, none of the type I pacemaker neurons are affected by FFA and no type II pacemaker neurons are affected by riluzole, which allows using such channel blockers to diminish the activity of a specific population of respiratory pacemaker neurons, without affecting others (Peña et al. 2004).

5. Role of pacemaker neurons in respiratory rhythm generation is state dependent

Although both riluzole and FFA may have several unspecific effects, mainly when used at high concentrations (Peña & Tapia 2000; Del Negro et al. 2005; Wang et al., 2006), both drugs have been used to test the role of specific pacemaker neurons on the activity of the preBötC. The evidence has shown that riluzole, at the concentration that blocks most of type I pacemaker neurons, affects but does not abolishes the generation of fictive eupnea (Del Negro et al. 2002; Peña et al. 2004). Certainly riluzole abolishes generation of fictive sighs (Peña et al. 2004; Table 1). A similar effect was observed when FFA was applied, at the concentration that blocks most of type II pacemaker neurons (elimination of sighs but maintenance of fictive eupnea generation, Peña et al. 2004, Table 1). However when both drugs are applied, no rhythm activity is recorded in the PreBötC (Peña et al. 2004; Del Negro et al. 2005). Even though a report showed that rhythmic activity can be restored upon application of substance P (Del Negro et al. 2005), we failed to consistently reproduce this finding (Tryba et al. 2006; Ben-Mabrouk & Tryba, 2008). In fact, we have been able to reproduce all our findings *in vivo*, where we found that neither riluzole nor FFA were able to block eupnea by themselves but abolished respiration when applied simultaneously (Peña & Aguileta, 2007). Furthermore we found that substance P was not able to recorver eupnea generation *in vivo* (Peña & Aguileta, 2007). Taken together, the evidence suggests that eupnea produced by the PreBötC *in vitro* can be maintained if one population of pacemaker neurons is blocked either with riluzole or with FFA, but when most type I and type II pacemaker neurons are blocked with both drugs, the PreBötC is not longer able to produce any physiologically meaningful rhythmic activity (Peña et al. 2004; Tryba et al. 2006).

Another seems to be the scenery during gasping generation. As previously mentioned, the PreBötC undergoes a reconfiguration process during hypoxia to generate gasping (Lieske et al. 2000; Peña, 2009). Three major changes occur during hypoxic conditions in this network: The first involves a generalized reduction of inhibitory synaptic transmission (Richter et al., 1991; Lieske et al. 2000), the second involves the shutdown of most of the non-pacemaker neurons (Ballanyi et al., 1994; Thoby-Brisson & Ramirez 2000), and the third involves a differential effect of hypoxia on pacemaker neurons. Type II (or Cd^{2+}-sensitive) pacemaker neurons cease to produce rhythmic bursting activity in hypoxic conditions, whereas a major subset of type I (or Cd^{2+}-insensitive) pacemaker neurons maintain their bursting activity in hypoxia (Thoby-Brisson & Ramirez 2000; Peña et al. 2004; Tryba et al. 2006; Table 1). This evidence suggests that type I (or Cd^{2+}-insensitive) pacemaker neurons may play a major role in the generation of gasping in hypoxia (Thoby-Brisson & Ramirez 2000; Peña et al. 2004;

Tryba et al. 2006). Consistent with this idea we showed that riluzole, but not FFA, specifically blocks gasping generation both *in vitro* (Peña et al. 2004) and *in vivo* (Peña & Aguileta, 2007). Our conclusion that riluzole-sensitive pacemaker activity is necessary for gasping generation, but not eupnea, has been corroborated in the *in situ* preparation as well as *in vivo* by other authors (Paton et al. 2006; St. John et al., 2006). This leads to some important conclusions: First, type I (or Cd^{2+}-insensitive) pacemaker neurons cannot be considered as the principal drivers of the more complex respiratory network operating during normoxia, but they become the sole drivers of gasping. Second, hypoxia renders the respiratory network more vulnerable to the blockade of a single ionic mechanism: namely, the persistent Na^+ current (Peña & Ramirez 2002; Tryba et al. 2006). Gasping is an important autoresuscitation mechanism that seems to fail in victims of sudden infant death syndrome (SIDS, Poets et al., 1999; Sridhar et al., 2003). Consistent with a change in configuration of the respiratory network, SIDS victims breathe normally during normoxia, but do not gasp effectively when exposed to hypoxic conditions (Poets et al., 1999; Sridhar et al. 2003).

6. Respiratory pacemaker neurons as targets of neuromodulation

Respiratory function, as most of brain functions are regulated by neuromodulatory systems, which change the functionality of the respiratory rhythm generator and more specifically the activity of respiratory pacemaker neurons (Peña et al. 2002; 2004; Ramirez et al., 2004; Doi & Ramirez, 2008; 2010). It has been shown that pacemaker neurons are differentially regulated by several neuromodulators, including serotonin (5-HT) (Peña et al. 2002; Peña & Ramirez, 2004; Viemari & Ramirez, 2006; Tryba et al., 2008). As reported for motoneurons in the spinal cord (Harvey et al., 2006a, b), activity of the persistent sodium current, in the preBötC, is regulated by tonic activation of $5\text{-}HT_{2A}$ receptors (Peña & Ramirez 2002). We reported that type I (or Cd^{2+}-insensitive) pacemaker neurons require endogenous activation of $5\text{-}HT_{2A}$ receptors to maintain bursting activity; whereas type II (or Cd^{2+}-sensitive) pacemaker neurons do not (Peña & Ramirez 2002; Tryba et al. 2006, Table 1). Interestingly, pharmacological blockade of $5\text{-}HT_{2A}$ receptors resemble the actions of riluzole (Peña & Ramirez 2002; Peña et al. 2004; Tryba et al. 2006). Namely, bath application of $5HT_{2A}$ antagonists specifically inhibits type I (or Cd^{2+}-insensitive) pacemaker neurons, eliminates sigh activity and affects eupneic activity without producing apnea (Peña & Ramirez 2002; Tryba et al. 2006). As reported for riluzole, $5HT_{2A}$ antagonists abolished gasping generation in hypoxia and produce apnea in normoxia when they were applied in conjunction with FFA (Tryba et al. 2006). Data suggest that endogenous $5HT_{2A}$ receptor activation is essential for type I pacemaker activity and gasping generation *in vitro* (Peña & Ramirez 2002; Tryba et al. 2006). This finding may have important implications for understanding the failure of autoresuscitation in SIDS since serotonergic abnormalities have been reported in the brainstem of SIDS victims (Ozawa & Takashima 2002; Sridhar et al. 2003; Weese-Mayer et al., 2003; Weese-Mayer et al, 2003; Kinney et al., 2003).

Other neuromodulator that differentially affects pacemaker activity in the PreBötC is substance P (Peña & Ramirez 2004; Ben-Mabrouk & Tryba, 2008). We have shown that substance P produce a generalized PreBötC excitation by activating a TTX-insensitive sodium current, possibly a TRP channel (Crowder et al., 2007; Mironov, 2008; Ben-Mabrouk & Tryba, 2008), in all recorded respiratory neurons. In particular we observed that whereas substance P increased burst frequency of type I (or Cd^{2+}-insensitive) pacemaker neurons, it potently enhanced bursting activity in type II (or Cd^{2+}-sensitive) pacemakers (Peña &

Ramirez 2004), which seems to contribute to the increase in the regularity of the rhythm induced by this neuromodulator (Ben-Mabrouk & Tryba, 2008). A similar effect is observed with noradrenaline. Viemari & Ramirez (2006) have shown that noradrenaline depolarizes most respiratory neurons and increases burst frequency of type I (or Cd^{2+}-insensitive) pacemaker neurons but, as reported for SP, noradrenaline potently enhances bursting activity in type II (or Cd^{2+}-sensitive) pacemaker activity (Viemari & Ramirez 2006). This differential modulation of pacemaker properties might be important to differentially modulate shape and stability of respiratory activity (Peña & Ramirez 2002; 2004; Viemari & Ramirez 2006; Doi & Ramirez, 2008; 2010).

In conclusion we can affirm that the journey to understand the basic mechanisms involved in respiratory rhythm generation is at the beginning. This challenge is complicated by the fact that pacemaker neurons in the PreBötC constitute a highly heterogeneous population regarding its intrinsic properties, sensitivity to oxygen concentration and response to neuromodulators. All these factors must be taken into account if we really want to understand this circuit. It is important never to forget that such diversity is there and that might contribute to respiratory rhythm generation in a state-dependent manner.

7. Acknowledgements

This work was supported by Conacyt-59187, México.

8. References

Arshavsky, Y.I. (2003) Cellular and network properties in the functioning of the nervous system: from central pattern generators to cognition. *Brain Res. Brain Res. Rev.* 41, 229–267.

Ballanyi, K., Volker, A. & Richter D.W. (1994) Anoxia induced functional inactivation of neonatal respiratory neurones in vitro. *Neuroreport.* 6, 165-168.

Ben-Mabrouk, F. & Tryba AK. (2010) Substance P modulation of TRPC3/7 channels improves respiratory rhythm regularity and ICAN-dependent pacemaker activity. *Eur. J. Neurosci.* 31,1219-1232.

Bianchi, A.L., Denavit-Saubie, M. & Champagnat, J. (1995) Central control of breathing in mammals: neuronal circuitry, membrane properties, and neurotransmitters. *Physiol. Rev.* 75,1-45.

Buzsaki, G. & Draguhn, A. (2004) Neuronal oscillations in cortical networks. *Science* 304, 1926–1929.

Cardin, J.A., Palmer, L.A. and Contreras, D. (2005) Stimulus-dependent gamma (30-50 Hz) oscillations in simple and complex fast rhythmic bursting cells in primary visual cortex. *J. Neurosci.* 25, 5339-5350.

Crowder, E.A., Saha, M.S., Pace, R.W., Zhang, H., Prestwich, G.D., Del Negro, C.A. (2007) Phosphatidylinositol 4,5-bisphosphate regulates inspiratory burst activity in the neonatal mouse preBötzinger complex. *J. Physiol.* 582, 1047-1058.

Cunningham, M.O., Whittington, M.A., Bibbig, A., Roopun, A., LeBeau, F.E., Vogt, A., Monyer, H., Buhl, E.H., & Traub, R.D. (2004) A role for fast rhythmic bursting neurons in cortical gamma oscillations in vitro. *Proc. Natl. Acad. Sci. U. S. A.* 101, 7152-7157.

Del Negro, C.A.; Morgado-Valle, C. & Feldman, J.L. (2002) Respiratory rhythm: an emergent network property? *Neuron*. 34, 821-830.

Del Negro, C.A., Morgado-Valle, C., Hayes, J.A., Mackay, D.D., Pace, R.W., Crowder, E.A. & Feldman JL. (2005) Sodium and Calcium Current-Mediated Pacemaker Neurons and Respiratory Rhythm Generation. *J. Neurosci*. 25, 446-453.

Del Negro, C.A. & Feldman, J.L. (2006) Looking for inspiration: new perspectives on respiratory rhythm. *Nat. Rev. Neurosci*. 7,232-242.

Doi, A. & Ramirez, J.M. (2008) Neuromodulation and the orchestration of the respiratory rhythm. *Respir. Physiol. Neurobiol*. 1641,96-104.

Doi, A. & Ramirez, J.M. (2010) State-dependent interactions between excitatory neuromodulators in the neuronal control of breathing. *J. Neurosci*. 30,8251-8262.

Egorov, A.V., Hamam, B.N., Fransen, E., Hasselmo, M.E. & Alonso, A.A. (2002) Graded persistent activity in entorhinal cortex neurons. *Nature*. 420, 173-178.

Elsen, F.P. & Ramirez, J.M. (1998) Calcium Currents of Rhythmic Neurons Recorded in the Isolated Respiratory Network of Neonatal Mice. *J. Neurosci*, 18,10652-10662

Freund, T.F. & Antal, M. (1988) GABA-containing neurons in the septum control inhibitory interneurons in the hippocampus. *Nature*. 336, 170-173.

Feldman, J.L. (1995) Neurobiology of breathing control. Where to look and what to look for. *Adv. Exp. Med. Biol*. 393,3–5.

Gray, P.A.; Janczewski, W.A., Mellen, N., McCrimmon, D.R. & Feldman, J.L. (2001) Normal breathing requires preBotzinger complex neurokinin-1 receptor-expressing neurons. *Nat. Neurosci*. 4, 927-930.

Greer, J.J., Funk, G.D. & Ballanyi, K. (2006) Preparing for the first breath: Prenatal maturation of respiratory neural control. *J. Physiol*. 570,437–444.

Harris-Warrick, R.M. & Marder, E. (1991) Modulation of neural networks for behavior. *Annu. Rev. Neurosci*. 14, 39-57.

Harvey, P.J., Li, X., Li, Y. & Bennett DJ. (2006) Endogenous monoamine receptor activation is essential for enabling persistent sodium currents and repetitive firing in rat spinal motoneurons. *J. Neurophysiol*. 96, 1171-1186.

Harvey, P.J., Li, X., Li, Y. & Bennett DJ. (2006) 5-ht2 receptor activation facilitates a persistent sodium current and repetitive firing in spinal motoneurons of rats with and without chronic spinal cord injury. *J. Neurophysiol*. 96, 1158-1170.

Janczewski, W.A., & Feldman J.L. (2006) Distinct rhythm generators for inspiration and expiration in the juvenile rat. *J. Physiol*. 570, 407-420.

Johnson, S.M., Koshiya, N. & Smith, J.C. (2001) Isolation of the kernel for respiratory rhythm generation in a novel preparation: the pre-Botzinger complex "island". *J. Neurophysiol*. 85, 1772-1776.

Johnson, B.R., Kloppenburg, P. & Harris-Warrick, R.M. (2003) Dopamine modulation of calcium currents in pyloric neurons of the lobster stomatogastric ganglion, *J. Neurophysiol* 90, 631–643.

King, C., Recce, M. & O'Keefe, J. (1998) The rhythmicity of cells of the medial septum/diagonal band of Broca in the awake freely moving rat: relationships with behaviour and hippocampal theta. Eur. J. Neurosci. 10, 464-477.

Kinney, H.C., Randall, L.L., Sleeper, L.A., Willinger, M., Belliveau, R.A., Zec, N., Rava, L.A., Dominici, L., Iyasu, S., Randall, B., Habbe, D., Wilson, H., Mandell McClain, M. &

Welty, T.K. Serotonergic brainstem abnormalities in Northern Plains Indians with the sudden infant death syndrome. *J. Neuropathol. Exp. Neurol.* 62, 1178-1191.

Koshiya, N. & Smith, J.C. (1999) Neuronal pacemaker for breathing visualized in vitro. Nature. 400, 360-363.

Leresche, N., Lightowler, S., Soltesz, I., Jassik-Gerschenfeld, D. & Crunelli V. Low-frequency oscillatory activities intrinsic to rat and cat thalamocortical cells. *J. Physiol.* 441, 155-174.

Lieske, S.P., Thoby-Brisson, M., Telgkamp, P. & Ramirez, J.M. (2000) Reconfiguration of the neural network controlling multiple breathing patterns: eupnea, sighs and gasps *Nat. Neurosci.* 3, 600-607.

Llinas, R. & Sugimori, M. (1980) Electrophysiological properties of in vitro Purkinje cell somata in mammalian cerebellar slices. *J. Physiol.* 305, 171-195.

Llinas, R.R. (1988) The intrinsic electrophysiological properties of mammalian neurons: insights into central nervous system function, *Science* 242, 1654–1664.

Mellen, N.M. & Mishra, D. (2010) Functional anatomical evidence for respiratory rhythmogenic function of endogenous bursters in rat medulla. *J. Neurosci.* 30,8383-8392.

Mironov, S.L. (2008) Metabotropic glutamate receptors activate dendritic calcium waves and TRPM channels which drive rhythmic respiratory patterns in mice. *J. Physiol.* 586, 2277-2291.

Onimaru, H., Arata, A. & Homma, I. (1989) Firing properties of respiratory rhythm generating neurons in the absence of synaptic transmission in rat medulla in vitro. *Exp. Brain Res.* 76, 530-536.

Onimaru, H. & Homma, I. (2003) A novel functional neuron group for respiratory rhythm generation in the ventral medulla. *J. Neurosci.* 23,1478-1486.

Onimaru, H. & Homma, I. (2006) Point:Counterpoint: The parafacial respiratory group (pFRG)/pre-Botzinger complex (preBotC) is the primary site of respiratory rhythm generation in the mammal. Point: the PFRG is the primary site of respiratory rhythm generation in the mammal. *J. Appl. Physiol.* 100, 2094-2095.

Ozawa, Y. & Takashima, S. (2002) Developmental neurotransmitter pathway in the brainstem of sudden infant death syndrome: a review and sleep position. *Forensic Sci. Int.* 30, S53-S99.

Pagliardini, S., Ren, J. & Greer, J.J. (2003) Ontogeny of the pre-Bötzinger complex in perinatal rats. *J. Neurosci.* 23,9575–9584.

Paton, J.F., Abdala, A.P.L., Koizumi, H., Smith, J.C. & St-John, W. (2006) Respiratory rhythm generation during gasping depends on persistent sodium current. *Nature Neurosci.* 9, 311-313.

Peña, F. & Tapia, R. (2000) Seizures and neurodegeneration induced by 4-aminopyridine in rat hippocampus in vivo: role of glutamate- and GABA-mediated neurotransmission and of ion channels. *Neuroscience.* 101, 547-561.

Peña, F., Bargas, J. & Tapia, R. (2002) Paired pulse facilitation is turned into paired pulse depression in hippocampal slices after epilepsy induced by 4-aminopyridine in vivo. *Neuropharmacology.* 42, 807-812.

Peña, F., Ramirez, J.M. (2002) Endogenous Activation of Serotonin-2A Receptors Is Required for Respiratory Rhythm Generation In Vitro *J. Neurosci.* 22, 11055-11064

Peña, F., Ramirez, J.M. (2004) Substance P-mediated modulation of pacemaker properties in the mammalian respiratory network. *J. Neurosci.* 24, 7549-7556.

Peña, F., Parkis, M.A., Tryba, A.K. & Ramirez, J.M. (2004) Differential contribution of pacemaker properties to the generation of respiratory rhythms during normoxia and hypoxia. *Neuron.* 43, 105-117.

Peña, F. & Ramirez, J.M. (2005) Hypoxia-induced changes in neuronal network properties. *Mol. Neurobiol.* 32, 251-283.

Peña, F., Gutierrez-Lerma, A.I., Quiroz-Baez, R. & Arias, C. (2006) The role of beta-amyloid protein in synaptic function: Implications for Alzheimer's disease therapy. *Curr. Neuropharmacol.* 4, 149-163.

Peña, F. & Aguileta, M.A. (2007) Effects of riluzole and flufenamic acid on eupnea and gasping of neonatal mice in vivo. *Neurosci. Lett.* 30,288-293.

Peña, F. (2008) Contribution of pacemaker neurons to respiratory rhythms generation in vitro. *Adv. Exp. Med. Biol.* 605,114-118.

Peña, F. (2009) Neuronal network properties underlying the generation of gasping. *Clin. Exp. Pharmacol. Physiol.* 36,1218-1228.

Poets, C.F., Meny, R.G., Chobanian, M.R. & Bonofiglo, R.E. (1999) Gasping and other cardiorespiratory patterns during sudden infant deaths. *Pediatr. Res.* 45, 350-354.

Ramirez, J.M., Quellmalz, U.J. & Richter, D.W. (1996) Postnatal changes in the mammalian respiratory network as revealed by the transverse brainstem slice of mice. *J. Physiol.* 491, 799-812.

Ramirez, J.M., Telgkamp, P., Elsen, F.P., Quellmalz, U.J. & Richter, D.W. (1997) Respiratory rhythm generation in mammals: synaptic and membrane properties. *Respir. Physiol.* 110, 71-85.

Ramirez, J.M., Schwarzacher, S.W., Pierrefiche, O., Olivera, B.M. & Richter, D.W. (1998) Selective lesioning of the cat pre-Botzinger complex in vivo eliminates breathing but not gasping. *J. Physiol.* 507, 895-907.

Ramirez, J.M. & Lieske, S.P. (2003) Commentary on the definition of eupnea and gasping. *Respir. Physiol. Neurobiol.* 139, 113-119.

Ramirez, J.M., Tryba, A.K. & Peña F (2004) Pacemaker neurons and neuronal networks: an integrative view. *Curr. Opin. Neurobiol.* 14, 665-674.

Rekling, J.C. & Feldman, J.L. (1998) PreBotzinger complex and pacemaker neurons: hypothesized site and kernel for respiratory rhythm generation. *Annu. Rev. Physiol.* 60, 385-405.

Richter, D.W. (1982) Generation and maintenance of the respiratory rhythm. *J. Exp. Biol.* 100,93–107.

Richter, D.W., Bischoff, A., Anders, K., Bellingham, M. & Windhorst, U. (1991) Response of the medullary respiratory network of the cat to hypoxia. *J. Physiol.* 443, 231-256.

Richter, D.W. & Spyer, K.M. (2001) Studying rhythmogenesis of breathing: comparison of in vivo and in vitro models. *Trends Neurosci.* 24, 464-472.

Schwindt, P.C. & Crill, W.E. (1982) Factors influencing motoneuron rhythmic firing: results from a voltage-clamp study. *J. Neurophysiol.* 48, 875-890.

Selverston, A. (1999) What invertebrate circuits have taught us about the brain. *Brain Res. Bull.* 50, 439-440.

Shu, Y., Hasenstaub, A. & McCormick, D.A. (2003) Turning on and off recurrent balanced cortical activity. *Nature.* 423, 288-293.

Shu, Y., Hasenstaub, A., Duque, A., Yu, Y. & McCormick DA. (2006) Modulation of intracortical synaptic potentials by presynaptic somatic membrane potential. *Nature*. 441, 761-765.

Sipila, S.T., Huttu, K., Soltesz, I., Voipio, J. & Kaila, K. (2005) Depolarizing GABA acts on intrinsically bursting pyramidal neurons to drive giant depolarizing potentials in the immature hippocampus. *J. Neurosci.* 25, 5280-5289.

Smith, J.C., Ellenberger, H.H., Ballanyi, K., Richter, D.W. & Feldman, J.L. (1991) Pre-Botzinger complex: a brainstem region that may generate respiratory rhythm in mammals. *Science*. 254, 726-729.

Sotty, F., Danik, M., Manseau, F., Laplante, F., Quirion, R. & Williams, S. (2003) Distinct electrophysiological properties of glutamatergic, cholinergic and GABAergic rat septohippocampal neurons: novel implications for hippocampal rhythmicity. *J. Physiol*. 551, 927-943.

Sridhar, R., Thach, B.T., Kelly, D.H. & Henslee, J.A. (2003) Characterization of successful and failed autoresuscitation in human infants, including those dying of SIDS. *Pediatr. Pulmonol*. 2003 36, 113-122.

St-John, W.M., Waki, H., Dutschmann, M. & Paton JF. (2006) Maintenance of eupnea of in situ and in vivo rats following riluzole: A blocker of persistent sodium channels. *Respir. Physiol. Neurobiol*. 155,97-100.

Stewart, M. & Fox, S.E. (1989) Two populations of rhythmically bursting neurons in rat medial septum are revealed by atropine. *J. Neurophysiol*. 61, 982-993.

Stewart, M. & Fox, SE. (1990) Do septal neurons pace the hippocampal theta rhythm? *Trends Neurosci*. 13, 163-168.

Steriade, M. (2004) Neocortical cell classes are flexible entities. *Nat. Rev. Neurosci* 5, 121–134.

Thoby-Brisson, M. & Ramirez, J.M. (2000) Role of inspiratory pacemaker neurons in mediating the hypoxic response of the respiratory network in vitro. *J. Neurosci*. 20, 5858-5866.

Thoby-Brisson, M. & Ramirez, J.M. (2001) Identification of two types of inspiratory pacemaker neurons in the isolated respiratory neural network of mice. *J. Neurophysiol*. 86,104-112.

Thoby-Brisson, M., Trinh, J.B., Champagnat, J. & Fortin, G. (2005) Emergence of the pre-Bötzinger respiratory rhythm generator in the mouse embryo. *J. Neurosci*. 25,4307–4318.

Traub, R.D., Buhl, E.H., Gloveli, T. & Whittington, M.A. (2003) Fast rhythmic bursting can be induced in layer 2/3 cortical neurons by enhancing persistent Na^+ conductance or by blocking BK channels, *J. Neurophysiol*. 89, 909–921.

Tresch, M.C. & Kiehn, O. (2000) Motor coordination without action potentials in the mammalian spinal cord. *Nat. Neurosci*. 3, 593-599.

Tryba, A.K., Peña, F. & Ramirez, J.M. (2006) Gasping activity in vitro: a rhythmic behavior dependent on 5HT2A receptors. *J. Neurosci*. 26, 2623-2634.

van den Top, M., Lee, K., Whyment, A.D., Blanks, A.M. & Spanswick, D. (2004) Orexigen-sensitive NPY/AgRP pacemaker neurons in the hypothalamic arcuate nucleus, *Nat. Neurosci* 7, 493–494.

Vergara, R., Rick, C., Hernandez-Lopez, S., Laville, J.A., Guzman, J.N., Galarraga, E., Surmeier, D.J. & Bargas, J. (2003) Spontaneous voltage oscillations in striatal projection neurons in a rat corticostriatal slice. *J. Physiol*. 553, 169-182.

Viemari, J.C. & Ramirez, JM. (2006) Norepinephrine Differentially Modulates Different Types of Respiratory Pacemaker and Nonpacemaker Neurons. *J. Neurophysiol.* 95, 2070-2082

Wang, X.J. (2002) Pacemaker neurons for the theta rhythm and their synchronization in the septohippocampal reciprocal loop. *J. Neurophysiol.* 87, 889-900.

Wang, D., Grillner, S. & Wallen, P. (2006) Effects of flufenamic acid on fictive locomotion, plateau potentials, calcium channels and NMDA receptors in the lamprey spinal cord. *Neuropharmacology.* 51,1038-1046.

Wenninger, J.M., Pan, L.G., Klum, L., Leekley, T., Bastastic, J., Hodges, M.R., Feroah, T.R., Davis, S. and Forster, H.V. (2004) Large lesions in the pre-Botzinger complex area eliminate eupneic respiratory rhythm in awake goats. *J. Appl. Physiol.* 97, 1629-1636.

Weese-Mayer, D.E., Zhou, L., Berry-Kravis, E.M., Maher, B.S., Silvestri, J.M. & Marazita, ML. (2003) Association of the serotonin transporter gene with sudden infant death syndrome: a haplotype analysis. *Am. J, Med. Genet.* A. 122, 238-245.

Weese-Mayer, D.E., Berry-Kravis, E.M., Maher, B.S., Silvestri, J.M., Curran, M.E. & Marazita ML. (2003) Sudden infant death syndrome: association with a promoter polymorphism of the serotonin transporter gene. *Am. J. Med. Genet.* A. 117, 268-274.

Yuste, R., MacLean, J.N., Smith, J. & Lansner, A. (2005) The cortex as a central pattern generator. *Nat. Rev. Neurosci.* 6, 477-483.

26

Diaphragmatic Pacemaker

Salim Surani, MD, MPH, MSHM, FACP, FCCP, FAASM
Assistant Professor, Baylor College of Medicine, Houston
Assistant Professor, Texas A&M University
Texas

1. Introduction

The diaphragm is a major respiratory muscle and plays an integral part in normal respiration. It is supplied by the phrenic nerve, which originates mainly from the fourth cervical nerve, but also receives contribution from the third and fifth cervical nerves. The phrenic nerve contains sensory, motor, and sympathetic nerve fibers, and it supplies motor supply to the diaphragm and sensory supply to the central tendon. Both phrenic nerves runs along the scalene anterior muscle deep to the carotid sheath. The right phrenic nerve passes over the brachiocephalic artery and posterior to the subclavian vein and over the right atrium. It enters the diaphragm at the level of T8th verbetrae. The left phrenic nerve also runs posterior to the left subclavian vein and passes over the pericardium of the left ventricle and penetrates the left hemidiaphragm separately.

The diaphragm, on the other hand, is an elliptical cylindroid structure that is capped by the fibrous dome. The central tendon, which is the highest part of the diaphragm, consists of interwoven collagenous fibers; whereas, the cylindrical portion of the diaphragm consists of a continuous muscle fiber band, the majority of which is directly in contact with the inner surface of the lower ribs. Injury to the central nervous system, phrenic nerve, or diaphragm can lead to an impairment of diaphragm function and lead to respiratory impairment, resulting in a decrease in tidal volume, minute ventilation, and abnormal gas exchange. Injuries to the nerve can be of various types, as described in Table 1 [1, 2]. Diaphragmatic pacing (phrenic nerve pacing) can lead to significant improvements in quality of life and decrease complications along with the savings in a mechanical ventilator dependent patients. In the current chapter of this book we will discuss the role of a diaphragmatic pacemaker (Phrenic nerve stimulator).

2. History of diaphragmatic pacemaker

In 1987, Duchenne [3] was the first to discover that direct stimulation of the phrenic nerve can lead to the contraction of diaphragm and imitate normal respiration (Figure 1); however, discussion about electrically stimulating the diaphragm and heart dates back almost two hundred years. In 1777, Cavallo was the first to suggest electricity as a means for artificial respiration, and in 1818 Andrew Ure claimed that life could be restored in cases of suffocation, hanging, and drowning by stimulating the phrenic nerve [4]. In the late 1800s, it was reported that electrical impulses cause the heart to beat. Hufeland [5], in 1873, was the first person to suggest that electrical stimulation of the phrenic nerve can lead to artificial respiration and can treat asphyxia.

There was a long pause in work of phrenic nerve pacing despite the earlier success, which is mainly attributed to the advent of positive pressure ventilation. The first step in the direction of positive pressure ventilation was taken by Friedrich Trendelenburg in 1871 when the cuffed tube was introduced. He invented the devise to prevent aspiration during larynx surgery [6]. A decade later, Samuel Meltzer and Charles Elsberg described the use of ventilator equipment for anesthesia, which marked an era of positive pressure ventilation [6]. During the first half of the twentieth century, both the positive pressure ventilating device and the negative pressure ventilating device (iron lung) were in use. In 1940s Sarnoff et al. from Harvard University suggested that the absence of rhythmic diaphragmatic contractions can alter minute ventilation and henceforth result in an increase in carbon dioxide and a decrease in oxygen concentration. He described the new means of artificial respiration in which one or both phrenic nerves are stimulated by electrical current. He applied the current via a Grass stimulator set to deliver 40 impulses per second, with each impulse having a duration of two seconds. "The current was fed through a rotating potentiometer which describes an arc, the length of which can be set by an adjustable lever." (7) The voltage can be regulated, and a gradual increase in voltage results in a smooth diaphragmatic contraction, which produces respiration. He also was able to perform 52 hours of phrenic nerve stimulation as an only means of artificial respiration in a five-year-old patient with cerebral aneurysm leading to respiratory paralysis [7].

In 1950s, on the other hand, the first cardiac pacemaker was developed, which was not internally implanted as the current pacemakers are. The device was powered by A/C and had small electrical leads that were implanted in the heart. By 1957 a fully functional battery-operated cardiac pacemaker was developed by Rune Elqvist (Figure 2). In 1960 the first cardiac pacemaker that was totally implanted into the body was invented [8]. William Glenn (Figure 3) from Yale University, along with his colleague, was the first to create the first practical application of phrenic nerve pacing. Their first clinical application of radiofrequency stimulation was done in 1964; it was a short-term application in the immediate postoperative period [9]. Glenn and colleague mentioned phrenic nerve pacing in their paper in 1966 [10], though their seminal work on this topic was published in JAMA in 1968 on the use of radio-frequency electrophrenic respiration, a long-term application to a patient with primary hypoventilation syndrome [11].

In collaboration with Dr. Glenn and Roger E. Avery, Glenn's prototype was brought into commercial distribution by Avery Laboratories, Inc. in the early 1970s [12]. Flageole et al. [13] in 1995 described their experience with inserting phrenic nerve pacemakers in three children. In 2006 Hunt et al. [14] published their experience from Children Memorial Hospital in Chicago, Illinois, USA, of phrenic nerve pacemaker implantation among 34 infants and children since 1976. In 2002 Shaul et al. [15] described the thoracoscopic technique for phrenic nerve pacemaker implantation among nine children from 1997-2000. So far approximately 330 diaphragmatic pacemakers have been implanted among infants and children, and a total of approximately 2,000 diaphragmatic pacemakers have been implanted in over 20 countries. For approximately two decades, Dr. Onders and colleague from Cleveland clinic initiated the implantation of the diaphragmatic pacer. Christopher Reeve, who played Superman, was his first success story. Onders used the device NeuRx Diaphragm Pacing stimulation (DPS) [16]. NeuRx DPS ™ has developed over the past 22 years via the joint effort of several institutions including Case Western Reserve University, University Hospital, and VA Medical Center. It achieved its IDE status in October 2005 for use in clinical trials in amyotrophic lateral sclerosis (ALS) patients. Over 150 spinal cord injury patients, including Christopher Reeves have been treated with NeuRx DPS TM (DPS: Diaphragmatic Pacing System) system in the USA. Onders et al. [17, 18] reported the data of 88 patients' experiences on the use of NeuRx DPS.

3. Introduction to diaphragmatic pacemaker

The initial diaphragmatic pacemaker was developed by Dr. Glenn at Yale University. It consisted of an external battery-powered transmitter with an antenna placed on the skin and a radio receiver placed subcutaneously beneath the antenna. A platinum electrode was used to surround and conduct current to the phrenic nerve [19]. Even after half a century the design of the diaphragmatic pacemaker remains almost the same. Today, it still consists of an external transmitter and antenna, a subcutaneously implanted receiver and electrodes (Figure 4). The external transmitter and antenna send the radiofrequency energy to the subcutaneous receiver, which in turn converts the radio frequency waves into stimulating pulses, which are transmitted from electrodes to the phrenic nerve, resulting in the contraction of the diaphragm. The earlier versions were limited by the battery life, with fresh 9-volt alkaline battery providing enough energy to pace for almost 40 hours. The newer Mark IV transmitter was approved by the U.S. Food and Drug administration (FDA) in 1988 and received approval from European Active Implantable Medical Device Directives in 1994. The current subcutaneous receiver is approximately 1″ x ¼″. The electrodes are highly flexible stainless steel wire, which is insulated by silicone rubber, and have a platinum nerve contact on one end, and a connector to connect with the receiver on the other end. The antenna is worn externally over the implanted devise (Figure 5). It is suggested by the manufacturer to replace the antenna every six months. The current devises are compatible for remote trans-telephonic monitoring. In the earlier models, the most common challenge other than the short battery life was the failure of the radio receiver. Impending failure was usually heralded by sharp pain over the electrode site in the neck or by erratic pacing. With the advent of newer models and significant improvements in technology and designed along with bilateral redundancy lead to introduction of a safer device. The transmitters do not require complicated external programmers to configure, and they use standard, alkaline batteries [12]. An alternate to the phrenic nerve stimulator, the DPS has been used to stimulates the diaphragm to help restore normal negative pressure breathing. It consists of four electrodes implanted in the diaphragm to stimulate the muscle. The fifth electrode is placed under the skin to complete the circuit. In addition a connector holder, a cable, and an external battery-powered pulse generator are used. The timing and control of stimuli to regulate movement in the diaphragm are provided by the pulse generator, which creates a negative pressure and allows the air to enter the lungs (Figure 6). [16]

4. Outcome data in adults

In an appropriately selected individual, the diaphragmatic pacemaker provides an opportunity for liberation from mechanical ventilation, either completely or partially. Moreover, by providing an opportunity for the normal negative pressure ventilation, and henceforth eliminating the adverse effects of positive pressure ventilation.

Glenn et al. [19] reported their initial experience with phrenic nerve stimulation of 37 patients with quadriplegia in 1975. Full-time pacing was achieved in 13 patients, and in other ten patients ventilation was provided by pacing at least 50% of the time. In the remaining 14 patients in the series, ventilator support for 50% of the day could not be achieved. Eight of those patients died mainly from the complications of positive pressure ventilation. The main cause of failure to support ventilation was due to injury and subsequent damage to one or both phrenic nerves either from the initial trauma or operative manipulation. Malfunction of the pacemaker due to shorting of electronic components and antenna connector breakage also contributed to failure to pace or ineffective pacing.

Another work by Glenn and colleague [20], reviewed the records of 477 patients who had undergone diaphragm pacemaker implantation for chronic hypoventilation. The data were from 1966 to 1988. Out of 477 patients, 165 patients were from multicenter study patients, 203 were from non-center study patients, and 109 patients were from non-study patients. Cervical cord injury and brain stem injury patients made the majority of patients (Table 2). 47.27% of patients had success, whereas 34.54% of patients had significant support, and approximately 16% of patients had failure or minimal support.

In another paper by Glenn et al. [21], they reported the long-term follow-up of pacing of the conditioned diaphragm in twelve quadriplegic patients. All twelve patients were successfully conditioned and they all were able to achieve full ventilation. In 1998 Garrido-Garcia et al. [22] described a series of 22 patients who underwent placement of diaphragmatic pacemaker for the treatment of chronic respiratory failure. Thirteen of them had quadriplegia, five were status post-surgical treatment of intracranial lesion, and four patients had central alveolar hypoventilation syndrome. In their series, 81.8% of patients achieved permanent diaphragmatic paced breathing, whereas in 18.2% of patients it was done during sleep. On the long-term follow-up only two of the twenty-two patients were considered as failure. Garrido=Garcia et al. felt diaphragmatic pacemakers promote complete stable ventilation and improve the quality of life for patients. They used two types of diaphragmatic pacemakers—the monopolar stimulation model (Avery Lab, Framingdale, NY) with an S-242 transmitter in two cases and the S-232 transmitter in six cases. They used an Atrostim (Atro-tech, Finland), which was a multipolar sequential stimulation model with either a Pekka transmitter in three cases or a Jukka transmitter in 11 cases. In 2002, Elefteriades and colleagues [23] reviewed the data on twelve patients who underwent implantation procedures between 1981 and 1987. They reported that 50% continued to pace full time with a mean duration of 14.8 years. Two (16%) patients died, one (8%) patient paced part-time, and three (25%) patients stopped pacing. Recently, Khong et al. [24] published an Australian series of 19 patients. Of those, 14 required phrenic nerve pacing due to quadriplegia, one had central hypoventilation syndrome, one had encephalitis, and the information on the remaining three was not known. Currently, 11 of the pacers are known to be actively implanted to date with a mean duration of 13 years.

5. Outcome data in children

From the information available, the first breathing pacemaker occurred on August 23, 1974 at St. Mary's Hospital (Mayo Clinic) in Rochestor, Minnesota, [25] in a fifteen-year-old quadriplegic patient who is still being paced to date. In 1983 Brouilette et al. [26] reported the case series of nine infants and children who underwent phrenic nerve pacing; five of those were less than one year of age. Seven of those were still alive at the time of publication. From August 1974 to June 2006, 324 diaphragmatic pacemakers have been implanted in children under the age of 18. Congenital central alveolar hypoventilation syndrome and quadriplegia account for approximately 75% of cases. Table 3 gives the breakdown of the indication and average implant days among the pediatric population [25]. Approximately 71% of the patients still have active working pacemakers, whereas 18% of the patients are deceased, as shown in Table 3 [25].

6. Indication

The diaphragmatic pacemaker is mainly indicated for patients with central lesion above the second and third cervical level. For functioning of the phrenic nerve pacemaker, one needs to have functioning nerve cell bodies in C3-C5 level. In contrast, trauma to the central nervous system at the level of C3-C5 does not allow pacing due to the damage of phrenic nerve cell bodies. Table 5 illustrates the disorder of the diaphragm due to either central, phrenic nerve, or diaphragm dysfunction and the etiologies related to it. Phrenic nerve injury can occur during open heart surgery or as a result of trauma, radiation, or neuropathic injury. The central or upper motor neuron disorders leading to diaphragm dysfunction are treated by mechanical ventilation or phrenic nerve pacing, whereas phrenic nerve dysfunction or lower motor neuron disorders are usually treated with non-invasive positive pressure ventilation, intercostals nerve grafting/pacing, and diaphragm placation. The diaphragm placation is usually reserved for non-functional phrenic nerves or disorders leading to contractile dysfunction of diaphragm. The ideal candidates for pacing with a phrenic nerve stimulator are the patients with complete cervical spine injuries at C1 and C2 level, congenital or acquired central alveolar hypoventilation syndrome, brainstem injury (tumor, trauma, bleed, infarct), or basilar meningitis [20, 24, 27].

Diaphragmatic pacing has been used for other indications as Arnold Chiari malformation, meningomyelocele, neurofibromatosis (with multiple meningiomas), complete tetraplegia , patients with C3-C4 incomplete fracture, C4-C5 fracture with ascending paralysis to C2-C3 level, radiation induced phrenic nerve injury [24, 26, 28]. In a twenty-year experience of phrenic nerve stimulation for diaphragmatic pacing, Glann and colleague used the pacing in 2% of patients with chronic obstructive pulmonary disease (COPD). The details are shown in Table 6 [27].

Disease of the lower motor neurons as amyotrophic lateral sclerosis (ALS) and poliomyelitis have been considered as contraindications for the placement of diaphragmatic pacemakers, but there have been case reports with the successful use of the diaphragmatic pacemaker in patients with poliomyelitis (29). Onders et al. [17, 18] from Cleveland Clinic reported their data on a multi-center study on the implantation of the diaphragmatic pacemaker in ALS and spinal cord injury (SCI) patients. From March 2000 to September 2007, they implanted the device in 88 patients (50 SCI and 38 ALS). They found that ALS patients had much weaker diaphragms, which were identified during surgery. They required trains of stimulation during mapping to identify motor points. They found no perioperative mortality even in patients with forced vital capacity (FVC) less than 50%. They found that ALS patients were able to delay their need for mechanical ventilation by 24 months.

7. Evaluation

Patients who need to be considered as candidates should be carefully evaluated. The patients should meet the indication for implantation. Furthermore, the patients should have severe, chronic respiratory insufficiency requiring mechanical ventilation or respiratory insufficiency for more than three months [17, 28-30]. They should have respiratory insufficiency for more than three months after the onset of injury and viable motor neurons (exception cases of those in ALS and Poliomyelitis as mentioned earlier). Failure of the diaphragmatic contraction after the stimulation of the phrenic nerve is considered a contraindication. On the other hand, there have been reports of intercostals to phrenic anastomosis in patients with anterior spinal artery syndrome [31]. Krieger et al. [32] reported a case series of ten nerve transfers from intercostals to phrenic nerves in six patients. Eight of ten transfers had more than three months to allow for axonal regeneration. 100% of those nerve transfers achieved successful diaphragmatic pacing [32].

8. Viability of phrenic nerve

The fundamental requirement of successful pacing is the viability of the phrenic nerve. It is usually assessed by percutaneous electrical stimulation of the phrenic nerve at the level of the neck where the nerve passes over the scalene muscle. This technique was initially employed by Sarnoff et al. [33)]. They mentioned that quick hiccup-like contractions of the diaphragm on the stimulated side were evidence of nerve integrity. If most nerves were viable, then contractions were vigorous. Currently, fluoroscopy is used to detect diaphragmatic function [34]. It is important to assess the diaphragmatic movement under fluoroscopy, as there have been misdiagnoses in detecting diaphragmatic contractions without it [35]. Garrido-Garcia et al. [22], considered the conduction time of 4-12 msec as normal. Brouillette et al. [26], found the phrenic nerve conduction time to be between 2.7 msec to 7.8 msec in the pediatric population. The phrenic nerve conduction time appeared to be shorter in the pediatric population [36-38]. They also found that phrenic nerve conduction time was significantly shorter after intrathoracic stimulation when compared to cervical stimulation. They also found that phrenic nerve conduction timing increased in correlation with age.

The best time to test phrenic nerve viability is a controversial subject, but the general consensus is to wait for three months after an injury. Versteegh et al. found that when tested early, the phrenic nerves were responsive but later became unresponsive; whereas, it is also possible that the nerves may be initially unresponsive but may become responsive up to a year after the injury [39]. It is extremely important not to reject the patient for phrenic nerve stimulator placement if nerves were unresponsive initially. It is suggested that testing the viability of the nerves may be repeated again up to two years later.

9. Diaphragmatic action potential amplitude

In the study by Brouillette et al. [26], the diaphragmatic action potential amplitude after supramaximal stimulation of the phrenic nerve varies from 0.08 to 4.1 mV. They also found that unlike the phrenic nerve conduction timing, diaphragmatic action potential amplitudes vary significantly on serial testing of the phrenic nerve.

10. Surgical implantation techniques

The initial technique for the placement of phrenic nerve stimulator was described by Glenn et al. [19]. Adults were given a four inch transverse incision above and parallel to the clavicle under local anesthesia. Glenn and colleague then isolated the phrenic nerve where it crosses the scalenus anterior muscle and they placed electrode cuff around it. Children under 12 years of age whose necks were too short to accommodate the cuff required the placement of the cuff by thoracotomy approach, as far from the heart as possible.

In 2002, Shaul et al. [40] described the thoracoscopic technique for the placement of phrenic nerve electrodes. The description of surgical detail is beyond the scope of this chapter and is described in detail in their manuscript [40].

Briefly in the cervical approach, a horizontal incision is made and the sternocleidomastoid muscle is retracted medially. The phrenic nerve is identified and the electrode is applied. In the thoracic approach, the procedure can be performed either by thoracotomy or thoracoscpically. The lungs are deflated on one side and the phrenic nerve is identified and mobilized. The electrode is positioned below the nerve and sutured. The leads are then brought through the thoracic cavity and tunneled into the subcutaneous pocket inferior to the 12th rib and the receiver is placed into the pocket [24, 41].

During surgery, after securing the electrodes and connecting to the receiver, the device is tested to ensure good contact with the nerve and stimulation via the receiver results in good contraction of the diaphragm. Device implantation is carried out on each side—two separate procedures performed two weeks apart. Intra-operative diaphragm function can be confirmed by visual observation of the chest wall, palpation of the costal margin, and observation of CO2 changes or fluoroscopy.

As far as the NeuRx DPS system is concerned, it can be implanted by using the laparoscopic technique by creating four small openings in the abdominal region and inserting the laparoscope through the incisions. Electrodes are placed in the area near the phrenic nerves, which control the diaphragmatic contractions. The implanted electrodes are connected to the four channel external stimulator, which is placed at the percutaneous exit site. The stimulator provides biphasic balanced stimulation to each of the electrodes with a common indifferent electrode that is placed subcutaneously. The stimulator controls the charge, which is delivered via the clinician's pre-programmed parameters of pulse duration, pulse amplitude, pulse frequency, pulse ramp, respiratory rate, and inspiratory time. The users just connect the device and turn it on for the use. For the patients with spinal cord injury, the DPS is set to provide the tidal volume 15% over the basal need. For the ALS patients, an amplitude setting of 25 mA, a frequency below 20 Hz, and pulse width below 200 microseconds is recommended. ALS patients undergo diaphragmatic conditioning five times per day for 30 minutes [17].

11. Pacemaker setting & diaphragm conditioning

Signals are generated by the transmitter, and the subcutaneously implanted receiver picks up the radiofrequency energy and converts it to electrical impulses. Electrical pulses of 150 microsecond duration are delivered with varying amplitude, based on the patient's requirements. A pulse train of 1.3 second and 0.9 second is used for adult and pediatric patients respectively [21]. In order to allow time for the postoperative edema to subside, the diaphragm conditioning is not initiated for at least 12 days after implantation of the second unit. The diaphragm is conditioned by increase in duration of pacing time per hour during the day and rest at night. During the rest period, the patient is placed on positive pressure ventilation.

12. Benefits of the breathing pacemaker

Mechanical ventilation, or positive pressure breathing, is associated with significantly higher costs than normal negative pressure breathing. Moreover, positive pressure ventilation is associated with an increase in cost related to the use of the intensive care unit, or if at home, high cost associated with home health, and durable medical equipment, higher demand on the patient's family, decreased mobility for the patient, and higher rate of complications. Positive pressure ventilation is also associated with poor quality of life, increased risk of deep venous thrombosis and pulmonary embolism due to limited activity. In contrast, the diaphragmatic pacemaker is associated with the natural breathing pattern. Patients are ambulatory (if not quadriplegic or CNS deficit limiting mobility) due to not being attached to the mechanical ventilation system for their breathing needs. The patients are also able to talk and eat normally and perform the normal activities associated with everyday living, as well as their job in many instances. In addition, the patient also is able to breathe through the nose, which offers protection against the bacteria which can bypass the body's defense system when one breathes through a tracheal tube. There have also been reports of long-term recovery of diaphragmatic function in patients with phrenic nerve pacing [47].

13. Complications

Complications may include risk associated with anesthesia and surgery; infection, bleeding, hypoxia, injury to the phrenic nerve, and injury to surrounding structures, among others. In the Australian study, eight out of 19 patients had repeat operations for replacement/reimplantation of hardware. The original I-107 receiver had a life span of three to five years, whereas the battery life of the current receiver is as long as that of the patient [24]. In the pediatric population of a study by Shaul et al. [40], two patients developed postoperative atelectasis, and one patient had pneumonia. One patient had pneumothorax, and one patient had liver laceration. In their twenty-year phrenic nerve implantation experience, Glenn et al. found the major complication to be iatrogenic injury to the phrenic nerve. They also observed injury to the diaphragm by overstimulation. In addition, there have been reported incidences of diaphragmatic pacemaker failure due to twisting of the phrenic nerve wires following the manipulation of the implanted receiver

[42, 43]. Diaphragmatic origin of the pacemaker sound has also been described in literature [44-46].

14. Conclusion

Over last fifty years, significant progress has been made in the area of breathing pacemakers in the area of phrenic nerve stimulation and the diaphragmatic pacemaker. The surgical technique has also evolved from open thoracotomy to new laparoscopic procedures. Breathing pacemakers, which can delay the need for mechanical ventilation by approximately two years, should be offered to all patients with spinal cord injury, central alveolar hypoventilation syndrome, and even in patients with ALS. This in turn can lead to improvements in patients' physical, mental, and psychological qualities of life. Future studies should be undertaken to develop a simpler and more redundant system.

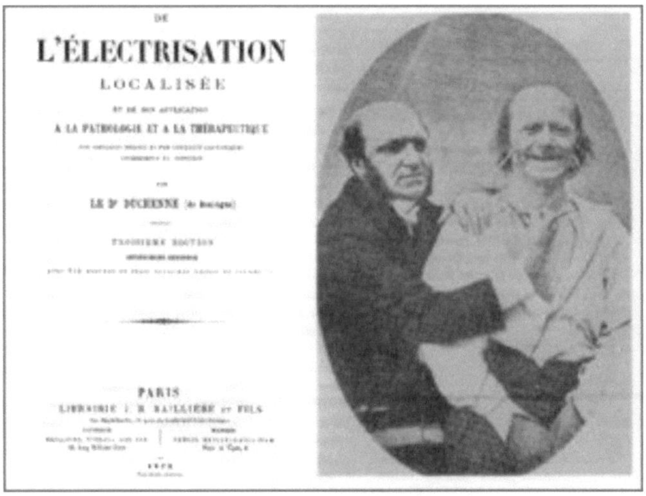

Fig. 1. Duchenne's seminal work on electrical stimulation
(Published with Permission from Avery Biomedical Device, Inc)

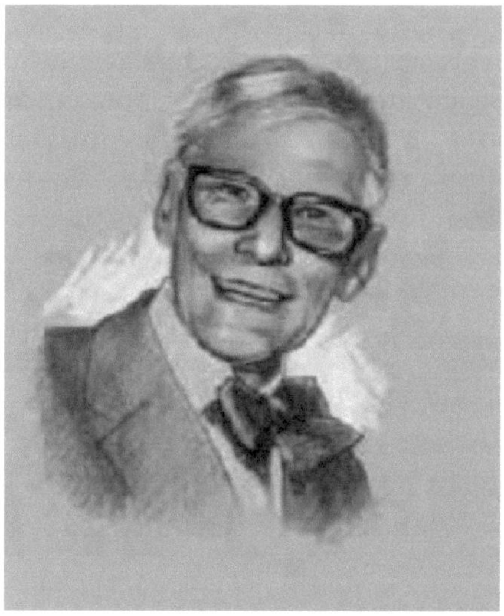

Fig. 2. Rene Elmqvist

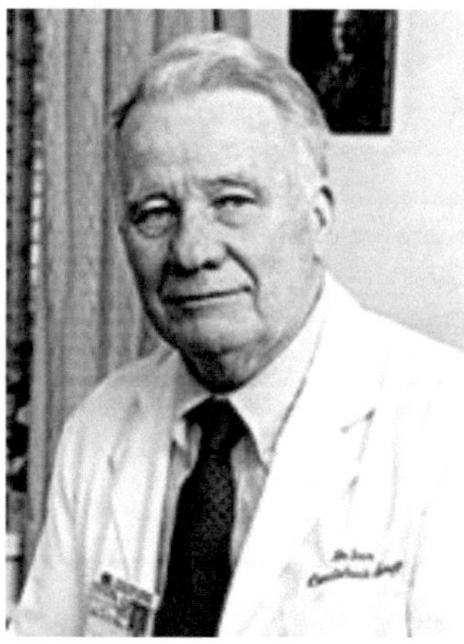

Fig. 3. William W. L. Glenn, MD

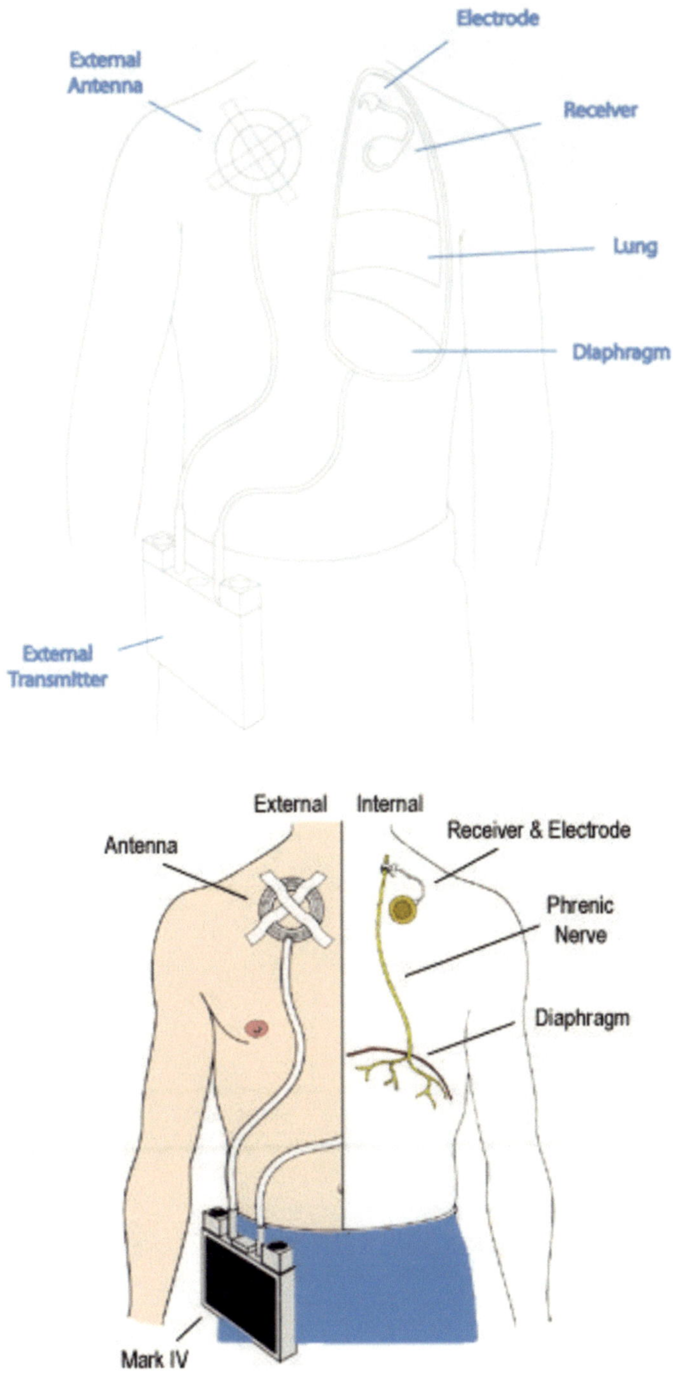

Fig. 4. Diaphragmatic Pacemaker System. Published with permission from Avery Biomedical Device, Inc

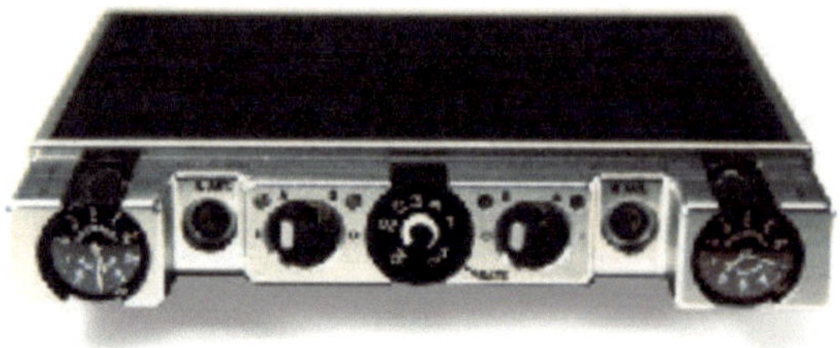

Fig. 5A. Mark IV Transmitter

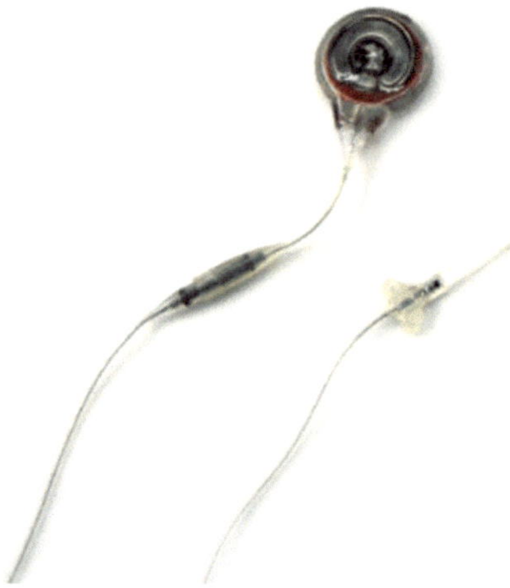

Fig. 5B. Receiver and Electrode

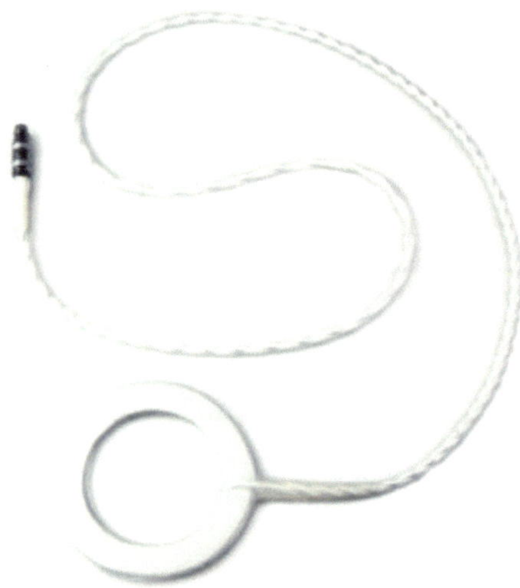

Fig. 5C. External Antenna

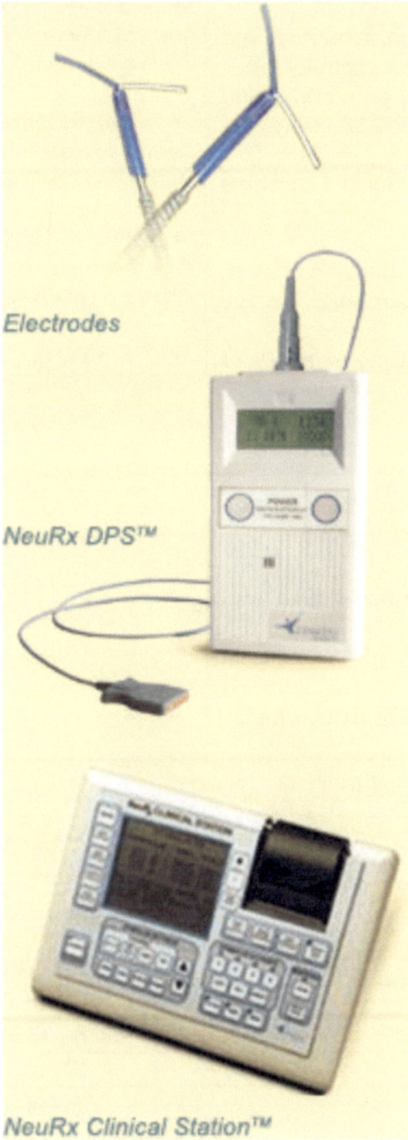

Fig. 6. NeuRx DPS. Copied with Permission from Synapse Biomedical Inc.

Seddon's	Sutherland
Neuropraxia • Injury to the myelin sheath • Larger nerves covered by greater amounts of myelin are most susceptible to this injury. • Reflexes, muscle function, vibratory, and two-point discrimination are typically lost • Repair may take days to months and healing is usually perfect, as only the sheath needs to be repaired. • Corresponds to Sutherland's 1st Degree injury. **Axonotmesis** • Involves disruption of the nerve itself, but the surrounding and supportive nerve myelin sheath is affected. • Causes include long or severe periods of compression, pulling or loss of blood flow to the nerve. • All nerve types may be affected. • Recovery is usually good. • Corresponds to a 2nd or 3rd degree injury in Sutherland's system. **Neurotmesis** • Disruption of both the nerve fiber and the supportive myelin sheath. • Healing is usually poor without surgical repair. • Corresponds to a 4th or 5th degree injury in Sutherland's system.	• First Degree: Injury with only local changes to the nerve sheath (myelin). • Second Degree: Incomplete injury to the nerve axons Nerve is intact. • Third Degree: Severe axonal injury with scar tissue. Nerve may be injured but is still intact. • Fourth Degree: Complete disruption of axon. Nerve is severely injured but is still intact. • Fifth Degree: Complete transaction of the nerve.

Table 1. Nerve injury Classification

	Center	Non-Center	Non-Study
	165	203	109
Diagnosis			
Cervical Cord Injury	55 (33.33%)	114 (56.16%)	
Brain Stem Injury	50 (30.3%)	54 (26.6%)	
Idiopathic	31 (18.79%)	17 (8.37%)	
Congenital	27 (16.36%)	8 (3.94%)	
Peripheral Lesion	2 (1.21%)	10 (4.93%)	
Numbers of Years Paced			
Up to 5 years	108 (67.9%)	155 (86.1%)	
5-10 years	31 (19.5%)	24 (13.3%)	
10-15 years	16 (10.1%)	1 (.6%)	
15-20 years	4 (2.5%)		

Table 2. Chronic Ventilatory Insufficiency Treated by Diaphragm Pacing. Adapted from Glen WW et al (14)

Diagnosis	Number of Patients	Percentage of Population	Youngest Implant Age (Days)	Average Implant Age (Years)
CCHS	134	41	56	5.6
Quadriplegia	110	34	204	9.8
Brain Injury/Tumor	7	2	756	8.6
Arnold Chiari	7	2	714	6.9
Other	10	3	89	7.1
Unknown	56	17	98	8.8
Totals:	324	100%	56	7.7

Table 3. Phrenic Pacemaker Implanted in Pediatric Population (With Permission from Avery Biomedical Lab, Inc)

Active	230	71
Deceased1	57	18
Inactive -Explanted	4	1
Inactive -Implanted	5	2
Inactive -Unknown	28	9
Totals	324	100

Table 4. Phrenic Nerve Stimulator Device Status. (With Permission from Avery Biomedical Lab, Inc)

Disorders Leading to Diaphragm Dysfunction		
Central (Upper Motor Neuron Lesion)	Phrenic Nerve (Lower Motor Neuron Lesion)	Diaphragmatic Contractile Dysfunction
• Central Alveolar Hypoventilation (CAH) • - Stroke • - Tumor • - Infection • - Vascular • Lesions/trauma of C1 or C2 • Congenital Central Hypoventilation Syndrome (CCHS/Ondine's Curse)	• Spinal pathology (C3, 4, 5) • Neuropathies (idiopathic, ALS, viral) • Trauma: Surgical damage, resection, itrogenic • Tumor • Idiopathic • Radiation Injury	• Muscular dystrophy • Disuse atrophy • Myositis

Table 5. Causes of Diaphragm Dysfunction

Etiology	Percentages
Lesion of Brain Stem or above	
CVA	11%
Tumor or cyst	4%
Encephalitis	9%
Other infections	3%
Shy dragger Syndrome	2%
Other	3%
Lesions of Upper Cervical Cord	
Trauma	22%
Tumor or cyst	1%
Poliomyelitis	3%
Syrinx	1%
Cervical cordotomy	1%
Atlanto-occipital deformity	2%
Others	1%
Idiopathic Central Alveolar Hypoventlation	
Congenital	1%
Undetermined	15%
Peripheral respiratory insufficiency	
COPD	2%

Table 6. Diaphragmatic Pacemaker placement by etiology

15. References

[1] Seddon HJ. Three types of nerve injury. Brain 1943; 66(4): 238-288.
[2] Sutherland S. Classification of peripheral nerve injuries producing loss of function. Brain 1951; 74: 491
[3] Duchene GB. De L'electrisation localisee et de son application a la pathologie et a le therapeutique par courants induits et par courants galvaniques interrompus et continues per le dr. Duchenne. Paris, Bailliere 1872.
[4] Spartacus Educational. www.spartacus.school.co.uk/IRue.htm. Accessed on 7/17/2010.
[5] Hufeland CW. De use vis electricae in asphyxia experimentis illustrato. Inaugraldissert. Gottingae 1873.
[6] Gedeon A. Mechanical ventilation, a historical perspective. Clinical window web journal # 22. Dec 2006. www.clinicalwindow.net. Accessed 7/4/2010
[7] Sarnoff SJ, hardenbergh E, Whittenberger JL. Electrophrenic Respiration. Science 1948; 108: 482.
[8] History of pacemakers. Http://www.medtronic.com/brady/patients/pacemakerhistory.html. Accessed on 7/5/2010.

[9] Glenn WW, Holcomb BE, Bernard J, Gee L, Rath R. Central hypoventilation; Long term ventilator assistance by radiofrequency electrophrenic respiration. Ann of Surg 1970; 172 94): 755-773).

[10] Glenn WW, Anagnostopoulos CE. Electronic pacemakers of the heart, gastrointestinal tract, phrenic nerve, bladder, and carotid sinus: Current status. Surgery, 1996; 60 (2): 480-494.

[11] Glenn WW, Judson JP. Radio-frequency electrophrenic respiration. Long-term application to a patient with primary hypoventilation. Journal of the Am Med Ass 1968; 203 (12): 1033-1037.

[12] Breathing Pacemaker. www.averylabs.com/breathing-pacemakers/introduction.html. Accessed on 7/4/2010.

[13] Flageole H, Adolph VR, Davis M, Laberge JM, Nguyen LT, Guttman FM. Diaphragmatic pacing in children with congenital central alveolar syndrome. Surgery 1995; 118 (1): 25-28.

[14] Hunt CE, Brouillette RT, Weese-Mayer DE, Morrow A, Ilbawi MN. Diaphragm pacing in infants and children. PACE 2006; 11 (11); 2135-2141.

[15] Shaul DB, Danielson PD, McComb JG, Keens TG. Thoracoscopic placement of phrenic nerve electrodes for diaphragm pacing in children. J Ped Surg 2002; 37 (7): 974-978

[16] The NeuRx DPS. www.synapsebiomedical.com/products/neurx.shtml. Accessed on 7/12/2010.

[17] Onders RP, Elmo M, Khansarinia S, Bowman B, Yee J, et al. Complete worldwide operative experience in laparoscopic diaphragm pacing: results and differences in spinal cord injured patients and amyotrophic lateral sclerosis patients. Surg Endosc 2009; 23 (7): 1433-1440.

[18] Onders RP, Carlin AM, Elmo M, Sivashankaran SB, Schilz R. Amyotrophic lateral sclerosis: the Midwestern surgical experience with the diaphragm pacing stimulation system shows that general anesthesia can be safely performed. Am J Surg 2009; 197 (3): 386-390.

[19] Glenn WL, Holcomb BE, Shaw RK, Hogan JF. Long term ventilator support by diaphragm pacing in quadriplegia. Ann Surg 1976; 183 (5): 566-576.

[20] Glenn WL, Brouillette RT, Dentz B, Fodstad H, Hunt CE, Keens TG, Marsh HM, et al. Fundamental considerations in pacing of the diaphragm for chronic ventilator insufficiency: A multi-center study. PACE 1988; 11: 2121-2128.

[21] Elefteriades JA, Quin JA, Hogan JF, Holcomb WG, Letsou GV, Chlosta WF, Glenn WW. Long-term followup of pacing of the conditioned diaphragm in quadriplegia. PACE 2002; 25 (6): 897-906.

[22] Garrido-Garcia H, Alvarez JM, Escribano PM, Ganuza JR, Banda FL et al. Treatment of chronic ventilator failure using a diaphragmatic pacemaker. Spinal Cord 1998; 36: 310-314.

[23] Elefteriades J, Quin J. Diaphragm Pacing. Ann Thorac Surg 2002; 73: 691-692

[24] Khong P, Lazzaro A, Mobbs R. Phrenic nerve stimulation: The Australian experience. J of Clin Neuroscience 2010; 17: 205-208.

[25] Avery Biomedical Laboratory Company records. Avery Biomedical Devices Inc.

[26] Brouillette RT, Ilbawi MN, Hunt CE. Phrenic nerve pacing in ingants and children: A review of experience and report on the usefulness of phrenic nerve stimulation studies. The Journal of Pediatrics 1983; 102 (1): 32-39.

[27] Glenn WL, Phelps ML, Elefteriades JA, Dentz B, Hogan JF. Twenty years of experience in phrenic nerve stimulation to pace the diaphragm. PACE 1986; 9: 780-784.

[28] Surani S, Afzal A, Elizabeth EE, Varon J. Unilateral diaphragmatic pacing: An innovative solution for unilateral diaphragm paralysis. Critical Care and Shock 2007; 10 (3): 108-110.
[29] Taslimuddin M, Islam S, Islam Q, Islam S. Breathing pacemakers in poliomyelitis- A case report. Indian journal of Physical Med and Rehab 2003; 14: 1-4.
[30] Huttl TP, Wichmann MW, Reichart B, et al. Laparoscopic diaphragmatic placation: Long-term results of a novel surgical technique for postoperative phrenic nerve palsy. Surg Endosc 2004; 18: 547.
[31] Krieger AJ, Gropper MR, Alder RJ. Electrophrenic respiration after intercostals to phrenic anastomosis in a patient with anterior spinal artery syndrome: Technical case report. Neurosurgery 1994; 35 (4): 760-764.
[32] Krieger L, Krieger A. The intercostals to phrenic nerve transfer: An effective means of reanimating the diaphragm in patients with high cervical spine injury. Plastic and reconst surg 2000; 103(4): 1255-1261.
[33] Sarnoff SJ, Sarnoff LC, Whittenberger JL. Electrophrenic respiration. VII. The motor point of the phrenic nerve in relation to external stimulation. Surg Gynecol Obstet 1951; 93: 190.
[34] Haller J, Pickard L, Tepas J, et al. Management of diaphragmatic paralysis in infants with special emphasis on selection of patients for operative placation. J Pediatr Surg 1979; 14: 779.
[35] Ciccolella DE, Dally BD, Celli BR. Improved diaphragmatic function after surgical placation for unilateral diaphragmatic paralysis. Am Rev respire Dis 1992; 146: 797.
[36] Davis JN. Phrenic nerve conduction in man. J Neurol Neurosurg Psychiatry 1967; 88: 969.
[37] MacLean IC, Mattioni TA. Phrenic nerve conduction studies: A new technique and its application in quadriplegic patients. Arch Phys Med Rehabil 1981; 62: 70.
[38] Shaw RK, Glen WW, Hogan JF, Phelps ML. Electrophysiological evaluation of phrenic nerve function in candidates for diaphragm pacing. J Neurosurg 1980; 53: 345.
[39] Versteegh MI, Braun J, Voigt PG, et al. Diaphragm placation in adult patients with diaphragm paralysis leads to long term improvement of pulmonary function and level of dyspnea. Eur J Cardiothorac surg 2007; 32: 449.
[40] Shaul DB, Danielson PD, McComb GJ, Keens TG. Thoracoscopic placement of phrenic nerve electrodes for diaphragmatic pacing in children. J of Pediatric Surg 2002; 37 (7): 974-978.
[41] Sandham J, Shaw D, Guenter C. Acute supine respiratory failure due to bilateral diaphragmatic paralysis. Chest 1977; 72: 96.
[42] Fitzgerald D, Davis MG, Gottesman R, Fecteau A, Guttman F. Diaphragmatic pacemaker failure in congenital central hypoventilation syndrome: A tale of two twiddlers. Pediatric Pulmonology 1996; 22: 319-321.
[43] Weese-Meyers DE, Morrow AS, Brouillette RT, Ilbawi MN, Hunt CE. Diaphragm pacing in infants and children. A life table analysis of implanted components. Am Rev Respir Dis 1989; 139; 974-979.
[44] Gaidula JJ, Barold SS. Diaphragmatic origin of the pacemaker sound. Chest 1972; 61: 195-198.
[45] Massumi RA. An unusual complication of the transvenous pacemaker catheter. Am Heart J 1970; 81: 259-263.
[46] Misra KP, Korn M, Chahramani AR et al. Auscultatory findings in patients with cardiac pacemakers. Ann Intern Med 1971; 74: 245-250.
[47] Surani S, Ayala EE, McMillam M, Sablonte E, Acosta P. Long term recovery of diaphragmatic function in patients with unilateral diaphragmatic pacemaker.

Part 6

Future Technologies

27

Optical Techniques for Future Pacemaker Technology

Yasuaki Kumamoto, Nicholas Isaac Smith, Katsumasa Fujita, Jun Ando and Satoshi Kawata
Osaka University
Japan

1. Introduction

Current muscle pacemaker technology mostly relies on electrical techniques. The electrical method is well understood and established, however, the electricity is difficult to localize and has a risk of interfering with intact cells, tissues, and organisms, affecting their electrophysiology.

Light has the potential to be a novel medium in future pacemaker technology. Light is typically minimally invasive and has low interactivity with biological tissues. Depending on the wavelength, this unique property allows its use to access deep inside biological tissues and opens up potential extension of light and photonics technology to a variety of applications in biosciences, such as in vivo manipulation of biological functions. Combined with nonlinear optical technology, only light technology allows location-selective manipulation deep inside tissues with minimum disturbance to the surrounding areas. Other light properties, such as an inherent sterility and the fact that it does not interfere with measurement instruments, makes the technology attractive.

In this chapter, we describe light-based techniques that may be used for future muscle pacemaker technology. Recently we presented femtosecond laser pacemaker for heart muscle cells through nonlinear light technology. This chapter describes details of light interaction with cells and in particular muscle cells, including experimental and modeling studies. Besides nonlinear light technology, other light-based techniques for manipulating muscle activities are reviewed. These techniques may not be able to pace muscle activities, but are still worth considering since they can change the beat rate. In the latter part, this chapter also includes indirect light-tissue interactions mediated by implanted pacemaker devices, such as rechargeable battery and transcutaneous telemetry systems for both deliverying power to an implanted pacemaker and also for monitoring pacemaker function. The light-driven and light-mediated implanted devices may in the future play an important role in developing implanted pacemaker technology.

Light-based pacemaker technology has just started recently and the interaction effect is partially unclear and needs to be studied more precisely. The light-based technology, however, has significant and perhaps surprising potential for pacemaker technology. In the future, light-based techniques may not only shed light on the future development of pacemaker technology but can also help understandings of basic underlying science in fatal cardiac arrhythmia caused by unexpected local distortion of the beating rhythm, which can also be controlled by light.

2. Overview of light-tissue interactions for pacemaker technology

2.1 Slow acting or non-localized approach to optical pacing

Light typically has low interactivity with biological tissues. Depending on the wavelength, this unique property allows its use to access deep inside biological tissues and opens up potential extension of light and photonics technology to a variety of applications in biosciences, such as in vivo manipulation of biological functions. Additionally, light is inherently sterile, reducing the chance of infectious deseases.

Through the interaction with pigments, such as flavin and cytochrome C (Karu, T, 1999) in the visible spectral range, and aromatic compounds and water in the ultraviolet (UV), light can efficiently manipulate biological tissues. Manipulation based on linear absorption by chromophores is reported for different types of cells. The nerve cell is one of the most frequently studied types of cells regarding light-based manipulation technology and photostimulation of nerve cells by both visible (Fork, 1971) and UV (Oxford & Pooler, 1975; Schwarz and Fox, 1977) light excitation are reported. In these papers, the electrical activity is manipulated by laser exposure. In mast cells, an increase in calcium ion concentration by visible light exposure has been shown (Yang *et al.*, 2007). The calcium ion plays crucial and different roles in many types of cells, and light-based calcium manipulation is then one compelling indicator of the potential for light technology to stimulate and control biological functions.

Regarding the pacing of muscle beating, several studies have been carried out, which are not directly pacemaker technology, but still have potential to modulate the muscle contraction activity. Gimeno *et al.* first reported the acceleration of heart beating rate by exposure to visible light (Gimeno *et al.*, 1967). They simply measured the beat rate of 2-5 day old embryo chick heart cells while changing the illumination intensity (set to high or low) and isolating the irradiation from different wavelength ranges between 450 and 650 nm. The heart beat rate is modified by changing the illumination intensity. Interestingly, this switching seems to be reversible in their report. Salet *et al.* showed an increase in the beating rate of myocardial cells following laser irradiation under the absence of ATP in culture medium (Salet *et al.*, 1979). Alteration of membrane electrical activity in rat myocardial cells as well as changes in the contractility by laser irradiation was also demonstrated (Kitzes *et al.*, 1977). Nathan *et al.* showed that UV (260-310 nm) illumination could also modulate the beat rate of embryo chick heart cells as well as the electrical properties (Nathan *et al.*, 1976). In their measurement, the heart beat rate was increased to a maximum plateu level, up to approximately 200% of the original frequency, followed by fatal cessation, over a one minute time scale. Salet at al. reported a temporary increase in the beating frequency of myocardial cells due to UV (254 nm) micro-irradiation of the cytoplasm, especially mitochondria (Salet *et al.*, 1976), although it should be noted that using UV irradiation does not allow for the precise targeting of particular parts of the cell since photons are linearly absorbed throughout the focused light cone. A recent study also shows that near UV radiation modifies the membrane sodium current in Guinea-pig ventricular myocytes (La *et al.*, 2006).

The issue of these light interactions for pacemaker technology is the use of single photon absorption and usually a corresponding interaction with the whole cell or indeed whole heart, which means that it is difficult to precisely manipulate cells. Additionally, use of

wavelengths with high single-photon interactivity with cells, can lead to unwanted harm, and poor accessibility to deep regions in the tissue is another critical issue to be solved before applying those techniques for future pacemaker technology.
Quite recently, a report used infrared light to affect the beating of an embryonic heart, in vivo (Jenkins *et al.*, 2010). The use of infrared light is a different regime to affect the heart beat while still utilizing a presumably single-photon interaction. While the precise mechanism is not yet clear, the use of infrared light appears to reversibly modify the membrane condition, causing contraction. This approach may provide a path to optical pacing using single-photon interactions, and will no doubt be followed with interest. Although this chapter is focused on optical methods (including different regimes of interactions), there is another method with the potential for remote and sterile pacing of the intact heart.. Lee *et al.* have proposed the use of ultrasound to entrain the intact heart (Lee *et al.*, 2007), and although ultrasound and light have different interactions, if the final result of the interaction is transient heating of ion channels in the cell membrane (Dalecki *et al.*, 2004), the ultrasound and infrared single-photon absorption pacemaking methods may be mediated in the same manner.

2.2 Nonlinear, fast and local approach to optical pacing

Although most of the above-mentioned work using single-photon interactions was not specifically targeted towards pacemakers, it shows the interactions that can be used to modify heart muscle cells or a whole heart. In doing so, we can turn to a different optical interaction which can target specific parts of cells and can be used to trigger biophysical effects in the cells that can be applied to pacemaking. In nonlinear light technology, visible or near infrared (NIR) light can effectively and locally interact with tissues via multiphoton absorption process (Vogel & Venugopalan, 2003). When the photon density is sufficiently high and the resonant molecular absorption energy corresponds to a multiple of photon energy, a number of photons are simultaneously absorbed by single molecule. Tissues contain a large number of UV or near UV absorbing chromophores, such as DNA, proteins, and even water, therefore several photons absorption can occur in the tissues if the incident light has the right wavelength and sufficient intensity. As well as the two-photon absorption, as Vogel *et al.* have shown, more complicated nonlinear absorption processes, such as inverse Bremsstrahlung absorption, leads to avalanche ionization of water and biomolecules (Vogel *et al.*, 2005).
Nonlinear absorption can occur in the tissues by high photon density irradiation. Currently established ultrashort pulse laser technology allows us to easily achieve high photon density conditions. Ultrashort pulses have an almost instantaneous (several hundred femtosecond duration) rise in intensity, followed by a period of no irradiation that is, relatively, much longer at a duration of tens of nanoseconds. This, together with tight focusing by suitable objective lenses results in instantaneous high photon density in a local volume. Because the volume of high photon density is limited to the tightly-focused space, the multiphoton absorption occurs only in the sub-femtolitre volume. When NIR light, which can generally pass through biological tissues, is used, the total modification volume is limited to femtolitre scale (Heisterkamp *et al.*, 2005; Niioka *et al.*, 2008; Shen *et al.*, 2005).
Multiphoton absorption by biological tissues is employed to manipulate biological functions, such as inter-/intra-cellular calcium ion waves (Iwanaga *et al.*, 2006b; Smith *et al.*, 2001), and electrical activities, such as hyperpolarization, depolarization, firing action

potential (Ando *et al.*, 2009; Hirase *et al.*, 2002; Daria *et al.*, 2009), in different types of living cells, including neurons.

These studies used NIR light pulse trains with ~76 or 82 MHz repetition rate, ~100 femtosecond duration, and up to 70 mW in average power. When the cytoplasm is exposed to the tightly focused light for a short time, intracellular calcium ion concentration was increased (Iwanaga *et al.*, 2006b; Smith *et al.*, 2001). Figure 1 shows calcium-indicator fluorescence images of HeLa cells before (a), just after (b), and following (c-f) exposed to an ultrashort pulse trains for 8 ms. The exposure time was controlled by a mechanical shutter. The cells are stained with fluorescent dye, fluo-4/AM, plasma membrane permeable free calcium ion indicator. The fluorescence intensity, indicating relative calcium ion concentration in the cell, increases with time after the irradiation. Similar, but faster, calcium ion activity evoked by femtosecond laser irradiation was reported in nerve cells (Smith *et al.*, 2005) and astrocytes (Zhao *et al.*, 2009)

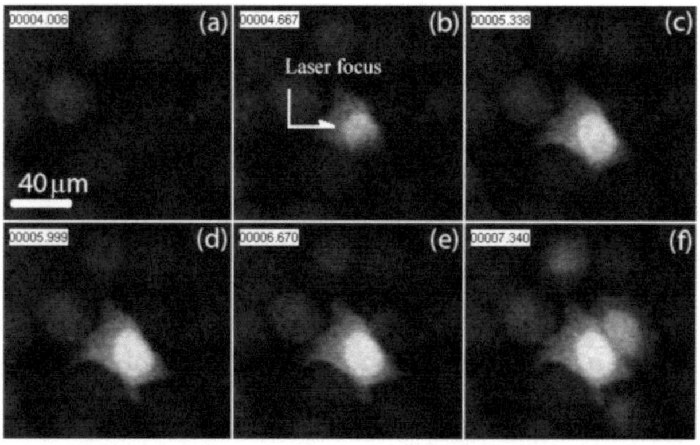

Fig. 1. Calcium indicator fluorescence images of HeLa cells (a) before, (b) just after, and (c-f) over the next two seconds after exposure to 8 ms NIR pulse trains. The time in seconds is noted in each frame. The calcium ion concentration rise is observed in the targeted cell. The laser was focused in the intracellular space outside of the nucleus.

The underlying mechanism of intracellular calcium ion concentration rise was studied (Iwanaga *et al.*, 2005; Iwanaga *et al.*, 2006a). Calcium ion stores such as endoplasmic reticulum (ER) and mitochondria play a central role in the phenomena. They are distributed in the cytoplasm, particularly near the nucleus. In the normal (non-irradiated) situation, the ER plays a role of regulating the intracellular calcium ion concentration by pumping into the ER or by releasing calcium ions via ion channels into the cytoplasm. To rapidly regulate calcium ion dynamics, the so-called calcium-induced calcium release process occurs, where released calcium ions stimulate further calcium release from ER via ligand activation calcium ion channel receptors in the ER. When the cell is irradiated, light can both directly and indirectly interact with ER and mitochondria. Indirect interaction can be mediated by multiphoton absorption, causing generation of reactive oxygen species in a localized area, where they can modify membrane permeability to release calcium ions to the cytosol. This light-induced calcium release provides the initial trigger for calcium-induced calcium release by the ER.

Under the same laser irradiation conditions, Hirase *et al.* and Ando *et al.* observed activation of electrical activities of (excitable) nerve cells (Hirase *et al.*, 2002) and (non-excitable) HeLa cells (Ando *et al.*, 2009). Among these studies, Ando *et al.* studied the relationship between intracellular calcium and electrical behaviors by simultaneously probing calcium ion concentration by fluo-4 and membrane potential by the patch clamp technique. The cell responses to near NIR light exposure are different depending on the irradiation position. When the cytoplasm was exposed to femtosecond light pulses, the membrane was rapidly hyperpolarized and then gradually recovered, consistent with the intracellular calcium ion concentration manner. This is shown in figure 2. The calcium induction by laser irradiation seems to trigger calcium-sensitive potassium ion channels in the plasma membrane, causing the hyperpolarization. When the membrane is irradiated, membrane depolarization (where the membrane potential goes to 0 mV) occurs almost instantaneously, consistent with a very rapid change in permeability (i.e. microablation) of the plasma membrane. However, the depolarization was in some cases followed by unstable repolarization of the membrane potential or in some cases restoration of the membrane potential failed to occur. Regarding the calcium dynamics, when the membrane potential did not recover after irradiation, the calcium concentration also showed incomplete recovery and did not return to pre-irradiation levels. These results indicate that the membrane irradiation can cause a hole in the plasma membrane, which may or may not be recoverable.

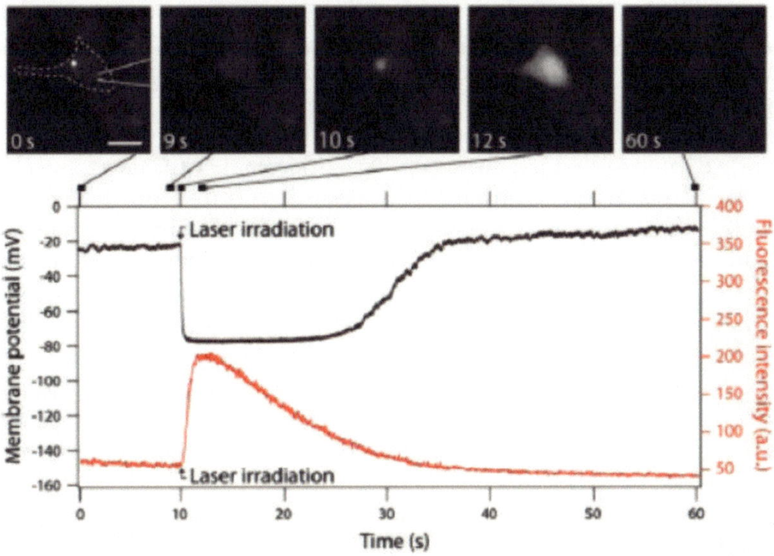

Fig. 2. Calcium indicator fluorescence images of HeLa cells before (a,b), during (c), and after (c-e) exposure to NIR femtosecond pulse trains for 8 ms, and temporal evolution of the intracellular calcium ion concentration and membrane potential of the irradiated cell. The laser was focused in the intracellular space outside of the nucleus. The glass micro-pipette was attached to the membrane of targeted cell in the whole-cell patch configuration. (Reprinted with permission from Ando *et al.*, 2009).

It is important to note the effect of femtosecond laser irradiation on cell viability and photodamage. According to the research described above, very few of the irradiated cells were killed when the laser power is carefully tuned and cytoplasm region was irradiated (Iwanaga *et al.*, 2006b), while high power or membrane irradiation resulted in low viability or abnormal electrical activity. So long as membrane functionality was not collapsed, the multiphoton interaction based manipulation can be used, with high spatial selectivity to control cell dynamics, without necessarily causing damage to the cells, and without any interaction at all with regions outside the focal zone, which is related to the fact that light-tissue interaction is so spatiotemporally limited.

Calcium ion concentration and electrical activity play important roles in the regulation of muscle contraction. Previous work from our group, as well as a report by another group (Koester *et al.*, 1999), indicates that the femtosecond laser light can independently provide sufficient stimulus to perturb and possibly control the contraction dynamics of a cardiomyocyte. By applying multiphoton light technology, we have recently demonstrated a femtosecond laser pacemaker for heart muscle cells. The detail will be described in the following section.

3. Light-based pacemaker of muscle cells through multiphoton interaction

3.1 Laser synchronization in single heart muscle cells

Calcium ions play a central role in muscle contractile activity. Calcium ion binding to troponin protein initiates the contraction of actin myosin filaments. According to the sliding filament theory, the calcium ion concentrations regulate the contractile length. In natural physiological conditions, the cytosolic calcium ion concentrations are regulated through calcium-induced calcium release, initiated by a triggering small increase of cytosolic calcium concentrations via calcium uptake from the outside of the cell. The increased calcium in the cytosol is then reduced via uptake by the sarcoplasmic reticulum (SR) and pumping to the outside of the cell via ion channels and ion pumps.

We have recently demonstrated a femtosecond laser pacemaker for heart muscle cells (Smith *et al.*, 2008). The neonatal rat ventricular muscle cell cultured for 2~4 days were used. Ventricular muscle cells extracted from neonatal rat spontaneously beat because the cells are not perfectly differentiated and separated from pacemaker parts. The spontaneous beating cultured heart muscle cell is periodically exposed (at 1 Hz) to tightly focused femtosecond pulse trains. The laser power was 25 mW. Each exposure duration was 8 ms. We probed the relative cytosolic calcium ion concentration with fluo-4/AM fluorescent dye as well as measuring the contraction itself for some experiments to confirm that the calcium concentration was correlated with the contraction. Figure 3 shows a calcium fluorescence image of the targeted cell and the temporal change in fluorescence intensity averaged

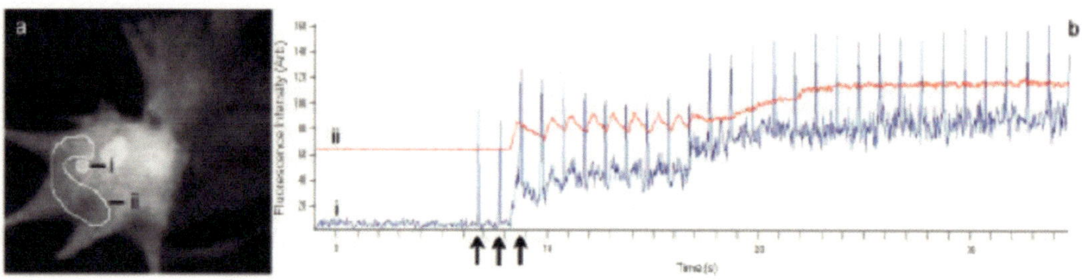

Fig. 3. (a). Heart muscle cell loaded with Fluo-4 calcium indicator. The region 'i' shows the laser focal spot. Region 'ii' encapsulates the surrounding area of the cell. (b) shows fluorescence intensity of region (i) and (ii). The laser is visible as a series of spikes in the fluorescence signal in trace 'i'. The first 3 laser exposures are indicated by vertical allows. (Reprinted from Smith *et al.*, 2008. Copyright Optical Society of America).

through the circled cytoplasmic regions. The fluorescence intensity, representing the relative calcium ion concentration in the cytosol, is synchronized with the laser irradiation following 2 exposures to the laser pulse train. We also succeeded in synchronizing the cell with higher (2 Hz) frequency periodic exposure with the same laser irradiation conditions except for the frequency of laser irradiation.

3.2 Laser synchronization in heart muscle cells group

Cultured heart muscle cells undergo spontaneous contractions that depend on substrate properties (Schweitzer & Seliktar, 2007), proximity of surrounding cells (Kaneko *et al.*, 2007), as well as other conditions (Vetter *et al.*, 1998). Cultured cell samples in our experiments exhibited spontaneous contractions of between 0.2 Hz and 1.5 Hz, depending predominantly on the number and location of surrounding cells.

For target cells with such a pre-existing contraction cycle, periodic laser exposure did not immediately cause the cells to begin contracting with the same periodicity as the irradiation, and the laser pacemaker effect was observed to compete with the spontaneous contraction, where the target cell was entrained by the contraction periodicities of the surrounding cells. In some cases, however, the laser irradiation could be seen to dominate the contraction periodicities of all cells and act as a pacemaker not only for the target cell but also for the surrounding cells. An example of this is shown in figure 4, where a small group of cells contract in phase with each other, at a rate of approximately 0.2 Hz before laser irradiation. Following periodic 1 Hz laser exposures of 8 ms and 20 mW (shown by trace i), the contractions in all cells begin to synchronize with the exposure periodicity (traces ii-v). The synchronization is clear after the 22nd exposure to laser irradiation, and continues until the laser irradiation is ceased. The calcium level then decreases without cell contraction, for approximately 5 seconds after irradiation is ceased, showing that the laser was driving the contraction of all cells. Finally, spontaneous contraction restarts, with a periodicity that is

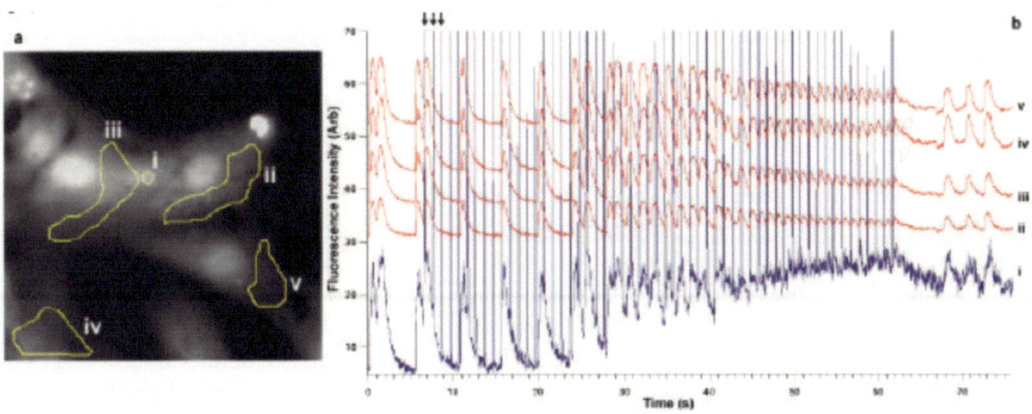

Fig. 4. (a). Heart muscle cells group loaded with Fluo-4 calcium indicator. The group consists of more than 6 cells, spontaneously contracting in synchronization. The region 'i' shows the laser focal spot. Region ii-v encapsulates the cytoplasm area of the target cell and surrounding cells. (b) shows fluorescence intensity of regions i-v. The laser is visible as a series of spikes in the fluorescence signal in trace 'i'. The first 3 laser exposures are indicated by vertical allows. (Reprinted from Smith *et al.*, 2008. Copyright Optical Society of America).

unrelated to the periodicities before, and during irradiation. The fluorescence intensity in all cells decreases over several seconds following the final laser exposure before contraction spontaneously restarts, showing that the cells can respond to laser exposure periodicities that are faster than the spontaneous contraction rates for these samples.

3.3 Mechanism of synchronization

The SR may play a central role in the laser-pacemaker effect as does the ER in the calcium ion waves observed in HeLa cells. SR contains a much larger amount of calcium ions compared with the amount present in the cytosol. If the interaction between laser and calcium is the same for cardiomyocytes as it is for non-excitable cells (such as HeLa cells) then the femtosecond laser irradiation causes SR calcium release and activates calcium-induced calcium release in whole cell. One significant difference between cardiomyocytes and non-excitable cell case is the inward calcium current via plasma membrane calcium ion channels. These calcium ion channels can be activated by membrane potential depolarization. As Ando *et al.* reported, light-induced membrane potential change can occur in non-excitable cells. Presumably it also occurs in a similar manner in excitable cells such as cardiomyocytes, although here it is more difficult to measure the light effect since the membrane potential dynamics are fast and complex in excitable cells. Certainly, such effects do occur in neurons (e.g. Hirase *et al.*, 2002) and in the case of cardiomyocytes the laser effect on membrane potential depolarization may be also play a role in the laser pacemaking effect. In the report by Ando *et al.*, the laser seemed to directly the cell membrane only when the laser focus overlapped the cell membrane. When the laser was focused in the cytoplasm, the membrane potential change seems to result rather from the laser induced change in intracellular calcium, which can itself drastically alter the permeability of the ion channels in the membrane. In short, when the laser was not focused on the cell membrane, the laser had only an indirect effect on the membrane potential.

This implies that the method of synchronization is mediated by calcium release, although we should remember that the direct comparison across cell types is not straightforward, because electrical activity and rates of change in intracellular calcium in muscle cells is more active and dynamic. Regardless, the result showing the synchronization of a group of cells necessarily implies that the cell to cell propagation of the synchronization occurs via action potential generation because laser-induced calcium dynamics of all cells have the same phase. The immediate laser interaction is localized at the laser focus, inside one cell, and the synchronization across groups of cells must then occur via gap-junction or other electrical connection between cells.

Additionally, in contrast to calcium wave generation in non-excitable cells, to evoke the pacemaker effect we need to irradiate a muscle cell repeated times. One single large irradiation could force the cell to raise intracellular calcium and subsequently contract but this method did not provide a means to periodically trigger contraction. Rather, the laser power was reduced and the repeated exposure was observed to entrain the contraction of the target cell as well as neighboring cells.

The accumulation of irradiation may cause a different degree and manner of photodamage. Following irradiation, the minimum level of calcium ion concentration was sometimes observed to increase and the dynamic range of calcium ion concentration during subsequent contraction was reduced. After stopping the laser irradiation, the beating rhythms do not simply return to the conditions before laser manipulation, this may be due to the fact that the dynamic of the entrained system of cells has been shifted to a different but stable regime, or it may be simply due to the fact that the laser has had a (possibly harmful) effect on the cells. What is clear is that when the laser power was raised further, or the irradiation repeated for a sufficiently long time, the calcium ion concentration in the target cell (but not surrounding cells) became high. There are several possible ways that the laser could harm the cell, the SR permeability may be increased, restricting the uptake of calcium ions, the plasma membrane permeability might be affected, or perhaps the ATP-driven pumping mechanisms are temporarily (or permanently) exhausted. In summary, the laser can affect the cell and overdrive the calcium dynamics. Nevertheless, it is predictable that accumulating photodamage can be minimized if exposure conditions are carefully set. Because the laser focus volume is as small as femtolitre or even less, but the optical pacemaker effect can spread over regions as large as several hundred micrometers in diameter, the photodamage issue can be minimized, possibly by scanning the laser over different targets, and allowing some recovery time for each individual focus region. It may then be possible to apply this technology to clinical and medical applications in the future. It is also worth noting that even a damaging interaction is still a new method with which to modify the normal heart system and study the effects of aberrant contractions around the laser focus on the function of the whole heart. This would require the method to be able to entrain or modify the contraction of cells even when the cells were otherwise entrained by a normal electrical signal as is the case in a normally functioning heart. This point will be discussed further below in Section 3.5.

3.4 Statistic analysis of laser power dependency

We statistically studied the laser power dependency of the femtosecond laser pacemaker phenomena.

In total, over 200 laser-heart muscle cell synchronization trials were performed in the experiments reported here with different laser powers and periodicities. The synchronization of the cell contraction periodicity with the laser exposure periodicity occurred in approximately 25% of all trials for average laser powers of between 15 to 30 mW (measured at the sample) at a laser periodicity of 1 Hz. To quantify the relationship, we restricted the definition of synchronization so that around 5 or more consecutive beats were required to follow the laser periodicity in frequency and phase. With this definition of synchronization, we recorded the results shown in figure 5, over a total of 181 cells using 1 Hz irradiation periodicity. The number of cells were counted that exhibited synchronization and also the number that exhibited some calcium response to the irradiation and/or showed indications of synchronization that did not fit our definition of synchronization as given above. The data necessarily includes experiments from different days, which means that there is a degree of variability in the cell culture conditions. This, as well as the difficulty in achieving large amounts of data where only one parameter is changing, probably accounts for the variation in probabilities across adjacent laser powers.

The data shows that the synchronization generally occurs at the onset of an observable response in the heart muscle cells and shows that while synchronization can be repeatedly induced, more work needs to be done to clarify the precise optical and/or biological parameters that govern the interaction of the cell's spontaneous contraction rate and the external periodicity of the laser influence on the cell dynamics. The data are then further divided into two constituent groups: experiments where a single isolated cell was irradiated, and experiments where one cell within a group of 2-14 connected cells was targeted and irradiated. While the data is insufficient to conclude the distinction between isolated cells and those within a group, it does point to an interesting possibility; the cell synchronization of an entire group of 2-14 heart muscle cells may be more probable than the synchronization of a single heart muscle cell. More research will be required to determine if this is the case, and this may have implications for the onset of new and often undesirable contraction periodicities in groups of heart muscle cells.

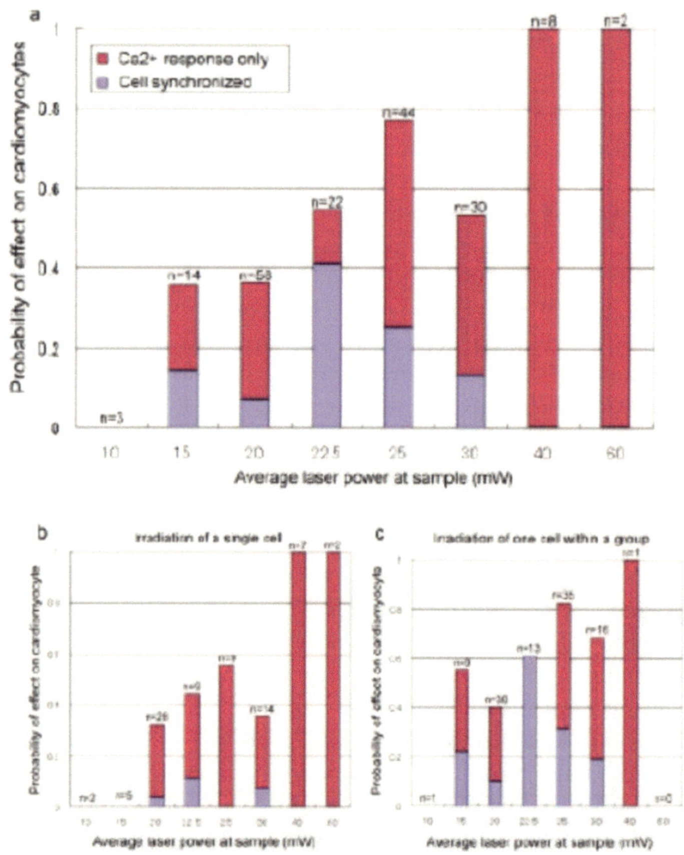

Fig. 5. The probability of generating a synchronized cell response or a calcium response without synchronization. The graph in (a) shows for all data sets of laser irradiation periodicity of 1Hz. In (b), the graph shows the cases where the targeted cell was an isolated heart muscle cell, and (c) shows the cases where the targeted cell was within a group of 2-14 cells. For synchronization to occur in cases shown in (c), all cells in the group were seen to synchronize with the laser periodicity. Conditions necessary to merit the term "synchronization" are described in the main text. (Reprinted from Smith *et al.*, 2008. Copyright Optical Society of America).

3.5 Laser effect on electrically regulated heart muscle cells

When electrical voltage is repeatedly and periodically applied on heart muscle cells, the beating of cells is well-regulated. Optical pacing may become a powerful tool in the study or treatment of a system of electrically regulated cells, tissues, or organs, due to its ability to perturb existing dynamics in a group of cells or whole heart. We confirmed a perturbation of electrically regulated beating rhythm by transient laser irradiation. Figure 6 shows the temporal change in fluorescence intensity, representing calcium dynamics, of electrically regulated heart muscle cells. The short femtosecond pulse trains of 8 ms duration, represented by a red dashed line, evoked calcium ion concentration increase in the irradiated cell. This result demonstrates that optical pacing can also modify the activity of electrically regulated heart muscle cells. The light-based pacemaker effect can then be stronger than the electrical regulation of the heartbeat. In Figure 6, note that the calcium level in subsequent electrically regulated contractions has a lower peak then the contractions prior to the laser irradiation.

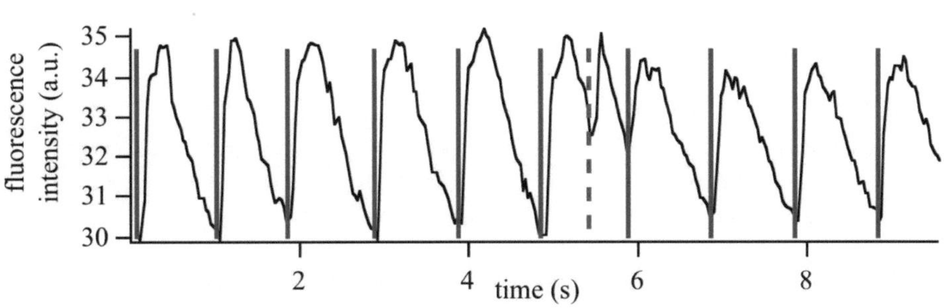

Fig. 6. Fluorescence intensity of an electrically regulated heart muscle cell, which represents the intracellular whole cell calcium concentration. Solid (blue) vertical line shows the timing of electrical stimulation, and dashed (red) line shows the transient laser irradiation, forcing the cell to undergo an abrupt change in contraction dynamics.

3.6 Modeling of the pacemaker effect

In experiments, it is difficult to further study the precise dependence of the optically-controlled activity on the exposure parameters such as the phase and frequency. This is because the spontaneous beating is not perfectly periodic and also because it depends on the individual heart muscle cell conditions, such as rat growth, cell culturing time, and cell density in the dish. Quantifying all of them and their relation to the optical pacing effect requires an extremely large number of experiments using animal-based samples, which is not ideal.

An alternative approach to study the phase and frequency dependency is the use of numerical modeling. We modeled the optically-controlled beating dynamics of heart muscle cells by simultaneous differential equations, based on perturbations to a modified form heart muscle cell model based on the sinoatrial node KYOTO model (Sarai *et al.*, 2003). The KYOTO model represents different type of cells (adult rat sinoatrial node) from the one we used in experiments. The reason we chose this model to be modified for modeling laser pacemaker effect is 1) a model of the neonatal rat heart muscle cell is not available because it is not well understood, and 2) the KYOTO model can similarly represent the calcium activity of our specimen, and can exhibit spontaneous oscillation of calcium ion concentration.

The KYOTO model has 50 ordinary differential rate equations for representing intracellular ion concentrations, ion channels dynamics, membrane potentials, and contractile activity.

Without reproducing the large number of equations in full, it is still worth showing some of the essential equations which are most relevant:

$$\frac{d[Na^+]i}{dt} = \frac{-I_{Na\_efflux} - I_{Na\_influx}}{FV} \tag{1}$$

$$\frac{d[K^+]i}{dt} = \frac{-I_{K\_efflux} - I_{K\_influx}}{FV} \tag{2}$$

$$\frac{d[Ca^{2+}]i}{dt} = \frac{-I_{Ca\_efflux} - I_{Ca\_influx} + I_{RyR} - I_{SR\_uptake} + I_{SR\_leak}}{2FV} + \frac{d[Ca^{2+}{}_{buffer}]_{free}}{dt} \tag{3}$$

$$\frac{dV_m}{dt} = \frac{I_{ext} - I_{ion}}{C_m} \tag{4}$$

In the above equations, $[X]_i$ stands for the cytosolic ion concentration of X ($X=Na^+$, K^+, Ca^{2+}), $[Ca^{2+}{}_{buffer}]_{free}$ for free calcium ion cytosolic concentrations, I_{X_efflux} and I_{X_influx} for inward and outward X currents over plasma membrane, respectively, I_{RyR} for current flows via ryanodine receptors, I_{SR_uptake} for current flow over SR CaATPase, I_{SR_leak} for leak currents via the ryanodine receptor site, V_m for membrane potential, F for the Faraday constant, V for the cell volume, C_m for the plasma membrane capacity, I_{ion} for total membrane ion currents and I_{ext} for the externally applied current.
To model the laser effect, we added a laser term to the calcium ion rate equation:

$$\frac{d[Ca^{2+}]i}{dt} = \frac{-I_{Ca\_efflux} - I_{Ca\_influx} + I_{RyR} - I_{SR\_uptake} + I_{SR\_leak}}{2FV} + \frac{d[Ca^{2+}{}_{buffer}]_{free}}{dt} + \left(\frac{d[Ca^{2+}]}{dt}\right)_{laser} \tag{5}$$

Because the laser effect is localized and must behave differently from any other calcium ion flux, the laser-induced calcium term is added separately to the term containing the other combined calcium related factors.
To simulate the laser effect, we chose a Gaussian function over more typical wave forms such as delta and rectangular functions. Experimentally, the femtosecond laser induces a local increase in the intracellular calcium ions, followed by diffusion of those ions in time through the cell via calcium-induced calcium release manner (Smith *et al.*, 2001). The KYOTO model does not contain any spatial dimensions. Therefore, a Gaussian function to simulate the rise and then diffusion of the calcium ion concentration may be the best approximation of the actual geometry of calcium trigger for the model.
By carefully setting Gaussian function constants, the model could successfully represent the laser-beating synchronization. Here, the definition of synchronization is that the period of calcium dynamics is within 1% of laser periodicity and that the phase is locked by laser irradiation. Figure 7(a) shows a simulated result of intracellular calcium ion concentration. Laser irradiation was periodically performed at time points 1512 and thereafter at multiples of 353xN (where N = 0,1,2,....,20) ms, as shown by red dotted lines. As is seen in figure 7(b), the period of calcium dynamics was entrained by the of laser irradiation periodicity after the eighth laser irradiation. The modeling result shows the calcium ion dynamics after laser irradiation stops.

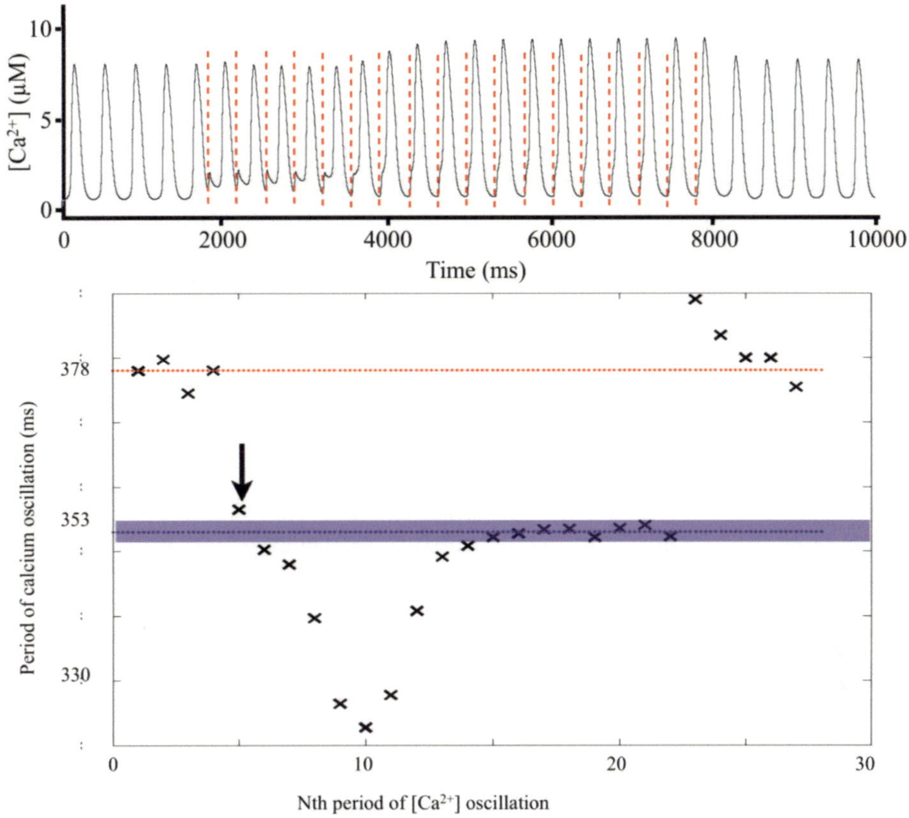

Fig. 7. (a) Simulated intracellular calcium ion concentration modified by 18 periodic exposures to laser irradiation, indicated as dotted vertical lines. (b) shows the evolution of the synchronization, shown as the time interval of the peak in calcium ion concentration. The arrow indicates the period of calcium oscillation just after the first laser irradiation. The blue area in the middle is for the periods of synchronization. After the 11 th irradiation, calcium oscillation is to be synchronized with periodic laser irradiation.

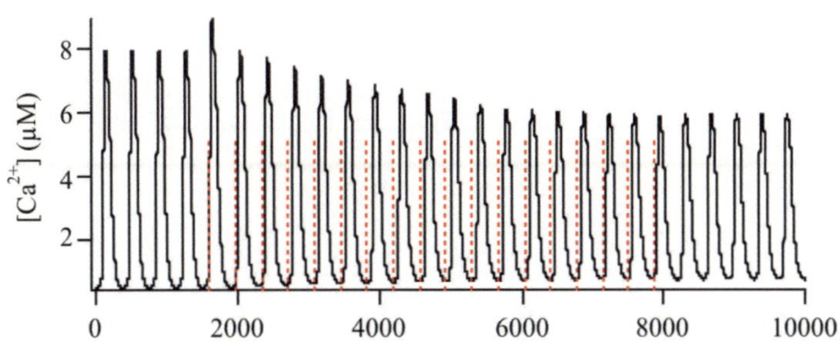

Fig. 8. Intracellular calcium ion concentration model of the heart muscle cell, modified to simulate 18 perioidic exposures to laser irradiation, indicated as dotted vertical lines, when the accumulation effect of SR calcium ion leakage is included in the model.

To better reproduce the empirically observed calcium ion dynamics, we modeled calcium ion leakage from SR, with a slight accumulation effect following repeated exposure, reflecting possible photodamage. The leakage is represented in the model as another accumulating term in the differential equation for calcium ion. Figure 8 shows the calculated temporal change in intracellular calcium ion concentrations. The oscillation range of the calcium ion concentration gradually becomes small with accumulation of calcium leakage amount. After stopping radiation, the level of calcium ion concentration and its dynamics are not observed to recover. This is very similar to our experimental results, indicating that the calcium ion leakage from SR may really accumulate in our experiments using optical pacing. It is also predictable from the model that either repeating exposures further, or increasing the laser power will cause degradation of the cell activities, as was seen in experiments.

3.7 Model study of the frequency and phase dependency

The modeling approach is useful for a quantitative analysis of the phenomena. The femtosecond laser-induced calcium dynamics were simulated, varying the phase and frequency of the periodic irradiation. The phase is determined to be 0 at the time when $[Ca^{2+}]_i$ is a local maximum. The phase is varied between - 140 and 230 ms, and the frequency ranges over between 298 and 428 ms. In this simulation for investigating frequency and phase parameters, the accumulation of SR calcium ion leakage was excluded due to the overbearing complexity when the number of variables is too high.

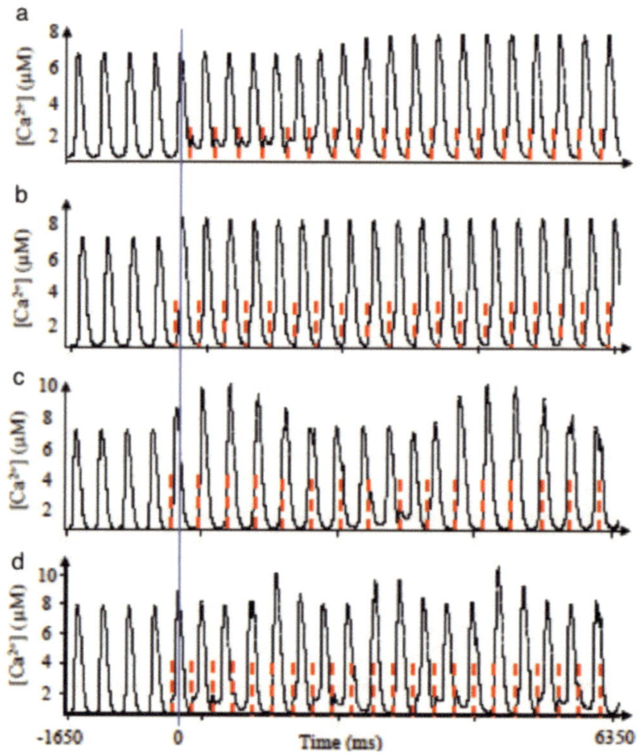

Fig. 9. Simulated intracellular calcium ion concentration modified with modeled periodic laser irradiation, indicated as dotted vertical lines. The dashed vertical line indicates the benchmark of phase of periodic laser irradiation. (a) "delayed synchronization," (b) "complete synchronization," (c) "partial synchronization," and (d) no synchronization.

By simulating the laser-induced calcium dynamics, 4 types of calcium dynamics are obtained. Figure 9 shows 3 types of synchronization (delayed synchronization, complete synchronization, and partial synchronization), as well as the case where no synchronization occured. In delayed synchronization, the synchronization takes time to start. In complete synchronization, increases in cytoplasmic calcium ion required for cell contraction follows all laser irradiation. In partial synchronization, calcium fluctuation partially synchronizes with laser irradiation.

The phase and frequency dependency of the laser pacemaker effect can be visualized in a synchronization map, giving a clue to the dependency on the choice of frequency and starting time for optical pacing experiments While the comparison between the model and experiment is not without complications, the resulting calculated phase and frequency synchronization map do show that there is a strong dependence on both phase and frequency. The strong correlation among the parameters is shown in figure 10.

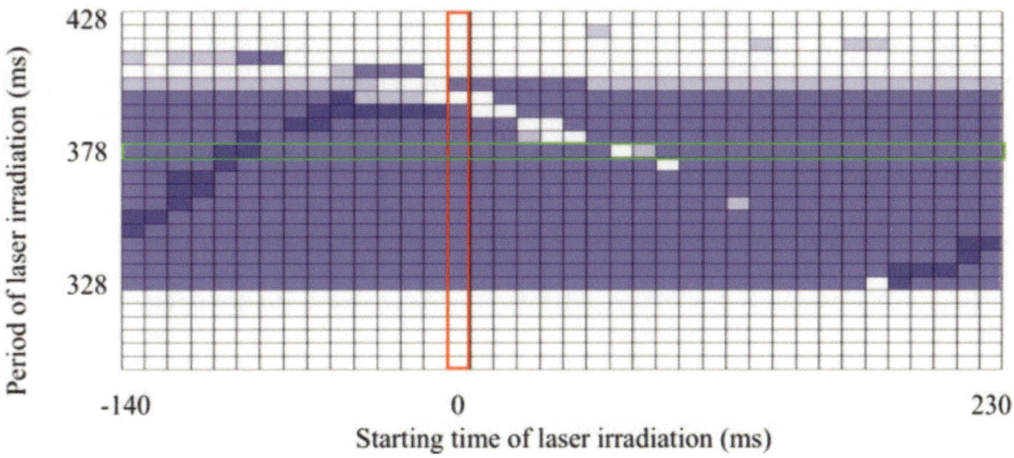

Fig. 10. A map visualizing a relationship between the effect of laser irradiation and both frequency and phase of laser irradiation. The red column outline indicates the baseline for the phase of laser irradiation (0 ms). The green row outline indicates the period of spontaneous calcium oscillation in the model that would occur if there were no laser irradiation. Each color in the map, dark-blue, blue, light-blue, and white, corresponds to 'complete ', 'delayed', and 'partial' synchronization, and no synchronization, that are represented in figure 9. The model shows that even for the choice of laser periodicity which completely matches the spontaneous beat rate, the laser phase should be chosen such that the laser irradiation comes before the peak of the calcium during the contraction process.

In the model, the synchronization only occurs for a restricted range of periodic laser frequency. This was predictable, but it is interesting to quantitatively discuss this result. The region of synchronization spreads from the natural beating frequency. However the distribution of synchronization is different between the upper and lower of natural beating period, the distribution of synchronization in the upper region is less than that in the lower region. This follows from the fact that for longer period laser irradiation, the self-excitation of the cell stimulates the calcium fluctuation before laser irradiation can trigger the cell. The effect is derived from the cardiac refractory stage where action potentials are not generated in order to maintain cellular homeostasis.

The complete synchronization is sensitive to both the phase and frequency, which is related to the refractory stage and the strength of the first laser-induced calcium release. When the first laser irradiation was administered during the cardiac refractory stage, the calcium concentration does not increase sufficiently to cause contraction. Furthermore, when the first laser induced calcium increase causes the intracellular calcium level to rise higher than it does during spontaneous contraction, the refractory stage duration becomes elongated.

Even within the frequency range of synchronization, at some phases, the modeled cell is not synchronized with laser irradiation. When both the period of laser irradiation was close to those of natural calcium oscillation and the starting time of laser irradiation was just after contraction, rhythm of [Ca^{2+}] oscillation did not correspond with rhythm of laser irradiation. These results could be understood from the refractory property of heart muscle cells excitation. However it is interesting that the critical laser irradiation period and starting time are related.

The synchronization map shows interesting interdependencies as well as providing information about which periodicities and starting times are suitable for synchronization. If the simulation times are longer than 10,000 ms, the shape of the map will change. However, since if the goal is synchronization for optical pacing, then the optical parameters of most interest will result in synchronization in less than 10,000 ms so that the current map is already useful. A more serious issue which should be considered is the discrepancy between the spontaneous beat frequency in the model and that observed in typical experiments using cultured cardiomyotyces. Other limitations of the model exist and are discussed below. The current model does not contain spatial dimensions The laser effect must be varied depending on the irradiation position and laser-induced calcium behavior in space is important in the pacemaker effect. Alternative models do exist but we selected the above model for its established performance in at least reproducing known and complex calcium behaviour in cardiomyocytes. The model does not contain parameters regarding surrounding conditions such as substrate type and whether groups of cells or single cells are present, and the type of cell represented in the model is slightly different from the one we used in the experiments.

Nevertheless, the current results already provide information about how to optimize optical pacing. A good starting point suggested from the simulations would be to use the minimum laser power necessary to cause an observable change, to use a frequency slightly higher than the spontaneous beat frequency, and to start the laser irradiation approximately 90 degrees out of phase, and before the calcium concentration peak during spontaneous contraction.

3.8 Perspective for femtosecond laser pacemaker

The laser-induced calcium based technique is unique because of 3-dimensional location-selectivity of the interaction without invasive interactions with surrounding areas. Near infrared light is only marginally absorbed via single photon processes in biological tissues, because there are very few chromophores absorbing NIR light in biological tissues. NIR pulses can only interact with tissues at the tightly focused volume, which is of femtolitre scale, via the multiphoton absorption process. Other orthodox techniques such as electrical, pharmaceutical, and mechanical technique, cannot access deep inside the tissue without interacting with surroundings of a targeted area. While optical technology is not yet ready to replace existing techniques it may develop into a clinical method in the future. In the short-term future it is already well-placed to provide a tool to control and study the contraction of cardiomyocytes.

Recent studies also show femtosecond-laser-induced contraction of smooth muscle cells (Choi *et al.*, 2010) and whole live body (Santos *et al.*, 2010). These researches support the potential of femtosecond-laser-based optical pacing in different types of muscle cells and in vivo and in situ conditions.

The technique is powerful also because exposure duration and phase can be easily and precisely regulated. A simple mechanical shutter can easily select periodicity and phase of the irradiation.

In the future, femtosecond laser-based techniques (as well as optical technologies utilizing single photon interactions mentioned above) should continue to be employed to discover new groundbreaking interactions and to be used for effective and efficient regulation of cell contraction. This indicates the techniques will open the possibility for not only developing pacemaker technology but also understandings of basic underlying science in fatal cardiac arrhythmia caused by unexpected local distortion of the beating rhythm.

4. Light technology for powering and monitoring implanted electrical devices

In the previous sections, we reviewed the light technology for pacemaker development using direct light-tissue interactions, i.e. using light as the pacemaker itself. Light technology can also be used to drive implanted medical devices for muscle pacemaker.

Implanted medical devices have several requirements which can be improved with the use of emerging light technology. One of the most important requirements is continuity of the device. Essentially for a pacemaker device, its sudden breakdown can cause fatal arrhythmia in the patient. Second, radio-frequency waves used for communication with the implanted device are subject to interference by nearby instruments with potentially very serious consequences.Implantable devices are expected to be compact, wireless, and free from causing or receiving electromagnetic disturbances due to radio-frequency waves, which most of today's implanted devices rely on for power supply or signal transmission.

Light technology has the potential to improve these issues. In terms of the robustness of the device, light is readily available, and can be used to wirelessly provide power for implanted devices containing a solar cell. Using near-infrared light, which easily penetrates biological tissues including skin, implanted devices deep inside the tissues can be used without the concern of removing them to recharge or replace batteries. Apart from the advantage of high transmission in biological tissue, the near-infrared light falls into a spectral range in which photoelectric cells such as solar cells exhibit a high light to electrical power conversion rate. In addition, light techniques have little chance to interfere with nearby instruments. Finally, light-based devices are typically compact. This is because they can be constructed from very small photo diodes and employ light-emitting diodes as receiver and transmitter.

As an aid to future implantable pacemakers, near-infrared light driven wireless power supplies have already been developed (Goto *et al.*, 2001a). The implantable device is composed of photodiodes and driven devices, such as a rechargeable battery and an LED as a transmitter. Photodiodes can drive a device as long as the exposure to near-infrared light is sufficient. In demonstrating the implantable power supply system in an adult rat, the light power sufficient to drive implantable devices increased the skin temperature by only around 2 degrees, which is not large enough to cause significant problems for the skin. This result demonstrates that the power supply technology based on a photodiode array can be used for driving an implanted pacemaker device.

By using the wireless power supply technique, two types of prototype devices were demonstrated. One of them is an optically rechargeable battery (Goto *et al.*, 2001a). This device is composed of assembled photodiodes with a rechargeable lithium battery. Lithium batteries are appropriate for implantation due to their compact size (e.g. 25mm in diameter, 3.2mm in thickness) and have sufficiently high voltage (~3V) to driving implanted devices. Figure 11 shows a schematic diagram of the near infrared power supply system. The NIR light emitted from the laser diode is collimated and exposed to the photodiode array embedded under the skin. The photodiode array converts the light energy to electric power and supplies the current to a rechargeable battery, which is connected to an implanted device. If the battery is fully charged it can then be used to drive a typical cardiac pacemaker for 6 months without any recharge. Additionally, more than 6000 charge/discharge cycles can be expected for 0.5 % discharge, which corresponds to operating a 20-μ-A-consuming cardiac pacemaker for 24 h. This means that if the battery is recharged once every day, over 100 years of continuous use of the pacemaker is possible, while the lifetime of conventional pacemaker batteries is within the 5-10 years range. The specifications of battery technology, photodiode efficiency and pacemaker current draw will only improve over time, and optical technology for delivering wireless power to implanted devices is already feasible and should become more attractive in the future.

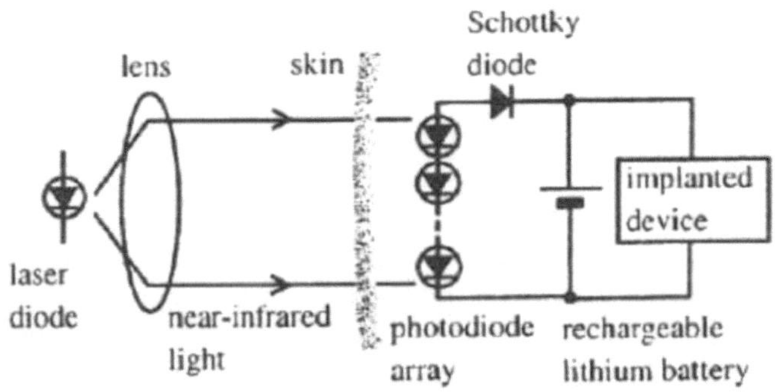

Fig. 11. Schematic diagram of the NIR power supply system. (Reprinted from Goto *et al.*, 2001. Copyright IEEE).

The other device we proposed using the power supply technique is transcutaneous telemetry system (Goto *et al.*, 2001b). The device uses photodiode arrays for directly driving LEDs used to transmit information to a detector outside the body. Figure 12 shows a schematic diagram of the telemetry system. In this system, an intensity-modulated laser diode is used to drive the photodiode arrays. The photodiode array is then to both drive the LED and for sending a carrier wave to the phase modulator. The carrier wave is phase-modulated by a baseband signal, corresponding to the biological signal. The phase-modulated carrier wave modulates the light emitted from the LED, which is received by external photodiode with lock-in-detection. This technology is unique because power supply and signal transmission is done by only light.

In the published report, the transmitter device is not actually compact since the system requires lenses. Our research group has demonstrated a compact transcutaneous photocoupler-like telemetry system for transmission of biological signals such as directly monitoring electromyograms (Goto *et al.*, 2002). In that system, once the LED array is externally driven, the biopotentials can be detected by the receiver. The electronics

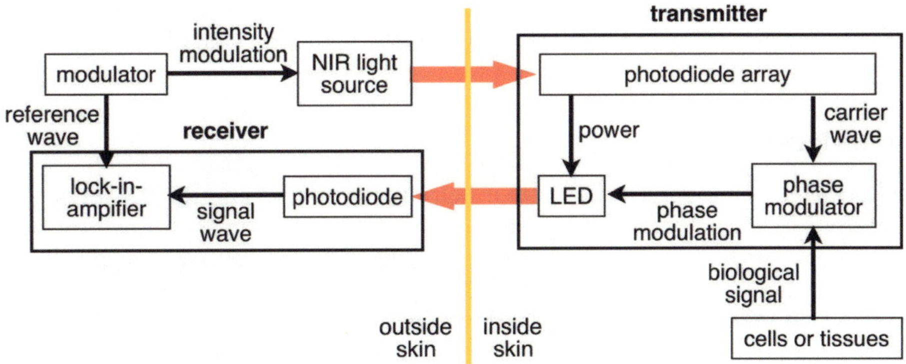

Fig. 12. Block diagram of the all optical telemetry system.

necessary for detecting and amplifying biopotentials can be incorporated into the transmitter. Using this system, biopotentials were obtained from living rats. This compact device is promising for optically recording muscle electrical activities in vivo with safe, wireless, and interference free telemetry.

5. Future perspective

The emerging optical pacemaker technology has the potential to be used as a pacemaker itself, and also to be used to investigate the mechanisms of unwanted arrhythmia and the breakdown of normal contraction conditions. Besides the clinical applications, the light technology can adaptively target new locations inside target tissue, and in the future may possibly even react in real time to counteract the onset of abnormal contraction within the heart. Light-based techniques may not only drive the future development of pacemaker technology but can also help the understanding of the basic underlying science in fatal cardiac arrhythmia caused by unexpected local distortion of the beating rhythm.

This chapter has emphasized femtosecond, localized interactions for studying optical pacing. Other light techniques mentioned in the previous sections based on single-photon light-tissue interactions are not comparable to femtosecond laser irradiations in terms of the speed and localization of the laser-cell interactions and until recently were not advantageous in terms of the invasive nature of using green light which is damaging and non-specifically absorbed throughout the cell. The recent proposal of infrared light-based single-photon optical pacing is also showing promise.

Regardless of the interaction mechanism, the optical pacing results are not only phenomenologically interesting but also attractive for pacemaker technology because of inherent sterility and property of low-interference with other signals or devices. Similarly sterile and interference-free, the use of light for driving and sending a power and telemetry signals to and from implanted-devices has high potential for practical clinical applications. The continuous operation and communication with implantable devices is already achievable.

Most experiments discussed in this chapter have used laser light. The use of LED light or low threshold laser diodes could replace the laser irradiation. As we have shown, implanted LEDs may themselves be driven by externally applied optical irradiation. By combining these concepts with already fully-developed technology, we can conceive of an optically powered, optical pacemaker, running on power by external light or sunlight, driving the power source for LEDs or tiny laser diodes which generate the pacemaking effect in the heart. These developments in light-based pacemaker technology should drive innovation in general pacemaker technology.

6. Acknowledgment

The authors sincerely thank Dr K. Goto for helpful discussions and for his previous work in our laboratory. We also thank Prof. T. Takamatsu and Dr. H. Tanaka for helpful advice and discussion on cardiology as well as for technical advice in electrophysiological measurement, Dr S. Iwanaga and Mr T. Uchiyama for help with the patch-clamp experimental setup. Finally, we thank Dr. H. Niioka for useful discussion and Ms. L. Gravitz for bringing the work with ultrasound pacemakers to our attention.

7. References

Ando, J; Smith, N, I; Fujita, K & Kawata, S. (2009). Photogeneration of membrane potential hyperpolarization and depolarization in non-excitable cells. *European Biophysics Journal*, 38, 2, 255-262, 0175-7571

Choi, M; Yoon, J & Choi, C. (2010). Label-free optical control of arterial contraction. *Journal of Biomedical Optics*, 15, 1, 015006, 1083-3668.

Dalecki, D. (2004) Mechanical bioeffects of ultrasound. *Annual Review of Biomedical Engineering*, 6, 229-248.

Daria, V,R; Stricker, C; Bowman, R; Redman, S; & Bachor, H,-A. (2009). Arbitrary multisite two-photon excitation in four dimensions. *Applied Physics Letters*, 95 (9), 093701.

Fork, R, L. (1971). Laser stimulation of nerve cells in aplysia. *Science*, 171, 3974, 907-908, 0036-8075

Gimeno, M, A; Roberts, C, M & Webb, J, L. (1967). Acceleration of rate of early chick embryo heart by visible light. *Nature*, 214, 3, 1014-1016, 0028-0836

Goto, K; Nakagawa, T; Nakamura, O & Kawata, S. (2001a). An implantable power supply with an optically rechargeable lithium battery. *IEEE Transactions on Biomedical Engineering*, 48, 7, 830-833, 0018-9294

Goto, K; Nakagawa, T; Nakamura, O & Kawata, S. (2001b). Near-infrared light transcutaneous telemetry system having an implantable transmitter driven by external laser irradiation. *Review of Scientific instruments*, 72, 7, 3079-3085, 0034-6748

Goto, K; Nakagawa, T; Nakamura, O & Kawata, S. (2002). Transcutaneous photocoupler for transmission of biological signals. *Optics Letters*, 27, 20, 1797-1799, 0146-9592

Heisterkamp, A; Maxwell, I, Z; Mazur, E; Underwood, J, M; Nickerson, J, A; Kumar, S & Ingber, D, E. (2005). Pulse energy dependence of subcellular dissection by femtosecond laser pulses. *Optics Express*, 13, 10, 3690-3696, 1094-4087

Hirase, H; Nikolenko, V; Goldberg, J, H & Yuste, R. (2002). Multiphoton stimulation of neurons. *Journal of Neurobiology*, 51,3, 237-247, 0022-3034

Iwanaga, S; Smith, N, I; Fujita, K & Kawata, S. (2006a). Slow Ca^{2+} wave stimulation using low repetition rate femtosecond pulsed irradiation. *Optics Express*, 14, 2, 717-725, 1094-4087

Iwanaga, S; Kaneko, T; Fujita, K; Smith, N; Nakamura, O; Takamatsu, T & Kawata, S. (2006b). Location dependent photogeneration of calcium waves in HeLa cells. *Cell Biochemistry and Biophysics*, 45, 2, 167-176. 1085-9195

Jenkins, M, W; Duke, A, R; Gu, S; Doughman, Y; Chiel, H, J; Fujioka, H; Watanabe, M; Jansen, E, D & Rollins, A, M. (2010). Optical pacing of the embryonic heart. *Nature Photonics*, in press, DOI: 10.1038/NPHOTON.2010.166

Kaneko, T; Kojima, K & Yasuda, K. (2007). Dependence of the community effect of cultured cardiomyocytes on the cell network pattern. *Biochemical and Biophysical Research Communications*, 356, 2, 494-498, 0006-291X

Karu, T. (1999). Primary and secondary mechanisms of action of visible to near-IR radiation on cells. *Journal of Photochemistry and Photobiology B: Biology*, 49, 1, 1-17, 1011-1344

Kitzes, M; Twiggs, G & Berns, M, W. (1977). Alteration of membrane electrical activity in rat myocardial cells following selective laser microbeam irradiation. *Journal of Cellular Physiology*, 93, 1, 99-104, 0021-9541

Koester, H, J; Baur, D; Uhl, R & Hell, S, W. (1999). Ca^{2+} fluorescence imaging with pico- and femtosecond two-photon excitation; signal and photodamage. *Biophysical Journal*, 77, 4, 2226-2236, 0006-3495

La, C; You, P; Zhabyeyev, P; Pelzer, D, J & McDonald, T, F. (2006). Ultraviolet photoalteration of late Na^+ current in guinea-pig ventricular myocytes. *Journal of Membrane Biology*, 210, 1, 43-50, 0022-2631

Lee, K,L; Lau, C,-P; Tse, H,-F; Echt, D,S; Heaven, D; Smith, W; Hood, M. (2007). First Human Demonstration of Cardiac Stimulation With Transcutaneous Ultrasound Energy Delivery. Implications for Wireless Pacing With Implantable Devices. *Journal of the American College of Cardiology*, 50 (9), 877-883

Nathan, R, D; Pooler, J, P; DeHaan, R, L. (1976). Ultraviolet-Induced Alterations of Beat Rate and Electrical Properties of Embryonic Chick Heart Cell Aggregates. *The Journal of General Physiology*, 67, 1, 27-44, 0022-1295

Niioka, H; Smith, N. I; Fujita, K; Inouye, Y & Kawata, S. (2008). Femtosecond laser nano-ablation in fixed and non-fixed cultured cells. *Optics Express*, 16, 19, 14447-14495, 1546-2048

Oxford, G, S & Pooler, J, P. (1975). Ultraviolet Photoalteration of ion channels in voltage-clamped lobster giant axons. *Journal of Membrane Biology*, 20, 1,13-30, 0022-2631

Salet, C; Moreno, G & Vinzens, F. (1976). A study of beating frequency of a single myocardial cell II. Ultraviolet micro-irradiation of the nucleus and of the cytoplasm. *Experimental Cell Research*,100, 2, 365-373, 0014-4827

Salet, C; Moreno, G & Vinzens, F. (1979). A study of beating frequency of a single myocardial cell : III. Laser micro-irradiation of mitochondria in the presence of KCN or ATP. *Experimental Cell Research*,120, 1, 25-29, 0014-4827

Santos, S, I, C; Mathew, M & Alvarez, P, L-. (2010). Real time imaging of femtosecond laser induced nano-neurosurgery dynamics in C. elegans. *Optics Express*, 18, 1, 364-377, 1094-4087

Sarai, N; Matsuoka, S; Kuratomi, S; Ono, K & Noma, A. (2003). Role of individual ionic current systems in the SA node hypothesized by a model study. *The Japanese Journal of Physiology*, 53, 2, 125-134, 0021-521X

Schwarz, W & Fox, J, M. (1977). Ultraviolet-induced alterations of the sodium inactivation in myelinated nerve fibers. *Journal of Membrane Biology*, 36, 1, 297-310, 0022-2631

Schweitzer, K, S-. & Seliktar, D. (2007). Matrix stiffness affects spontaneous contraction of cardiomyocytes cultured within a PEGylated fibrinogen biomaterial. *Acta Biomaterialia*, 3, 1, 33-41, 1742-7061

Shen, N; Datta, D; Schaffer, C, B; LeDuc, P; Ingber, D, E & Mazur, E. (2005). Ablation of cytoskeletal filaments and mitochondria in live cells using a femtosecond laser nanoscissor. *Mechanics and Chemistry of Biosystems*, 2, 1, 17-25, 1546-2048

Smith, N, I; Fujita, K; Kaneko, T; Katoh, K; Nakamura, O & Kawata, S. (2001). Generation of calcium waves in living cells by pulsed-laser-induced photodisruption. *Applied Physics Letters*, 79, 8, 1208-1210, 0003-6951

Smith, N, I; Iwanaga, S; Beppu, T; Fujita, K; Nakamura, O & Kawata, S. (2005). Photostimulation of two types of Ca^{2+} waves in rat pheochromocytoma PC12 cells by ultrashort pulsed near-infrared laser irradiation. *Laser Physics Letters*, 3, 3, 154-161, 1612-2011

Smith, N. I; Kumamoto, Y; Iwanaga, S; ando, J; Fujita, K & Kawata, S. (2008). A femtosecond laser pacemaker for heart muscle cells. *Optics Express*, 16, 12, 8604-8616, 1094-4087

Vetter, R; Monika, K; Wolfgang, S & Rupp, H. Influence of different culture conditions on sarcoplasmic reticular calcium transport in isolated neonatal rat cardiomyocytes. *Molecular and Cellular Biochemistry*, 188, 1-2, 177-185, 0300-8177

Vogel, A & Venugopalan, V. (2003). Mechanisms of Pulsed Laser Ablation of Biological Tissues. *Chemical Reviews*, 103, 2, 577-644, 0009-2665

Vogel, A; Noack, J; Huettman, G & Paltauf, G. (2005). Mechanisms of femtosecond laser nanosurgery of cells and tissues. *Applied Physics B*, 81, 8, 1015-1047, 0946-2171

Yang, W, Z; Chen, J, Y; Yu, J, T & Zhou, L, W. (2007). Effects of Low Power Laser Irradiation on Intracellular Calcium and Histamine Release in RBL-2H3 Mast Cells. *Photochemistry and Photobiology*, 83, 4, 979-984, 0031-8655

Zhao, Y., Zhang, Y., Liu, X., Lv, X., Zhou, W., Luo, Q., Zeng, S. (2009). Photostimulation of astrocytes with femtosecond laser pulses. Optics Express, 17 (3), pp. 1291-1298.

28

Creation of a Biopacemaker: Lessons from the Sinoatrial Node

A. Dénise den Haan, Arie O. Verkerk and Hanno L. Tan
Heart Failure Research Center, University of Amsterdam, Amsterdam
The Netherlands

1. Introduction

The sinoatrial (SA) node is the normal pacemaker of the mammalian heart and generates the electrical impulse for the regular, rhythmic contraction of the heart. SA node dysfunction and high-grade atrioventricular block may lead to failing impulse generation or propagation towards the ventricles. The resulting bradycardia may be life-threatening and is currently treated with implantation of an electronic pacemaker. Shortcomings of this technique include limited autonomic responsiveness, suboptimal cardiac activation pathways, limited battery life, magnetic interference, and risk of infections. In order to avoid these drawbacks research has focused on the development of genetically engineered biological pacemakers (biopacemakers).

To date, various approaches have been used to create biopacemakers. However, the biopacemaker in its current state is not applicable in humans. Before biopacemakers may find their way to the bedside, various issues need to be resolved for long-term function, including the ratio between upregulated inward currents and downregulated outward currents, the optimal site in the heart for genetic modification or implantation, optimal cell mass, and optimal electrical coupling to surrounding tissues.

A logical approach to improve the biopacemaker would be to implement our knowledge about the way in which the physiological pacemaker, the SA node, functions. In this chapter, we focus on function, structure, and regulation of the SA node in relation to the creation of a biopacemaker.

2. Ionic currents in the SA node

The action potential of SA nodal myocytes differs from that found in atrial or ventricular cells. Firstly, there is a slow diastolic depolarization (phase 4 depolarization), where cells depolarize spontaneously towards the action potential threshold. Secondly, the action potential upstroke (phase 0) is slow compared to the upstroke in atrial and ventricular myocytes. Thirdly, SA node cells have a less negative maximal diastolic potential (MDP).

The SA node action potential is a result of a complex interaction of multiple inwardly and outwardly directed ion currents, which are summarized in Figure 1 (for reviews see Boyett et al., 2000; Dobrzynski et al., 2007; Irisawa et al., 1993; Mangoni & Nargeot, 2008).

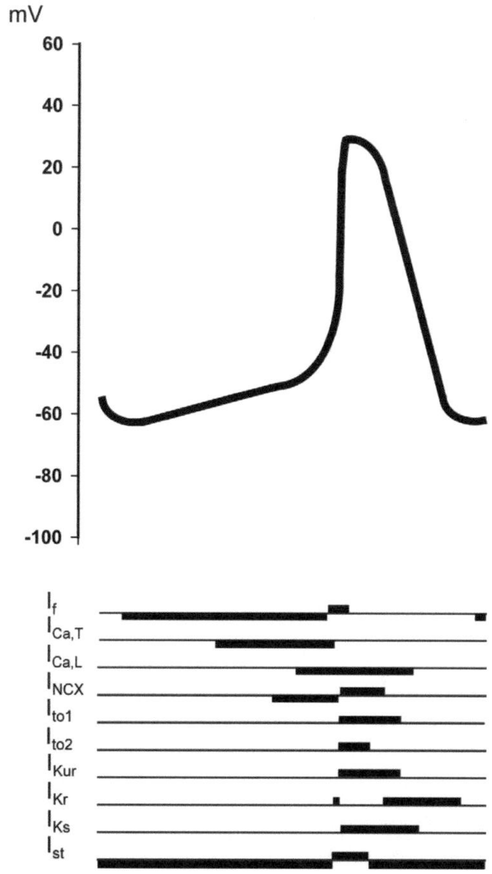

Downward bars indicate inward currents, upward bars outward currents. I_f = hyperpolarisation-activated current; $I_{Ca,T}$ = transient type Ca^{2+} current; $I_{Ca,L}$ = long lasting Ca^{2+} current; I_{NCX} = Na^+-Ca^{2+} exchange current; I_{to1} = transient outward current type 1; I_{to2} = transient outward current type 2; I_{Kur} = ultra-rapid component of the delayed rectifier current; I_{Kr} = rapid component of the delayed rectifier current; I_{Ks} = slow component of the delayed rectifier current; I_{st} = sustained inward current.

Fig. 1. SA node myocytes action potential and ionic currents.

2.1 Hyperpolarization-activated current (funny current, I_f)

Before the discovery of the hyperpolarization-activated current, the diastolic depolarization was thought to result from the decay of an outward K^+ current (Noble & Tsien, 1968). However, in 1979 this decaying outward current was shown to be an inward current activated upon hyperpolarization (Brown et al., 1979). Figure 2A, left panel, shows a typical example of the hyperpolarization-activated current in a rabbit SA node cell. Due to its activation upon hyperpolarization and mixed permeability to Na^+ and K^+, this current was named the funny current (I_f). The voltage-gated ion channels responsible for I_f are encoded by four gene isoforms: *HCN1* through *HCN4* (Ludwig et al., 1998; Stieber et al., 2004). All of these are found in the heart, with *HCN4* mRNA being most prevalent in human (Chandler et al., 2009) and rabbit SA node (Brioschi et al., 2009; Chandler et al., 2009). The physiological relevance of there being multiple isoforms may lie in their distinct kinetics and their different responsiveness to autonomic stimulation, with half-maximal activation voltages being more negative for *HCN4* than for *HCN2*, and *HCN4* having a larger increase in rate of activation in the presence of cAMP (Verkerk et al., 2009a). However, none of these isoforms seem to be capable of forming homomers that have properties corresponding to those of native I_f in rabbit SA node cells (Altomare et al., 2003) or (neonatal) rat ventricular cells (Qu et al., 2002; Qu et al., 2001). This led to the hypothesis that different isoforms could form heteromers with intermediate characteristics. By both expressing *HCN1* and *HCN2* in equal amounts, and by expressing a concatenated *HCN1-HCN2* construct, Ulens and Tytgat provided evidence that these subunits could spontaneously form heteromeric subunits (Jackson et al., 2007; Ulens & Tytgat, 2001).

In human SA node cells, I_f activates at potentials negative to –50 mV, with a reversal potential of -22.1±2.4 mV, due to its mixed permeability to both Na^+ and K^+ (Verkerk et al., 2007a). In rabbit SA node cells, I_f was found to reverse around -24 mV with a half-maximal activation at -76.1 mV (van Ginneken & Giles, 1991). Figure 2A, right panel, shows the average current-voltage (I-V) relationship of I_f in rabbit SA node cells during hyperpolarization (I_{step}) and upon stepping back to the holding potential of –40 mV (I_{tail}). I_{tail} is used to analyze the voltage dependency of current activation. The speed of activation and the voltage dependency of activation of HCN channels is influenced by a variety of factors (for review see Verkerk et al., 2009a), including both sympathetic and parasympathetic stimulation (Baruscotti et al., 2005). Direct interaction of cAMP with the cyclic nucleotide binding domain of HCN shifts the voltage dependence of activation towards more depolarized potentials (Wainger et al., 2001) and speeds up current activation. Furthermore, increased phosphorylation can cause an increase in I_f by increasing maximal conductance in a voltage independent way, and by increasing sensitivity to β-adrenergic stimulation (Accili et al., 1997).

Qu et al. showed that the kinetics of I_f are also context dependent with a less negative threshold of activation for *HCN2* and *HCN4* in neonatal ventricular myocytes than in HEK 293 cells (Qu et al., 2002). Factors possibly regulating I_f are auxiliary subunits (Decher et al., 2003) and cellular characteristics (Barbuti et al., 2004).

Properties that make I_f a likely current to be responsible for automaticity include the initiation of an inward current during diastolic, hyperpolarized potentials, its sensitivity to autonomous modulation, and its presence in pacemaking cells. However, due to other properties the role of I_f in cardiac automaticity remains a matter of debate (see Verkerk et al., 2009a and primary refs cited therein). The continuing debate on the physiological significance of I_f in SA node pacemaking is strongly related to the intrinsically slow activation kinetics and negative activation profile of I_f relative to the time scale and the voltage range of diastolic depolarization in the SA node. Other arguments are the fact that even though blocking I_f with drugs decreases beating rate, it does not completely block spontaneous activity, and that conditional *HCN4* knock out mice still show sinus rhythm (for review see Lakatta & DiFrancesco, 2009).

2.2 Ca^{2+} currents

2.2.1 T-type Ca^{2+} current ($I_{Ca,T}$)

So far, three different genes have been found that encode transient type (T-type) Ca^{2+} channels: $Ca_v3.1$ through $Ca_v3.3$, encoded by *CACNA1G* through *CACNA1I* (Perez-Reyes, 1999). Both $Ca_v3.1$ and $Ca_v3.3$ mRNA were found in the human SA node, with $Ca_v3.1$

mRNA and protein being more prevalent in the SA node than right atrium (Chandler et al., 2009). However, in murine SA node, no $Ca_v3.3$ mRNA has been identified, while $Ca_v3.2$ is present (Bohn et al., 2000; Marionneau et al., 2005).

When first characterized in rabbit SA node, T-type Ca^{2+} current ($I_{Ca,T}$) was found to activate at -47±2.4 mV with a voltage of half maximal activation at -23 mV (Hagiwara et al., 1988). Figure 2B shows a typical example and I-V relationship of $I_{Ca,T}$ in rabbit SA node cells. However, overexpression of different subtypes of Cav3.x in HEK293 cells showed a more hyperpolarized activation threshold and more hyperpolarized half maximal activation values. Activation thresholds were found to be -70 mV for $Ca_v3.1$, -55 mV for $Ca_v3.2$, and -80 mV for $Ca_v3.3$, with voltages of half maximal activation of -51.73, -43.15, and -60.7 mV respectively (McRory et al., 2001).

While, at first, $I_{Ca,T}$ was thought to be insensitive to neuromediators, several neuromediators, including norepinephrine and phenylephrine, were found to influence $I_{Ca,T}$ (Vassort & Alvarez, 1994). These effects have been found in different cell types, while the only mediator investigated in SA node, isoproterenol, did not show any effect (Hagiwara et al., 1988).

Bean was the first to hypothesize about the role of $I_{Ca,T}$ in automaticity, suggesting that fast Ca^{2+} channels would be useful in cells capable of generating spontaneous activity, since they will be activated at negative potentials and will help depolarize the cells, while the Na^+ channels are inactivated due to their more hyperpolarized inactivation curve (Bean, 1985). Indeed, blocking $I_{Ca,T}$ with 40 μM Ni^{2+} was shown to have a negative chronotropic effect on rabbit SA node cells by slowing the late phase of the diastolic depolarization (Hagiwara et al., 1988). When blocking $I_{Ca,T}$ specifically with R-efonidipine, this finding could not be reproduced completely, as this led to a clear increase in cycle length in mice, but not in rabbit (Tanaka et al., 2008).

The role of $I_{Ca,T}$ in murine SA node automaticity was confirmed in vivo by a slowing of mean heart rate in $Ca_v3.1^{-/-}$ mice, associated with a decrease in $I_{Ca,T}$. Patch clamp experiments of SA node cells of these mice showed a decrease in $I_{Ca,T}$, 37% slowing in cellular beating rate, and a decrease in depolarization slope of 44% (Mangoni et al., 2006). Since $Ca_v3.2$ was shown not to activate at voltages negative to -55 mV, with a voltage of half maximal activation of -43.15 (McRory et al., 2001), a considerable role in diastolic depolarization is not to be expected. Knock-out of $Ca_v3.2$, as predicted, had no significant effect on heart rate (Chen et al., 2003). This is also in agreement with SA node gene expression studies that show a higher level of $Ca_v3.1$ mRNA in SA node than other regions of the heart, but no difference in level of $Ca_v3.2$ mRNA (Chandler et al., 2009; Marionneau et al., 2005).

2.2.2 L-type Ca^{2+}current ($I_{Ca,L}$)

The cardiac long lasting type (L-type) Ca^{2+} channel consists of different subunits: α1-, β-, and α2-δ (Benitah et al., 2010). The α1-subunit forms the ion pore, and is selective for Ca^{2+} due to a high affinity binding site for Ca^{2+} within the pore (Yang et al., 1993). Different genes encode for different isoforms of the α1-subunit, with Cav1.2 (*CACNA1C*) and Cav1.3 (*CACNA1D*) mRNA being present in the human SA node. While Cav1.2 mRNA is more prevalent in atrial and nodal tissue, Cav1.3 is the only subtype more prevalent in SA node tissue than in atrial tissue (Chandler et al., 2009; Marionneau et al., 2005). When overexpressed in combination with a β-subunit, Cav1.3 channels were shown to activate at more hyperpolarized membrane potentials (-55 mV versus -35 mV), and were less sensitive to dihydropyridines than Cav1.2 channels (Xu & Lipscombe, 2001).

Of the different β-subunits identified, Gao and coworkers only detected the β2-subunit in rabbit myocytes by immunoblotting (Gao et al., 1997). However, in human and canine ventricular tissue, Foell and colleagues demonstrated the presence of 18 different mRNA splice forms of all 4 β-subunit families (Foell et al., 2004). In human SA node, mRNA of the β2-, and, to a lesser extent, β1- and β3-subunits was found (Chandler et al., 2009). The function of β-subunits has partly been elucidated. Firstly, these subunits alter channel kinetics and voltage dependence (Benitah et al., 2010). Secondly β-subunits can bind to the part of the α1-subunit which is involved in retention to the endoplasmic reticulum, thereby relieving the inhibition of trafficking and thus causing increased channel incorporation into the cell membrane (Bichet et al., 2000). Furthermore, it was shown that an increase in cAMP is associated with an increase in phosphorylation of the β-subunit, while there is no change in phosphorylation of the α1-subunit. This implies that autonomic control of the L-type Ca2+ channel is regulated via the β-subunit (Haase et al., 1993). By overexpressing β1b, β2a, β3, and β4-subunits in adult rat ventricular myocytes, Colecraft and colleagues showed that different β-subunits have different functions. Overexpression of β2a and β4-subunits caused the biggest increase in current density and largest decrease in rate of inactivation. Cells overexpressing β2a showed predominant subunit localization to the cell membrane, while overexpression of β4-subnits showed staining of transverse elements and the nucleus (Colecraft et al., 2002).

The α_2-δ-subunit is a transmembrane subunit composed of 2 subunits encoded by the same gene, connected to each other by a disulfide bond (De Jongh et al., 1990). Singer and colleagues investigated the effect of the α_2-δ-subunit on the L-type Ca^{2+} current ($I_{Ca,L}$) by overexpression of different combinations of subunits in Xenopus oocytes (Singer et al., 1991). Addition of the α_2-δ subunit to the α_1-subunit resulted in an increase in current amplitude, sensitivity to the dihydropyridine agonist Bay K 8644, voltage sensitivity of inactivation, and faster activation.

The upstroke of the action potential in SA node cells depends on $I_{Ca,L}$. Figure 2B shows a typical example of $I_{Ca,L}$ in rabbit SA node cells. Since one of the characteristics that distinguishes L-type Ca^{2+} channels from T-type Ca^{2+} channels is their opening at relatively depolarized potentials (Fig. 2B, right panel), their role in diastolic depolarization was long considered to be negligible. However, $Ca_v1.3$ opens at more hyperpolarized potentials than other isoforms (Xu & Lipscombe, 2001; Xue et al., 2002), and thus could play a more substantial role in automaticity. The difficulty in studying the importance of $I_{Ca,L}$ in diastolic depolarization lies in the fact that depolarization of SA node cells depends on this current, instead of the Na^+ current, and thus inhibition of $I_{Ca,L}$ will invariably influence automaticity. Verheijck and colleagues avoided this problem by applying a depolarizing pulse to rabbit SA node cells that had lost spontaneous activity due to 5 μM nifedipine, to a degree that subsequent repolarization and diastolic depolarization resembled those during spontaneous activity (Verheijck et al., 1999). This way, they showed that depolarization from a holding potential of -90 to -60 mV could already activate $I_{Ca,L}$. Consequently this current could serve as an inward current during the entire diastolic depolarization. These findings were later confirmed in $Ca_v1.3$ knock out mice (Mangoni et al., 2003; Zhang et al., 2002b).

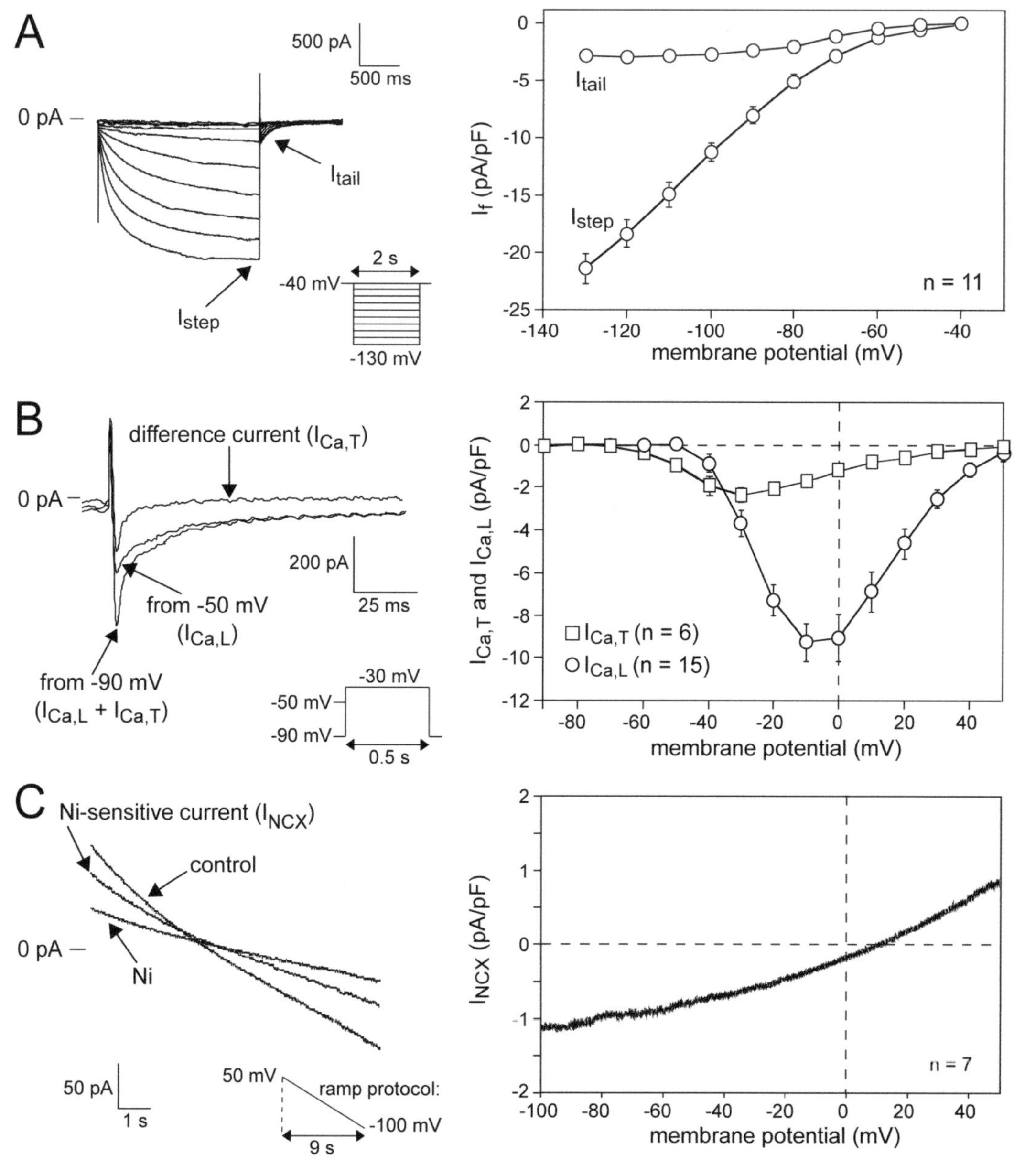

A, Typical examples (left) and average current-voltage (I-V) relation (right) of I_f. Inset, Voltage clamp protocol used. B, Typical examples (left) and average I-V (right) relation of $I_{Ca,T}$ and $I_{Ca,L}$. Inset, Voltage clamp protocol used. Please note that current traces were elicited by depolarizing voltage steps from -90 for combined measurements of $I_{Ca,L}$ and $I_{Ca,T}$ and -50 mV for measurements of only $I_{Ca,L}$. $I_{Ca,T}$, if present, was obtained as the difference current. C, Typical example (left) and average I-V relationship (right) of I_{NCX}. Inset, Voltage clamp protocol used. I_{NCX} was measured as Ni-sensitive current during a descending voltage clamp ramps. For cell isolations and experimental details, see Verkerk et al., 2003.

Fig. 2. Inward currents in rabbit SA node cells.

2.2.3 Ca^{2+} release activated Na^{+}-Ca^{2+} exchange current (I_{NCX})

In recent years, low-voltage activated Ca^{2+} releases (LVCRs) from the sarcoplasmic reticulum have attracted a lot of attention (for review see Lakatta et al., 2010). This Ca^{2+} release could increase the subsarcolemmal Ca^{2+} concentration, thereby activate the Na^{+}-Ca^{2+} exchanger (NCX) and thus generate an inward current (I_{NCX}) by extruding one Ca^{2+} in exchange for three Na^{+} (Blaustein & Lederer, 1999). In 1993 Zhou and colleagues showed that after activation of $I_{Ca,L}$, there was a second inward current which was due to I_{NCX} (Zhou & Lipsius, 1993). Figure 2C shows a typical example and I-V relationship of I_{NCX} in rabbit SA node cells. This finding was further explored and led to a theory on spontaneous release from the sarcoplasmic reticulum as being the oscillator responsible for SA node automaticity (Maltsev et al., 2006). Conflicting evidence has been found regarding the spontaneous occurrence of these Ca^{2+} releases, with Huser and colleagues showing that LVCRs no longer occur when feline latent pacemaker cells are voltage clamped at a hyperpolarized resting potential (-70 mV), and only occur in the presence of depolarization, starting at a membrane potential of –57 mV. They also demonstrated that LVCRs depend on $I_{Ca,T}$, as they disappear when $I_{Ca,T}$ is blocked with 50 µM Ni^{+} (Huser et al., 2000). However, in rabbit SA node cells, addition of 50 µM Ni^{+} did not stop the occurrence of LVCRs, nor did voltage clamping these cells at -10 mV. At more negative holding potentials, LVCRs ceased due to a decrease in sarcoplasmic Ca^{2+} as a result of extrusion of Ca^{2+} following NCX activity after each Ca^{2+} release (Vinogradova et al., 2004).

2.3 Transient outward currents

2.3.1 Transient outward K^{+} current, type 1 (I_{to1})

Two transient outward current components are found in cardiac cells, one carried by K^{+} (I_{to1}), the other by Cl^{-} ions (I_{to2}) (Nerbonne & Kass, 2005). The pore-forming α-subunit of the transient outward K^{+} current I_{to1} is formed by different members of the Kv family. *KCND2* (Kv4.2) and *KCND3* (Kv4.3) encode $I_{to,fast}$, which recovers rapidly from inactivation, while *KCNA4* encodes Kv1.4, which recovers slowly from inactivation ($I_{to,slow}$) (Nerbonne & Kass, 2005). Similar to other channels from the Kv family, channels are formed by tetramerization. Multiple β-subunits have been proposed, including KChiPs (Kuo et al., 2001), MiRP1 (*KCNE2*) and MiRP2 (*KCNE3*) (Roepke et al., 2008; Zhang et al., 2001b), Kvβ (Aimond et al., 2005), and DPP6 (Radicke et al., 2005).

In human SA node, mRNA for Kv4.2, Kv1.4 and, in particular, Kv4.3 was found (Chandler et al., 2009); all these transcripts were also found in murine SA node (Marionneau et al., 2005).

Upon membrane depolarization, I_{to1} exhibits fast activation, followed by fast inactivation (Nerbonne & Kass, 2005). The influence of this current differs among different species and different parts of the heart. In ventricular tissue of most mammals, except for guinea pig (Sanguinetti & Jurkiewicz, 1990) and pig (Li et al., 2003), I_{to1} is responsible for the early phase of repolarization. Differences in I_{to1} density and composition between epicardium and endocardium may in part explain the difference in action potential waveform and duration in these different areas of the heart (Liu et al., 1993).

Investigation of the role of I_{to1} in SA node function is hampered by the lack of a specific blocker. In older studies 4-aminopyridine (4-AP) was used as a specific blocker for I_{to1} (Thompson, 1977). However, more recent studies have shown that 4-AP also blocks the ultra-rapid, rapid, and slow components of the delayed rectifier K^+ current (I_{Kur}, I_{Kr}, and I_{Ks}, respectively) at concentrations used to analyze the role of I_{to1} (Li et al., 1996; Ridley et al., 2003; Arechiga-Figueroa et al., 2010). As will be discussed later, block of these currents influences SA node function. In addition, 4-AP stimulates $I_{K,Ach}$ (Arechiga-Figueroa et al., 2010).

Whether or not I_{to1} is present in SA node cells still remains to be resolved. The current was first described in cells from the crista terminalis of rabbit heart in 1985 (Giles & van Ginneken, 1985). This current was completely blocked by 4-AP, and activated between -20 and +10mV with a reversal potential around –75 mV. In 2000, Lei et al characterized the current in rabbit SA node (Lei et al., 2000). Using a holding potential of –80 mV and 200 ms pulses between -40 and 60 mV, they showed a rapidly activating (within 10 ms) current that inactivated within 200 ms, with a voltage of half maximal activation of -11 mV and a fast and a slow inactivating component (10 vs 107 ms). In the presence of an extremely high concentration of 4-AP (10 mM), the outward current was abolished. The effect of 4-AP on spontaneous activity of SA node cells was studied in small and large cells, under the assumption that small cells originate from the center of the SA node, while larger cells are situated more in the periphery. In small cells, 4-AP decreased action potential amplitude, increased action potential duration, decreased maximum diastolic potential, and increased cycle length. In large cells, spontaneous activity ceased. These observations seem to correspond with blockade of I_{Kur}, I_{Kr}, and I_{Ks}, which are also blocked by 4-AP (see below). Based on these experiments, it is not possible to distinguish between the effects of these different currents.

In a letter to the editor based on this paper, Verkerk and Van Ginneken discuss the interference of I_f tail current when measuring I_{to1} (Verkerk & van Ginneken, 2001). Even in the presence of drugs that block I_f there will be interference due to the fact that these drugs will block the current more efficiently at hyperpolarized membrane potentials than during depolarization. In a study on ionic remodelling of SA node cells during heart failure by Verkerk et al., no I_{to1} was found to be present in rabbit SA node (Verkerk et al., 2003).

To our knowledge, no data have been published regarding the heart rate in genetically modified mice lacking I_{to1}.

2.3.2 Ca^{2+} activated Cl^- current ($I_{Cl(Ca)}$ or I_{to2})

In 2002 the Ca^{2+} activated Cl^- current ($I_{Cl(Ca)}$), also known as the 4-AP insensitive part of I_{to}, or I_{to2}, was found to be present in one third of spontaneously beating rabbit SA node cells (Verkerk 2002). Figure 3A, left panel, shows a typical example of $I_{Ca(Cl)}$ in rabbit SA node cells. This current, which is sensitive to 4,4,-diisothiocyanostilbene-2,2,-disulphonic acid (DIDS), is a transient outward current activated by Ca^{2+} release of the sarcoplasmic reticulum and is present at potentials positive to –20 mV with a peak at 40 mV (Fig. 3A, right panel). By decreasing $I_{Cl(Ca)}$, DIDS increased action potential overshoot and prolonged APD20, without affecting diastolic depolarization rate, MDP, action potential duration at 50% repolarization (APD_{50}), or cycle length. In the presence of norepinephrine, $I_{Cl(Ca)}$ density doubled, but also under these circumstances inhibition did not influence beating rate. Incorporation into in silico models of SA node cells also showed a limited role in pacemaker synchronization and conduction from SA node to atrium.

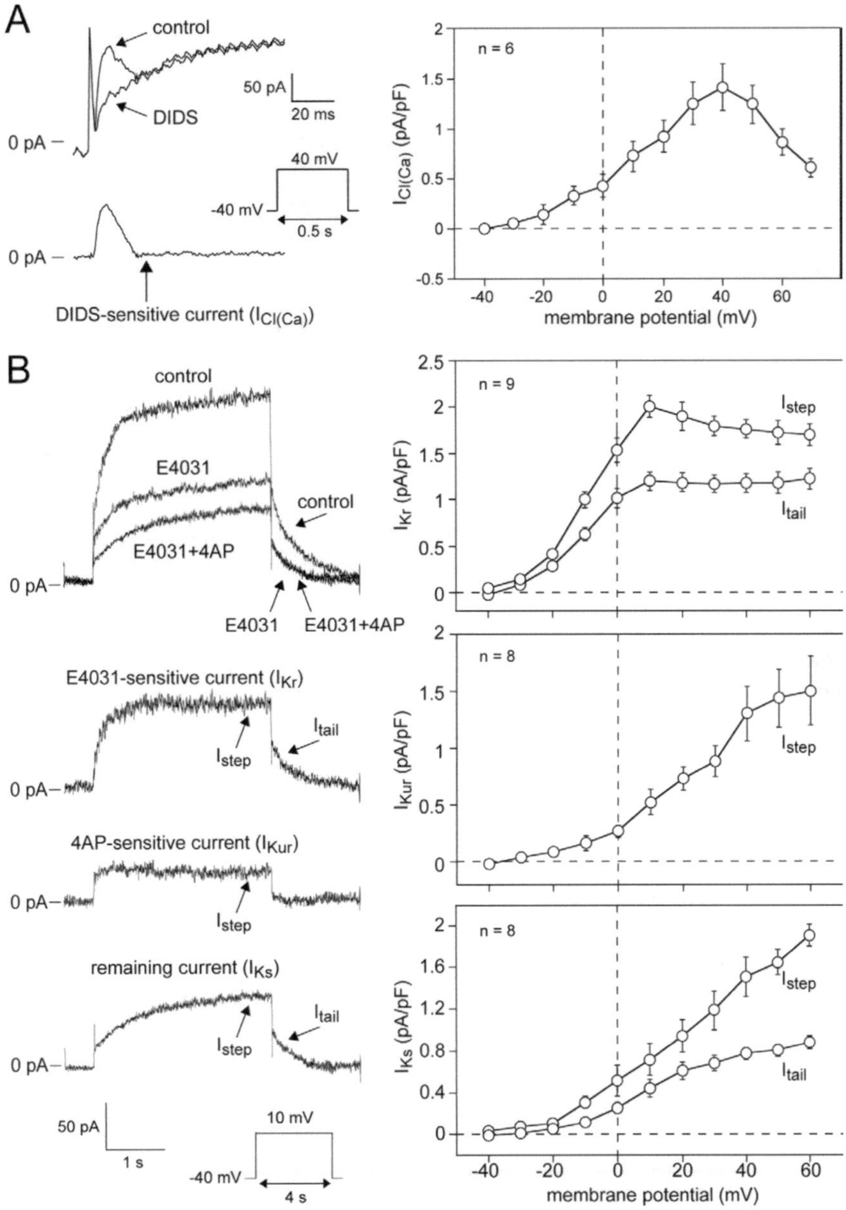

A, Typical example (left) and average I-V relationship (right) of the Ca^{2+}-activated Cl^- current ($I_{Cl(Ca)}$). Inset, Voltage clamp protocol used. $I_{Cl(Ca)}$ was measured as current sensitive for 4,4,-diisothiocyanostilbene-2,2,-disulphonic acid (DIDS) B, Typical examples (left) and average I-V relationships of the delayed rectifier K^+ currents (right). Inset, Voltage clamp protocol used. Currents were measured in control conditions, in presence of E4031 and in combined presence of E4031 and 4AP. E4031-sensitive current was defined as I_{Kr}, 4AP-sensitive current was defined as I_{Kur}, and remaining time-dependent current was defined as I_{Ks}. For cell isolations and experimental details, see Ref (Verkerk et al., 2003).

Fig. 3. Outward currents in rabbit SA node cells.

2.4 Delayed rectifier K^+ currents

The delayed rectifier K^+ current (I_K), first described in Purkinje fibers in 1968 (Noble & Tsien, 1968), is composed of three different components: the ultra-rapid (I_{Kur}), rapid (I_{Kr}), and slow (I_{Ks}) components. Figure 3B, shows typical examples and I-V relationships of the various I_K components in rabbit SA node cells. I_{Kur}, I_{Kr}, and I_{Ks} can be identified by their gating kinetics and difference in sensitivity to drugs. In 1976, Noma and Irisawa described the presence of these currents in rabbit SA node cells (Noma & Irisawa, 1976).

I_K currents are responsible for repolarization, but the role of the different I_K components in the SA node varies between species. I_{Kr} seems to play an important role in rabbits, while, in guinea pig, I_K is mainly composed of I_{Ks} (Matsuura et al., 2002); in pig, I_{Kr} appears to be absent altogether (Ono et al., 2000). Functional data about I_K in human SA node are lacking, but mRNA for all three channels has been found in human SA node (Chandler et al., 2009).

2.4.1 Ultra-rapid component of the delayed rectifier K^+ current (I_{Kur})

Of the different components of I_K, least is known about the presence, function and role of the ultra-rapid component (I_{Kur}) in SA node. In 2000, Dobrzynski et al. proved the presence of Kv1.5, the α-subunit of the channel encoded by *KCNA5*, in guinea pig SA node by Western blotting and immunolabeling (Dobrzynski et al., 2000). As discussed previously, mRNA for Kv1.5 is present in human SA node.

This rapidly activating and non-deactivating current was first described in 1991 (Boyle & Nerbonne, 1991) and has since then been referred to as I_{ss} (steady-state), I_{sus} (sustained), and I_{Kur} (ultra-rapid) (Nerbonne, 2000). I_{Kur} activates around –40 mV and is blocked effectively with low concentrations of 4-AP (Boyle & Nerbonne, 1991). In 2003, the current was described in SA node of healthy and heart failure rabbits (Verkerk et al., 2003). Block of I_{Kur} with low concentrations of 4-AP (too low to block I_{to}) prolonged murine SA node cycle length by 20% (from 272±25 to 328±31 ms) (Nikmaram et al., 2008).

2.4.2 Rapid component of the delayed rectifier K^+ current (I_{Kr})

The α-subunit of I_{Kr} is encoded by Kv11.1 (also known as *hERG* or *KCNH2*). Mutations in this gene are found in patients with long QT syndrome type 2 (Curran et al., 1995). While expression of *hERG* in Xenopus oocytes confirmed the hypothesis that this gene encodes the α-subunit of I_{Kr}, differences between the expressed current and native current still existed (Sanguinetti et al., 1995). The role of the proposed β-subunit MiRP1 (minK related peptide 1, *KCNE2* gene) remains controversial (Abbott et al., 1999).

I_{Kr} shows inward rectification, meaning that the channel passes current more easily in the inward direction than the outward direction. This rectification is caused by very rapid inactivation that develops after activation of the channel by depolarization. Thus, very little I_{Kr} exists during the plateau phase of the action potential. During repolarization, there is recovery from inactivation causing an outward current responsible for late repolarization, followed by slow deactivation (Ono & Ito, 1995).

In rabbit SA node cells, I_{Kr} activation starts around –50 mV with a voltage of half maximal activation of -17.4 mV (Lei & Brown, 1996). Adrenergic stimulation of I_{Kr} has a dual effect. On the one hand, phosphorylation by PKA causes a reduction in current amplitude, faster deactivation and a depolarizing shift in voltage-dependence of activation. On the other hand, direct binding of cAMP to Kv11.1 causes a hyperpolarizing shift in voltage-dependence of activation. Whether this results in an increase or decrease of net current

depends on the presence of accessory proteins. In the absence of MiRP1, there is a decrease in current, while there is an increase in the presence of MiRP1 (Cui et al., 2000).
As mentioned above, the role of I_{Kr} differs between species. *ERG1B* knock out mice did not display a reduction in overall heart rate, but 6 out 21 mice did show abrupt and spontaneous bradycardias that were never seen in control littermates (Lees-Miller et al., 2003). In rabbit and mouse SA node cells, blockade of I_{Kr} with E-4031 prolonged cycle length and action potential duration, and depolarized the MDP (Clark et al., 2004; Verheijck et al., 1995). Since I_{Kr} is absent from pig SA node, blocking of I_{Kr} did not have any affect on the action potential or cycle length in this species (Ono et al., 2000).

2.4.3 Slow component of the delayed rectifier K^+ current (I_{Ks})

Until 1996, there was controversy about the proteins responsible for generating I_{Ks}. In 1988, the gene *IsK*, also known as minK (*KCNE1*), was cloned into Xenopus oocytes, resulting in a K^+ current resembling I_{Ks} (Takumi et al., 1988). Expression in other cell lines, however, did not result in the generation of a similar current, leading to the hypothesis that minK coassembles with other proteins present in Xenopus oocytes to form I_{Ks}. When a new K^+ channel was identified through positional cloning (Kv7.1), this channel was found to produce a current resembling I_{Ks} when co-expressed with its β-subunit, minK protein (Barhanin et al., 1996; Sanguinetti et al., 1996).
The α-subunit Kv7.1, encoded by *KCNQ1*, is formed by tetramerization of four 6-transmembrane segments (Nerbonne & Kass, 2005). Together with 2 minK proteins and the protein Yotiao, this tetramer forms a macromolecular complex (Lin et al., 1998). Apart from regulating current kinetics, interaction between Kv7.1 and minK within the endoplasmic reticulum stabilizes newly synthesized channels (Peroz et al., 2009).
In guinea pig ventricular myocytes, I_{Ks} activates slowly upon depolarization to potentials positive to -30 mV, with a voltage of half maximal activation around 26 mV (Balser et al., 1990). In rabbit SA node cells, a voltage of half maximal activation of 15.6 mV was found (Lei & Brown, 1996).
In 1991, Sanguinetti et al. reported experiments in which they showed that isoproterenol increases I_{Ks} in guinea pig ventricular myocytes (Sanguinetti et al., 1991). This responsiveness to β-adrenergic stimulation requires the presence of the β-subunit, minK protein, and Yotiao (Kurokawa et al., 2003; Marx et al., 2002), and involves phosphorylation of Kv7.1 by protein kinase A (Walsh & Kass, 1988). The increase in I_{Ks} upon β-adrenergic stimulation also augments its role in spontaneous activity: while blocking I_{Ks} in rabbit SA node cells has negligible effects on cycle length or MDP in control conditions, blockade during stimulation with isoproterenol led to an increase in cycle length, a depolarized MDP and slower diastolic depolarization (Lei et al., 2002). An increase in I_{Ks} due to β-adrenergic stimulation is also partly due to an increase in heart rate, since there is incomplete deactivation at high rates (Jurkiewicz & Sanguinetti, 1993).
The role of I_{Ks} in SA node function in human can only be deduced from patients with long QT syndrome type 1 (mutations in *KCNQ1*). Not only do these patients exhibit prolonged QT intervals, causing arrhythmias during exercise due to prolonged repolarization in ventricular tissue, they also have a diminished increase in heart rate upon exercise (Haapalahti et al., 2006). No I_{Ks} has been found in mouse SA node (Cho et al., 2003), and, as expected, *KCNQ1* knock out mice do not show prolongation of cycle length (Knollmann et al., 2004). Since I_{Ks} is the only I_K present in pig, spontaneous activity ceased on blocking I_{Ks} with chromanol 293B (Ono et al., 2000).

2.5 Inward rectifier K^+ current current (I_{K1})

The α-subunit of the inward rectifier K^+ current current (I_{K1}) is formed by tetramerization of four 2-membrane spanning domains that do not include a voltage sensor (Hibino et al., 2010). The α-subunit can be formed by homomerization or heteromerization of members of the Kir2.x subfamily. Kir2.1, the major component of the cardiac α-subunit of I_{K1}, is encoded by *KCNJ2* (Plaster et al., 2001).

I_{K1} is an inward rectifier which is blocked at potentials more positive than the equilibrium for K^+ (E_K), which lies at around -85 mV, by Mg^{2+} and polyamines (Lopatin et al., 1994; Matsuda et al., 1987). Figure 4A, left panel, shows a typical examples in an isolated rabbit left ventricular myocyte; the arrow indicates E_K. Due to the inward rectifying properties, I_{K1} is reduced during depolarization (Fig. 4B); this allows the action potential plateau phase to exists. During repolarization, the current is unblocked (Fig. 4B) and I_{K1} further repolarizes the membrane towards E_K. Importantly, negative and positive to E_K, I_{K1} is an inward and outward current, respectively. Consequently, I_{K1} will stabilize the membrane potential around E_K.

This current, which at first glance appears to antagonize spontaneous activity, is not present in rabbit SA node (Irisawa et al., 1993), and is negligibly small in murine and rat SA node cells (Cho et al., 2003; Shinagawa et al., 2000). Figure 4A, right panel, shows typical current traces in a rabbit SA node cell measured with a similar voltage clamp protocol and solutions as in the ventricular myocyte (left panel). Note the absence of I_{K1} in the SA node cell (arrow), which is also summarized in the I-V relationships in Figure 4B. Due to the fact that I_{K1} is absent or functionally negligibly small, SA node cells have a relatively positive MDP, at around -60 mV (Mangoni & Nargeot, 2008)

Knock-out of Kir2.1 in mouse resulted in no detectable I_{K1}, longer action potentials, and spontaneous activity in 70% of isolated ventricular cells. Knock-out of Kir2.2 resulted in a 50% reduction of I_{K1} without other abnormalities (Zaritsky et al., 2001). Since these mice died at young age due to cleft palate, mice expressing a dominant-negative construct were designed. These mice, who did not show facial abnormalities, showed a 90% reduction in I_{K1}. This was associated with a decrease in heart rate of 31% (McLerie & Lopatin, 2003). Whether this is a consequence of the reduction in I_{K1} in SA node cells or results from reduced electrical load imposed by the atrium remains to be resolved.

In 2009, Chan et al. proposed that I_{K1} may act to increase heart rates by enhancing I_f through its effect to maintain membrane potentials within a range where HCN channels can most effectively operate. By overexpressing *HCN1* and *KCNJ2,* both independently and together, in quiescent guinea pig ventricular myocytes, they showed that I_{K1} further increased automaticity that was already induced by *HCN1* overexpression (Chan et al., 2009). Not only was there an increase in beating rate (320 bpm vs 181 bpm), but there was also a more hyperpolarized MDP and an increase in I_f.

2.6 Voltage dependent Na^+ current (I_{Na})

The α-subunits of the voltage dependent Na^+ channels contains four homologous domains, all containing six transmembrane segments. Of the different α-subunits, several have been found to be present in murine SA node, including neuronal isoforms (Lei et al., 2004; Maier et al., 2003). In human SA node, Nav1.5 (*SCN5A*) mRNA was detected, although at lower levels than in paranodal and right atrial tissue. Nav1.2 (*SCN2A*) and Nav1.4 (*SCN4A*) mRNA was also identified in the SA node, but at negligible levels (Chandler et al., 2009).

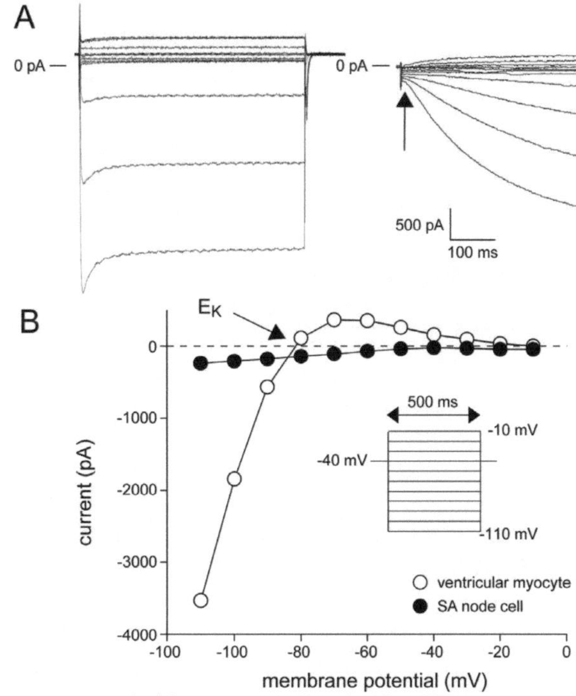

A, Typical current traces recorded between -110 and -10 mV in a ventricular (left) and SA node (right) cell of rabbit. Please note the absence of a prominent I_{K1} in the SA node cell (arrow). B, I-V relationships of the current measured in the beginning of the voltage clamp steps. The arrow indicates the reversal of current (E_K) in the ventricular myocyte. Inset, Voltage clamp protocol used.

Fig. 4. Inward rectifier K^+ current (I_{K1}) in ventricular and SA node cells.

However, in canine SA node, mRNA for Nav1.1 (*SCN1A*), 1.2, 1.3 (*SCN3A*), and 1.5 is present (Haufe et al., 2005). Expression of only α-subunits leads to functional Na^+ current (I_{Na}), but co-expression of β-subunits influences gating kinetics and current amplitude. So far, 4 different β-subunits (*SCN1B* to *SCN4B*) have been identified (Isom et al., 1995; Isom et al., 1992; Morgan et al., 2000; Yu et al., 2003).

Cardiac Na^+ channels open upon depolarizaton, allowing an influx of Na^+ ions, responsible for the rapid upstroke of the atrial and ventricular action potential. In 1975, Kreitner reported experiments in rabbit SA node preparations. She showed that tetrodotoxin (TTX), a blocker of I_{Na}, only negligibly affected spontaneous rate and action potential waveform. Carbamylcholine, a cholinergic agonist, hyperpolarized the MDP and increased the rate of rise of the action potential, suggesting a role for I_{Na} at more negative membrane potentials. Indeed, adding TTX after addition of carbamylcholine caused a decrease in the slope of depolarization. It was concluded that I_{Na} is present in the SA, but is inactivated under normal conditions, due to the relatively depolarized membrane potential of SA node cells (Kreitner, 1975). More recent studies, however, indicate a role for Na^+ channels in SA node pacemaking in newborn rabbit (Baruscotti et al., 2000).

In 2004, Lei et al investigated the role of the different α-subunits in adult mouse SA node cells. They showed that the I_{Na} present in these cells consisted of two components: one that is blocked by nanomolar concentrations of TTX and one that is blocked by micromolar concentrations. The neuronal isoforms are known to be more sensitive to block by TTX. In

intact preparations, both high and low concentrations caused an increase in cycle length, while only at high concentrations activity in the periphery ceased. Immunostaining showed the neuronal isoform Nav1.1 to be present in small and large cells throughout the SA node. Nav1.5, on the other hand, was not present in the center of the SA node. In 2010, Protas et al. showed that I_{Na} is present in 80% of canine SA node cells, with greater current densities at younger age. Due to inactivation at relatively negative potentials this current would be unavailable at physiological potentials, but might be recruited in case of hyperpolarization (Protas et al., 2010). Verkerk et al. had the opportunity to study ion currents in human SA node cells and showed that, upon switching off a hyperpolarizing pulse, there was a large inward current that rapidly activated and inactivated, probably I_{Na} (Verkerk et al., 2009b).
The notion that there is a role for I_{Na} in human SA node is further supported by the fact that mutations in *SCN5A* are known to influence sinus rate. Loss of function mutations in *SCN5A* have been associated with sick sinus syndrome (Benson et al., 2003).
Moreover, there is an overlap in I_{Na} activation and inactivation curves resulting in a window Na^+ current. It is suggested that such a Na^+ window current can be present at potentials found in SA node (Attwell et al., 1979; Muramatsu et al., 1996). Accordingly, late or persistent Na^+ current ($I_{Na,L}$), due to mutations in the *SCN5A* gene (Tan et al., 2003) may affect SA node function significantly. $I_{Na,L}$ due to mutation in SCN5A or drug use, induced SA node pacemaker slowing due to action potential prolongation and depolarization of the MDP (Veldkamp et al., 2003; Wu et al., 2008)
While homozygous *SCN5A* knock-out is embryonically lethal (Papadatos et al., 2002), heterozygous deletion of *SCN5A* in mouse results in lower heart rate and sino-atrial block (Lei et al., 2005)

2.7 Sustained inward current (I_{st})

Relatively little is known about the sustained inward current (I_{st}), a current first described in rabbit SA node in 1995 (Guo et al., 1995). So far, the molecular structure of the channels is unknown. I_{st} is an inward current that is activated upon depolarization to -60 mV and that shows pharmacological characteristics resembling those of the voltage-gated Ca^{2+} channels, including sensitivity to nicardipine and resistance to TTX, but is carried by Na^+ (Guo et al., 1995). The first single channel measurements followed a few years later, showing the current to be absent from quiescent cells, to activate at potentials positive to -80mV, and to reverse at 13 mV (Mitsuiye et al., 2000).
β-Adrenergic stimulation shifts the threshold for activation and the potential of maximum amplitude to more negative potentials (Cho et al., 2003; Huang et al., 2008; Toyoda et al., 2005). Acetylcholine (ACh) does not have an inhibitory effect in an unstimulated situation, but, after stimulation with isoproterenol, ACh causes a reduction in amplitude (Toyoda et al., 2005).
The role in spontaneous activity is difficult to assess, considering the overlap with $I_{Ca,L}$ in drug sensitiviy. Taurine, which increases I_f and $I_{Ca,T}$ but decreases I_{st} and $I_{Ca,L}$, inhibits spontaneous activity in rat SA node cells, implying that the decrease in I_{st} and $I_{Ca,L}$ is more important than increase in I_f and $I_{Ca,T}$ in controlling beating rate (Satoh, 2003).
Action potential clamp studies show I_{st} to be present in control conditions over the entire voltage rage of guinea pig SA node cells, with a maximum around -20 mV. Since this inward current is present within the voltage range of the diastolic depolarization, part of the depolarization seems to be caused by I_{st}. In silico models of SA cells consistently show an

increase in beating rate upon incorporation of I_{st}, varying from an increase of 0.8% to 20% (Zhang et al., 2002a).

2.8 Other currents

2.8.1 Background current (I_{Ba})

The equilibrium for K^+ lies around -85mV and the SA node MDP is less negative, suggesting a greater conductance for Na^+ than K^+. In the absence of I_{K1}, there is indeed a low permeability for K^+. In 1995, a background current carried by Na^+ (I_{Ba}) was shown in rabbit SA. After inhibition of K^+ currents, I_f, I_{NCX}, Ca^{2+} currents and the Na^+/K^+ pump, this background current was inward at potentials negative to -21 mV (Hagiwara et al., 1992).

2.8.2 Na^+-K^+ pump current (I_p)

This current, generated by the electrogenic Na^+/K^+ pump (I_p), is responsible for keeping intracellular Na^+ concentration low and the K^+ concentration high by extruding 3 Na^+ from the cell in exchange for 2 K^+. In a solution containing 5 mM K^+, rabbit SA node strips had an MDP of -58 mV. Upon exchanging this fluid for a K^+-free solution, there was depolarization with initially an increase in beating rate, eventually resulting in oscillation. When again K^+ was added again to a concentration of 5 mM, hyperpolarization occurred and spontaneous activity resumed. Ouabain, a Na^+/K^+ pump blocker, or replacement of Na^+ with Li^+, prevented this hyperpolarization, suggesting a role for I_p (Noma & Irisawa, 1975; Noma & Irisawa, 1974). With a voltage of half maximal activation of -52 mV and a current magnitude of 22.5 pA, this outward current could partly control normal pacemaking by counterbalancing inward currents (Sakai et al., 1996).

2.8.3 ACh-activated K^+ current ($I_{K,ACh}$)

The K^+ current activated by ACh ($I_{K,ACh}$) is involved in the negative chronotropic effect of ACh by hyperpolarizing the cell (Noma & Trautwein, 1978). The proteins responsible for the tetramers, Kir3.1 (KCNJ3) and Kir3.4 (*KCNJ5*), were indeed identified by immunofluorescence in rat SA node (Dobrzynski et al., 2001). Apart from the direct and short lasting hyperpolarizing effect of $I_{K,ACh}$ on the SA node, the increase in $I_{K,ACh}$ in surrounding atrial muscle leads to a longer lasting effect on the SA node by electrotonic interaction (Kodama et al., 1996).

2.8.4 ATP-sensitive current ($I_{K,ATP}$)

Activation of ATP sensitive current $I_{K,ATP}$ by depletion of ATP or by $I_{K,ATP}$ openers (pinacidil, cromakalim, nicorandil) hyperpolarizes the diastolic membrane potential by activation of an outward K^+ current with a reversal potential around E_K which is sensitive to the $I_{K,ATP}$ blocker glibenclamide (Han et al., 1996; Satoh, 2003). Knock out of Kir6.2 (*KCNJ11*), the α-subunit of $I_{K,ATP}$ channels, results in a diminished response to hypoxia both in Langendorff perfused hearts and in isolated SA node cells. The decrease in beating rate seen in wild type mice can presumably prevent against ischemia induced damage (Fukuzaki et al., 2008).

3. Anatomy of the SA node

3.1 Location of the SA node

After the location of the SA node was first described in 1907 (Keith & Flack, 1907), the anatomy of this structure has been found to vary among species. While the node is always identified at the junction of the right atrium and superior caval vein, there is considerable variation. In human, dog, and pig the SA node lies epicardially, while in rabbit it covers the entire thickness of the intercaval region and part of the endocardial surface of the crista terminalis (Boyett et al., 2000; Opthof, 1988). Additionally, while man, monkey, dog, pig, and horse have a central SA node artery, there is none in rabbit, guinea pig, and cat (Opthof, 1988). In man, the SA node artery originates from the right coronary artery in 55% of cases, and from the circumflex branch of the left coronary artery in the remainder. In rat, blood supply comes from the internal mammary artery, which is a very relevant aspect to take into account when studying Langendorff perfused hearts (James, 2002).

3.2 Different cells within the SA node

The SA node exhibits changes in electrophysiological characteristics from center to periphery. The cause of this heterogeneity has led to some debate (for review see Boyett et al., 2000). Whether there is a gradual change in cell type from SA node center to atrium (gradient model) or a change in composition of cells (mosaic model), still remains to be resolved. The mosaic model states that there are no differences between single cells isolated from the center or periphery of the SA node, but that the differences found in intact preparations are based on the differences in the amount of atrial cells within the tissue, with 41% of cells in the center, and 63% of cells in the periphery being atrial atrial cells. Supporting this hypothesis are the findings that not all myocytes within the SA node stain with neurofilament antibody (used to characterize SA node cells), and that cell isolation within the intercaval region results in typical SA node cells and atrial cells (Verheijck et al., 1998). In their response to this article, Zhang et al. consider a few arguments ontradicting this theory (Zhang et al., 2001a). Firstly, they use data from three different studies showing that, when the SA node and surrounding atrial tissue are intact, the leading pacemaker site is the center of the SA node, while, when different parts are separated, the more peripheral regions show faster spontaneous activity. This argument, however, does not account for the fact that, according to the mosaic model, these parts contain more atrial cells, and the hyperpolarizing effect of these cells might increase beating rate, just like overexpression of I_{K1} can increase beating rate (Chan et al., 2009). Under normal conditions, the extra load of the attached atrial muscle might prevent a more peripheral start of activation by electrotonic influence. However, when the mosaic model was tested in silico, by making two square lattices of 20x20 cells filled with nodal cells and either 41 or 63% atrial cells with a coupling conductance between cells of 0 to 25 nS, a faster intrinsic rate was found in the more central (41% atrial cells) than peripheral (63% atrial cells) lattice (Zhang et al., 2001a). Other data supporting the gradient cell model are the differences in electrophysiological characteristics found in small and large cells, originating from the center and periphery of the SA node, respectively. Action potential amplitude, MDP, take-off potential, action potential upstroke velocity, rate of diastolic depolarization, and spontaneous beating rate are faster in larger cells, combined with a larger density in I_f and I_{Na} (Honjo et al., 1996).

Within the SA node, there is a remarkable amount of connective tissue: islands of nodal cells are separated by connective tissue (De Maziere et al., 1992). While, at first, myocytes were thought to be electrically isolated from non-excitable cells, immunohistochemical labelling has shown that fibroblasts surrounded by other fibroblasts express connexin40, while fibroblasts adjacent to nodal cells express connexin45. Moreover, functional testing showed occasional spread of Lucifer yellow between adjacent myocytes and fibroblasts (Camelliti et al., 2004). The functional role of the connections between nodal cells and fibroblasts needs further studying, but, theoretically, fibroblasts could have different functions in the SA node. To begin with, they can function as a current sink, possibly affecting spontaneous activity. Secondly, because cardiac fibroblasts are thought to be mechanosensitive, they are thought to play a role in the positive chronotropic response to stretch of the right atrium (Kohl et al., 1994). Finally, although not being electrically active themselves, fibroblasts can conduct an electrical signal between myocytes (Kohl et al., 2005).

3.3 Coupling within the SA node and between SA node and right atrium

Despite the fact that the SA node is relatively small and the atrium is more hyperpolarized, the SA node is capable of generating impulses and propagating these to the surrounding tissue. The question how the SA node is capable of doing this was first studied using in vitro models. It was shown that a low coupling resistance between SA node and atrium would inhibit impulse generation by electrotonic interaction. On the other hand, if coupling resistance becomes too high, the SA node will be able to generate impulses, but these impulses will not be propagated to the atrium. Optimal pacemaking and conduction was reached with a low conductance within the SA node and a gradual increase of coupling towards the periphery (Joyner & van Capelle, 1986). Interdigitation of atrial strand within the SA node was found by immunolabeling (Oosthoek et al., 1993; ten Velde et al., 1995). This interdigitation was shown to have beneficial effects on impulse conduction from SA node to atrium (Winslow & Varghese, 1995). The intermingling of strands of atrial tissue within the SA node prevents the SA node from too strong a hyperpolarizing influence, while the atrial strands can propagate the action potential.

The electrotonic effect of the atrium can also protect the SA node. Blocking I_{Kr} results in a depolarization of the SA node, without affecting atrial resting membrane potential. This never results in pacemaker arrest. When the atrium is removed, blocking I_{Kr} results in pacemaker arrest, showing a beneficial effect of the electrotonic influence of the atrium (Verheijck et al., 2002).

The question is how well SA node cells are coupled to each other and to atrial cells. First of all, very little coupling is necessary between two SA node cells for entrainment (Verheijck et al., 1998; Wilders et al., 1996). Since two rabbit SA node cells with a 26% difference in interbeat interval require a coupling conductance of only 0.17 nS for frequency entrainment, and conductance of sinatrial node gap junctional channels can be ~75 pS, only 3 gap junctional channels would suffice (Verheijck et al., 1998). The slow conduction velocity within the SA node and the low space constant are signs of the limited electrical coupling between the cells (Boyett et al., 2000).

Gap junction channels allow for intercellular cytoplasmic communication. Connexins (Cx) form hemichannels called connexons. In the heart, several different connexins are found, including Cx43 in working myocardium, and Cx40 and Cx45 in conduction system. These different connexins can generate a variety of gap junctions with different properties, including conductance (Veenstra et al., 1992). Studies on the different connexins present in SA node are contradictory, but most studies have not shown Cx43 in rabbit SA node, and have found Cx40 and Cx45. These studies are complicated by the difficulty in finding subtype specific antibodies and the scarcity of the amount of connexins within the SA node. In human SA node, mRNA of Cx40, Cx43, Cx45 and negligible amounts of Cx31.9 were identified (Chandler et al., 2009).

4. Autonomic modulation of the SA node

Almost all of the ionic currents discussed so far are sensitive to autonomic modulation. However, the response of the SA node to different stimuli cannot be easily predicted due to the heterogeneity of, and interaction between, the cells. Basic heart rate results from a balance between sympathetic and parasympathetic input, which may differ between species. In rabbit, like in rodents, sympathetic tonus dominates, since the beating rate of isolated right atrium is much lower than in vivo rate. In dog and human, parasympathetic tonus prevails (Opthof, 2000). When studying (para-) sympathetic stimulation, it is always relevant to realize that addition of a substance, for example adrenalin, might give a very different response than nerve stimulation (Choate et al., 1993).

4.1 Sympathetic stimulation

Activation of the β-adrenergic receptor (β-AR) by catecholamines can give rise to a multitude of changes. Activation of the β-ARs, a G-protein coupled receptor, leads to stimulation of the stimulatory G-protein (G_s), whereby adenylyl cyclases are activated and cAMP is formed. CAMP can either bind directly to ion channels or influence their function by activating protein kinase A (PKA). PKA can in turn, by phosphorylation, influence the function of other proteins, including ion channels,.

Both β1- and β2-adrenergic receptors are present in SA node (Hedberg et al., 1980), differing in their coupling to G-proteins en localization within the cell membrane. While β1-ARs are coupled to only stimulatory G-proteins, β2-ARs are coupled to both stimulatory and inhibitory G-proteins (Xiao et al., 1999). This can account for the shorter duration of the positive chronotropic effect of β2-adrenergic stimulation compared to stimulation of the β1-AR (Devic et al., 2001). Furthermore β2-adrenergic receptors have been found to localize to caveolae, specific regions of the cell membrane, while β1-ARs do not (Barbuti et al., 2004).

The changes induced by β-adrenergic stimulation include an increase in I_f, $I_{Ca,L}$, I_{Kr}, I_{Ks}, and I_{st}, and an increase in spontaneous Ca^{2+} releases from the sarcoplasmic reticulum, all supporting either faster diastolic depolarization or a shorter action potential duration, causing an increase in beating rate.

The response to β-adrenergic stimulation is not equal among different areas of the SA node, causing a shift in site of earliest activation upon stimulation (Mackaay et al., 1980).

4.2 Parasympathetic stimulation

Parasympathetic modulation not only involves modulation of the currents usually active by decreasing the cAMP concentration, but as mentioned previously also involves activation of $I_{K,ACh}$ (Noma & Trautwein, 1978).

After stimulation of the M2-receptor, different phases in heart rate response can be detected: first there is a decrease in rate, followed by a short increase, and afterwards again a decrease. The first decrease is thought to be the result of a direct effect of ACh on SA node, the second decrease a result of the hyperpolarizing effect of the atrium upon the SA node. The effect of ACh is exaggerated in the presence of noradrenalin (Levy, 1971).

As with sympathetic stimulation, the response to parasympathetic stimulation is also not homogeneous within the SA node. While the primary pacemaker is very sensitive and will increase cycle length considerably, other parts that have a lower intrinsic frequency are less sensitive and will take over as the site of earliest activation (Mackaay et al., 1980). This heterogeneity prevents too slow bradycardia or asystole from occurring.

5. Creation of a biopacemaker

When working on the creation of a biopacemaker, several issues need be kept in mind. To begin with, the goal should not be the recreation of an SA node. Apart from the simple fact that a complicated structure like the SA node can not easily be reconstructed, this might not be necessary. The biopacemaker is not required to generate a rhythm in the same way the SA node does, as long as it generates a stable rhythm. For instance, while the biopacemaker is a therapy to be used in clinical situations where the heart is no longer paced sufficiently by the SA node, it does not need to be capable of generating a heart rhythm during the development of the heart. Secondly, longevity is required. This is especially relevant when choosing a delivery strategy, as will be discussed in paragraph 5.2. Also, the biopacemaker should be responsive to autonomic modulation, as is the SA node. Finally, and most importantly, safety should be a priority when considering gene or cell therapy.

5.1 How to generate rhythm

As is clear from the previous paragraphs, the SA node cells contains multiple ion channels that can facilitate the generation of spontaneous activity. However, not only SA node cells contain these ion channels. Although the rate of automatic activity might be slower, spontaneous activity is also present in cells from the atrium, atrioventricular (AV) node, and Purkinje fibers. And even though ventricular cells might not be active, the machinery to generate spontaneous activity is present, albeit repressed by a high activity of I_{K1}.

The first study published on biopacemaking used the spontaneous activity already present. By injection of a plasmid carrying human β2-adrenergic receptor cDNA into the right atrium of mice, heart rate temporarily increased (Edelberg et al., 1998). Others have used the intrinsic capacity of ventricular cells to generate rhythm by increasing the level of cAMP in the cell by temporary overexpression of adenylyl cyclase VI (Ruhparwar et al., 2010). After injection of adenovirus containing the AC-VI gene in the left ventricle of pig, and after ablation of the AV node, all animals showed an escape rhythm coming from the left ventricle after rapid ventricular pacing and administration of isoprenalin, while, in control animals, right ventricular escape rhythms were observed. Maybe the most elegant way of using the cells' own ability to generate a rhythm so far has been to inhibit the cells own suppression on spontaneous activity, i.e., I_{K1}. Overexpression of a Kir2.1 dominant negative construct led to a 80% reduction in I_{K1} and spontaneous beating in cells originating from the left ventricle (Miake et al., 2002).

Another way to generate spontaneous activity is the introduction of depolarizing currents into normally quiescent cells. The most obvious target is I_f, as this current activates at potentials negative to -50 mV and this means the current is active at normal atrial and ventricular resting membrane potentials (Verkerk et al., 2007b).

This started when in 2001 Qu et al. overexpressed murine *HCN2* in spontaneously beating neonatal ventricular myocyte cell cultures, leading to a more regular and faster rhythm, due to diastolic phase 4 depolarization (Qu et al., 2001). In 2003, they described experiments in which they used this adenoviral construct in order to overexpress *HCN2* in the left atrial appendage in dog. Several days after subepicardial injection of the construct, dogs underwent vagal stimulation in order to suppress sinus rhythm. During vagal stimulation, all dogs injected with Ad-*mHCN2* showed spontaneous activity originating from the atrium, which was not seen in control dogs (Ad-GFP) (Qu et al., 2003). The introduction of a mutant *HCN2* channel in left ventricle by Bucchi et al. in dogs with permanent AV-block showed a

modest advantage of the mutant channel regarding response to catecholamines (Bucchi et al., 2006).
Since *HCN4* is the predominant isoform of I_f in the SA node, Boink et al. overexpressed this gene in rat cardiac myocytes using a lentiviral vector (Boink et al., 2008). In cell cultures, this led to an increase in beating rate, responsive to autonomic stimulation by cAMP.
A novel approach was used by Xiao et al who interfered in the microRNA pathway in order to overexpress *HCN2* and *HCN4* in vitro (Xiao & Sigg, 2007). MicroRNAs are small non-coding RNAs that bind to mRNA, thereby decreasing translation. *HCN2* and *HCN4* translation are regulated by miR-1 and miR-133. By masking the microRNA binding sites with gene specific oligodeoxynucleotides on *HCN2/HCN4* mRNA, protein expression of *HCN2* increased by 70% and *HCN4* by 45% in cultured ventricular myocytes, causing an increase in beating rate of monolayer culture.
As previously discussed, the synergistic effect of overexpression of I_{K1} and I_f leads to an increased beating rate in isolated guinea-pig ventricular cells compared to only overexpression of I_f, due to maintenance by I_{K1} of the voltage range wherein I_f can function optimally (Chan et al., 2009).
Other currents that can be considered are $I_{Ca,T}$, $I_{Ca,L}$, I_{NCX}, and I_{st}. Regarding $I_{Ca,T}$: as mentioned above, the different isoforms of $I_{Ca,T}$ show different activation kinetics, with Cav3.3 activating at potentials positive to -80 mV (McRory et al., 2001). This might make it useful in cells with a relatively depolarized resting membrane potential, but in ventricular cells with a stable resting membrane potential around -85 mV, the contribution might be negligible. The same is true for $I_{Ca,L}$, which activates at potential positive to -60 mV (Verheijck et al., 1999), but the advantage of this current is its sensitivity to β-adrenergic stimulation. Since the theory of the 'Ca^{2+} clock' states that spontaneous activity depends on spontaneous Ca^{2+} releases from the sarcoplasmic reticulum (Maltsev et al., 2006), it could be possible that overexpression of proteins involved in either sarcoplasmic Ca^{2+} loading (e.g., sarco/endoplasmic reticulum Ca^{2+}-ATPase - SERCA) or Ca^{2+} release (the Ryanodine receptor - RyR) increase spontaneous activity. *NCX1* transgene mice showed a 2,5-fold higher protein level of *NCX1* expression without alterations in SERCA, the Na^+/K^+ pump, phospholamban, and ryanodine receptor. This led to a 42% increase in *NCX1* current amplitude and a higher SR Ca^{2+} content, but no change in heart rate (Wang et al., 2009). A similar study using overexpression of *SERCA2A* also did not show an effect on basic heart rate or heart rate after isoproterenol (He et al., 1997). However, these studies were done in animals with normal SA node function. When it comes to I_{st}, there might be another problem. I_{st} seems to be a good candidate when it comes to activation kinetics. However, since the molecular background remains to be clarified, it is currently not a reasonable option.
While it might seem easiest to use one of the ion channels already present in SA node, it is, of course, also possible to modify existing proteins to generate a current suitable for biopacemaking. This can be done by making small adjustments, like using a modified *HCN2* channel with faster activation kinetics (Plotnikov et al., 2008), but bigger adjustments are also possible. By changing both kinetics and ion selectivity, Kashiwakura et al. turned the human Kv1.4 depolarization-activated K^+ channel into a hyperpolarization-activated, nonselective channel (Kashiwakura et al., 2006). Gene transfer to ventricular myocytes indeed initiated spontaneous activity.

5.2 Gene therapy, cell therapy, or both?

Most studies discussed so far have used adenovirus as the vector transferring the cDNA into the host cells (for a review on the use of viral vectors in cardiac therapy see Gray & Samulski, 2008). While adenovirus has advantages, e.g., high titers, the capability to transduce both dividing and non-dividing cells, and the capability to transfer large cDNA molecules, there are also downsides. Most importantly, it cannot be used for long-term expression, since the cDNA is not incorporated into the host genome. This might not make it useful for long-term expression, but the fast transgene expression makes it very useful for short-term proof-of-principle studies. Apart from the lack of genome incorporation, high immunogenicity also poses a big problem, especially since it is a common pathogen. Other viral vectors that can be used are adeno-associated virus vectors and lentiviral vectors. Advantages of adeno-associated virus are the capacity to transduce dividing and non-dividing cells, cardiac tropism of certain subtypes, its mild immunogenicity and relatively long-lasting expression. A major restriction is the limited size of 4.6 kb (Grieger & Samulski, 2005). By their larger packaging size, lower immunogenicity, and their capability to integrate their genome into the host genome, lentiviruses seem to evade the limitations of the other types of viral vectors. The integration of viral DNA within the host genome at the same time forms the chief concern: that of carcinogenicity.

To circumvent these obstacles, Potapova et al. used genetically engineered human mesenchymal stem cells (hMSCs) transfected with murine *HCN2* to deliver pacemaker current (Potapova et al., 2004). Since hMSCs lack necessary ion channels, they are not capable of generating an action potential themselves. However, they are capable of spreading the depolarizing current to connected cardiomyocytes, which may cause an action potential in these coupled myocytes. As anticipated, co-cultures with canine ventricular myocytes and hMSCs overexpressing *HCN2* showed a higher spontaneous beating rate and a less negative MDP than control cultures with hMSCs overexpressing EGFP. When injected into canine heart, *HCN2* overexpressing hMSCs induced a faster ventricular escape rhythm, mapped to the site of cell injection, than seen in controls.

While the hMSCs are not spontaneously active, one could also use spontaneously active embryonic stem cells (Kehat et al., 2004) or fetal cardiomyocytes (Ruhparwar et al., 2002). By transplanting fetal atrial and SA nodal myocytes in the left ventricle of dogs that later underwent AV node ablation, a ventricular escape rhythm originating from the transplantation site was seen. Transplanted cells could later be identified by dystrophin immunoreactivity because they were coming from wildtype dogs, while host dogs did not express dystrophin. Expression of connexin 43 between donor and host cells suggests not only survival, but also electrical integration. However, with cell therapy, carcinogenicity remains a risk. Apart from that, the duration of the effect is not certain, one can imagine that stem cells which are coupled to adult myocytes differentiate and would lose their ability to generate spontaneous action potentials.

5.3 Location

The site of biopacemaker creation has varied between the different studies, including atrium, the ventricular conduction system, and a distinct region in the left ventricular free wall; also a more generalized approach with pacemaker creation throughout the left ventricle was published. Placement of a biopacemaker in the atria has an important limitation in that it depends on intact AV-node function. Advantages are intact atrio-ventricular synchronization, the fact that atrial cells already show spontaneous activity, albeit at low frequency, and extensive innervation of the atria. This means only small modifications might be needed in order to generate a stably functioning biopacemaker sensitive to autonomic modulation. This advantage is shared by cells from the ventricular conduction system, while circumventing the disadvantage that normal AV node function is required. If the biopacemaker is placed relatively high in the conduction system, for instance the His bundle, this would also ensure a normal sequence of activation of the ventricles, maximizing cardiac output. So far, most studies have chosen injection of either cells or virus in the left ventricular free wall, probably because of the relatively easy access, especially relevant when using small animals.

5.4 Autonomic modulation

In the SA node, there is a heterogeneous response to sympathetic and parasympathetic stimulation. Due to this heterogeneous response, the SA node is capable of functioning within a wide range of heart rates. Since the cells with the lowest spontaneous rate are least sensitive to ACh, they serve as a back-up when the faster cells are made slower or even quiescent in the presence of ACh. The biopacemaker will most probably not be so heterogeneous, and for this reason it is of the utmost importance that it is not too sensitive to parasympathetic stimulation. As discussed in a review by Opthof, this makes I_f an appropriate target (Opthof, 2007), since it is mainly the opening of $I_{K,Ach}$ that decelerates rate and not a decrease in I_f during parasympathetic stimulation.

While sensitivity to parasympathetic stimulation should be limited, the great advantage of the biopacemaker should be its ability to increase rate upon physical or emotional stress.

6. Conclusion

As discussed in this chapter, the electrophysiology and anatomy or the SA node are complex. Therefore, it is not feasible to create a biopacemaker with all features of a native pacemaker. The most important issue for the creation of a biopacemaker is, that by adding an inward, or by reducing an outward current, working myocytes will be capable of stable action potential formation and propagation to the ventricles. While various approaches have been tried, so far a long-living biopacemaker suitable for clinical use, has not been developed. Further studies are required.

7. Reference

Abbott, G.W. et al. (1999). MiRP1 forms IKr potassium channels with HERG and is associated with cardiac arrhythmia. Cell, 97, 2, 175-187,

Accili, E.A. et al. (1997). Differential control of the hyperpolarization-activated current (i(f)) by cAMP gating and phosphatase inhibition in rabbit sino-atrial node myocytes. J. Physiol, 500 (Pt 3), 643-651,

Aimond, F. et al. (2005). Accessory Kvbeta1 subunits differentially modulate the functional expression of voltage-gated K+ channels in mouse ventricular myocytes. Circ. Res., 96, 4, 451-458,

Altomare, C. et al. (2003). Heteromeric HCN1-HCN4 channels: a comparison with native pacemaker channels from the rabbit sinoatrial node. J. Physiol, 549, Pt 2, 347-359,

Arechiga-Figueroa, I.A. et al. (2010). Multiple effects of 4-aminopyridine on feline and rabbit sinoatrial node myocytes and multicellular preparations. Pflugers Arch., 459, 3, 345-355,

Attwell, D. et al. (1979). The steady state TTX-sensitive ("window") sodium current in cardiac Purkinje fibres. Pflugers Arch., 379, 2, 137-142,

Balser, J.R. et al. (1990). Time-dependent outward current in guinea pig ventricular myocytes. Gating kinetics of the delayed rectifier. J. Gen. Physiol, 96, 4, 835-863,

Barbuti, A. et al. (2004). Localization of pacemaker channels in lipid rafts regulates channel kinetics. Circ. Res., 94, 10, 1325-1331,

Barhanin, J. et al. (1996). K(V)LQT1 and lsK (minK) proteins associate to form the I(Ks) cardiac potassium current. Nature, 384, 6604, 78-80,

Baruscotti, M. et al. (2005). Physiology and pharmacology of the cardiac pacemaker ("funny") current. Pharmacol. Ther., 107, 1, 59-79,

Baruscotti, M. et al. (2000). Na(+) current contribution to the diastolic depolarization in newborn rabbit SA node cells. Am. J. Physiol Heart Circ. Physiol, 279, 5, H2303-H2309,

Bean, B.P. (1985). Two kinds of calcium channels in canine atrial cells. Differences in kinetics, selectivity, and pharmacology. J. Gen. Physiol, 86, 1, 1-30,

Benitah, J.P. et al. (2010). L-type Ca(2+) current in ventricular cardiomyocytes. J. Mol. Cell Cardiol., 48, 1, 26-36,

Benson, D.W. et al. (2003). Congenital sick sinus syndrome caused by recessive mutations in the cardiac sodium channel gene (SCN5A). J. Clin. Invest, 112, 7, 1019-1028,

Bichet, D. et al. (2000). The I-II loop of the Ca2+ channel alpha1 subunit contains an endoplasmic reticulum retention signal antagonized by the beta subunit. Neuron, 25, 1, 177-190,

Blaustein, M.P. & Lederer, W.J. (1999). Sodium/calcium exchange: its physiological implications. Physiol Rev., 79, 3, 763-854,

Bohn, G. et al. (2000). Expression of T- and L-type calcium channel mRNA in murine sinoatrial node. FEBS Lett., 481, 1, 73-76,

Boink, G.J. et al. (2008). Engineering physiologically controlled pacemaker cells with lentiviral HCN4 gene transfer. J. Gene Med., 10, 5, 487-497,

Boyett, M.R. et al. (2000). The sinoatrial node, a heterogeneous pacemaker structure. Cardiovasc. Res., 47, 4, 658-687,

Boyle, W.A. & Nerbonne, J.M. (1991). A novel type of depolarization-activated K+ current in isolated adult rat atrial myocytes. Am. J. Physiol, 260, 4 Pt 2, H1236-H1247,

Brioschi, C. et al. (2009). Distribution of the pacemaker HCN4 channel mRNA and protein in the rabbit sinoatrial node. J. Mol. Cell Cardiol., 47, 2, 221-227,

Brown, H. et al. (1979). Cardiac pacemaker oscillation and its modulation by autonomic transmitters. J. Exp. Biol., 81, 175-204,

Bucchi, A. et al. (2006). Wild-type and mutant HCN channels in a tandem biological-electronic cardiac pacemaker. Circulation, 114, 10, 992-999,

Camelliti, P. et al. (2004). Fibroblast network in rabbit sinoatrial node: structural and functional identification of homogeneous and heterogeneous cell coupling. Circ. Res., 94, 6, 828-835,

Chan, Y.C. et al. (2009). Synergistic effects of inward rectifier (I) and pacemaker (I) currents on the induction of bioengineered cardiac automaticity. J. Cardiovasc. Electrophysiol., 20, 9, 1048-1054,

Chandler, N.J. et al. (2009). Molecular architecture of the human sinus node: insights into the function of the cardiac pacemaker. Circulation, 119, 12, 1562-1575,

Chen, C.C. et al. (2003). Abnormal coronary function in mice deficient in alpha1H T-type Ca2+ channels. Science, 302, 5649, 1416-1418,

Cho, H.S. et al. (2003). The electrophysiological properties of spontaneously beating pacemaker cells isolated from mouse sinoatrial node. J. Physiol, 550, Pt 1, 169-180,

Choate, J.K. et al. (1993). Effects of sympathetic nerve stimulation on the sino-atrial node of the guinea-pig. J. Physiol, 471, 707-727,

Clark, R.B. et al. (2004). A rapidly activating delayed rectifier K+ current regulates pacemaker activity in adult mouse sinoatrial node cells. Am. J. Physiol Heart Circ. Physiol, 286, 5, H1757-H1766,

Colecraft, H.M. et al. (2002). Novel functional properties of Ca(2+) channel beta subunits revealed by their expression in adult rat heart cells. J. Physiol, 541, Pt 2, 435-452,

Cui, J. et al. (2000). Cyclic AMP regulates the HERG K(+) channel by dual pathways. Curr. Biol., 10, 11, 671-674,

Curran, M.E. et al. (1995). A molecular basis for cardiac arrhythmia: HERG mutations cause long QT syndrome. Cell, 80, 5, 795-803,

De Jongh, K.S. et al. (1990). Subunits of purified calcium channels. Alpha 2 and delta are encoded by the same gene. J. Biol. Chem., 265, 25, 14738-14741,

De Maziere, A.M. et al. (1992). Spatial and functional relationship between myocytes and fibroblasts in the rabbit sinoatrial node. J. Mol. Cell Cardiol., 24, 6, 567-578,

Decher, N. et al. (2003). KCNE2 modulates current amplitudes and activation kinetics of HCN4: influence of KCNE family members on HCN4 currents. Pflugers Arch., 446, 6, 633-640,

Devic, E. et al. (2001). Beta-adrenergic receptor subtype-specific signaling in cardiac myocytes from beta(1) and beta(2) adrenoceptor knockout mice. Mol. Pharmacol., 60, 3, 577-583,

Dobrzynski, H. et al. (2007). New insights into pacemaker activity: promoting understanding of sick sinus syndrome. Circulation, 115, 14, 1921-1932,

Dobrzynski, H. et al. (2001). Distribution of the muscarinic K+ channel proteins Kir3.1 and Kir3.4 in the ventricle, atrium, and sinoatrial node of heart. J. Histochem. Cytochem., 49, 10, 1221-1234,

Dobrzynski, H. et al. (2000). Presence of the Kv1.5 K(+) channel in the sinoatrial node. J. Histochem. Cytochem., 48, 6, 769-780,

Edelberg, J.M. et al. (1998). Enhancement of murine cardiac chronotropy by the molecular transfer of the human beta2 adrenergic receptor cDNA. J. Clin. Invest, 101, 2, 337-343,

Foell, J.D. et al. (2004). Molecular heterogeneity of calcium channel beta-subunits in canine and human heart: evidence for differential subcellular localization. Physiol Genomics, 17, 2, 183-200,

Fukuzaki, K. et al. (2008). Role of sarcolemmal ATP-sensitive K+ channels in the regulation of sinoatrial node automaticity: an evaluation using Kir6.2-deficient mice. J. Physiol, 586, Pt 11, 2767-2778,

Gao, T. et al. (1997). Identification and subcellular localization of the subunits of L-type calcium channels and adenylyl cyclase in cardiac myocytes. J. Biol. Chem., 272, 31, 19401-19407,

Giles, W.R. & van Ginneken, A.C. (1985). A transient outward current in isolated cells from the crista terminalis of rabbit heart. J. Physiol, 368, 243-264,

Gray, S.J. & Samulski, R.J. (2008). Optimizing gene delivery vectors for the treatment of heart disease. Expert. Opin. Biol. Ther., 8, 7, 911-922,

Grieger, J.C. & Samulski, R.J. (2005). Packaging capacity of adeno-associated virus serotypes: impact of larger genomes on infectivity and postentry steps. J. Virol., 79, 15, 9933-9944,

Guo, J. et al. (1995). A sustained inward current activated at the diastolic potential range in rabbit sino-atrial node cells. J. Physiol, 483 (Pt 1), 1-13,

Haapalahti, P. et al. (2006). Ventricular repolarization and heart rate responses during cardiovascular autonomic function testing in LQT1 subtype of long QT syndrome. Pacing Clin. Electrophysiol., 29, 10, 1122-1129,

Haase, H. et al. (1993). Phosphorylation of the L-type calcium channel beta subunit is involved in beta-adrenergic signal transduction in canine myocardium. FEBS Lett., 335, 2, 217-222,

Hagiwara, N. et al. (1988). Contribution of two types of calcium currents to the pacemaker potentials of rabbit sino-atrial node cells. J. Physiol, 395, 233-253,

Hagiwara, N. et al. (1992). Background current in sino-atrial node cells of the rabbit heart. J. Physiol, 448, 53-72,

Han, X. et al. (1996). Identification and properties of an ATP-sensitive K+ current in rabbit sino-atrial node pacemaker cells. J. Physiol, 490 (Pt 2), 337-350,

Haufe, V. et al. (2005). Contribution of neuronal sodium channels to the cardiac fast sodium current INa is greater in dog heart Purkinje fibers than in ventricles. Cardiovasc. Res., 65, 1, 117-127,

He, H. et al. (1997). Overexpression of the rat sarcoplasmic reticulum Ca2+ ATPase gene in the heart of transgenic mice accelerates calcium transients and cardiac relaxation. J. Clin. Invest, 100, 2, 380-389,

Hedberg, A. et al. (1980). Differential distribution of beta-1 and beta-2 adrenergic receptors in cat and guinea-pig heart. J. Pharmacol. Exp. Ther., 212, 3, 503-508,

Hibino, H. et al. (2010). Inwardly rectifying potassium channels: their structure, function, and physiological roles. Physiol Rev., 90, 1, 291-366,

Honjo, H. et al. (1996). Correlation between electrical activity and the size of rabbit sino-atrial node cells. J. Physiol, 496 (Pt 3), 795-808,

Huang, J. et al. (2008). Novel mechanism for suppression of hyperpolarization-activated cyclic nucleotide-gated pacemaker channels by receptor-like tyrosine phosphatase-alpha. J. Biol. Chem., 283, 44, 29912-29919,

Huser, J. et al. (2000). Intracellular Ca2+ release contributes to automaticity in cat atrial pacemaker cells. J. Physiol, 524 Pt 2, 415-422,

Irisawa, H. et al. (1993). Cardiac pacemaking in the sinoatrial node. Physiol Rev., 73, 1, 197-227,

Isom, L.L. et al. (1992). Primary structure and functional expression of the beta 1 subunit of the rat brain sodium channel. Science, 256, 5058, 839-842,

Isom, L.L. et al. (1995). Structure and function of the beta 2 subunit of brain sodium channels, a transmembrane glycoprotein with a CAM motif. Cell, 83, 3, 433-442,

Jackson, H.A. et al. (2007). Evolution and structural diversification of hyperpolarization-activated cyclic nucleotide-gated channel genes. Physiol Genomics, 29, 3, 231-245,

James, T.N. (2002). Structure and function of the sinus node, AV node and His bundle of the human heart: part I-structure. Prog. Cardiovasc. Dis., 45, 3, 235-267,

Joyner, R.W. & van Capelle, F.J. (1986). Propagation through electrically coupled cells. How a small SA node drives a large atrium. Biophys. J., 50, 6, 1157-1164,

Jurkiewicz, N.K. & Sanguinetti, M.C. (1993). Rate-dependent prolongation of cardiac action potentials by a methanesulfonanilide class III antiarrhythmic agent. Specific block of rapidly activating delayed rectifier K+ current by dofetilide. Circ. Res., 72, 1, 75-83,

Kashiwakura, Y. et al. (2006). Gene transfer of a synthetic pacemaker channel into the heart: a novel strategy for biological pacing. Circulation, 114, 16, 1682-1686,

Kehat, I. et al. (2004). Electromechanical integration of cardiomyocytes derived from human embryonic stem cells. Nat. Biotechnol., 22, 10, 1282-1289,

Keith, A. & Flack, M. (1907). The Form and Nature of the Muscular Connections between the Primary Divisions of the Vertebrate Heart. J. Anat. Physiol, 41, Pt 3, 172-189,

Knollmann, B.C. et al. (2004). Isoproterenol exacerbates a long QT phenotype in Kcnq1-deficient neonatal mice: possible roles for human-like Kcnq1 isoform 1 and slow delayed rectifier K+ current. J. Pharmacol. Exp. Ther., 310, 1, 311-318,

Kodama, I. et al. (1996). Regional differences in the response of the isolated sino-atrial node of the rabbit to vagal stimulation. J. Physiol, 495 (Pt 3), 785-801,

Kohl, P. et al. (2005). Electrical coupling of fibroblasts and myocytes: relevance for cardiac propagation. J. Electrocardiol., 38, 4 Suppl, 45-50,

Kohl, P. et al. (1994). Mechanosensitive fibroblasts in the sino-atrial node region of rat heart: interaction with cardiomyocytes and possible role. Exp. Physiol, 79, 6, 943-956,

Kreitner, D. (1975). Evidence for the existence of a rapid sodium channel in the membrane of rabbit sinoatrial cells. J. Mol. Cell Cardiol., 7, 9, 655-662,

Kuo, H.C. et al. (2001). A defect in the Kv channel-interacting protein 2 (KChIP2) gene leads to a complete loss of I(to) and confers susceptibility to ventricular tachycardia. Cell, 107, 6, 801-813,

Kurokawa, J. et al. (2003). Requirement of subunit expression for cAMP-mediated regulation of a heart potassium channel. Proc. Natl. Acad. Sci. U. S. A, 100, 4, 2122-2127,

Lakatta, E.G. & DiFrancesco, D. (2009). What keeps us ticking: a funny current, a calcium clock, or both? J. Mol. Cell Cardiol., 47, 2, 157-170,

Lakatta, E.G. et al. (2010). A coupled SYSTEM of intracellular Ca2+ clocks and surface membrane voltage clocks controls the timekeeping mechanism of the heart's pacemaker. Circ. Res., 106, 4, 659-673,

Lees-Miller, J.P. et al. (2003). Selective knockout of mouse ERG1 B potassium channel eliminates I(Kr) in adult ventricular myocytes and elicits episodes of abrupt sinus bradycardia. Mol. Cell Biol., 23, 6, 1856-1862,

Lei, M. & Brown, H.F. (1996). Two components of the delayed rectifier potassium current, IK, in rabbit sino-atrial node cells. Exp. Physiol, 81, 5, 725-741,

Lei, M. et al. (2002). Role of the 293b-sensitive, slowly activating delayed rectifier potassium current, i(Ks), in pacemaker activity of rabbit isolated sino-atrial node cells. Cardiovasc. Res., 53, 1, 68-79,

Lei, M. et al. (2005). Sinus node dysfunction following targeted disruption of the murine cardiac sodium channel gene Scn5a. J. Physiol, 567, Pt 2, 387-400,

Lei, M. et al. (2000). Characterisation of the transient outward K+ current in rabbit sinoatrial node cells. Cardiovasc. Res., 46, 3, 433-441,

Lei, M. et al. (2004). Requirement of neuronal- and cardiac-type sodium channels for murine sinoatrial node pacemaking. J. Physiol, 559, Pt 3, 835-848,

Levy, M.N. (1971). Sympathetic-parasympathetic interactions in the heart. Circ. Res., 29, 5, 437-445,

Li, G.R. et al. (2003). Calcium-activated transient outward chloride current and phase 1 repolarization of swine ventricular action potential. Cardiovasc. Res., 58, 1, 89-98,

Li, G.R. et al. (1996). Evidence for two components of delayed rectifier K+ current in human ventricular myocytes. Circ. Res., 78, 4, 689-696,

Lin, J.W. et al. (1998). Yotiao, a novel protein of neuromuscular junction and brain that interacts with specific splice variants of NMDA receptor subunit NR1. J. Neurosci., 18, 6, 2017-2027,

Liu, D.W. et al. (1993). Ionic bases for electrophysiological distinctions among epicardial, midmyocardial, and endocardial myocytes from the free wall of the canine left ventricle. Circ. Res., 72, 3, 671-687,

Lopatin, A.N. et al. (1994). Potassium channel block by cytoplasmic polyamines as the mechanism of intrinsic rectification. Nature, 372, 6504, 366-369,

Ludwig, A. et al. (1998). A family of hyperpolarization-activated mammalian cation channels. Nature, 393, 6685, 587-591,

Mackaay, A.J. et al. (1980). Interaction of adrenaline and acetylcholine on cardiac pacemaker function. Functional inhomogeneity of the rabbit sinus node. J. Pharmacol. Exp. Ther., 214, 2, 417-422,

Maier, S.K. et al. (2003). An unexpected requirement for brain-type sodium channels for control of heart rate in the mouse sinoatrial node. Proc. Natl. Acad. Sci. U. S. A, 100, 6, 3507-3512,

Maltsev, V.A. et al. (2006). The emergence of a general theory of the initiation and strength of the heartbeat. J. Pharmacol. Sci., 100, 5, 338-369,

Mangoni, M.E. et al. (2003). Functional role of L-type Cav1.3 Ca2+ channels in cardiac pacemaker activity. Proc. Natl. Acad. Sci. U. S. A, 100, 9, 5543-5548,

Mangoni, M.E. & Nargeot, J. (2008). Genesis and regulation of the heart automaticity. Physiol Rev., 88, 3, 919-982,

Mangoni, M.E. et al. (2006). Bradycardia and slowing of the atrioventricular conduction in mice lacking CaV3.1/alpha1G T-type calcium channels. Circ. Res., 98, 11, 1422-1430,

Marionneau, C. et al. (2005). Specific pattern of ionic channel gene expression associated with pacemaker activity in the mouse heart. J. Physiol, 562, Pt 1, 223-234,

Marx, S.O. et al. (2002). Requirement of a macromolecular signaling complex for beta adrenergic receptor modulation of the KCNQ1-KCNE1 potassium channel. Science, 295, 5554, 496-499,

Matsuda, H. et al. (1987). Ohmic conductance through the inwardly rectifying K channel and blocking by internal Mg2+. Nature, 325, 7000, 156-159,
Matsuura, H. et al. (2002). Rapidly and slowly activating components of delayed rectifier K(+) current in guinea-pig sino-atrial node pacemaker cells. J. Physiol, 540, Pt 3, 815-830,
McLerie, M. & Lopatin, A.N. (2003). Dominant-negative suppression of I(K1) in the mouse heart leads to altered cardiac excitability. J. Mol. Cell Cardiol., 35, 4, 367-378,
McRory, J.E. et al. (2001). Molecular and functional characterization of a family of rat brain T-type calcium channels. J. Biol. Chem., 276, 6, 3999-4011,
Miake, J. et al. (2002). Biological pacemaker created by gene transfer. Nature, 419, 6903, 132-133,
Mitsuiye, T. et al. (2000). Sustained inward current during pacemaker depolarization in mammalian sinoatrial node cells. Circ. Res., 87, 2, 88-91,
Morgan, K. et al. (2000). beta 3: an additional auxiliary subunit of the voltage-sensitive sodium channel that modulates channel gating with distinct kinetics. Proc. Natl. Acad. Sci. U. S. A, 97, 5, 2308-2313,
Muramatsu, H. et al. (1996). Characterization of a TTX-sensitive Na+ current in pacemaker cells isolated from rabbit sinoatrial node. Am. J. Physiol, 270, 6 Pt 2, H2108-H2119,
Nerbonne, J.M. (2000). Molecular basis of functional voltage-gated K+ channel diversity in the mammalian myocardium. J. Physiol, 525 Pt 2, 285-298,
Nerbonne, J.M. & Kass, R.S. (2005). Molecular physiology of cardiac repolarization. Physiol Rev., 85, 4, 1205-1253,
Nikmaram, M.R. et al. (2008). Characterization of the effects of ryanodine, TTX, E-4031 and 4-AP on the sinoatrial and atrioventricular nodes. Prog. Biophys. Mol. Biol., 96, 1-3, 452-464,
Noble, D. & Tsien, R.W. (1968). The kinetics and rectifier properties of the slow potassium current in cardiac Purkinje fibres. J. Physiol, 195, 1, 185-214,
Noma, A. & Irisawa, H. (1974). Electrogenic sodium pump in rabbit sinoatrial node cell. Pflugers Arch., 351, 2, 177-182,
Noma, A. & Irisawa, H. (1975). Contribution of an electrogenic sodium pump to the membrane potential in rabbit sinoatrial node cells. Pflugers Arch., 358, 4, 289-301,
Noma, A. & Irisawa, H. (1976). A time- and voltage-dependent potassium current in the rabbit sinoatrial node cell. Pflugers Arch., 366, 2-3, 251-258,
Noma, A. & Trautwein, W. (1978). Relaxation of the ACh-induced potassium current in the rabbit sinoatrial node cell. Pflugers Arch., 377, 3, 193-200,
Ono, K. & Ito, H. (1995). Role of rapidly activating delayed rectifier K+ current in sinoatrial node pacemaker activity. Am. J. Physiol, 269, 2 Pt 2, H453-H462,
Ono, K. et al. (2000). Properties of the delayed rectifier potassium current in porcine sino-atrial node cells. J. Physiol, 524, Pt 1, 51-62,
Oosthoek, P.W. et al. (1993). Immunohistochemical delineation of the conduction system. I: The sinoatrial node. Circ. Res., 73, 3, 473-481,
Opthof, T. (2007). Embryological development of pacemaker hierarchy and membrane currents related to the function of the adult sinus node: implications for autonomic modulation of biopacemakers. Med. Biol. Eng Comput., 45, 2, 119-132,
Opthof, T. (1988). The mammalian sinoatrial node. Cardiovasc. Drugs Ther., 1, 6, 573-597,

Opthof, T. (2000). The normal range and determinants of the intrinsic heart rate in man. Cardiovasc. Res., 45, 1, 177-184,

Papadatos, G.A. et al. (2002). Slowed conduction and ventricular tachycardia after targeted disruption of the cardiac sodium channel gene Scn5a. Proc. Natl. Acad. Sci. U. S. A, 99, 9, 6210-6215,

Perez-Reyes, E. (1999). Three for T: molecular analysis of the low voltage-activated calcium channel family. Cell Mol. Life Sci., 56, 7-8, 660-669,

Peroz, D. et al. (2009). LQT1-associated mutations increase KCNQ1 proteasomal degradation independently of Derlin-1. J. Biol. Chem., 284, 8, 5250-5256,

Plaster, N.M. et al. (2001). Mutations in Kir2.1 cause the developmental and episodic electrical phenotypes of Andersen's syndrome. Cell, 105, 4, 511-519,

Plotnikov, A.N. et al. (2008). HCN212-channel biological pacemakers manifesting ventricular tachyarrhythmias are responsive to treatment with I(f) blockade. Heart Rhythm., 5, 2, 282-288,

Potapova, I. et al. (2004). Human mesenchymal stem cells as a gene delivery system to create cardiac pacemakers. Circ. Res., 94, 7, 952-959,

Protas, L. et al. (2010). Age-dependent changes in Na current magnitude and TTX-sensitivity in the canine sinoatrial node. J. Mol. Cell Cardiol., 48, 1, 172-180,

Qu, J. et al. (2002). Functional comparison of HCN isoforms expressed in ventricular and HEK 293 cells. Pflugers Arch., 444, 5, 597-601,

Qu, J. et al. (2001). HCN2 overexpression in newborn and adult ventricular myocytes: distinct effects on gating and excitability. Circ. Res., 89, 1, E8-14,

Qu, J. et al. (2003). Expression and function of a biological pacemaker in canine heart. Circulation, 107, 8, 1106-1109,

Radicke, S. et al. (2005). Expression and function of dipeptidyl-aminopeptidase-like protein 6 as a putative beta-subunit of human cardiac transient outward current encoded by Kv4.3. J. Physiol, 565, Pt 3, 751-756,

Ridley, J.M. et al. (2003). Inhibition of HERG K+ current and prolongation of the guinea-pig ventricular action potential by 4-aminopyridine. J. Physiol, 549, Pt 3, 667-672,

Roepke, T.K. et al. (2008). Targeted deletion of kcne2 impairs ventricular repolarization via disruption of I(K,slow1) and I(to,f). FASEB J., 22, 10, 3648-3660,

Ruhparwar, A. et al. (2010). Adenylate-Cyclase VI transforms ventricular cardiomyocytes into biological pacemaker cells. Tissue Eng Part A, 16, 6, 1867-1872,

Ruhparwar, A. et al. (2002). Transplanted fetal cardiomyocytes as cardiac pacemaker. Eur. J. Cardiothorac. Surg., 21, 5, 853-857,

Sakai, R. et al. (1996). Sodium--potassium pump current in rabbit sino-atrial node cells. J. Physiol, 490 (Pt 1), 51-62,

Sanguinetti, M.C. et al. (1996). Coassembly of K(V)LQT1 and minK (IsK) proteins to form cardiac I(Ks) potassium channel. Nature, 384, 6604, 80-83,

Sanguinetti, M.C. et al. (1995). A mechanistic link between an inherited and an acquired cardiac arrhythmia: HERG encodes the IKr potassium channel. Cell, 81, 2, 299-307,

Sanguinetti, M.C. & Jurkiewicz, N.K. (1990). Two components of cardiac delayed rectifier K+ current. Differential sensitivity to block by class III antiarrhythmic agents. J. Gen. Physiol, 96, 1, 195-215,

Sanguinetti, M.C. et al. (1991). Isoproterenol antagonizes prolongation of refractory period by the class III antiarrhythmic agent E-4031 in guinea pig myocytes. Mechanism of action. Circ. Res., 68, 1, 77-84,

Satoh, H. (2003). Taurine on sino-atrial nodal cells: Ca2+-dependent modulation. Adv. Exp. Med. Biol., 526, 17-23,

Shinagawa, Y. et al. (2000). The sustained inward current and inward rectifier K+ current in pacemaker cells dissociated from rat sinoatrial node. J. Physiol, 523 Pt 3, 593-605,

Singer, D. et al. (1991). The roles of the subunits in the function of the calcium channel. Science, 253, 5027, 1553-1557,

Stieber, J. et al. (2004). Pacemaker channels and sinus node arrhythmia. Trends Cardiovasc. Med., 14, 1, 23-28,

Takumi, T. et al. (1988). Cloning of a membrane protein that induces a slow voltage-gated potassium current. Science, 242, 4881, 1042-1045,

Tan, H.L. et al. (2003). Genetic control of sodium channel function. Cardiovasc. Res., 57, 4, 961-973,

Tanaka, H. et al. (2008). Species difference in the contribution of T-type calcium current to cardiac pacemaking as revealed by r(-)-efonidipine. J. Pharmacol. Sci., 107, 1, 99-102,

ten Velde, I. et al. (1995). Spatial distribution of connexin43, the major cardiac gap junction protein, visualizes the cellular network for impulse propagation from sinoatrial node to atrium. Circ. Res., 76, 5, 802-811,

Thompson, S.H. (1977). Three pharmacologically distinct potassium channels in molluscan neurones. J. Physiol, 265, 2, 465-488,

Toyoda, F. et al. (2005). Responses of the sustained inward current to autonomic agonists in guinea-pig sino-atrial node pacemaker cells. Br. J. Pharmacol., 144, 5, 660-668,

Ulens, C. & Tytgat, J. (2001). Functional heteromerization of HCN1 and HCN2 pacemaker channels. J. Biol. Chem., 276, 9, 6069-6072,

van Ginneken, A.C. & Giles, W. (1991). Voltage clamp measurements of the hyperpolarization-activated inward current I(f) in single cells from rabbit sino-atrial node. J. Physiol, 434, 57-83,

Vassort, G. & Alvarez, J. (1994). Cardiac T-type calcium current: pharmacology and roles in cardiac tissues. J. Cardiovasc. Electrophysiol., 5, 4, 376-393,

Veenstra, R.D. et al. (1992). Multiple connexins confer distinct regulatory and conductance properties of gap junctions in developing heart. Circ. Res., 71, 5, 1277-1283,

Veldkamp, M.W. et al. (2003). Contribution of sodium channel mutations to bradycardia and sinus node dysfunction in LQT3 families. Circ. Res., 92, 9, 976-983,

Verheijck, E.E. et al. (1995). Effects of delayed rectifier current blockade by E-4031 on impulse generation in single sinoatrial nodal myocytes of the rabbit. Circ. Res., 76, 4, 607-615,

Verheijck, E.E. et al. (1999). Contribution of L-type Ca2+ current to electrical activity in sinoatrial nodal myocytes of rabbits. Am. J. Physiol, 276, 3 Pt 2, H1064-H1077,

Verheijck, E.E. et al. (2002). Atrio-sinus interaction demonstrated by blockade of the rapid delayed rectifier current. Circulation, 105, 7, 880-885,

Verheijck, E.E. et al. (1998). Pacemaker synchronization of electrically coupled rabbit sinoatrial node cells. J. Gen. Physiol, 111, 1, 95-112,

Verkerk, A.O. et al. (2007a). Single cells isolated from human sinoatrial node: action potentials and numerical reconstruction of pacemaker current. Conf. Proc. IEEE Eng Med. Biol. Soc., 2007, 904-907,

Verkerk, A.O. & van Ginneken, A.C. (2001). Considerations in studying the transient outward K(+) current in cells exhibiting the hyperpolarization-activated current. Cardiovasc. Res., 52, 3, 517-520,

Verkerk, A.O. et al. (2009a). Pacemaker activity of the human sinoatrial node: role of the hyperpolarization-activated current, I(f). Int. J. Cardiol., 132, 3, 318-336,

Verkerk, A.O. et al. (2003). Ionic remodeling of sinoatrial node cells by heart failure. Circulation, 108, 6, 760-766,

Verkerk, A.O. et al. (2007b). Pacemaker current (I(f)) in the human sinoatrial node. Eur. Heart J., 28, 20, 2472-2478,

Verkerk, A.O. et al. (2009b). Is sodium current present in human sinoatrial node cells? Int. J. Biol. Sci., 5, 2, 201-204,

Vinogradova, T.M. et al. (2004). Rhythmic ryanodine receptor Ca2+ releases during diastolic depolarization of sinoatrial pacemaker cells do not require membrane depolarization. Circ. Res., 94, 6, 802-809,

Wainger, B.J. et al. (2001). Molecular mechanism of cAMP modulation of HCN pacemaker channels. Nature, 411, 6839, 805-810,

Walsh, K.B. & Kass, R.S. (1988). Regulation of a heart potassium channel by protein kinase A and C. Science, 242, 4875, 67-69,

Wang, J. et al. (2009). Induced overexpression of Na+/Ca2+ exchanger transgene: altered myocyte contractility, [Ca2+]i transients, SR Ca2+ contents, and action potential duration. Am. J. Physiol Heart Circ. Physiol, 297, 2, H590-H601,

Wilders, R. et al. (1996). Model clamp and its application to synchronization of rabbit sinoatrial node cells. Am. J. Physiol, 271, 5 Pt 2, H2168-H2182,

Winslow, R.L. & Varghese, A. (1995). Modeling the Functional Role of SA Node - Atrial Interdigitation. 649-652,

Wu, J. et al. (2008). Sinus node dysfunction in ATX-II-induced in-vitro murine model of long QT3 syndrome and rescue effect of ranolazine. Prog. Biophys. Mol. Biol., 98, 2-3, 198-207,

Xiao, R.P. et al. (1999). Recent advances in cardiac beta(2)-adrenergic signal transduction. Circ. Res., 85, 11, 1092-1100,

Xiao, Y.F. & Sigg, D.C. (2007). Biological approaches to generating cardiac biopacemaker for bradycardia. Sheng Li Xue. Bao., 59, 5, 562-570,

Xu, W. & Lipscombe, D. (2001). Neuronal Ca(V)1.3alpha(1) L-type channels activate at relatively hyperpolarized membrane potentials and are incompletely inhibited by dihydropyridines. J. Neurosci., 21, 16, 5944-5951,

Xue, T. et al. (2002). Dominant-negative suppression of. Circ. Res., 90, 12, 1267-1273,

Yang, J. et al. (1993). Molecular determinants of Ca2+ selectivity and ion permeation in L-type Ca2+ channels. Nature, 366, 6451, 158-161,

Yu, F.H. et al. (2003). Sodium channel beta4, a new disulfide-linked auxiliary subunit with similarity to beta2. J. Neurosci., 23, 20, 7577-7585,

Zaritsky, J.J. et al. (2001). The consequences of disrupting cardiac inwardly rectifying K(+) current (I(K1)) as revealed by the targeted deletion of the murine Kir2.1 and Kir2.2 genes. J. Physiol, 533, Pt 3, 697-710,

Zhang, H. et al. (2001a). Gradient model versus mosaic model of the sinoatrial node. Circulation, 103, 4, 584-588,

Zhang, H. et al. (2002a). Sustained inward current and pacemaker activity of mammalian sinoatrial node. J. Cardiovasc. Electrophysiol., 13, 8, 809-812,

Zhang, M. et al. (2001b). minK-related peptide 1 associates with Kv4.2 and modulates its gating function: potential role as beta subunit of cardiac transient outward channel? Circ. Res., 88, 10, 1012-1019,

Zhang, Z. et al. (2002b). Functional Roles of Ca(v)1.3 (alpha(1D)) calcium channel in sinoatrial nodes: insight gained using gene-targeted null mutant mice. Circ. Res., 90, 9, 981-987,

Zhou, Z. & Lipsius, S.L. (1993). Na(+)-Ca2+ exchange current in latent pacemaker cells isolated from cat right atrium. J. Physiol, 466, 263-285,

29

Advances in Research on Pacemaking Function of Interstitial Cell of Cajal in Gastrointestinal Tract

Wen Xie Xu
Department of Physiology, Shanghai Jiaotong University School of Medicine, Shanghai, 200240, China

1. Introduction

Most visceral smooth muscles, especially gastrointestinal (GI) smooth muscle, display spontaneous rhythmic contractions in the absence of neuronal or hormonal stimulation, which are associated with their physiological functions. The contractile behavior of gastrointestinal (GI) smooth muscles depends to a considerable extent on the intrinsic electrical activities of the muscles. This is particularly true of the phasic portions of the GI tract where cyclic depolarizations and repolarizations, referred to as slow waves, determine contractile frequency and maintain the phasic nature of contractions. Slow waves are of great functional importance because they determine the rate and timing of GI smooth muscle activity, and their impairment is likely to cause various motility disorders.

GI smooth muscles exhibit a wide range of electrical behaviors (Szurszewski, 1987), and understanding the mechanisms of these events has been the goal of physiologists for more than half a century. Electrical activity can vary from slow changes in membrane potential, to hyperpolarization and depolarization responses to neurotransmitters, to oscillatory slow wave activity, to fast Ca^{2+} action potentials. All this behavior can be recorded during impalements of a single smooth muscle cell, which suggests that a plethora of ionic conductances and regulatory mechanisms are at play in GI muscles. Such diversity is almost unprecedented in other excitable cells. Diversity, the small size of smooth muscle cells, and the structural complexities of GI muscles have slowed progress toward understanding the ionic basis for electrical rhythmicity. The electrical output of GI muscles is a product of contributions from two electrically coupled cell types, smooth muscle cells and interstitial cells of Cajal (ICC) (Sanders,1996). These cells have distinct electrical missions and express different types of ionic conductances to accomplish those tasks. ICC generate slow waves and conduct them into adjacent smooth muscle cells to generate spontaneous contractions (Sanders, 1996; Thuneberg et al, 1982; Huizinga et al, 1995; Koh et al, 1998; Sanders et al, 1999). Smooth muscle cells respond to the depolarization/repolarization cycle imposed by ICC.

Regulatory input from nerves, hormones, and paracrine substances are superimposed upon the ongoing myogenic activity. Responses to biologically active substances result from modulations of ionic conductances that are already active and going through dynamic changes in open probability during the slow wave cycle and from activation of new conductances that do not participate in basal electrical activity (Sanders et al, 1999). The conductances affected by regulatory substances could be expressed in either smooth muscle cells or ICC. Finally, the conductance of both cell types mutually affects the electrical behavior of the total syncytium.

2. Morphological and physiological properties of ICC in gastrointestinal tract

Morphological studies have shown that each of the pacemaker regions in the GI tract contains ICC (Dickens et al, 1999; Suzuki et al, 1986; Burns et al, 1996; Thuneberg, 1982). To anatomists, the morphological features of ICC suggested that ICC may serve as pacemaker cells (Thuneberg, 1982; Faussone Pellegrini et al, 1997). Two types of ICC are found in the guinea-pig gastric antrum, namely ICC-MY and ICC-IM (Burns et al., 1997). Both ICC-MY and ICC-IM express Kit receptors on their cell membrane and can be identified by ACK2 (neutralizing Kit antibody) (Torihashi et al., 1995; Komuro et al., 1996; Burns et al., 1997). ICC-MY which lie in the plane of the myenteric plexus between the circular and longitudinal muscle layers (Sanders et al, 2006) have triangular or irregularly shaped cell bodies with multiple processes which interconnect to form a dense network with other ICC-MY (Burns et al., 1997; Dickens et al., 1999). There are also ICC in the small intestine near the submucosal surface of the circular muscle layer in close association with the nerve terminals in the deep muscular plexus (DMP) which cells are called ICC-DMP (Sanders et al,1999; Ward and Sanders, 2006). Pacemaker cells in the colon along the submucosal surface of the circular muscle layer are referred to as ICC-SM. The gastric antrum and pylorus also have populations of ICC-SM (Horiguchi, 2001; Ward, 1998), but the physiological roles of these ICC have not been described. There are important differences in the organization of electrical pacemaker activity between the small and large intestine. In the small bowel, electrical slow waves are generated by ICC-MY; slow waves in the colon, in contrast to the small intestine, originate in ICC-SMs and actively propagate along the submucosal surface into the circular muscle (Lee et al, 2009).

Intracellular recordings made from the guinea-pig gastric antrum revealed a rhythmic generation of pacemaker potentials with a fast rising phase followed by plateau components, slow waves with triangular form and square shaped follower potentials, each from ICC-MY, circular and longitudinal smooth muscle, respectively (Dickens et al., 1999). The amplitude and maximum rate of rise (dV/dtmax) of pacemaker potentials are larger than those of either slow waves or follower potentials, while the frequency and duration of pacemaker potentials and potentials recorded from smooth muscle cells are similar (Dickens et al., 1999, 2000; Hirst and Edwards, 2001; Kito and Suzuki, 2003). Simultaneous recordings of the electrical responses from ICC-MY and smooth muscle cells show that pacemaker potentials appear prior to slow waves or follower potentials, suggesting that the signals are generated in ICC-MY and are propagated to smooth muscle cells, possibly through gap junctions (Dickens et al., 1999; Hirst and Edwards, 2001). Thus, the potentials produced in the smooth muscle cells are largely passive, as an electrotonic potential of the pacemaker potentials. The difference between the active and passive properties of the potential is apparent when the membrane is hyperpolarized by a group of chemicals which open ATP-sensitive K+-channels (K-channel openers), in that the amplitude of the pacemaker potentials is increased while that of the slow waves is decreased. The latter is due to inhibition of the first component, probably because the decrease of input resistance induced by hyperpolarization decreases the amplitude of the passive electrical responses (Kito and

Suzuki, 2003). On rare occasions, discharges of membrane noise (unitary potentials) are generated during the interval between pacemaker potentials (Hirst and Edwards, 2001; Kito et al., 2002). The frequency of the generation of unitary potentials increases with time after the cessation of the pacemaker potentials, suggesting that depolarization of the membrane due to summation of unitary potentials then triggers pacemaker potentials (Hirst and Edwards, 2001; Kito et al., 2002). Pacemaker potentials recorded from ICC-MY in the mouse gastric antrum also showed properties similar to those of the guinea-pig stomach (Hirst et al., 2002). Immuno-histochemical studies have shown that the density of ICC-MY is highest in the greater curvature, while the population is reduced successively towards the lesser curvature and that they are either absent or distributed very sparsely in the lesser curvature (Hirst et al., 2002).

Additionally, colon and stomach have ICC intermixed with smooth muscle fibers. These intramuscular ICC are referred to as ICC-IM which are critical for inputs from enteric motor neurons (Ward and Sanders, 2006; Horiguchi, 2001). In contrast to ICC-MY, the ICC-IM are spindle shaped cells with bipolar processes that run parallel to the direction of the smooth muscle cells (Burns et al., 1997; Dickens et al., 2001; Hirst et al., 2002). In isolated bundles of the circular smooth muscle layer of the mouse gastric antrum, transmural nerve stimulation evokes two types of inhibitory junction potentials (IJP), both fast-IJP and slow-IJP, with a following depolarizing excitatory junction potential (EJP)(Suzuki et al., 2003). Since atropine and Nω-nitro-L-arginine (nitroarginine) inhibit the EJP and slow-IJP, respectively, it is likely that the former is generated in response to released acetylcholine and the latter is generated by the release of nitric oxide (Suzuki et al., 2003). On the other hand, the EJP and slow-IJP are absent in the antrum region of *W/WV* mice which lack ICC-IM. Therefore, ICC-IM may be transducing both cholinergic and nitrergic nerve signals to circular smooth muscle cells in the mouse gastric antrum (Suzuki et al., 2003). Similar results are also obtained in smooth muscle isolated from the fundus region of *W/WV* mutant mice and *steel* mutant mice (Burns et al., 1996; Beckett et al., 2002). In the small intestine, ICC-IM are replaced by a dense network of ICC located at the level of deep muscular plexus; ICC-DMP are intimately associated with the enteric nerve terminals (Torihashi, et al, 1993). The enteric nerve terminals appear to form synapses preferentially with ICC-DMP rather than the smooth muscle cells (Wang et al, 1999). In an ultrastructure study, it was found that ICC-DMP were innervated by both cholinergic and nitrergic nerves and were the only cells to possess specialized synapse-like junctions with nerve varicosities and gap junction contacts with the smooth muscle cells (Wang et al, 2003; Ward and Sanders, 2006). The functional role of ICC-DMP is difficult to prove since they persist in the small intestine of W/Wv and Sl/Sld mutants. However, the loss of ICC-DMP by blocking Kit was shown to cause loss of cholinergic and nitrergic neural responses (Ward et al, 2006), suggesting that in the small intestine, ICC-DMP play a critical role in the cholinergic and nitrergic neurotransmission.

2.1 Pacemaking activity in ICC

ICC are unique cells that generate electrical pacemaker activity in gastrointestinal (GI) smooth muscles. Many previous studies have attempted to characterize the conductances responsible for pacemaker current and slow waves in the GI tract, but the precise mechanism of electrical rhythmicity is still debated. ICC are pacemaker cells in the small bowel, and therefore this cell type must express the mechanism responsible for slow wave activity. Koh et al (1998) early demonstrated that isolated ICC cultured for 1~3 days from the murine small intestine were rhythmically active, producing regular slow wave depolarizations with waveforms and properties similar to slow waves in intact tissues. The spontaneous activity of ICC was inhibited by reduced extracellular Na^+, gadolinium, and reduced extracellular Ca^{2+}. Voltage clamp studies showed rhythmic inward currents that were probably responsible for the slow wave activity. The subsequent experiments also indicated that both the whole-cell currents and single-channel currents reversed at 0 mV when the equilibrium potentials of all ions present were far from 0 mV(Koh et al, 2002). The recordings from on-cell patches revealed oscillations in unitary currents at the frequency of pacemaker currents in ICC. Voltage-clamping cells to -60 mV did not change the oscillatory activity of channels in on-cell patches. Depolarizing cells with high external K+ caused loss of resolvable single-channel currents, but the oscillatory single-channel currents were restored when the patches were stepped to negative potentials. This conductance may contribute to the pacemaker current and generation of electrical slow waves in GI muscles. ICC have been studied after chemical isolation and under culture conditions, but concerns that these methods affect the intrinsic properties have hindered progress in our understanding of ICC. To overcome this problem, Wang et al (2008) developed a method to obtain electrophysiological recordings from ICC in situ. The critical feature is the ability to make high resistance seals onto cells that are embedded within tissue to obtain patch clamp recordings. Their results showed a prominent presence of a chloride channel, one of the proposed ICC pacemaker channels.

Microelectrode arrays (MEAs) are useful in spatiotemporal studies of pacemaker activity in the gut. Previously, MEA analysis was used to investigate neuronal activity in brain slices that generate action potentials with a high rate of increase. To record electrical slow waves originating from ICC in musculature preparations, microelectrodes with low impedance (<10 kU at 1 kHz) have been recently employed. In the guinea pig stomach (Nakayama et al., 2006), such a high-performance MEA system has revealed spontaneous electrical activity synchronised with resolving phase shifts over a range of several hundred micrometers. The electrical activity frequently propagates from the oral to the anal direction, even in the presence of tetrodotoxin (TTX). These observations indicate that the ICC-MY network also contributes to coordinated actions of gut motility and probably enables smooth contractions. In the small intestine of wild-type mice (Nakayama et al., 2009), the propagation of ICC electrical activity is also measurable over an area of 1 mm^2, although oral-to-anal and anal-to-oral propagations are both observed. In contrast, in W/Wv mice with a largely reduced population of ICC-MY in the small intestine, electrical activity is significantly smaller and fluctuates with no clear propagating direction.

It has been demonstrated that ICCs are pacemakers in the gastrointestinal tract using neutralizing antibody to block the development of ICCs and animals with gene mutation. ICC-MY in these animals were decreased dramatically or devoid, meanwhile slow waves and associated spontaneous activities were also inhibited significantly (Huizinga et al, 1995; Maeda et al, 1992; Torihashi et al, 1995). In the stomach and small bowel (Dickens et al., 1999; Kito et al, 2003), two kinds of electrical activities with similar frequencies were recorded by using microelectrode technique: pacemaker potentials and slow waves. Pacemaker potentials were proved to be generated by ICC-MY, while slow waves were generated by smooth muscle cells. Compared to slow waves, pacemaker potentials display greater amplitude and longer duration and usually precede slow waves. Pacemaker potentials generated by ICC-MY were passively propagated to the smooth muscle cells to generate slow waves. All these results demonstrate that ICC-MY is the pacemaker trigging spontaneous activities in gastrointestinal tract. The most direct evidences to support this hypothesis are that both freshly isolated and cultured ICCs generate spontaneous rhythmic electrical activity as it is recorded in intact tissues.

3. Mechanisms Involved in generation of ICC pacemaker currents

3.1 Intracellular calcium activities

It has been still controversial about the mechanism of generating pacemaker currents by far, but the role of intracellular calcium in the generation has been widely proved (Nakayama et al., 2007). Simultaneous recordings of intracellular calcium and electrical activity in ICCs revealed that intracellular calcium oscillations in ICCs were synchronized with slow waves, which indicates the close relationship between the intracellular calcium oscillations and the pacemaker activities of ICCs (Liu et al, 2005a; Liu et al, 2005b). Similar activities were also observed in ICCs of murine stomach and rabbit urethra (Johnston et al, 2005). Moreover, the evidence which 1,2-bis (2-aminophenoxy) ethane- N,N,N',N'-tetraacetic acid acetoxymethyl ester (BAPTA-AM), an intracellular calcium chelator inhibited both pacemaker potentials and slow waves of murine intestine demonstrates the crucial role of intracellular calcium in the generation of pacemaker activities in ICCs (Kito et al, 2003). The major pacemaker current is presumed to be generated by Ca^{2+}-activated ion channels. Specifically, intracellular Ca^{2+} ($[Ca^{2+}]i$) oscillations periodicallyactivate plasmalemmal Ca^{2+}-activated ion channels such as Ca^{2+}-activated Cl^- channels (Dickens et al., 1999; Huizinga et al., 2002; Tokutomi et al., 1995) and/or non-selective cation channels (Goto et al., 2004; Koh et al., 1998; Kim et al., 2002; Thomsen et al., 1998; Walker et al., 2002); however, it remains unclear which Ca^{2+}-activated ion channels make a predominant contribution.

Generally, intracellular calcium level are controled by calcium influx from extracellular circumstances and calcium release or uptake by calcium stores and mitochondrion. It was demonstrated that extracellular calium influx is important for the pacemaker activities of ICCs because both removal of extracellular calcium and replacement of extracellular calcium with equimolar Mn^{2+} abolished intracellular calcium oscillations and spontaneous electrical activities (Koh et al, 1998; Sergeant et al, 2000; Torihashi et al, 2002; Johnston et al, 2005). Unlike cardiac pacemaker cells that utilize voltage-gated ion channels to produce spontaneous rhythmicity, intracellular Ca^{2+} dynamics play a crucial role in ICC-MY pacemaking (Torihashi et al., 2002; Yamazawa and Iino, 2002). However, it is very interesting that L-type calcium channels blocker, for example, nicardipine did not affect to slow waves, intracellular calcium oscillations and spontaneous electrical activities of ICCs (Dickens et al., 1999; Torihashi et al, 2002; Johnston et al, 2005; Liu et al, 2005a), but both Ni^{2+} and mibefradil inhibited the upstroke component of pacemaker potentials (Kito et al, 2003). These phenomenon strongly suggest that L-type calcium channels are not involved in the pacemaker activities but a voltage-dependent dihydropyridine-resistant calcium channel may be involved in the pacemaker activity.

Intracellular calcium oscillations induced by calcium release or uptake by calcium stores and mitochondrion is very important factor for generation of pacemaker currents in ICCs. Sanders et al (Sanders et al, 2006) suggest that 'pacemaker unit' comprised of inositol1,4,5,-trisphosphate (IP_3)-operated calcium stores, adjacent mitochondrion and ion channels in the plasma membrane is the basic structure to generate pacemaker currents. The generation of pacemaker currents is initiated by calcium released from IP_3-operated calcium stores and intracellular high calcium induce calcium uptake by nearby mitochondrion. Calcium oscillations activate ion channels in the plasma membrane to generate pacemaker currents. In this process, calcium handling between calcium stores and adjacent mitochondria is considered as an important premise (Ward et al, 2000). Many studies have shown that thapsigargin and cyclopiazonic acid (CPA), inhibitors of calcium pump in the calcium stores, inhibited slow waves, calcium oscillations and pacemaker currents of ICCs (Torihashi et al, 2002; Ward et al, 2000; Hashitani et al, 2007). The results suggest that calcium store play an important role in the pacemaker activities. It is a common view that IP_3-operated calcium stores are involved in the pacemaker activities (Liu et al, 2005a; Ward et al, 2000), but the role of ryanodine receptor-operated calcium stores in the pacemaker activities have been still debatable. Ward et al (2000) found that ryanodine, an inhibitor of ryanodine receptor, had no significant effect on the pacemaker currents in ICCs, and Malysz et al (2001) also found that ryanodine had no significant effect on the frequency of slow waves. These results indicate that ryanodine receptor-operated calcium release may not be involved in the pacemaker activities in ICCs. However, Aoyama et al (2004) and Liu et al (2005b) reported that ryanodine abolished intracellular calcium oscillations in ICCs of murine intestine and stomach, respectively, and the expression of ryanodine receptor type3 has been confirmed by using RT-PCR technique. These result suggest that both IP_3-operated calcium stores and ryanodine-operated calcium stores are important for the pacemaker activities. In the rabbit urethra ryanodine-operated calcium stores are considered to be prominent in the pacemaker activities in ICCs. The studies demonstrated that ryanodine abolished the intracellular calcium oscillations and pacemaker currents in ICCs from rabbit urethra, whereas 2-APB, an inhibitor of IP_3 receptor, partially but not completely inhibited the amplitude of the intracellular calcium oscillations (Johnston et al, 2005). Moreover, the calcium uptake by mitochondrion is also important for ICCs pacemaker activities in both gastrointestinal tract and urethra, because disruption of the mitochondiral membrane potential with the electron transport chain inhibitors rotenone and antimycin A and mitochondrial uncoupler carbonyl cyanide p-(trifluoromethoxy) phenylhydrazone (FCCP) and carbonyl cyanide m-chlorophenylhydrazone (CCCP) abolished both intracellular calcium oscillations and pacemaker currents in ICCs (Ward et al, 2000).

Since intracellular calcium is a very important factor for pacemaking activity so what kind of channel is activated by intracellular calcium? There are still divergence of views about pacemaker channels and now two kinds of ionic channels are recognized as the candidates for pacemaker channels.

3.2 Non-selective cation channels

Many studies suggested that intracellular calcium level or calcium oscillation is the premise in the generation of ICCs pacemaker currents. However, it is still debatable which phase of calcium oscillations contribute to elicit pacemaker currents in ICCs. Consequently, it is a very important question which kind of channel is responsible for pacemaker currents and the pacemaker channels are sensitive to low caclium or high calcium. Koh et al (1998; 2002) found that pacemaker currents generated by cultured intestinal ICCs from murine could be abolished by removal of Na^+ in external solution. In succession, buffering intracellular calcium by BAPTA-AM induced persistent inward currents, which could be blocked by replacement of Na^+ in external media with equimolar $NMDG^+$. The open probability of the channels responsible for generating pacemaker currents was increased by the decrease of intracellular calcium using different configurations of patch clamp techniques. These results indicate that a calcium-inhibited non-selective cation channel is responsible for the generation of pacemaker currents in intestinal ICCs from murine. The current—voltage relationship showed that the spontaneous currents reversed at about +17 mV. These observations are consistent with the involvement of a non-selective cation current in the generation of slow waves, but do not rule out contributions from other conductances or transporters. Moreover, the conductance of single-channel was 13pS, and this channel could be strongly activated by calmodulin inhibitors in on-cell and excised patches. The channels were strongly activated by the calmodulin inhibitors calmidazolium and W-7 in on-cell and excised patches, and calmidazolium and W-7 also activated a persistent inward current under whole-cell conditions. Murine ICC express Ca^{2+}-inhibited, non-selective cation channels that are periodically activated at the same frequency as pacemaker currents (Koh et al, 2002).

Recently the electrophysiologic and pharmacologic study also demonstrated the evidences of non-selective cation channel (NSCC) is involved in generation of pacemaker currents in murine intestinal ICC. The application of flufenamic acid, a non-selective cation channel blocker, but not niflumic acid, abolished the generation of pacemaker currents induced by DA-9701. Then pretreatment with a Ca^{2+}-free solution and thapsigargin, a Ca^{2+}-ATPase inhibitor in the endoplasmic reticulum, abolished the generation of pacemaker currents. In addition, the tonic inward currents were inhibited by U-73122, an active phospholipase C inhibitor, but not by GDP-β-S, which permanently binds G-binding proteins. Furthermore, the protein kinase C inhibitors, chelerythrine and calphostin C, did not block the DA-9701-induced pacemaker currents. These results suggest that DA-9701 might affect gastrointestinal motility by the modulation of pacemaker activity in the ICC, and the activation is associated with the non-selective cationic channels via external Ca^{2+} influx, phospholipase C activation, and Ca^{2+} release from internal storage in a G proteinindependent and protein kinase C-independent manner (Choi et al 2009). The cells studied were identified by RT-PCR using cell-specific primers that included Myh11 (smooth muscle cells), Kit (ICC) and Uchl1 (enteric neurons) following electrophysiolgical recordings. Distinct ionic conductances were observed in Kit-positive cells. One group of ICC expressed a basal non-selective cation conductance that was inhibited by an increase in $[Ca^{2+}]_i$ in a calmodulin (CaM)-dependent manner (Takeda et al, 2008).

NSCC in both populations of ICC appear to be regulated by a Ca^{2+}–CaM-dependent process providing an insight into the cellular mechanisms underlying the generation of pacemaker activity and unitary/regenerative potentials. Since their discovery, a number of investigators have suggested that transient receptor potential (TRP) channels are the molecular candidates of NSCC. TRPC 1–7 (Tang et al., 2001; Clapham, 2003; Zhu, 2005), TRPV1 (Numazaki et al. 2003; Rosenbaum *et al.* 2004), V4 (Strotmann et al. 2003) and V6 (Niemeyer et al. 2001; Lambers et al. 2004), along with TRPM2 (Tong et al. 2006) and M4 (Nilius et al. 2005) have been shown to bind with CaM and are positively (facilitated) and negatively (inhibited) regulated in a Ca^{2+}–CaM-dependent manner. The Ca^{2+}–CaM regulation of the NSCC observed in the present study suggests that TRP channels may be involved in the Ca^{2+}–CaM-inhibited or -activated conductances expressed in gastric ICC. It has been suggested that TRPM7 encodes for the NSCC responsible for pacemaker activity in acutely cultured ICC from the small intestine (Kim et al. 2005). At the C-terminus, TRPM7 contains an *α*-kinase domain (chaK1), which negatively regulates channel activity when $[Mg^{2+}]_i$ increases (Schmitz et al. 2003). At physiological concentrations of Ca^{2+}, only Mg^{2+} and not other divalents can directly modulate TRPM7/ChaK1 kinase (Ryazanova et al.

2004). At high concentrations of [Ca^{2+}]i (>100 μm), CaM (5 μm) can inhibit ChaK1 phosphotransferase activity. Binding of CaM to its substrates or competitive inhibition of the α-kinase domain by CaM was suggested to inhibit the phosphotransferase activity (Ryazanova et al. 2004). Although the CaM binding sequence on TRPM7 has not been identified, it is known that Ca^{2+}–CaM inhibits ChaK1 and therefore it is possible that Ca^{2+}–CaM could enhance TRPM7 activity. Since pacemaking was activated by a reduction in [Ca^{2+}]i in ICC cultured from the small intestine (Koh et al. 2002), it is unlikely that TRPM7 activity is responsible for this pacemaker activity. A [Ca^{2+}]i-inhibited conductance expressed in one population of ICC was similar to the conductance previously described in cultured ICC from the small intestine. A conductance of this type appears to be responsible for spontaneous pacemaker activity in the small bowel and may serve the same function in the stomach. The properties of this calcium-inhibited non-selective cation channel are in analogy to those of TPRC4 in transient receptor potential (TRP) family, which is also regulated by intracellular calcium and calmodulin, and both channels have similar conductance (13 versus 17 pS) (Sander et al, 2006). The expression of TRPC4 has been confirmed in cultured ICCs clusters of murine intestine (Torihashi et al, 2002) and stomach (Liu et al, 2005a) by using immunohistochemistry and RT-PCR techniques. However, recently study demonstrated that human GI tract generated slow electrical waves and had ICCs which functioned as pacemaker cells an flufenamic acid, a nonselective cation channel blocker, and 2-APB (2-aminoethoxydiphenyl borate) and La^{3+}, TRPM7 channel blockers, inhibited the slow waves. Also, TRPM7 channels were expressed in ICCs in human tissue (Kim et al, 2009). They suggested that the physiological role of TRPM7 channels in ICCs in human GI tract requires more investigation. As a primary molecular candidate for the NSCC responsible for pacemaking activity in ICCs, TRPM7 may be a new target for pharmacological treatment of GI motility disorders.

3.3 Calcium activated chloride channels

Chloride channels have long been considered as just 'background' channels but recently they have been implicated in important physiological and pathophysiological processes related to blood pressure regulation, muscle tone, volume regulation, synaptic transmission, and cellular excitability. Up to now more and more evidences were demonsted that calcium activated chloride channels are responsible for ICCs pacemaker currents. In smooth muscle cells and, presumably, interstitial cells of Cajal (ICC), the Cl^- equilibrium potential is positive to the resting membrane potential, which makes it possible that selective opening of Cl^- channels contributes to cell depolarization (Kito et al, 2003). Many studies have implicated that inward (depolarizing) pacemaker currents were carried by chloride channels in ICC (Kito et al, 2003; Kito et al, 2002; Zhu et al, 2009).

Early study has been presented that Cl^- channels may contribute to the depolarization phase and the plateau phase of rhythmic membrane potential changes (slow waves) in ICC. First, pharmacological data suggested that Cl^- channels play a role in rhythmic inward currents generated by chemically isolated ICC (Tokutomi et al, 1995). As ICC in the urethra resembled ICC in the GI tract it was thought that they may share a common pacemaker mechanism. Under voltage clamp conditions ICC isolated from the rabbit urethra and networks of ICC cultured from the murine small intestine develop spontaneous transient inward currents (STICs) of similar amplitude and time courses (Koh et al, 1998; Sergeant et al, 2000). However, the ionic basis of pacemaker activity in both tissues appears to be fundamentally different. STICs in urethral ICC were inhibited in Ca2+-free medium and by the traditional chloride channel blockers A-9-C and niflumic acid (Sergeant et al, 2000). Recent study demonstrated that ICCs exhibite a specialized 'slow wave' current, for example, the reversal of tail current analysis showed this current was due to a Cl^- selective conductance in a new transgenic mouse with a bright green fluorescent protein and the ICC express ANO1, a Ca^{2+}-activated Cl^- channel (Zhu et al, 2009). Removal of extracellular Ca^{2+}, replacement of Ca^{2+} with Ba^{2+}, or extracellular Ni^{2+} blocked the slow wave current. Single Ca^{2+}-activated Cl^- channels with a unitary conductance of 7.8 pS were resolved in excised patches of ICC. Slow wave current was associated with transient depolarizations of ICC in current clamp, and these events were blocked by niflumic acid (Zhu et al, 2009). Most recently study proposed that $[Cl^-]i$ is seen to fluctuate in ICC explant clusters, possibly evoked by rhythmic changes in intracellular calcium. The intracellular chloride concentration in ICC fluctuates to keep its equilibrium potential constant (E_{Cl}). The identification of E_{Cl} as positive to the resting membrane potential of ICC indicates that opening of chloride channels will depolarize ICC (Zhu et al, 2010). These findings demonstrate a role for a Ca^{2+}-activated Cl^- conductance in slow wave current in ICC and are consistent with the idea that ANO1 participates in pacemaker activity.

4. Function of neurotransmission

How nerves transmit their signals to regulate activity of smooth muscle is of fundamental importance to autonomic and enteric physiology, clinical medicine and therapeutics. A traditional view of neurotransmission to smooth muscles has been that motor nerve varicosities release neurotransmitters that act on receptors on smooth muscles to cause their contraction or relaxation via electromechanical and phamacomechanical signaling pathways in the smooth muscle. In recent years, an old hypothesis that certain ICC may transduce neural signals to smooth muscle cells has been resurrected. This later hypothesis is based on indirect evidence of closer proximity and presence of synapses between the nerve varicosities and ICCs, gap junctions between ICC and smooth muscles and presence of receptors and signaling pathways for the neurotransmitters and ICCs (Daniel et al, 1984).

4.1 Morphologic evidence for ICC-IM mediate neurotransmission

Ultrastructural studies have identified membrane densifications between enteric nerve terminals and ICC-IM in different organs of the GI tracts from several species (Wang et al, 2000; Horiguchi et al, 2003; Sanmarti-Vila et al, 2000). The ultrastructure of these membrane specializations are unlike the nerve-to-nerve synapses that exist in the central nervous system (Kennedy et al, 2000; Aoki et al, 2001; Ruegg et al, 2001) or the structural arrangement of the skeletal neuromuscular junction (Aguado et al, 1999). Even less is known about these proteins that exist between nerve terminals and neuroeffector cells in the GI tract. It has been established that enteric motor nerve terminals in the rat oesophagus and small intestine and in the murine stomach contain members of the *N*-ethylmaleimide-sensitive fusion protein attachment protein receptors or SNAREs that are involved in the release of neurotransmitters from these terminals (Beckett et al, 2005; Sudhof et al, 1996). SNAREs are involved in neurovesicle docking to the presynaptic membrane, fusion of the neurovesicle and release of neurotransmitter in the synaptic cleft. Several of the SNARE proteins that have been identified to date in the murine stomach include synaptotagmin, syntaxin and SNAP-25 (Vannucchi et al, 1997). Each of these proteins has a specific role in the neurotransmitter release process (Lavin et al, 1998). Varicosities containing these

SNARE proteins were only observed in intimate association with ICC-IM and were not observed in close apposition to smooth muscle cells (Vannucchi et al, 1997). These data support the hypothesis that ICC-IM are directly innervated by active sites where neurotransmitter release occurs.

Transcripts for two postsynaptic scaffolding proteins PSD-93 and PSD-95 have been detected by RT-PCR in the murine stomach. Quantitative RT-PCR revealed that expression of PSD-93 and PSD-95 are decreased in the stomachs of W/W^V mutants that lack ICC-IM (Vannucchi et al, 1997). Finally, double-labelling immunohistochemical experiments using antibodies that recognize the PDZ domain of the PSD-95 family members (PSD-95 and PSD-93, and SAP 97) and Kit revealed the expression of PSD proteins on ICC-IM but not neighbouring smooth muscle cells (Vannucchi et al, 1997). These data suggest that ICC-IM express the necessary proteins to form postsynaptic proteins and further support the hypothesis that ICC-IM are directly innervated.

4.2 Functional evidence for ICC-IM mediate neurotransmission

ICCs possess a variety of receptors for neurotransmitters, hormones and paracrine substances, for example, NK1 receptors (Lavin et al, 1998; Epperson et al, 2000), VIP receptors (Patterson et al, 2001) and CCK-A receptors (Ward et al, 2000), and so on. More direct functional evidence for the primary role of ICCs in enteric motor neurotransmission came from experiments performed on the stomachs of W/W^V mutant mice that lack ICC-IM. In the absence of ICC-IM post-junctional neural responses to cholinergic excitatory and nitrergic inhibitory neurotransmission were absent or greatly attenuated within the circular muscle layers of the gastric fundus and antrum (Beckett et al, 2003; Suzuki et al, 2003; Song et al, 2005a). Although post-junctional cholinergic and nitrergic responses are absent or greatly attenuated in W/W^V mutant mice that lack ICC-IM, neural responses still persist. In the gastric antrum of wild-type animals, nerve stimulation evokes a complex series of post-junctional responses, consisting of an initial apamin-sensitive inhibitory junction potential (IJP) and a slower nitrergic IJP; the inhibitory responses are followed by an excitatory response that consists of both atropine-sensitive and at more sustained stimulation frequencies an insensitive excitatory response (Song et al, 2005b). In antrums of W/W^V mice the initial apamin-sensitive component still persists. Sustained stimulation of W/W^V mutant tissues also reveals a non-cholinergic excitatory response that is probably mediated through neurokinins (Iino et al, 2008). It is interesting that these post-junctional responses are still present but the cholinergic and nitrergic responses are absent when ICC-IM is absent.

A lot of studies indicated that soluble guanylate cyclae (sGC) is present in ICC-IM which are closely apposed to nitrergic neurons processes containing neuronal nitric oxide synthase (nNOS) (Iino et al, 2009; Wang et al, 2003). In guinea pig caecum, stimulation of nitrergic neurons or treatment with nitric oxide (NO) enhanced cyclic guanosine 3′,5′-monophospate (cGMP) which is a signal molecule in the NO signal pathway in ICC-IM (Wang et al, 2003), but the same phenomenon was not observed in the smooth muscle cells. These results indicate that ICC-IM may be the primary targets for NO released from neurons and mediate nitrergic signal transmission. In the murine antrum, transmural nerve stimulation evoked a fast inhibitory junction potential (IJP) followed by a long lasting inhibitory junction potential (slow-IJP) and a period of excitation. Slow-IJP and the excitatory component could be abolished by an inhibitor of NOS and atropine, respectively, which indicate that these two reactions were mediated by nitrergic and cholinergic neurons, respectively. But in the animals which lack ICC-IM, the nitrergic and cholinergic components were absent (Gillespie et al, 2004), which indicate the important role of ICC-IM in neurotransmission. It was also showed that ICC-IM were associated with cholinergic neurons containing vesicular acetylcholine transporter (VAChT) in the murine fundus. Fast excitatory junction potentials (EJP) which were blocked by atropine were induced by electrical field stimulation (EFS) in the smooth muscle. The neuronal responses were greatly reduced in the gene-mutation mouse in which ICC-IM were devoid (Beckett et al, 2003). These results suggest that ICC-IM also mediate cholinergic neurotransmission.

5. Pathophysiology of ICC in gastrointestinal tract

ICCs have, in the past 2 decades, been recognised as important elements in the regulation of gastrointestinal motility. Specifically, they have been shown to be critical for the generation and propagation of electrical slow waves that regulate the phasic contractile activity of gastrointestinal smooth muscle, and for mediating neurotransmission from enteric motor neurons to smooth muscle cells. These different functional roles are carried out by different phenotypic classes of ICC that have discrete distributions within the tunica muscularis. In humans, under certain pathophysiological conditions, loss or defects in ICC networks appear to play a role in the generation of certain motility disorders (Vanderwinden et al, 1999; Horisawa et al, 1998). Recent evidence suggests that loss of ICC is associated with numerous gastrointestinal disorders ranging from gastroparesis, pseudoobstruction and idiopathic constipation (Vanderwinden et al, 1999; Sanders et al, 1999; Burns et al, 2007; Rolle et al, 2007; Farrugia et al, 2008). An animal model of ICC loss, the W/WV mouse, has been used extensively to examine functional changes resulting from lesions in ICC (Maeda et al, 1992; Ward et al, 1994;. Huizinga et al, 1995) dense network of ICC in the region of the myenteric plexus (ICC-MY) is disrupted in the small intestine of these mice and ICC-MY are largely absent along the anti-mesenteric aspect. However, scattered remnants of ICC-MY networks can be found in the tunica muscularis of the small intestine (Ward et al, 1994). ICC-IM (which are concentrated in the region of the deep muscular plexus of the mouse and therefore are referred to as ICC-DMP) are preserved in the small bowel of the W/WV mouse (Ward et al, 1994), making this an ideal model to study the consequences of significant loss of the ICC-MY pacemaker network on motility.

5.1 Pathophysiology of ICC in diabetic gastroparesis

Gastric neuromuscular dysfunction occurs in up to 30–50% of patients after 10 years of type I or II diabetes. Symptoms of diabetic gastropathy can range from mild dyspepsia to recurrent vomiting, abdominal pain and gastroparesis (Mearin et al, 1995; De Block et al, 2006). Neither the pathophysiology of gastroparesis, nor the pathogenesis of patients's symptoms, is well understood; hence, medical therapy is generally not effective. A major symptom of gastroparesis is delayed gastric emptying although there is a poor correlation between symptom severity and the rate of gastric emptying (Koch et al, 2001). Numerous physiological studies have demonstrated that both enteric nerves and ICC play critical roles in gastric peristalsis (Koh et al, 1998; Thomsen et al, 1998; Hirst et al, 2002), a major determinant of gastric emptying (Vittal et al, 2007; Hirst et al, 2006). Another predominant symptom of gastroparesis is vomiting and nausea likely involving vagal afferent innervation (Andrews et al, 2002). ICCs are associated with vagal afferent nerves (Fox et al, 2000) and hence studies into the pathophysiology of ICC associated with gastroparesis may hold the key to advancing our understanding of the causes of gut motility disorders associated with diabetes. In some patients with severe diabetic gastroparesis, the number of ICC has been shown to be significantly reduced in different parts of gut using immunohistochemistry (He et al, 2001; Nakahara et al, 2002; Forster et al, 2005; Miller et al, 2008). Damage to ICC, pacemakers, and mediators of neuromuscular neurotransmission in the gastrointestinal tract contributes to the pathogenesis of diabetic gastroenteropathy in both patients and animal models. Viktor et al (2005) cultured murine gastric smooth muscle in normoglycemic or hyperglycemic basal media with or without insulin or IGF-I for 1–3 months, the time required for gastroparesis and ICC damage to develop in diabetic mice. Then they assessed ICC expression by c-Kit immunohistochemistry and quantitative analysis of c-kit expression. They found that ICC survived for at least 34 days in unsupplemented normoglycemic media, but their networks, c-kit expression, and slow waves were profoundly reduced after 68 days. These changes could be entirely prevented by insulin or IGF-I supplementation. ICC networks were completely resistant to hyperglycemia for at least 72 days. They suggested that hyperglycemia is unlikely to be responsible for the diabetes-associated depletion of ICC. In contrast, maintenance of ICC requires insulin or IGF-I, which are reduced or ineffective in diabetes. Insulin and IGF-I receptors were detected in smooth-muscle cells and myenteric neurons but not in ICC. The successive study (Horvath et al, 2006) showed that cell-surface expression of SCF was only found in smooth-muscle cells, and ICC depletion in diabetes was accompanied by smooth-muscle atrophy and reduced SCF, whereas neuron-specific gene expression remained unchanged. In organotypic cultures, prevention of ICC loss by insulin or IGF-I was paralleled by rescue of smoothmuscle cells and SCF expression but not of myenteric neurons. Immunoneutralization of endogenous SCF caused ICC depletion closely resembling that elicited by insulin/IGF-I deficiency. The results suggest that reduced insulin/IGF-I signaling in diabetes may lead to ICC depletion and its consequences by causing smooth-muscle atrophy and reduced SCF production. Thus, myopathy may play a more central role in diabetic gastroenteropathies than previously recognized.

ICC are associated with afferent innervation and peristalsis of the stomach suggestive of a key role in the pathophysiology of gastroparesis. Recently study was investigated that changes in the density and ultrastructure of ICC and enteric nerves in the streptozotocin-induced diabetes mellitus (STZ-DM) in Wistar rats using immunohistochemistry and electron microscopy (Wang et al, 2009). In the STZ-DM antrum, a marked reduction was observed in the density of the intramuscular ICC (ICC-IM) and ICC located at the submucosal border of the circular muscle layer of the antrum (ICC-SM). The surviving ICC showed lamellar bodies and partial vacuolation of the cytoplasm content, loss of connections between ICC-IM and nerves; it appeared that injured ICC-IM developed into fibroblast-like ICC. ICC associated with Auerbach's plexus (ICC-AP) in the antrum and ICC in the fundus were not affected significantly except for a loss of connections with nerve structures. Marked reduction in nerve tissue (Protein Gene Product-9.5 positivity) was also restricted to the muscle layers including nitrergic nerves (neuronal nitric oxide synthase positivity). In vivo assessed gastric emptying was markedly reduced in STZ-DM rats. These data demonstrate in the STZ-DM rat stomach a decreased density of ICC limited to the antrum and to ICC-IM and ICC-SM, and structural degeneration in ICC-IM and associated nerves with a special emphasis on loss of synaptic connections, accompanied by a decrease in gastric emptying.

5.2 Pathophysiology of ICC in other gastroenteropathy

The findings outlined above, obtained from laboratory animals, highlight the key roles played by ICCs in the regulation of GI motility, and suggest that alterations in ICC networks in humans also could have an impact on gut motility and/or GI diseases. Indeed, loss of ICCs or disruption of ICC networks has been reported in a wide range of GI diseases, including achalasia, chronic intestinal pseudoobstruction, Hirschsprung disease, inflammatory bowel diseases, slow transit constipation, and others (Vanderwinden et al, 1999; Sanders et al, 2002).

Intestinal obstruction may ensue from mechanical or functional causes and, when complete, it may represent a fatal complication of several gastrointestinal disorders. If partial, the stenosis progressively hinders the flow of ingesta, generating orally distension and thickening of the gut wall. Both motor and absorptivesecretory dysfunctions, along with widespread morphological and neurochemical changes, are reported to occur orally to the point of occlusion (Schuffler et al, 1993; Prommegger et al, 1997). Since ICC generate and propagate electrical slow waves in gastrointestinal muscles, Chang et al (2001) investigated whether the loss of ICC leads to loss of function in partial bowel obstruction. They observed that the populations of ICC decreased oral, but not aboral, to the site of obstruction, two weeks following the onset of a partial obstruction, as well as increased in diameter and hypertrophy of the tunica muscularis, oral to the obstruction site. ICC networks were disrupted oral to the obstruction, and this disruption was accompanied by the loss of electrical slow waves and responses to enteric nerve stimulation. Ultrastructural analysis revealed no evidence of cell death in regions where the lesion in ICC networks was developing. Cells with a morphology intermediate between smooth muscle cells and fibroblasts were found in locations that are typically populated by ICC. However, removal of the obstruction led to the redevelopment of ICC networks and recovery of slow wave activity within 30 days. These data describe the plasticity of ICC networks in response to partial obstruction. Chronic idiopathic intestinal pseudoobstruction (CIIP) has similarities to the neonatal form in that it presents with symptoms suggestive of intestinal obstruction due to abnormalities in intestinal transit, causing significant morbidity and mortality. Several studies have indicated that ICC are decreased or absent in some idiopathic CIIP patients (Jain et al, 2003; Streutker et al, 2003; Isozaki et al, 1997; Yamataka et al, 1998; Feldstein et al, 2003; Faussone-Pellegrini et al, 1999; Tong et al, 2004). There is also a second subgroup of CIIP patients with myocyte changes suggestive of visceral myopathy in whom ICC are absent in the dilated portion of the megaduodenum (Boeckxstaens et al, 2002). CIIP can also occur in the colon and electrophysiological studies show that these patients have absent or decreased slow wave rhythms (Shafik et al, 2003) and absent / decreased ICC are also demonstrable in some cases (Jain et al, 2003; Streutker et al, 2003) the changes in the ICC occur in a subpopulation of cases and are often focal.

Gastrointestinal tract is one of the most susceptible organ systems to ischaemia. Not only mucosal injury but also alterations of the intestinal motility and loss of ICC have been reported in response to ischaemia and reperfusion (I/R) (Shimojima et al, 2006). Most recently study demonstrated that gastric emptying was transiently delayed at 12 h after I/R, but returned to normal by 48 h, and expression of c-Kit protein of the smooth muscle layer was reduced at both 12 and 48 h after I/R. The expression of neuronal nitric oxide synthase (nNOS) protein was also decreased at 12 h after I/R, but was restored to normal by 48 h (Suzuki et al, 2010). These data suggest gastric I/R evokes transient gastroparesis with delayed gastric emptying, associated with disruption of the ICC network and nNOS-positive neurons.

6. Summary

Most region of the gastrointestinal (GI) tract generate an ongoing discharge of rhythmical electrical activity in the absence of neural or hormonal stimulation. ICCs are the pacemaking cells in gastrointestinal smooth muscles that generate the rhythmic oscillations in membrane potential known as slow waves. The ICC lie in the myenteric region (ICC-MY) are pacemaker cells. Individual ICC-MY form gap junctions with neighbouring ICC-MY forming a network of cells which is in turn electrically coupled to the adjacent muscle layers. Another ICC distributed through the muscle layers (ICC-IM) which similarly form gap junctions with surrounding smooth muscle cells, so presumably forming an electrical syncytium. Calcium release from inositol triphosphate (IP_3) is known to contribute to many important cellular functions, including generation of spontaneous rhythmicity in gastrointestinal motility. However, there are differences and contradictions what kind channel is involved in generation of pacemaker currents. One candidate for pacemaker current is intracellular low calcium-sensitive nonselective cation channels and another is calcium activated chloride channels. These two kinds of candidate channels have supported experimental evidences, respectively. ICC plays an important role in gut motility and absent or disordered ICC networks have been identified in a variety of motility disorders. Many evidences suggest that normal gastrointestinal motility depends on interactions among several cell types occurring within the smooth muscle layers. ICC just like other regulatory cell types, perform specialized functions and should retain their place among the key players. However, in order to explain the ICC pacemaking mechanism many studies are need to do further.

7. Reference

[1] Szurszewski JH. 1987. Electrical basis for gastrointestinal motility. In *Physiology of the Gastrointestinal Tract*, pp. 383–422. New York: Raven. 2nd ed.

[2] Sanders KM. A case for interstitial cells of Cajal as pacemakers and mediators of neurotransmission in the gastrointestinal tract. *Gastroenterology, 1996,* 111: 492–515.

[3] Thuneberg L. Interstitial cells of Cajal: intestinal pacemaker cells?[J] Advances in Anatomy, Embryology, and Cell Biology. 1982; 71: 1-130.

[4] Huizinga JD, Thuneberg L, Klüppel M, Malysz J, Mikkelsen HB, Bernstein A. W/kit gene required for interstitial cells of Cajal and for intestinal pacemaker activity. Nature. 1995, 373: 347-349.

[5] Koh SD, Sansers KM, Ward SM. Spontaneous electrical rhythmicity in cultured interstitial cells of Cajal from the murine small intestine. J Physiol. 1998, 513: 203-213.

[6] Sanders KM, Ordög T, Koh SD, Torihashi S, Ward SM. Development and plasticity of interstitial cells of Cajal[J]. Neurogastroenterology and Motility. 1999, 11: 311-338.

[7] Dickens EJ, Hirst GD, Tomita T. 1999. Identification of rhythmically active cells in guinea-pig stomach. *J. Physiol. London* 514:515–31

[8] Suzuki N, Prosser CL, Dahms V. 1986. Boundary cells between longitudinal and circular layers: essential for electrical slowwaves in cat intestine. *Am. J. Physiol.* 250:G287–94

[9] Burns AJ, Lomax AEJ, Torihashi S, Sanders KM, Ward SM. 1996. Interstitial cells of Cajal mediate inhibitory neurotransmission in the stomach. *Proc. Natl. Acad. Sci. USA.* 93:12008–13

[10] Faussone Pellegrini MS, Cortesini C, Romagnoli P. 1977. Ultrastructure of the tunica muscularis of the cardial portion of the human esophagus and stomach, with special reference to the so-called Cajal's interstitial cells. *Arch. Ital. Anat. Embriol.* 82:157–77

[11] Burns, A.J., Herbert, T.M., Ward, S.M. and Sanders, K.M. (1997). Interstitial cells of Cajal in the guineapig gastrointestinal tract as revealed by *c-kit* immunohistochemistry. *Cell Tiss. Res.1997,* 290: 11–20.

[12] Torihashi, J., Ward, S.M., Nishikawa, S., Nishi, S., Kobayashi, S. and Sanders, K.M. c-kit dependent development of interstitial cells and electrical activity in the murine gastrointestinal tract. *Cell Tissue Res.,1995,* 280: 97–111.

[13] Komuro, T., Tokui, K. and Zhou, D.S. (1996). Identification of the interstitial cells of Cajal. *Histol. Histopathol.* 11: 769–786.

[14] Sanders KM, Koh SD, Ward SM. Interstitial cells of Cajal as pace3makers in the gastrointestinal tract. Annu. Rev. Physiol. 2006. 68:307–343

[15] Ward SM, Sanders KM. Involvement of intramuscular interstitial cells of Cajal in neuroeffector transmission in the gastrointestinal tract. J Physiol. 2006; 576: 675-682.

[16] Horiguchi K, Semple GS, Sanders KM, Ward SM. Distribution of pacemaker function through the tunica muscularis of the canine gastric antrum. *J. Physiol. London,* 2001, 537:237–50

[17]Ward SM, Morris G, Reese L, Wang XY, Sanders KM. Interstitial cells of Cajal mediate enteric inhibitory neurotransmission in the lower esophageal and pyloric sphincters. *Gastroenterology, 1998,* 115:314–29

[18] Lee HT, Hennig GW, Park KJ, Bayguinov PO, Ward SM, Sanders KM. Heterogeneities in ICC Ca2t activity within canine large intestine. Gastroenterology 2009; 136:2226–2236.

[19] Hirst, G.D.S., Beckett, E.A.H., Sanders, K.M.and Ward, S.M. Regional variation in contribution of myenteric and intramuscular interstitial cells of Cajal to generation of slow waves in mouse gastric antrum. *J. Physiol. (Lond.) 2002,* 540: 1003–1012.

[20] Suzuki, H., Ward, S.M., Bayguinov, Y.R., Edwards, F.R. and Hirst, G.D.S. Involvement of intramuscular interstitial cells in nitrergic inhibition in the mouse gastric antrum. *J Physiol. (Lond.), 2003,* 546: 751–763.

[21] Dickens, E.J., Edwards, F.R. and Hirst, G.D.S. (2000). Vagal inhibition in the antral region of guinea pig stomach. *Am. J. Physiol.* 279: G388–G399.

[22] Hirst, G.D.S. and Edwards, F.R. Generation of slow waves in the antral region of guinea-pig stomach - a stochastic process. *J. Physiol. (Lond.), 2001,* 535: 165–180.

[23] Kito, Y. and Suzuki, H.Modulation of slow waves by hyperpolarization with potassium channel openers in antral smooth muscle of the guinea-pig stomach. *J. Physiol. (Lond.), 2003,* 548: 175–189.

[24] Kito Y, Suzuki H, Edwards FR. Properties of unitary potentials recorded from myenteric interstitial cells of Cajal distributed in the guinea pig gastric antrum. *J. Smooth Muscle Res., 2002,* 38: 165–179.

[25] Torihashi S, Kobayashi S, Gerthoffer WT, Sanders KM. Interstitial cells in deep muscular plexus of canine small intestine may be specialized smooth muscle cells. Am J Physiol. 1993; 265: G638–45.

[27] Wang XY, Sanders KM, Ward SM.Intimate relationship between interstitial cells of Cajal and enteric nerves in the guinea-pig small intestine. Cell Tissue Res. 1999; 295: 247–56.

[28] Wang XY, Paterson C, Huizinga JD. Cholinergic and nitrergic innervation of ICC-DMP and ICC-IM in the human small intestine. Neurogastroenterol Motil. 2003, 15: 531–43.

[29] Ward SM, McLaren GJ, Sanders KM.Interstitial cells of Cajal in the deep muscular plexus mediate enteric motor neurotransmission in the mouse small intestine. J Physiol. 2006; 573: 147–59.

[30] Wang BX, Kunze WA, Zhu Y, Huizinga JD. In situ recording from gut pacemaker cells. Pflugers Arch-Eur J Physiol. 2008, 457:243–251.

[31] Nakayama, S., Shimono, K., Liu, H.-N., Jiko, H., Katayama, N., Tomita, T., Goto, K., 2006. Pacemaker phase shift in the absence of neural activity in guinea-pig stomach: a microelectrode array study. J. Physiol. (Lond.) 576, 727e738.

[32] Nakayama, S., Ohishi, R., Sawamura, K., Watanabe, K., Hirose, K., 2009. Microelectrode array evaluation of gut pacemaker activity in wild-type and W/Wv mice. Biosens. Bioelectron. 25, 61e67.

[33] Maeda H, Yamagata A, Nishikawa S, Yoshinaga K, Kobayashi S, Nishi K, Nishikawa S. Requirement of c-kit for development of intestinal pacemaker system[J]. Development. 1992; 116(2): 369-375.

[34] Nakayama S, Kajioka S, Goto K, Takaki M, Liu HN. Calcium-associated mechanisms in gut pacemaker activity. J Cell Mol Med. 2007; 11(5): 958-968.

[35] Torihashi, S., Fujimoto, T., Trost, C., Nakayama, S., 2002. Calcium oscillation linked to pacemaking of interstitial cells of Cajal. J. Biol. Chem. 277, 19191-19197.

[36] Yamazawa, T., Iino, M., 2002. Simultaneous imaging of Ca2t signals in interstitial cells of Cajal and longitudinal smooth muscle cells during rhythmic activity in mouse ileum. J. Physiol. (Lond.) 538, 823e835.

[37] Huang, S.-M., Nakayama, S., Iino, S., Tomita, T. Voltage sensitivity of slow wave frequency in isolated circular muscle strips from guinea pig gastric antrum. Am. J. Physiol. Gastrointest. Liver Physiol, 1999, 276: G518-G528.

[38] Liu HN, Ohya S, Furuzono S, Wang J, Imaizumi Y, Nakayama S. Co-contribution of IP_3R and Ca^{2+} influx pathways to pacemaker Ca^{2+} activity in stomach ICC. J Biol Rhythms., 2005a, 20: 15-26.

[38] Liu HN, Ohya S, Wang J, Imaizumi Y, Nakayama S. Involvement of ryanodine receptors in pacemaker Ca2+ oscillation in murine gastric ICC. Biochem Biophy Res Com., 2005b, 328: 640-646.

[39] Johnston L, Sergeant GP, Hollywood MA, Thornbury KD, McHale NG. Calcium oscillations in interstitial cells of the rabbit urethra. J physiol., 2005, 565: 449-461.

[40] Kito Y, Suzuki H. Properties of pacemaker potentials recorded from myenteric interstitial cells of Cajal distributed in the mouse small intestine. J Physiol., 2003, 553:803-818.

[41] Huizinga, J.D., Zhu, Y., Ye, J., Molleman, A. High conductance chloride channels generate pacemaker currents in interstitial cells of Cajal. Gastroenterology, 2002, 123; 1627-1636.
[42] Tokutomi, N., Maeda, H., Tokutomi, Y., Sato, D., Sugita, M., Nishikawa, S., Nishikawa, S., Nakao, J., Imamura, T., Nishi, K., 1995. Rhythmic Cl^- current and physiological roles of the intestinal c-kit-positive cells. Pflügers Arch., 1995, 431; 169-177.
[43] Goto, K., Matsuoka, S., Noma, A.. Two types of spontaneous depolarizations in the interstitial cells freshly prepared from the murine small intestine. J. Physiol. (Lond.), 2004, 559: 411-422.
[45] Kim, Y.C., Koh, S.D., Sanders, K.M. Voltage-dependent inward currents of interstitial cells of Cajal from murine colon and small intestine. J. Physiol. (Lond.), 2002, 541: 797-810.
[46] Thomsen, L., Robinson, T.L., Lee, J.C.F., Farraway, L.A., Hughes, M.J.G., Andrews, D.W., Huizinga, J.D. Interstitial cells of Cajal generate a rhythmic pacemaker current. Nat. Med., 1998, 4: 848-851.
[47] Walker, R.L., Koh, S.D., Sergeant, G.P., Sanders, K.M., Horowitz, B. TRPC4 currents have properties similar to the pacemaker current in interstitial cells of Cajal. Am. J. Physiol. Cell Physiol., 2002, 283: C1637-C1645.
[48] Sergeant GP, Hollywood MA, McCloskey KD, Thornbury KD, McHale NG. Specialised pacemaking cells in the rabbit urethra. J Physiol, 2000, 526: 359-366.
[49] Ward SM, Ördög T, Koh SD, Baker SA, Jun JY, Amberg G, Monaghan K, Sanders KM. Pacemaking in interstitial cells of Cajal depends upon calcium handling by endoplasmic reticulum and mitochondria. J Physiol, 2000, 525: 355-361.
[50] Hashitani H, Suzuki H. Properties of spontaneous Ca2+ transients recorded from interstitial cells of Cajal-like cells of the rabbit urethra in situ. J physiol., 2007, 583: 505-519.
[51] Malysz J, Donnelly G, Huizinga JD. Regulation of slow wave frequency by IP(3)-sensitive calcium release in the murine small intestine. Am J Physiol Gastrointest Liver Physiol. 2001; 280: G439-48.
[52] Aoyama M, Yamada A, Wang J, Ohya S, Furuzono S, Goto T, Hotta S, Ito Y, Matsubara T, Shimokata K, Chen SR, Imaizumi Y, Nakayama S. Requirement of ryanodine receptors for pacemaker Ca2+ activity in ICC and HEK293 cells. J Cell Sci., 2004, 117: 2813-2825.
[53] *Choi S, Choi JJ, Jun JY, Koh JW, Kim SH, Kim DH.* Induction of Pacemaker Currents by DA-9701, a Prokinetic Agent, in Interstitial Cells of Cajal from Murine Small Intestine. Mol. Cells, 2009, 27: 307-312.
[54] Tang J, Lin Y, Zhang Z, Tikunova S, Birnbaumer L & Zhu MX. Identification of common binding sites for calmodulin and inositol 1,4,5-trisphosphate receptors on the carboxyl termini of Trp channels. *J Biol Chem, 2001,* 276: 21303–21310.
[55] Clapham DE. TRP channels as cellular sensors. *Nature, 2003,* 426: 517–524.
[56] Zhu MX. Multiple roles of calmodulin and other Ca2+-binding proteins in the functional regulation of TRP channels. *Pflugers Arch, 2005,* 451: 105–115.
[57] Numazaki M, Tominaga T, Takeuchi K, Murayama N, Toyooka H & Tominaga M. Structural determinant of TRPV1 desensitization interacts with calmodulin. *Proc Natl Acad Sci U S A, 2003,* 100: 8002–8006.

[58] Rosenbaum T, Gordon-Shaag A, Munari M & Gordon SE. Ca^{2+}/calmodulin modulates TRPV1 activation by capsaicin. *J Gen Physiol, 2004,* 123, 53-62.
[59] Strotmann R, Schultz G & Plant TD. Ca2+-dependent potentiation of the nonselective cation channel TRPV4 is mediated by a C-terminal calmodulin binding site. *J Biol Chem, 2003,* 278: 26541-26549.
[60] Niemeyer BA, Bergs C,Wissenbach U, Flockerzi V & Trost C. Competitive regulation of CaT-like-mediated Ca2+ entry by protein kinase C and calmodulin. *Proc Natl Acad Sci U S A, 2001,* 98: 3600-3605.
[61] Lambers TT,Weidema AF, Nilius B, Hoenderop JG & Bindels RJ. Regulation of the mouse epithelial Ca2+ channel TRPV6 by the Ca2+-sensor calmodulin. *J Biol Chem, 2004,* 279: 28855-28861.
[62] Tong Q, Zhang W, Conrad K, Mostoller K, Cheung JY, Peterson BZ & Miller BA. Regulation of the transient receptor potential channel TRPM2 by the Ca2+ sensor calmodulin. *J Biol Chem, 2006,* 281: 9076-9085.
[63] Nilius B, Prenen J, Tang J,Wang C, Owsianik G, Janssens A, Voets T, Zhu MX. Regulation of the Ca2+ sensitivity of the nonselective cation channel TRPM4. *J Biol Chem, 2005,* 280: 6423-6433.
[64] Schmitz C, Perraud AL, Johnson CO, Inabe K, Smith MK, Penner R, Kurosaki T, Fleig A & Scharenberg AM. Regulation of vertebrate cellular Mg^{2+} homeostasis by TRPM7. *Cell, 2003,* 114: 191-200.
[65] Ryazanova LV, Dorovkov MV, Ansari A & Ryazanov AG. Characterization of the protein kinase activity of TRPM7/ChaK1, a protein kinase fused to the transient receptor potential ion channel. *J Biol Chem, 2004,* 279: 3708-3716.
[66] Zhu MH, Kim TW, Ro S, Yan W, Ward SM, Koh SD, Sanders KM. A Ca^{2+}-activated Cl^{-} conductance in interstitial cells of Cajal linked to slow wave currents and pacemaker activity. J Physiol., 2009, 587: 4905-4918.
[67] Identification of TRPM7 channels in human intestinal interstitial cells of Cajal Byung Joo Kim, Kyu Joo Park, Hyung Woo Kim, Seok Choi, Jae Yeoul Jun, In Youb Chang, Ju-Hong Jeon, Insuk So, Seon Jeong Kim *World J Gastroenterol* 2009, 15: 5799-5804.
[68] Zhu Y, S. P. Parsons SP, Huizinga JD. Measurement of intracellular chloride ion concentration in ICC in situ and in explant culture. Neurogastroenterol Motil, 2010, 22: 704-709
[69] Watanabe H, Vriens J, Prenen J, Droogmans G, Voets T, Nilius B. Anandamide and arachidonic acid use epoxyeicosatrienoic acids to activate TRPV4 channels. Nature, 2003, 424: 434-8.
[70] Daniel EE, Posey-Daniel V. Neuromuscular structures in opossum esophagus: role of interstitial cells of Cajal. *Am J Physiol, 1984,* 246: G305-G315.
[71] Wang XY, Sanders KM, Ward SM. Relationship between interstitial cells of Cajal and enteric motor neurons in the murine proximal colon. *Cell Tissue Res, 2000,* 302: 331-342.
[72] Horiguchi K, Sanders KM, Ward SM. Enteric motor neurons form synaptic-like junctions with interstitial cells of Cajal in the canine gastric antrum. *Cell Tissue Res,* 2003, 311: 299-313.
[73] Sanmarti-Vila L, tom Dieck S, Richter K, Altrock W, Zhang L, Volknandt W, Zimmermann H, Garner CC, Gundelfinger ED, Dresbach T. Membrane association

of presynaptic cytomatrix protein bassoon. *Biochem Biophys Res Commun, 2000,* 275: 43–46.
[73] Kennedy MB. Signal-processing machines at the postsynaptic density. *Science, 2000,* 290, 750–754.
[74] Aoki C, Miko I, Oviedo H, Mikeladze-Dvali T, Alexandre L, Sweeney N, Bredt DS. Electron microscopic immunocytochemical detection of PSD-95, PSD-93, SAP-102, and SAP-97 at postsynaptic, presynaptic, and nonsynaptic sites of adult and neonatal rat visual cortex. *Synapse, 2001,* 40: 239–257.
[75] Ruegg MA . Molecules involved in the formation of synaptic connections in muscle and brain. *Matrix Biol, 2001,* 20: 3–12.
[76] Aguado F, Majo G, Ruiz-Montasell B, Llorens J, Marsal J, Blasi J. Syntaxin 1A and 1B display distinct distribution patterns in the rat peripheralnervous system. *Neuroscience,* 1999, 88: 437–446.
[77] Beckett EAH, Takeda Y, Yanase H, Sanders KM, Ward SM. Synaptic specializations exist between enteric motor nerves and interstitial cells of Cajal in the murine stomach. *J Comp Neurol, 2005,* 493: 193–206.
[78] Sudhof TC, Rizo J. Synaptotagmins: C2-domain proteins that regulate membrane traffic. *Neuron, 1996,* 17: 379–388.
[79] Vannucchi MG,De Giorgio R & Faussone-Pellegrini MS. NK1 receptor expression in the interstitial cells of Cajal and neurons and tachykinins distribution in rat ileum during development. *J Comp Neurol, 1997,* 383: 153–162.
[80] Lavin ST, Southwell BR, Murphy R, Jenkinson KM, Furness JB (1998). Activation of neurokinin 1 receptors on interstitial cells of Cajal of the guinea-pig small intestine by substance P. *Histochem Cell Biol, 1998,* 110: 263–271.
[81] Epperson A, Hatton WJ, Callaghan B, Doherty P,Walker RL, Sanders KM,Ward SM, Horowitz B. Molecular components expressed in cultured and freshly isolated interstitial cells of Cajal. *Am J Physiol Cell Physiol, 2000,* 279: C529–C539.
[82] Patterson LM, Zheng H,Ward SM & Berthoud HR. Immunohistochemical identification of cholecystokinin A receptors on interstitial cells of Cajal, smooth muscle, and enteric neurons in rat pylorus. *Cell Tissue Res, 2001,* 305: 11–23.
[83] Ward SM, Beckett EAH,Wang X-Y, Baker F, Khoyi M & Sanders KM. Interstitial cells of Cajal mediate cholinergic neurotransmission from enteric motor neurons. *J Neurosci, 2000,* 20: 1393–1403.
[84] Beckett EA, McGeough CA, Sanders KM, Ward SM. Pacing of interstitial cells of Cajal in the murine gastric antrum: neurally mediated and direct stimulation. J Physiol., 2003, 553: 545-559.
[85] Song G, Hirst GDS, Sanders KM, Ward SM. Regional variation in ICC distribution, pacemaking activity and neural responses in the longitudinal muscle of the murine stomach. *J Physiol, 2005a,* 564: 523–540.
[86] Song G, McKee JD, Dixon RE, Spencer EAH, Sanders KM & Ward SM (2005*b*). Neurokinin neural responses are preserved in the absence of ICC-IM in the stomach. *Neurogastro Mot, 2005b,* 17 (Suppl. 2): 6–7.
[87] Iino S, Horiguchi K, Nojyo Y. Interstitial cells of Cajal are innervated by nitrergic nerves and express nitric oxide-sensitive guanylate cyclase in the guinea-pig gastrointestinal tract. Neuroscience., 2008, 152: 437-448.

[88] Iino S, Horiguchi K, Nojyo Y, Ward SM, Sanders KM. Interstitial cells of Cajal contain signalling molecules for transduction of nitrergic stimulation in guinea pig caecum. Neurogastroenterol Motil. 2009; 21: 542-550.
[89] Gillespie JI, Markerink-van Ittersum M, de Vente J. cGMP-generating cells in the bladder wall: identification of distinct networks of interstitial cells. BJU international. 2004, 94: 1114-1124.
[90] Vanderwinden JM, Rumessen JJ. Interstitial cells of Cajal in human gut and gastrointestinal disease. Microsc Res Tech 1999, 47: 344–60.
[91] Burns AJ. Disorders of interstitial cells of Cajal. J Pediatr Gastroenterol Nutr 2007, 45: 103–6. 4
[92] Rolle U, Piaseczna-Piotrowska A, Puri P. Interstitial cells of Cajal in the normal gut and in intestinal motility disorders of childhood. Pediatr Surg Int 2007; 23: 1139–52.
[94] Farrugia G. Interstitial cells of Cajal in health and disease. Neurogastroenterol Motil 2008, 20: 54–63.
[95] Maeda H, Yamagata A, Nishikawa S et al. Requirement of c-kit for development of intestinal pacemaker system. Development 1992, 116: 369–75.
[96] Ward SM, Burns AJ, Torihashi S, Sanders KM. Mutation of the protooncogene c-kit blocks development of interstitial cells and electrical rhythmicity in murine intestine. J Physiol 1994, 480: 91–7.
[97] Huizinga JD, Thuneberg L, Klu¨ ppel M, Malysz J, Mikkelsen HB, Bernstein A. W/kit gene required for interstitial cells of Cajal and for intestinal pacemaker activity. Nature 1995, 373: 347–9
[98] Horisawa M, Watanabe Y, Torihashi S. Distribution of c-kit immunopositive cells in normal human colon and in Hirschsprung's disease. J Pediatr Surg 1998, 33:1209–14
[99] Mearin F, Malagelada JR. Gastroparesis and dyspepsia in patients with diabetes mellitus. Eur J Gastroenterol Hepatol 1995, 7: 717–23.
[100] De Block CE, De Leeuw I, Pelckmans PA, Van Gaal LF. Current concepts in gastric motility in diabetes mellitus. Curr Diabetes Rev 2006, 2: 113–30.
[101]Koch KL. Electrogastrography: physiological basis and clinical application in diabetic gastropathy. Diabetes Technol Ther 2001, 3: 51–62.
[102] Vittal H, Farrugia G, Gomez G, Pasricha PJ. Mechanisms of disease: the pathological basis of gastroparesis–a review of experimental and clinical studies. Nat Clin Pract Gastroenterol Hepatol 2007, 4: 336–46.
[103] Hirst GD, Edwards FR. Electrical events underlying organized myogenic contractions of the guinea pig stomach. J Physiol 2006, 576: 659–65.
[104] Andrews PL, Sanger GJ. Abdominal vagal afferent neurones: an important target for the treatment of gastrointestinal dysfunction. Curr Opin Pharmacol 2002, 2: 650–6.
[105] Fox EA, Phillips RJ, Martinson FA, Baronowsky EA, Powley TL. Vagal afferent innervation of smooth muscle in the stomach and duodenum of the mouse: morphology and topography. J Comp Neurol 2000, 428: 558–76.
[106] He CL, Soffer EE, Ferris CD, Walsh RM, Szurszewski JH, Farrugia G. Loss of interstitial cells of Cajal and inhibitory innervation in insulindependent diabetes. Gastroenterology 2001, 121: 427–34.
[107] Nakahara M, Isozaki K, Hirota S et al.Deficiency of KIT-positive cells in the colon of patients with diabetes mellitus. J Gastroenterol Hepatol 2002, 17: 666–70.

[108] Forster J, Damjanov I, Lin Z, Sarosiek I, Wetzel P, McCallum RW. Absence of the interstitial cells of Cajal in patients with gastroparesis and correlation with clinical findings. J Gastrointest Surg 2005, 9: 102–8.

[109] Miller SM, Narasimhan RA, Schmalz PF et al. Distribution of interstitial cells of Cajal and nitrergic neurons in normal and diabetic human appendix. Neurogastroenterol Motil 2008; 20: 349–57.

[110] Viktor J. Horva´ th,1 Harsha Vittal,1,2 and Tama´s O¨ rdo¨g1 Reduced Insulin and IGF-I Signaling, not Hyperglycemia, Underlies the Diabetes-Associated Depletion of Interstitial Cells of Cajal in the Murine Stomach. Diabetes, 2005, 54:1528–1533.

[111] Horvath VJ, Vital H, Lorincz A, Chen H, Almeida-Porda A, Redelman D, Ördog T. Reduced Stem Cell Factor Links Smooth Myopathy and Loss of Interstitial Cells of Cajal in Murine Diabetic Gastroparesis. Gastroenterol, 2006, 130:759–770.

[112] Wang XY, Huizinga JD, Diamond J, Liu LWC. Loss of intramuscular and submuscular interstitial cells of Cajal and associated enteric nerves is related to decreased gastric emptying in streptozotocin-induced diabetesNeurogastroenterol Motil, 2009, 21: 1095–1107.

[113] Sanders KM, Ordog T, Ward SM. Physiology and pathophysiology of the interstitial cells of Cajal: from bench to bedside. IV. Genetic and animal models of GI motility disorders caused by loss of interstitial cells of Cajal. Am J Physiol Gastrointest Liver Physiol 2002, 282: G747–56.

[114] Schuffler MD, Sinanan MN. Intestinal obstruction and pseudo-obstruction. In: Sleisenger MH, Fordtran JS, eds. Gastrointestinal Disease–Pathophysiology/ Diagnosis/Management. Philadelphia: WB Saunders, 1993: 898–916.

[115] Prommegger R, Marksteiner J, Wetscher G et al. Obstructive ileus of large bowel is associated to low tissue levels of neuropeptides in prestenotic bowel segment. Dig Dis Sci 1997, 7: 1513–8.

[116] Chang IY, Glasgow NJ, Takayama I, Horiguchi K, Sanders KM, Ward SM. Loss of interstitial cells of Cajal and development of electrical dysfunction in murine small bowel obstruction. *J* Physiol, *2001,* 536:*555–568.*

[117] Jain D, Moussa K, Tandon M, Culpepper-Morgan J, Proctor DD. Role of interstitial cells of Cajal in motility disorders of the bowel. Am. J. Gastroenterol. 2003, 98: 618–624.

[118] Streutker CJ, Huizinga JD, Campbell F, Ho J, Riddell RH. Loss of CD117 (c-kit)- and CD34-positive ICC and associated CD34-positive fibroblasts defines a subpopulation of chronic intestinal pseudo-obstruction. Am. J. Surg. Pathol. 2003, 27: 228–235.

[119] Isozaki K, Hirota S, Miyagawa J, Taniguchi M, Shinomura Y, Matsuzawa Y. Deficiency of c-kit+ cells in patients with a myopathic form of chronic idiopathic intestinal pseudo-obstruction. Am. J. Gastroenterol. 1997, 92: 332–334.

[120] Yamataka A, Ohshiro K, Kobayashi H et al. Abnormal distribution of intestinal pacemaker (C-KIT-positive) cells in an infant with chronic idiopathic intestinal pseudoobstruction. J. Pediatr. Surg. 1998, 33: 859–862.

[121] Feldstein AE, Miller SM, El Youssef M et al. Chronic intestinal pseudoobstruction associated with altered interstitial cells of Cajal networks. J. Pediatr. Gastroenterol. Nutr. 2003, 36: 492–497.

[122] Faussone-Pellegrini MS, Fociani P, Buffa R., Basilisco G. Loss of interstitial cells and a fibromuscular layer on the luminal side of the colonic circular muscle presenting as megacolon in an adult patient. Gut 1999, 45: 775–779.

[123] Tong WD, Liu BH, Zhang LY, Zhang SB, Lei Y. Decreased interstitial cells of Cajal in the sigmoid colon of patients with slow transit constipation. Int. J. Colorect. Dis. 2004, 19: 467–473.

[124] Shafik A, Shafik AA, El Sibai O, Mostafa RM. Electric activity of the colon in subjects with constipation due to total colonic inertia: an electrophysiologic study. Arch. Surg. 2003, 138:1007–1011.

[125] Boeckxstaens GE, Rumessen JJ, de Wit L, Tytgat GN, Vanderwinden JM. Abnormal distribution of the interstitial cells of cajal in an adult patient with pseudo-obstruction and megaduodenum. Am. J. Gastroenterol. 2002, 97: 2120–2126.

[126] Suzuki S, Suzuki H, Horiguchi K, ORIGUCHI, Tsugawa H, Matsuzaki J, Takagi T, Shimojima, Hibi T. Delayed gastric emptying and disruption of the interstitial cells of Cajal network after gastric ischaemia and reperfusion. Neurogastroenterol Motil, 2010, 22: 585–594.

[127] Shimojima N, Nakaki T, Morikawa Y et al. Interstitial cells of Cajal in dysmotility in intestinal ischemia and reperfusion injury in rats. J Surg Res 2006, 135: 255–61.

30

Biological Pacemaker – Main Ideas and Optimization

Han-Gang Yu and Yen-Chang Lin
Centre for Cardiovascular and Respiratory Sciences, Department of Physiology & Pharmacology
Robert C. Byrd Health Sciences Centre, West Virginia University, Morgantown, WV USA

1. Introduction

Electronic pacemaker, since its invention over five decades ago, has saved numerous lives and improved the life quality of patients suffering from cardiac arrhythmias. However, it has its own limitations. Over the past decade, rapid progress in the molecular studies of cardiac ion channels and stem cell biology has led to efforts for creating a biological pacemaker to supplement the widely used electronic pacemaker. We focus on the development of the ideas for creating a working biological pacemaker. The gene-based and cell-based approaches to meet the requirements of a working biological pacemaker will be reviewed. The important roles of the hyperpolarization-activated cyclic, nucleotide-modulated (HCN) channels, the inward rectifier Kir2.1 potassium channels, and the gap junctions in the biological pacemaker system will be discussed. Finally, recent development of cell-based strategy and precautions for creation of an effective biological pacemaker superior to the electronic counterpart will also be discussed.

2. Hierarchic organization of cardiac pacemakers

Throughout life, the heart beats close to 3 billion times (assuming 70 beats per minute with a mean life span of 80 years). The ability of the heart to beat spontaneously and continuously relies on its highly organized pacemaker system.

The cardiac pacemaker activity is originated in the sinoatrial node (SAN) located in the right atrium. The electrical impulses are transmitted to the atria, then the atria-ventricular (AV) node to the His/Purkinje conducting system, and to the working ventricles.

Pacemaker activity has also been found in regions outside the SA node, including atria, AV node, and Purkinje fibers. Under physiologic conditions, these regions have much slower intrinsic pacing rates, and thus are overdriven by the SA node. Pacemaker activity is absent in the adult mammalian ventricle, but is present in the cultured newborn ventricle. Abnormal pacemaker activity also appears in cardiomyopathies such as heart failure and hypertrophy.

Heart rate is subject to autonomic regulation. Sympathetic stimulation accelerates heart rate by activating β adrenergic receptors, whereas parasympathetic stimulation slows heart rate by activating muscarinic acetylcholine receptors. Through the G-protein/adenylate cyclase pathway, autonomic stimulation alters the intracellular cAMP levels, which in turn, changes the heart rate by altering the gating properties of membrane transporters including ion channels, exchangers and pumps. Increased cAMP levels enhance, while decreased cAMP levels reduce, the heart rate.

2.1 Cardiac pacemaker activity generation

Cardiac pacemaker activity begins with the diastolic (phase-4) depolarization, which is a slow time-dependent depolarizing process different from the rapid action potential firing (Figure 1). The major ionic mechanisms for the initiation of this diastolic depolarization have

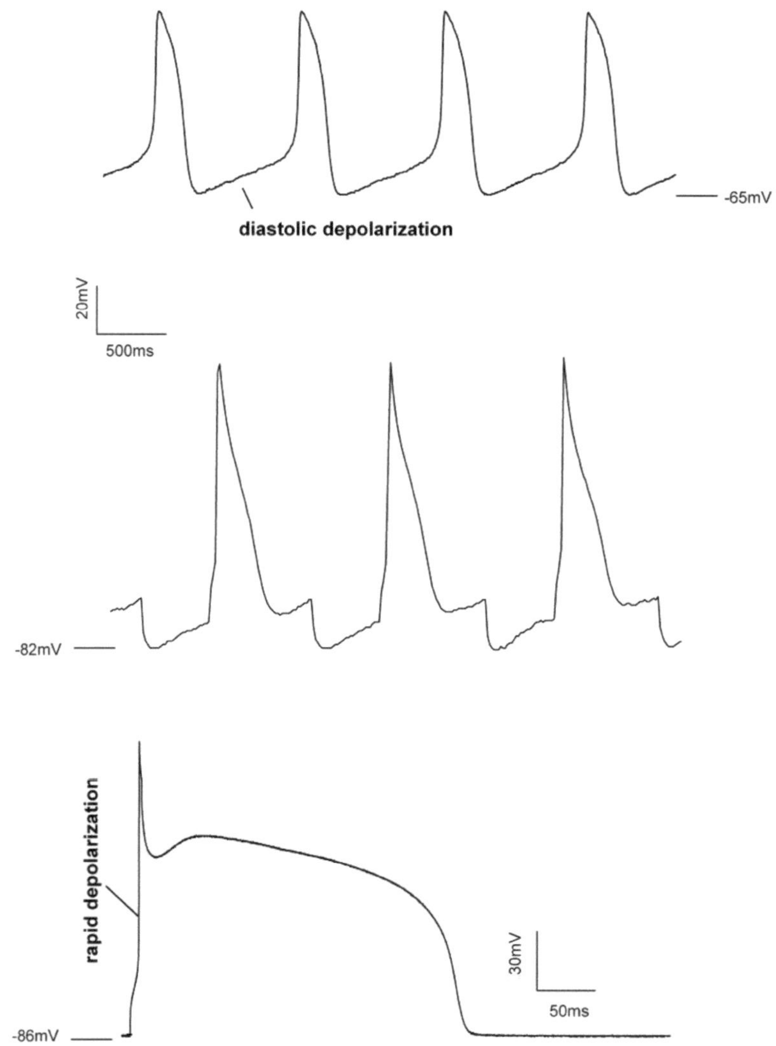

Fig. 1. Action potentials recorded from single myocytes isolated from rabbit SA node (A), canine Purkinje fiber (B), and canine ventricle. Current stimulus was used to generate action potentials in Purkinje and ventricular myocytes.

been debated for nearly three decades (Brown *et al.*, 1979; DiFrancesco, 1995; Vassalle, 1995; Liu *et al.*, 1998; Lipsius & Bers, 2003; Bers, 2006; Sanders *et al.*, 2006; Lakatta & DiFrancesco, 2009; DiFrancesco, 2010; Lakatta, 2010), reflecting the complex nature of this essential biological function. Despite its complicated mechanism, there is a widely accepted agreement that a *net* inwardly increasing current (net positive ions entering the cell) must contribute to this process. The *minimal* requirement for producing such a net inward current could be a combination of either a time-dependent outward current and a constant inward background current, or a time-dependent inward current and a time independent outward background current (Vassalle *et al.*, 1999). With regard to the biological pacemaker, we will mainly focus on the discussion of the latter combination. This, by no means, undermines other mechanisms such as Ca^{2+} clocks that also play important roles in cardiac pacemaker activity (Lakatta *et al.*, 2008; Lakatta & DiFrancesco, 2009; Lakatta *et al.*, 2010).

2.2 Action potentials and membrane currents of cardiac myocytes

Cardiac pacemaker activity is tissue-specific. Spontaneous action potentials can be readily recorded in single myocytes isolated from SA node (Figure 1, upper panel), but harder from isolated Purkinje myocytes. However, with current stimulus, phase-4 depolarization can be elicited in isolated Purkinje cells (Figure 1, middle panel). In isolated ventricular myocytes, phase-4 depolarization cannot be induced with stimulus under physiological conditions (Figure 1, lower panel). According to Ohm's law, these differential action potentials in different regions of the heart indicate different underlying ionic mechanisms. Figure 2 shows the membrane currents near the end of repolarization that are different in primary pacemaker tissue (SA node), conducting system (Purkinje fibers), and working ventricles. In response to a hyperpolarizing pulse to the indicated voltages, in the SA node, there is a strong time-dependent inward current, but little background potassium outward current, indicated by the lack of an instant jump at the beginning of the hyperpolarizing pulse (upper panel); in the Purkinje cells, in additional to the time-dependent inward current, there is a considerable amount of background potassium current (middle panel); in the ventricular myocytes, the background outward current is dominant with little time-dependent inward current (lower panel).

It is noted that if the time independent outward current is so small that it can be negligible, such as in the SA node, inducing diastolic depolarization requires only a few pA of time-dependent inward current (Vassalle *et al.*, 1999). On the other hand, if the time-dependent background outward current is large, a much larger time-dependent inward current is needed to initiate diastolic depolarization, such as in the Purkinje fibers (Figure 2, middle panel). Once the time independent outward current dominates over the time dependent inward current, diastolic depolarization cannot be elicited, which is the case in the ventricle (Figure 2, lower panel). Thus, generation and inhibition of diastolic depolarization can be achieved by adjusting the expression levels of the time independent outward current and/or the time dependent inward current.

3. Hyperpolarization-activated HCN, inward rectifier Kir2.x potassium channels, and gap junction channels in the sinus node and in the ventricles

Action potential is an electrical process that reflects the time dependent changes in charges across the cell membrane. Due to uneven distribution of ions inside and outside of the cell, ions crossing the cell membrane via ion channels alter the membrane potential in a dynamic manner. The time- and voltage-dependent inward current (e.g., Na^+ current) makes the membrane more positive (or less negative), whereas the time- and voltage-dependent outward current (e.g., K^+ current) drives the membrane potential toward more negative values. The delicate balance of inward and outward currents initiates and maintains the rhythmic heart beat under physiological conditions. Disruption of this ionic balance predisposes the heart to arrhythmias (irregular heart beat).

In this chapter, we focus on the properties of two ionic currents, the hyperpolarization-activated cation current, I_f, and the inward rectifier potassium current, I_{K1}. We also describe the gap junction channels in the heart due to their critical roles in electrically connecting the myocytes to produce synchronous cardiac contraction.

3.1 I_f and HCN channels

I_f is an important contributor to the cardiac pacemaker activity. Opened by hyperpolarization near the end of repolarization in the sinus node, I_f contributes significantly to the diastolic (phase-4) depolarization, which leads to the threshold of Ca-channel activation and firing of an action potential.

Unlike most voltage-gated ion channels that are activated by membrane depolarization, I_f is activated by membrane hyperpolarization at the end of repolarization (Figure 2, Figure 4B). I_f channels pass Na^+ and K^+ ions (DiFrancesco, 1993) and a tiny amount of Ca^{2+} ions (Yu *et al.*, 2004; Yu *et al.*, 2007). Under physiological conditions, mainly Na^+ ions go in and much less K^+ ions come out through the channel near maximum diastolic potential (MDP) (e.g., -60mV to -90mV), generating a time dependent inward current with a reversal potential around –20mV (DiFrancesco, 1993).

The threshold activation of I_f is closely associated with the tissue pacemaker activity. In the SA node, I_f activates near -50mV and the MDP is around -65mV (upper panels in Figures 1&2). In Purkinje fibers, I_f activates around -70mV and the MDP is near -85mV (middle panels in Figures 1&2). In the ventricle, I_f activates at potentials more negative than -100mV (Yu *et al.*, 1993, 1995; Robinson *et al.*, 1997), and the MDP is around -90mV (lower panels in Figures 1&2).

In adult mammalian ventricles, the threshold activation of I_f in ventricular myocytes is also species specific. It is extremely negative in guinea pig ventricles (more negative than -140mV) and a little more positive in canine ventricles (around -120mV) (Yu *et al.*, 1993, 1995). In rat ventricles, there are varying results with regard to I_f activation. Early studies showed a -110mV threshold activation of I_f in myocytes isolated from 3-month old rat ventricles (Robinson *et al.*, 1997). However, more positive threshold activation of I_f in rat ventricles within the physiological voltages has been reported in several other studies (Cerbai *et al.*, 1994, 1996; Ranjan *et al.*, 1998; Xiao *et al.*, 2007). It has been hypothesized that the potential contribution of I_f to the diastolic depolarization is masked by a large I_{K1} in the ventricular myocytes (see below).

In the newborn ventricles, I_f activates around -70mV (Robinson *et al.*, 1997). Diseased adult ventricles also increases I_f and shifts its threshold activation into the physiological voltages, near -55mV (Cerbai *et al.*, 1997; Cerbai & Mugelli, 2006). The molecular basis of this developmental and disease modulated voltage dependent activation remains unclear.

I_f is generated by HCN channels. Among the four isoforms that have been identified, three of them (HCN1, HCN2, HCN4) are differentially expressed in various regions of the heart.

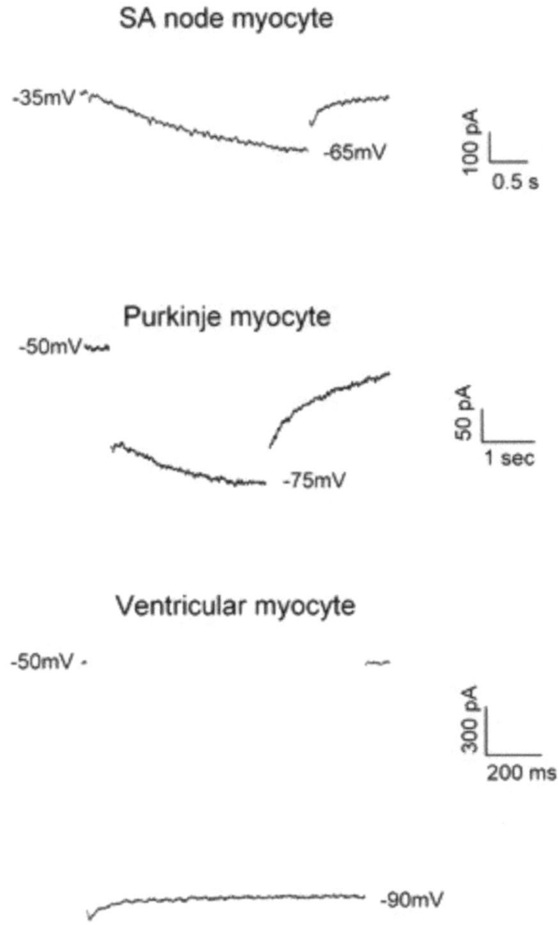

Fig. 2. Membrane currents recorded in single myocytes isolated from rabbit SA node (upper panel), canine Purkinje fibers (middle panel), and canine ventricle (lower panel). The holding potential was -35mV for SA node myocyte, and -50mV for Purkinje and ventricular myocytes. The hyperpolarizing pulse was applied to -65mV (SA node), -75mV (Purkinje), and -90mV (ventricle), respectively.

HCN total transcripts levels are the highest in the SA node, intermediate in the Purkinje fibers, and the lowest in the working ventricles (Shi *et al.*, 1999; Shi *et al.*, 2000). HCN4 is the dominant isoform in the SA node, representing about 80% of the total HCN transcripts. Equal amounts of HCN1 and HCN4 are present in the Purkinje fibers. In the ventricles, HCN2 expression levels are higher than HCN4, and no HCN1 has been detected (Shi *et al.*, 1999; Shi *et al.*, 2000; Han *et al.*, 2002).

When expressed in the heterologous expression systems (*Xenopus* oocytes, mammalian culture cells such as HEK and COS cells), HCN1, HCN2, and HCN4 channels displayed distinct properties. HCN1 activates at the least negative potential (near -50mV) associated with the fastest activation kinetics, mimicking the SA node I_f. HCN2 and HCN4 are activated at more negative potentials (-60mV to -80 mV) with much slower activation kinetics (Robinson & Siegelbaum, 2003). In addition, HCN1 is nearly insensitive to intracellular cAMP, while HCN2 and HCN4 activation curves can be shifted to depolarizing potentials by cAMP for more than 10mV. Binding of cAMP to the cyclic nucleotide binding domain in the C-terminus facilitates the gating of HCN channels (Wainger *et al.*, 2001).

3.2 I_{K1} and Kir2.1 channels

The inwardly rectifying potassium current, I_{K1}, is essential in the resting phase of ventricular action potential. Its reversal potential is close to the resting membrane potential. I_{K1} channels pass more inward current at potentials more negative than the potassium reversal potential (E_K), but much fewer outward current at potentials more positive than E_K; in the range of -40mV to 0mV, I_{K1} is negligibly small and close to zero (Dhamoon & Jalife, 2005).

I_{K1} is nearly absent in the sinus node, making the resting potential more positive (around -65mV) in comparison to that in the ventricular myocytes (around -86mV) (Fig. 1). The relatively depolarized membrane potential in the sinus node allows small but significant I_f inward current to slowly depolarize the membrane during diastole, which is critical in initiating the pacemaker activity (Figure 1, upper panel). In the ventricular myocytes, due to the presence of a large I_{K1} and low expression I_f, there is no diastolic depolarization under physiological conditions (Figure 1, lower panel).

I_{K1} is nearly undetectable in neonatal rat ventricular myocytes that have spontaneous pacemaker activity (Sekar *et al.*, 2009). Similarly, in failing ventricles I_{K1} is reduced (Beuckelmann *et al.*, 1993). Meantime, I_f activity is increased in neonatal (Robinson *et al.*, 1997) and in failing ventricles (Cerbai *et al.*, 1997; Hoppe *et al.*, 1998). A combination of reduced I_{K1} and an increased I_f predisposes the ventricle to generate unwanted diastolic depolarization (Cerbai & Mugelli, 2006).

I_{K1} is mainly produced by inward rectifier potassium Kir2.x (x=1,2,3,4) channels in the heart. In ventricular myocytes Kir2.1 is the predominant isoform, although Kir2.2 may also contribute to I_{K1} to some extent (Dhamoon & Jalife, 2005). Kir2.1 transcripts have been reported to be at the lower levels in the SA node and atria, but much higher in the ventricles (Gaborit *et al.*, 2007). During cardiac development, Kir2.1 is also found at the lowest levels in the mice SA node (Schweizer *et al.*, 2009). In neonatal rat ventricular myocytes, Kir2.1 protein expression is barely detected (Sekar *et al.*, 2009).

For both HCN and Kir2.1 channels, tetramers are formed as the functional channels. Different HCN or Kir2.x channel isoforms may form the functional heteromeric channels generating native I_f or I_{K1} in the heart.

3.3 Cardiac gap junction channels

Gap junctions allow direct passage of ions and small signaling molecules with molecular weight up to ~1000 Daltons between adjacent cells. Gap junctions are required in the orchestrated electrical activation of the heart. Spontaneous action potentials generated from the SA node are efficiently transmitted to the working ventricles due to electrical coupling among the myocytes in different regions of the heart. The coordinated muscle contraction depends upon normal gating of gap junction channels between myocytes.

Gap junctions are formed by two hemi-channels (connexons) with each expressed on the plasma membrane of adjacent myocytes. Each hemi-channel is assembled by six connexins (Cx) spanning the plasma membrane (Yeager, 1998). Their extracellular domains form the gap junction with their N- and C-termini in the intracellular space for channel regulation.

There are three main connexins identified in the heart: Cx40, Cx43, and Cx45. They can form either homomeric or heteromeric connexins (Yeager, 1998). When expressed in the heterologous expressing systems, they exhibit distinct single channel conductance that determines the propagation speed of electrical signals. Single channel conductance is large for Cx43 and Cx40, about 100pS and 158-198 pS, respectively, and small for Cx45, about 30pS (Gonzalez *et al.*, 2007).

Gap junctions with large conductance facilitate fast transmission of electrical signals such as Purkinje fibers and working ventricles. Gap junctions with small conductance are mainly restricted in the pacemaker tissues such as the SA node and AV node in which the electrical transmission is slow.

Cx43 is the dominant connexin in the working ventricles, co-expressed with Cx40 in atria, absent in the SA node and AV node. Cx45 is present in the atria including the SA node, AV node, His bundle and ventricles (Saez *et al.*, 2003; Severs *et al.*, 2008). All three connexins are present in Purkinje fibers (Severs *et al.*, 2008). In the slow conducting tissues, such as the SA node and AV node, only Cx45 is expressed. Redistribution and reduction in cell surface expression of gap junctions have been linked to severe arrhythmias associated with ischemia and failing heart (Severs *et al.*, 2008).

4. Need for biological pacemaker

When dysfunction of the SA node or blockade of the AV node occurs, generation of normal action potentials or the propagation of the normal electrical signals to the working ventricle is disrupted. The latent pacemakers in atria and Purkinje fibers will pace at their own rates (slower than the sinus rate). This creates an asynchronous rhythmic contraction of the heart muscle leading to a decreased blood pumping efficiency. It also predisposes the heart to more dangerous arrhythmias. To preserve the normal muscle contraction under SA node dysfunction, the standard surgical intervention is to implant an electronic pacemaker, which has become the industrial standard since its invention.

While extremely successful and widely used as a life-saving device, the electronic pacemaker has its own limitations. They include 1) battery life; it usually needs to be replaced every 5-7 years; 2) implantation sites of the leads which may affect the cardiac output; 3) in growing children, pacemaker lead length is problematic requiring multiple replacements in pediatric patients; 4) lack of physiological response to autonomic stimulations in exercise, although software has been developed to improve responses to varying heart rate in exercise; 5) potentially increased risk of heart failure for long-term use; 6) a separation of wires connecting the lead to the battery. In responding to these challenges, creating a biological pacemaker has been emerged as a promising supplement.

5. Implementation of biological pacemaker

Cardiac action potential is finely maintained by a number of channels, pumps, and exchangers (Figure 3). For discussion of biological pacemaker, we focus on the roles of I_{K1} and I_f currents that contribute to the membrane stability and diastolic depolarization.

Differential expression of HCN and Kir2.x channels and distinct properties of I_f and I_{K1} contribute to the different resting and action potentials in the sinus node and ventricular myocytes. As depicted in Figure 3, one of the characteristics in an electrically quiescent myocyte (such as a ventricular myocyte) is the abundant expression of I_{K1} and low expression of I_f. On the other hand, spontaneous myocytes (i.e., SA node cells) express high levels of I_f and no I_{K1}. Gap junction channels are needed to connect these two different types of myocytes for pacing at the same rate.

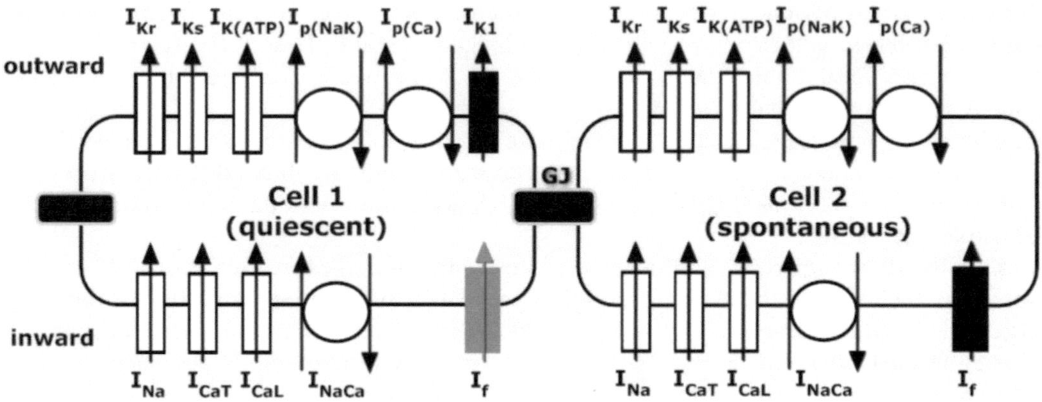

Fig. 3. Schematic illustration of major ion channels in quiescent and spontaneous cardiac myocytes. GJ= gap junction. Dark filled channels, I_{K1} and I_f, are the focuses in quiescent and spontaneous myocytes. I_f, I_{K1}, and gap junctions are essential requirements (among others) for enhancing, suppressing, and propagating the pacing activity throughout the entire heart. I_f in grey indicates much less physiological role in quiescent myocytes than in spontaneous myocytes.

A combination of an absent I_{K1} and an activated I_f at diastolic potential sets up the stage for the cardiac pacemaker activity in the sinus node (Fig. 4B). On the other hand, large I_{K1} and small I_f with negative activation mask the spontaneous pacemaker activity in the ventricle (Fig. 4A). These principles have been used as a working guidance in the development of the biological pacemaker. Therefore, enhancing HCN channel activity or inhibiting Kir2.1 channel activity or a combination of both should increase the spontaneous pacemaker activity in the ventricle.

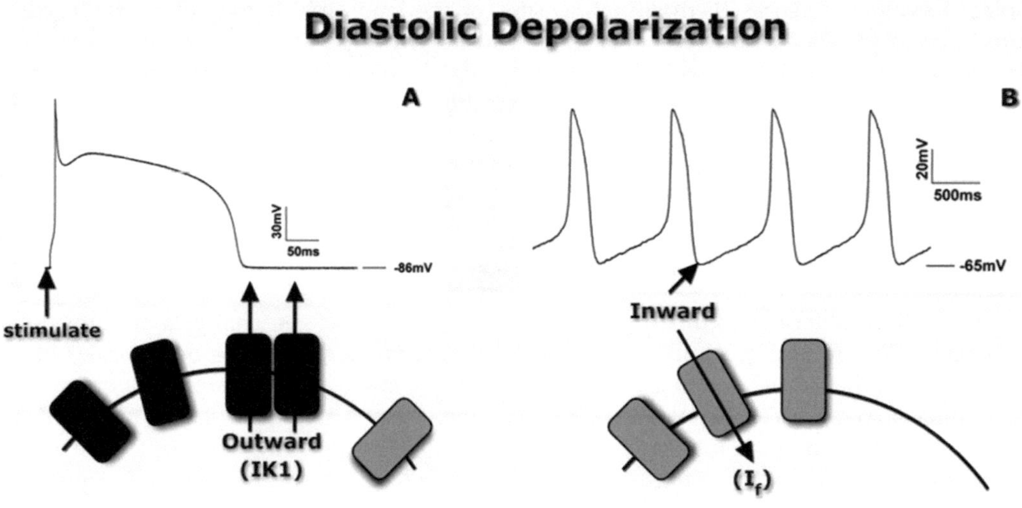

Fig. 4. Schematic illustration of roles for I_{K1} (dark) and I_f (grey) at diastolic depolarization of action potentials in a canine ventricular myocyte and in a spontaneous myocyte (e.g., rabbit sinus node cell).

Using a computer simulation of ventricular action potential (Figure 5), we had predicted that if I_{K1} conductance is reduced by 40% and the maximal conductance of I_f is increased by three-fold associated with a 40mV depolarized shift of the activation curve into the physiological voltages, the spontaneous pacemaker activity can be induced in the ventricles. These represent the minimal conditions to induce a ventricular spontaneous diastolic depolarization. In the past ten years the overexpression of either a dominant negative Kir2.1 or HCN channels have successfully induced spontaneous activity in the adult ventricular myocytes and in the hearts of intact animal models. The altered biophysical properties for both I_{K1} and I_f have far exceeded the simulation conditions shown in Figure 5.

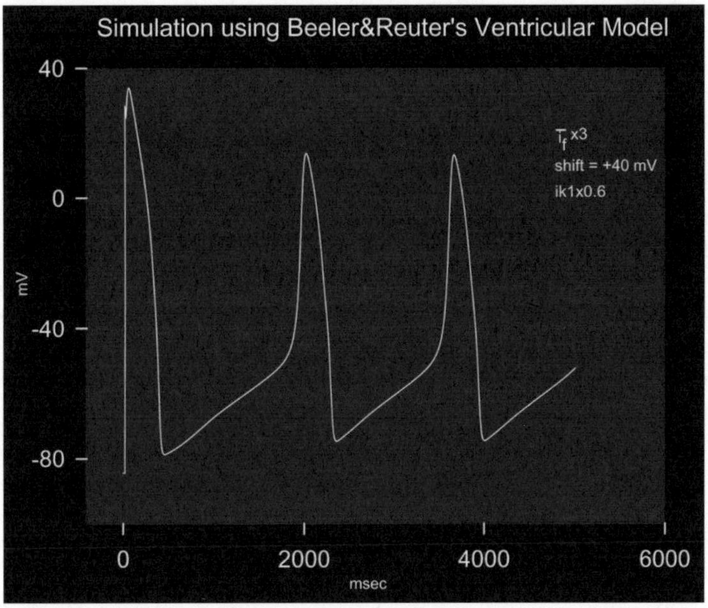

Fig. 5. Computer simulation of ventricular action potential using a Beeler and Reuter ventricular model (Beeler & Reuter, 1977). The parameters for I_{K1} and I_f were adjusted for minimal requirements to induce a ventricular pacing. I_f: maximal conductance. Shift: the voltage shift of the threshold activation.

Manipulation of HCN and Kir2.1 gene expression is a gene-based strategy for creation of a biological pacemaker. An alternative approach, a cell-based strategy, is to use the cells that have already had the desired ion channels for pacing (e.g., sinus node cells) or cells that are able to differentiate into the desired myocytes (e.g., stem cells). The advantages and disadvantages of these two approaches will be discussed below.

5.1 Gene-based approach

5.1.1 Overexpression of β-adrenergic receptors

The direct consequence of a sinus node dysfunction is the slow heart rate. Stimulation of β-adrenergic receptor can increase heart rate by increasing I_f (Brown *et al.*, 1979; DiFrancesco, 1986). Early studies in late 1990s demonstrated that overexpression of the β-adrenergic receptors in mouse embryonic and neonatal ventricular myocytes increased pacing rate (Edelberg *et al.*, 1998). Similar observation was made in a 6-week old intact mouse heart after

the right atria were injected with full-length β-adrenergic receptors plasmid (Edelberg *et al.*, 1998).
The cellular and ionic mechanisms that mediate the positive chronotropic effect of β-adrenergic receptors have been well documented. Stimulation of β-adrenergic receptors activates adenylate cyclase via G-proteins. Adenylate cyclase catalyzes ATP to cAMP which enhances I_f activity (DiFrancesco, 1993; Vassalle *et al.*, 1999). It is thus not surprising that overexpression of adenylate cyclase may also be able to pace the quiescent ventricle.

5.1.2 Overexpression of adenylate cyclase

In a pig AV-block model, Ruhparwar et al successfully converted the quiescent ventricular myocytes into the pacing cells near the injection site by overexpressing adenylate cyclase type VI (AC-VI) in the left ventricles (Ruhparwar *et al.*, 2010). The main idea was to boost the intracellular levels of cAMP that significantly increases the gating of HCN channels. The AC-VI in adenoviral vector was delivered into the left ventricle of a porcine heart. After 12 days, complete AV-block was induced by catheter ablation. After rapid ventricular pacing, an escape rhythm in the injection area was detected (Ruhparwar *et al.*, 2010).
Lack of normal ventricular diastolic depolarization is a result of large I_{K1} and small I_f. Although cAMP has been reported to cause a depolarizing shift of the I_f/HCN channel activation curves (DiFrancesco, 1986, 1993), it is unclear whether the dramatic increase of cAMP beyond the physiological level might also enhance the protein expression of HCN channels in the pig's ventricles. Another possibility is that rapid ventricular pacing may up-regulate HCN channel expression in the ventricle. A third possibility is that the basal level of intracellular cAMP is dramatically increased in AC-VI over-expressed ventricular myocytes (Ruhparwar *et al.*, 2010). Increased cAMP enhances the opening probability of HCN channels (Wainger *et al.*, 2001). However, the expression levels of both HCN2 and HCN4 are low in the ventricles under physiological conditions. Lack of diastolic depolarization of ventricular myocytes is well explained by a large I_{K1} and non-physiological threshold activation of I_f which are encoded by HCN2/HCN4 in the ventricles. Currently, it is unknown whether the dramatic increase in intracellular cAMP levels might also increase the functional HCN channels at the plasma membrane of the ventricular myocytes, which would make sense of converting quiescent ventricular myocytes into pacing myocytes by overexpression of AC-VI. Thus, how AC-VI overexpression is able to transform quiescent ventricular myocytes into spontaneously pacing myocytes remains an open question.
Adult cardiac myocytes are well differentiated and difficult in taking up exogenous proteins. One common method is to use virus-mediated infection. The gene of interest (HCN or Kir2.1) is inserted into a viral vector and viral particles containing the gene of interest are generated. Infected ventricular myocytes exhibit the spontaneous pacemaker activity under the condition in which either the Kir2.1 channel activity is inhibited or HCN channel activity is enhanced.

5.1.3 Inhibition of I_{K1}

The first evidence to demonstrate the feasibility of creating a biological pacemaker was to inhibit I_{K1} by overexpression of a dominant negative mutant of Kir2.1 (Kir2.1AAA) in guinea pig ventricular myocytes (Miake *et al.*, 2002). I_{K1} was inhibited by nearly 80%, leading to an increase in the resting membrane potential, action potential duration, and an induction of phase-4 depolarization (Miake *et al.*, 2002, 2003).

The idea of this approach is to remove I_{K1} suppression of the latent pacemaker activity for creation of a biological pacemaker in the quiescent adult ventricles. Later, studies have shown that strong inhibition of I_{K1} significantly reduced the membrane stability, and thus, can create large I_{K1} heterogeneity, which is pro-arrhythmogenic (Sekar *et al.*, 2009).

5.1.4 Enhancement of I_f

In both human atrial and ventricular myocytes, I_f has been detected at the physiological voltages (Hoppe & Beuckelmann, 1998; Hoppe *et al.*, 1998). Large I_{K1} suppresses the potential contribution of I_f to the pacemaker activity in these tissues. If reduced I_{K1} can unmask the pacemaker activity in ventricular myocytes as elegantly illustrated in the Kir2.1-AAA work, enhanced I_f should also be able to achieve the same goal.

HCN2 was first to be chosen to test an idea that overexpression of HCN2 in the adult ventricles can increase I_f activity leading to the spontaneous pacemaker activity. The reasons for choosing HCN2 among other HCN isoforms were HCN2's intermediate activation kinetics and its strong response to cAMP (Robinson *et al.*, 2006). HCN2 was overexpressed in the canine left atrium mediated by adenovirus (Qu *et al.*, 2003). After sinus arrest was achieved by vagal stimulation, spontaneous rhythm was detected in the left atrium. I_f amplitude was found more than 100-fold larger in HCN2-overexpressed atrial myocytes compared to native atrial myocytes or green fluorescent protein infected atrial myocytes by immunohistochemistry and Western blots. This work proved that it is feasible to create spontaneous pacemaker activity by increasing I_f current even in the presence of a large I_{K1}.

In a later study adenovirus containing HCN2 was injected to canine left bundle-branch. After two days, ventricular escape rhythms were recorded by 24-hour ECG monitoring during vagal stimulation (Plotnikov *et al.*, 2004). HCN2 overexpression was verified in the dissected tissues. The work provided strong evidence for a HCN2-based gene approach to induce a biological pacemaker within the left bundle-branch in the dog heart.

HCN1 has also been tested for creation of a biological pacemaker. A HCN1 mutant in which the S3-S4 linker was shortened by deleting three residues (HCN1- ΔΔΔ) in favor of channel gating was used to create an artificial SA node in a porcine model (Tse *et al.*, 2006). HCN1-ΔΔΔ was first overexpressed in the left ventricle of guinea pig to demonstrate its ability to pace the otherwise quiescent ventricular myocytes. Large I_f with physiological activation and fast activation kinetics, mimicking the SA node I_f, were detected in the adult guinea pig ventricular myocytes. This was to compare with the small I_f with very negative threshold activation (Yu *et al.*, 1993). The group then produced sinus node dysfunction by radiofrequency ablation to generate a sick sinus syndrome pig model (Tse *et al.*, 2006). At 10 to 14 days after injection of adenovirus containing HCN1-ΔΔΔ construct into the left atrial appendage, spontaneous atrial rhythm at a rate of 64 bpm was recorded. The advantage of using this HCN1 mutant is its fast activation kinetics similar to that of the native SA node I_f.

A recent study used HCN4 to create a biological pacemaker in the left ventricles of the pigs via an adenoviral gene transfer method (Cai *et al.*, 2007). In this research, one-month old pigs underwent catheter ablation for inducing a complete AV block after 3-4 days of adenoviral gene transfer of HCN4. ECG recordings detected idioventricular rhythm. HCN4 transcripts were not detected in non-infected ventricles, but abundantly expressed in Ad-HCN4 infected ventricles. Accordingly, large I_f-like current was recorded in the myocytes isolated from the Ad-HCN4 infected ventricles. The threshold activation was around -60mV with midpoint activation near -90mV. The I_f-like current activation curve was shifted to a more positive potential in response to 1μM isoproterenol, which was proposed as the cellular basis for the accelerated idioventricular rhythm (Cai *et al.*, 2007).

It is unclear why small I_f-like currents were also recorded in myocytes from saline treated ventricles of pigs with similar gating properties, presumably due to the presence of HCN2. I_f is encoded by both HCN2 and HCN4 in the ventricles (Shi *et al.*, 1999; Stillitano *et al.*, 2008). Recent evidence has shown that they can form heteromeric channels *in vitro* and *in vivo* producing an I_f with physiological activation (Much *et al.*, 2003; Whitaker *et al.*, 2007; Zhang *et al.*, 2009).

The respective roles for I_f and I_{K1} in the induced ventricular pacemaker activity have recently been evaluated in the guinea pig left ventricular myocytes overexpressing either HCN1-ΔΔΔ or Kir2.1 (Chan *et al.*, 2009). It was found that I_f activity is correlated with the slope of phase-4 depolarization and the firing frequency as well as the APD_{90}, whereas I_{K1} is correlated with APD90, but not the phase-4 slope and firing frequency (Chan *et al.*, 2009). The I_f functioning as a determinant for the basal firing frequency has also been observed in the neonatal rat ventricular myocytes (Chan *et al.*, 2010).

5.1.5 Creation of biological pacemaker by channel engineering

Recently, an alternative strategy has been used to create a biological pacemaker. Kv1.4 is a voltage dependent K^+ channel which is not present in the ventricle. It was converted into a hyperpolarization-activated, cation non-selective channel using site-directed mutagenesis (R447N, L448A, R431I in the S4 segment, and G528S in the pore region) (Kashiwakura *et al.*, 2006). Adenovirus-mediated gene transfer of this mutant channel into the left ventricle of guinea pig induced ectopic pacemaker activity in otherwise quiescent ventricle. This work provided additional supporting evidence for the requirement of time-dependent inward current, not necessarily from HCN channels, for the diastolic depolarization leading to the induction of pacemaker activity in adult heart ventricles.

5.2 Cell-based approach

5.2.1 Naturally pacing myocytes

Sinus node cells are natural cardiac pacemakers. The electrical impulses generated from the sinus node are transmitted to the neighboring atrial myocytes through gap junctions (Figure 6, upper panel). A fundamental question is how a SA node cell can pace its neighboring atrial myocytes, despite of the less negative MDP in SA node than in atrial myocytes? The upper panel in Figure 6 depicts a working principle (Robinson *et al.*, 2006), assuming the coupled SA node and atrial myocyte pair is at rest. The more negative membrane potential of the atrial myocyte hyperpolarizes the coupled SA node cell, leading to activation of HCN channels. The HCN inward current is a depolarizing current, which can pass through the gap junction and depolarize the atrial myocyte. When the HCN current is large enough to depolarize the membrane toward a threshold for further activation of the Na^+ channels, an action potential is fired in the atrial myocyte. After the SA node cell is depolarized, HCN channels will be deactivated. Thus, this working mechanism guarantees a depolarizing current only at diastole (Robinson *et al.*, 2006). This working principle also outlines the minimal requirements for creating a cell-base biological pacemaker. First, the implanted cells should be able to produce depolarizing current at the end of repolarization (i.e., at diastole). It does not matter whether the depolarizing current is a result of an enhanced

HCN current or a reduced I_{K1} current, or some other currents. Second, the implanted cells must be electrically coupled with the host cell via gap junctions. Third, the depolarizing current should not be needed after the action potential is fired in both the implanted and the host cells.

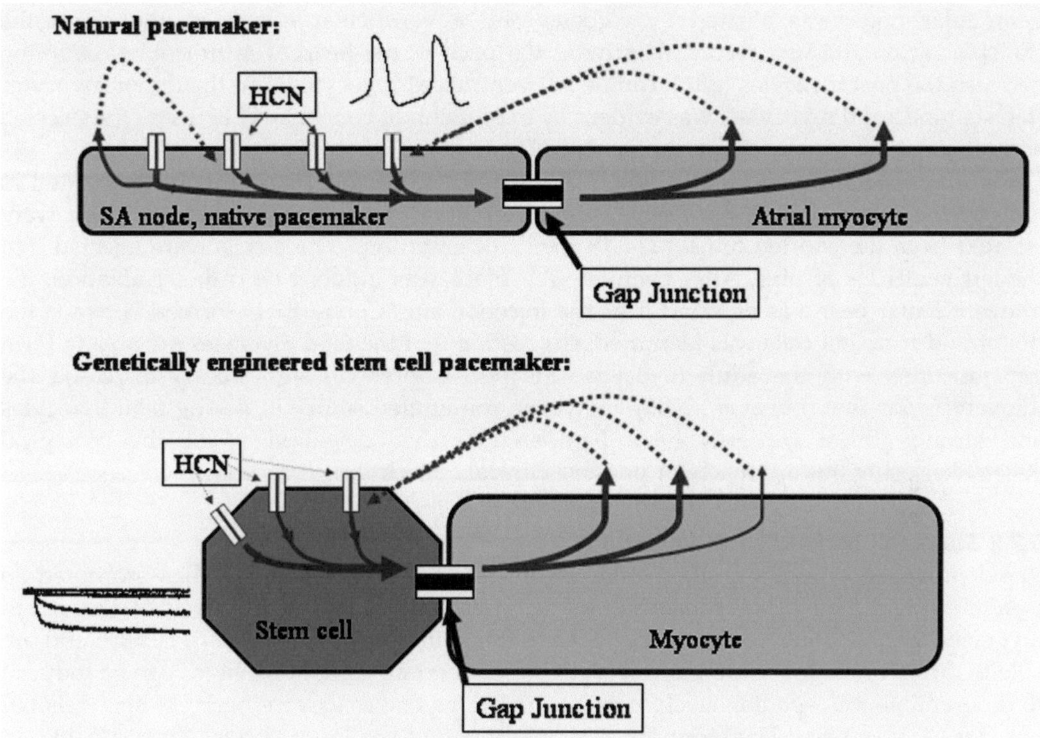

Fig. 6. Schematic illustration of using cell-based approach to deliver HCN channel genes into a ventricular myocyte. Upper panel: the native pacemaker cell (SA node cell) coupled to its adjacent myocyte (e.g., an atrial myocyte) for propagation of spontaneous action potentials via gap junction. Lower panel: engineered stem cell containing HCN channels to deliver HCN genes to a ventricular myocyte via formed gap junction for over-expression of HCN channels in the targeted myocyte. Reprinted with permission from (Rosen *et al.*, 2004).

In early 1990s, effort was made to first remove the SA node cells from a subject (the patient), then culture to generate a sufficient amount of healthy SA node cells, and finally implant these cells back to the right ventricle to provide pacing (King, 1992). This idea was to recreate a new working SA node in a new site. Although a great idea, the approach itself faced several challenges such as technical feasibility and working principles. First, growing adult human SA node cells to a critical mass represents a technical difficulty, although newborn rat SA node cells have been reported to culture for up to 4-5 days (Marvin *et al.*, 1984). Thus, feasibility of this approach is in question. Second, whether the reproduced SA nodal cells were able to form gap junctions with the ventricular myocytes was unclear. The native SA node cells are coupled with surrounding atrial cells through gap junctions. Without effective coupling between a spontaneous cell and a quiescent cell, the diastolic depolarization in the spontaneous cell cannot be transmitted to the quiescent cell for

triggering spontaneous pacing. Third, implantation in the right ventricle could represent a latent ectopic pacemaker that may trigger arrhythmia.
The proof-of-concept for creating a cell-based working biological pacemaker was first reported by transplanting the isolated fetal canine atrial myocytes including sinus node cells into the adult canine left ventricles (Ruhparwar *et al.*, 2002). After 3-4 weeks, atrial-ventricular node was ablated by catheter and a ventricular escape rhythm from the transplantation site was recorded, driving the pace of the heart. The functional coupling between the host myocytes (adult canine left ventricular myocytes) and the donor myocytes (fetal canine atrial myocytes) was evident by expression of connexin 43 between the injected and recipient myocytes (Ruhparwar *et al.*, 2002).
Using pacing fetal myocytes as a potential biological pacemaker has been further tested in the porcine model (Lin *et al.*, 2005). Human atrial myocytes containing sinus node were isolated from the aborted fetuses (14-19 weeks of gestation). These cells were injected into the left ventricles of pigs. After complete AV block was induced by catheter ablation, the idioventricular beat was detected near the injection site. Connexin 43 formed between the donor and recipient cells was identified, suggesting that the fetal myocytes are able to form gap junctions with the adult myocytes. Further, isoprenalin significantly increased the idioventricular rate (Lin *et al.*, 2005). However, the limited source of pacing fetal myocytes and strong ethical concerns have hampered further development of the biological pacemaker using this approach for possible clinical application.

5.2.2 Stem cell derived cardiomyocytes

Rapid progress on recent studies of embryonic stem cell differentiation has prompted an idea of creating a biological pacemaker using human embryonic stem cells (hESC) - derived myocytes. Human embryonic stem cells have the ability of proliferation in culture and are able to differentiate into different cell types. Under certain conditions, hESC can be induced to differentiate into spontaneously beating cardiac myocytes expressing HCN channels but not Kir2.1 channels. Therefore, the hESC-converted-beating-myocytes are capable of creating a biological pacemaker within the ventricles.
Human embryonic stem cells have been shown to differentiate into cardiac myocytes (He *et al.*, 2003). Various action potentials similar to those recorded in the SA node, atrial, and ventricular myocytes have been observed (He *et al.*, 2003). The isolated beating myocytes were shown to be able to functionally integrate into the neonatal rat ventricular myocytes to induce spontaneous rhythmic activity (Xue *et al.*, 2005). The hESC-derived beating myocytes were implanted into the left ventricle of guinea pig to initiate the spontaneous action potentials in otherwise quiescent ventricular myocytes, recorded by both ECG and optical mapping technique. In the beating hESC-derived myocytes, I_f has been recorded and HCN2 expression was detected (Satin *et al.*, 2004). Consistently, the I_f driven pacemaker activity has also been observed in mouse ESC-derived beating myocytes (Abi-Gerges *et al.*, 2000; Qu *et al.*, 2008; Barbuti *et al.*, 2009). Not surprisingly, in hESC-derived beating cardiomyocytes, the inward rectifier K^+ current, I_{K1}, and Kir2.1 protein expression were barely detected (Satin *et al.*, 2004). In a swine AV block model, injection of these spontaneously beating hESC-derived myocytes into the left ventricle induced a long-lasting ectopic ventricular rhythm (Kehat *et al.*, 2004).
While hESCs-derived beating myocytes hold promises for creating a biological pacemaker, its use is not without risks. Potential tumorigenesis, immuno-reactivity, and pro-arrhythmogenesis are major concerns (Gepstein, 2008). To bypass these concerns, adult

human mesenchymal stem cells have been used as an alternative strategy to deliver HCN genes to the ventricles.

It has been demonstrated that adult human mesenchymal stem cells can form gap junctions with the ventricular myocytes in the co-culture (Valiunas *et al.*, 2004). Using this property, HCN2 gene was introduced into the hMSC and via newly formed gap junctions to the coupled ventricular myocytes for triggering the spontaneous pacemaker activity in the host ventricular myocytes (Rosen *et al.*, 2008; Valiunas *et al.*, 2009).

6. Optimization of biological pacemaker

An effective biological pacemaker must meet the following minimal requirements: 1) a physiological heart rate that can change in response to metabolic needs, usually fulfilled via neurohumoral modulation, 2) the electrical integration of the donor cells with the host cells, 3) the control of ionic currents only during diastole to avoid pro-arrhythmic potential.

Gating of many cardiac ion channels is strongly dependent upon changes in membrane potential. HCN channels are activated at membrane hyperpolarization near diastolic potential, and are closed at membrane depolarization. Kir2.1 channels are not strongly dependent upon membrane potential. However, due to its inward rectifying property, Kir2.1 channels produce little currents in the voltage range from -40mV to 0mV.

Cardiac ion channel properties can also be altered by protein expression levels and post-translational modulation of the channel proteins at the plasma membrane. Signaling molecules such as norepinephrine, acetylcholine, adenosine, adenosine-5′- triphosphate (ATP) and cyclic adenosine monophosphate (cAMP) can all exert dramatic effects on ion channel functions. Sensitivity of the implanted biological pacemaker to cAMP is one of the requirements as the heart rate is modulated by β adrenergic receptor signaling pathway in which cAMP is the key signaling molecule.

Advancement in the cell biology of ion channel has significantly advanced our understanding of how ion channel forward trafficking to the plasma membrane for cell surface expression can critically affect the function of ion channels. Recently, a variety of cells has been differentiated into spontaneously beating myocytes. The potential technical issues as how to use these cells for a working biological pacemaker must be addressed.

6.1 Modulation of Kir2.x, HCN and Cx43 channel levels in the ventricle

Whether gene- or cell-based approach, the essential working principle is the *external* control of the relative levels of outward (I_{K1}) and inward (I_f) currents during diastole. Biophysics and molecular biology studies of I_{K1} and I_f in the past have significantly advanced our understanding how the Kir2.1 and HCN channels are modulated at the plasma membrane. More recently, microRNA studies have provided clues as how these channel transcripts are regulated. Enhanced understanding about regulation of Kir2.1 and HCN channel levels will offer new strategies to create *in vivo* biological pacemaker without the use of the full-length Kir2.1 and HCN channels.

6.2 Gene regulation of channels by microRNA

MicroRNAs (miRs) are small non-coding mRNA ~22nt in length. They bind to the 3′ untranslated region (3′-UTR) of the target genes and inhibit the transcription of the gene expression (Catalucci *et al.*, 2009). Although the working mechanisms of the miRs are still poorly understood, recent works have demonstrated a significant potential of the endogenous miRs in the treatment of heart diseases such as coronary artery disease and heart failure (Callis & Wang, 2008; van Rooij *et al.*, 2008; Catalucci *et al.*, 2009). The muscle specific forms of miR-1 and miR-133 have been demonstrated to be pivotal in the development of hypertrophy and arrhythmias (Care *et al.*, 2007; Yang *et al.*, 2007).

Overexpression of miR-1 has been detected in individuals with coronary artery disease (Yang *et al.*, 2007). Increased miR-1 has been shown to inhibit the gene expression of KCNJ2 (which encodes Kir2.1 channel proteins) and GJA1 (which encodes connexin 43) (Yang *et al.*, 2007). In the infarct rat hearts, the reduced Kir2.1 and Cx43 channels were linked to the arrhythmogenic potential by slowing conduction and depolarization of the resting membrane potential.

On the other hand, decreased levels of both miR-1 and miR-133 have been shown to enhance the HCN2/HCN4 protein expression and functional channels at the plasma membrane (Xiao *et al.*, 2007). These results suggested that regulation of Kir2.1, Cx3.2, and HCN gene expression by microRNAs may represent an alternative strategy for creation of a biological pacemaker.

6.3 Regulation of channel surface expression

The number of functional channels at the plasma membrane determines the contribution of current to the membrane potential. Decreased I_{K1} (Beuckelmann *et al.*, 1993; Kaab *et al.*, 1996), reduced number of Cx32 channels (Severs, 1994, 2002), and increased I_f as well as the number of HCN channels (Cerbai *et al.*, 1997; Hoppe *et al.*, 1998; Cerbai *et al.*, 2001; Stillitano *et al.*, 2008) have been reported in heart diseases such as ischemia and heart failure. Gene therapy aims primarily to change the number of functional channels. On the other hand, surface expression of ion channels can be regulated by endogenous mechanisms.

In the past ten years, surface expression of the ion channel has been realized as one of the effective ways to alter the function of ion channels. Molecular mechanisms that control the synthesized proteins to exit the endoplasmic reticulum (ER), move forward to the Golgi apparatus, and to the plasma membrane have been intensively investigated, particularly for potassium channel membrane trafficking. Defective membrane trafficking due to mutated Kir2.1/HCN channels has been linked to cardiac arrhythmias (Dhamoon & Jalife, 2005; Herrmann *et al.*, 2007; Baruscotti *et al.*, 2010). Furthermore, endogenous proteins, such as small GTPase Rho1/Rac1, have been found to modulate Kir2.1 surface expression (Boyer *et al.*, 2009).

We have recently discovered that tyrosine phosphorylation of HCN channels mediated by Src kinases and receptor protein tyrosine phosphatase alpha can significantly alter the surface expression of HCN2/HCN4 channels (Huang *et al.*, 2008; Lin *et al.*, 2009). The surface expression and current density of HCN2/HCN4 channels are increased via enhanced tyrosine phosphorylation mediated by Src kinases, and decreased through tyrosine dephosphorylation by RPTPα (Huang *et al.*, 2008; Lin *et al.*, 2009). Using this modulation mechanism, we have shown that Src kinases can restore the normal current and surface expression of a human HCN4 mutant with defective membrane trafficking (Lin *et al.*, 2009).

Future investigation of how the membrane trafficking of Kir2.1, HCN, and Cx43 channels are affected under pathologic conditions may provide novel strategies for efficiently controlling the pacemaker activity in the ventricle when the sinus node is dysfunctional.

6.4 Isolation of homogeneous ESCs-derived beating cardiomyocytes

In theory, ESC derived cardiomyocytes have the potential for arrhythmogenesis (Zhang *et al.*, 2002). At least three different types of action potentials have been recorded in cardiomyocytes derived from ESCs: the sinus node like spontaneously pacing action potential, the atrial like action potential with narrow action potential duration, and the ventricular like action potential.

Although SA node markers such as Cx45/Cx40 and HCN4 have been used to label SA node cells, it will remain a technical challenge to isolate "pure" ESCs derived cardiomyocytes that only exhibit the SA node like action potential. Inclusion of any other types of myocytes in the cell grafts will increase the arrhythmic risk to the host cells. In early-stage of cardiac development, HCN4 is also abundantly expressed in ventricular myocytes (Stieber *et al.*, 2003). More specific markers for SA node will facilitate the isolation of pure ESCs derive cardiomyocytes exhibiting SA node action potentials.

If ESCs-derived cardiomyocytes do express Cx45, an additional challenge would be the properties of possible heteromeric gap junction channels formed by Cx45 and Cx43 in the host ventricular myocytes. A potential solution can be a genetically modified ESC cell body that has suppressed Cx45 and enhanced the expression of Cx43.

6.5 Resources of stem cells for generation of beating cardiomyocytes

The main concerns for the use of hESC are the ethical issues, the anticipated immune rejection and the oncogenic risk. In 2006, mouse fibroblasts were reprogrammed by expression of four transcription factors (oct4, sox2, c-myc, and klf4) to produce cells with characteristics similar to those of the mouse ESCs including the most important pluripotent property (Takahashi & Yamanaka, 2006). These inducible pluripotent stem cells (iPSCs) can also differentiate into cardiomyocytes. In the human iPSCs derived beating myocytes, connexin 43 and HCN2 expression were detected (Zwi *et al.*, 2009). However, no Kir2.x expression was reported. The electrical properties of human iPSCs support the notion that the human iPSCs derived myocytes may represent a better choice than the hESCs derived myocytes for creation of a biological pacemaker.

6.6 Brown adipose tissue

Recently, Takahashi et al has reported the use of brown adipose tissue to create pacemaker like myocytes (Takahashi *et al.*, 2009). Brown adipose tissue (BAT) is one type of mesenchymal stem cells that have the potential to differentiate into several types of cells. Cultured cells isolated from the brown adipose tissue expressed key marker genes for cardiac conduction and pacemaker activity, such as connexins 40 and 45 (Cx40 and Cx45), and HCN1 to HCN4. These BAT-converted pacing cells were injected into the area around AV node of mice. After one week, complete AV block was improved in 50% of mice tested. Although this work is significant in terms of sources for biological pacemaker, the electrophysiology of these BAT-converted pacing cells is unclear. It was not reported whether an I_f-like current is present, I_{K1}-like current is absent or the gap junctions can be formed by the donor and recipients cells.

6.7 Mesoangioblasts

Mesoangioblasts (MABs) have been recently discovered as multipotent and self-renewing cells isolated from the aorta (Minasi *et al.*, 2002). MABs are also found in the small vessels of the mouse heart ventricle (Galvez *et al.*, 2008). A recent report showed that MABs can be converted into SAN-like pacing myocytes (Barbuti *et al.*, 2010). The MABs-derived myocytes expressed several proteins that characterize the pacemaker cells, such as HCN4 channels and connexin 45. Aggregates of these cells display stable pacemaker activity characterized by SAN-like action potential showing distinct phase-4 depolarization with the most negative potential around -60mV. These cells also exhibited an I_f-like current with threshold activation near -50mV and reversal potential around -20mV. In addition, there is also no I_{K1} in these myocytes.

Further, the pacemaker activity exhibited in these cells is modulated by neurotransmitters. Isoproterenol accelerated, while acetylcholine slowed down the action potentials (Barbuti *et al.*, 2010). These observations recapitulated the autonomous modulation of pacemaker activity in the SA node. These properties make MABs an alternative source for creation of biological pacemaker. It would be interesting to see whether MABs can induce an escape ventricular rhythm after being injected into the left ventricle of the heart in a large animal model such as canine or porcine.

6.8 Global gene transfer and electrical integration

It is known that cardiac ion channels are non-uniformly distributed in different regions of the heart. While the differential expression of ion channels is necessary for physiological heart function, it could also contribute to the pathologic genesis of electrophysiology under pathological conditions. In a neonatal rat ventricular myocyte monolayer model, I_{K1} heterogeneity has been shown to contribute to the generation of ventricular arrhythmias (Sekar *et al.*, 2009). Therefore, local gene transfer by injection not only is inefficient in terms of pacing the whole ventricle, but it could also be pro-arrhythmic. Recently, an improved approach for global gene transfer has been reported (Kikuchi *et al.*, 2005). In an effort to modify atrial electrophysiology without affecting ventricular function in atrial fibrillation, Kikuchi et al applied adenovirus containing HERG-G628S, a long-QT syndrome mutant, directly to the epicardial surface of the porcine atria, by using poloxamer gel to increase virus contact time, followed by using mild trypsin to increase virus penetration. The results showed a prolonged action potential duration and refractory period without changes in ventricular electrophysiology (Kikuchi *et al.*, 2005).

Membrane stability, diastolic depolarizing current and gap junction channels are the minimal requirement for an effective biological pacemaker that can pace the otherwise quiescent ventricles by electrically integrating the donor cells with the host cells. Without electrical integration, the donor cells can provoke the unwanted side effects, even the contractile performance can be improved. Clinical trial with skeletal myoblast has shown a high incidence of ventricular arrhythmias (Smits *et al.*, 2003). The possible reason is due to the lack of gap junction channels formed between the donor skeletal myoblasts and the ventricular myocytes, as skeletal muscle cells are electrically isolated without gap junction channels (Leobon *et al.*, 2003; Abraham *et al.*, 2005).

7. Summary

Cardiac arrhythmias have remained as the leading cause of mortality and morbidity in the developed countries and now also become a major public health problem in the developing countries. Electronic pacemaker has been working well and remains the industry standard. Numerous pharmacological tools have been developed to treat arrhythmias. However, due to the intrinsic limitations in each strategy, there is still a strong need for novel strategy to normalize these rhythmic disorders with fewer side effects. Advances in gene and cell therapy have made it possible for creation of a biological pacemaker that will be used to overcome the limitations of electronic pacemaker. While there are still many obstacles for an effective and long-lasting biological pacemaker, development of new technologies and more animal experiments for enhanced understanding of mechanisms that control the gene expression and coupling between the donor and host cells will make the use of biological pacemaker a clinical reality.

8. References

Abi-Gerges N, Ji GJ, Lu ZJ, Fischmeister R, Hescheler J & Fleischmann BK. (2000). Functional expression and regulation of the hyperpolarization activated non-selective cation current in embryonic stem cell-derived cardiomyocytes. *J Physiol* 523 Pt 2, 377-389.

Abraham MR, Henrikson CA, Tung L, Chang MG, Aon M, Xue T, Li RA, B OR & Marban E. (2005). Antiarrhythmic engineering of skeletal myoblasts for cardiac transplantation. *Circ Res* 97, 159-167.

Barbuti A, Crespi A, Capilupo D, Mazzocchi N, Baruscotti M & DiFrancesco D. (2009). Molecular composition and functional properties of f-channels in murine embryonic stem cell-derived pacemaker cells. *J Mol Cell Cardiol* 46, 343-351.

Barbuti A, Galvez BG, Crespi A, Scavone A, Baruscotti M, Brioschi C, Cossu G & DiFrancesco D. (2010). Mesoangioblasts from ventricular vessels can differentiate in vitro into cardiac myocytes with sinoatrial-like properties. *J Mol Cell Cardiol* 48, 415-423.

Baruscotti M, Bottelli G, Milanesi R, DiFrancesco J & DiFrancesco D. (2010). HCN-related channelopathies. *Pflügers Archiv European Journal of Physiology* in press, 1-11.

Beeler GW & Reuter H. (1977). Reconstruction of the action potential of ventricular myocardial fibres. *J Physiol* 268, 177-210.

Bers DM. (2006). The beat goes on: diastolic noise that just won't quit. *Circ Res* 99, 921-923.

Beuckelmann DJ, Nabauer M & Erdmann E. (1993). Alterations of K+ currents in isolated human ventricular myocytes from patients with terminal heart failure. *Circ Res* 73, 379-385.

Boyer SB, Slesinger PA & Jones SV. (2009). Regulation of Kir2.1 channels by the Rho-GTPase, Rac1. *J Cell Physiol* 218, 385-393.

Brown HF, DiFrancesco D & Noble SJ. (1979). How does adrenaline accelerate the heart? *Nature* 280, 235-236.

Cai J, Yi FF, Li YH, Yang XC, Song J, Jiang XJ, Jiang H, Lin GS & Wang W. (2007). Adenoviral gene transfer of HCN4 creates a genetic pacemaker in pigs with complete atrioventricular block. *Life Sci* 80, 1746-1753.

Callis TE & Wang DZ. (2008). Taking microRNAs to heart. *Trends Mol Med* 14, 254-260.

Care A, Catalucci D, Felicetti F, Bonci D, Addario A, Gallo P, Bang ML, Segnalini P, Gu Y, Dalton ND, Elia L, Latronico MV, Hoydal M, Autore C, Russo MA, Dorn GW, 2nd, Ellingsen O, Ruiz-Lozano P, Peterson KL, Croce CM, Peschle C & Condorelli G. (2007). MicroRNA-133 controls cardiac hypertrophy. *Nat Med* 13, 613-618.

Catalucci D, Gallo P & Condorelli G. (2009). MicroRNAs in cardiovascular biology and heart disease. *Circ Cardiovasc Genet* 2, 402-408.

Cerbai E, Barbieri M & Mugelli A. (1994). Characterization of the hyperpolarization-activated current, I(f), in ventricular myocytes isolated from hypertensive rats. *J Physiol* 481 (Pt 3), 585-591.

Cerbai E, Barbieri M & Mugelli A. (1996). Occurrence and properties of the hyperpolarization-activated current If in ventricular myocytes from normotensive and hypertensive rats during aging. *Circulation* 94, 1674-1681.
Cerbai E & Mugelli A. (2006). I(f) in non-pacemaker cells: role and pharmacological implications. *Pharmacol Res* 53, 416-423.
Cerbai E, Pino R, Porciatti F, Sani G, Toscano M, Maccherini M, Giunti G & Mugelli A. (1997). Characterization of the hyperpolarization-activated current, I(f), in ventricular myocytes from human failing heart. *Circulation* 95, 568-571.
Cerbai E, Sartiani L, DePaoli P, Pino R, Maccherini M, Bizzarri F, DiCiolla F, Davoli G, Sani G & Mugelli A. (2001). The properties of the pacemaker current I(F)in human ventricular myocytes are modulated by cardiac disease. *J Mol Cell Cardiol* 33, 441-448.
Chan YC, Siu CW, Lau YM, Lau CP, Li RA & Tse HF. (2009). Synergistic effects of inward rectifier (I) and pacemaker (I) currents on the induction of bioengineered cardiac automaticity. *J Cardiovasc Electrophysiol* 20, 1048-1054.
Chan YC, Tse HF, Siu CW, Wang K & Li RA. (2010). Automaticity and conduction properties of bio-artificial pacemakers assessed in an in vitro monolayer model of neonatal rat ventricular myocytes. *Europace* 12, 1178-1187.
Dhamoon AS & Jalife J. (2005). The inward rectifier current (IK1) controls cardiac excitability and is involved in arrhythmogenesis. *Heart Rhythm* 2, 316-324.
DiFrancesco D. (1986). Characterization of single pacemaker channels in cardiac sino-atrial node cells. *Nature* 324, 470-473.
DiFrancesco D. (1993). Pacemaker mechanisms in cardiac tissue. *Annu Rev Physiol* 55, 455-472.
DiFrancesco D. (1995). The pacemaker current (I(f)) plays an important role in regulating SA node pacemaker activity. *Cardiovasc Res* 30, 307-308.
DiFrancesco D. (2010). Funny channel-based pacemaking. *Heart Rhythm* 7, 276-279.
Edelberg JM, Aird WC & Rosenberg RD. (1998). Enhancement of murine cardiac chronotropy by the molecular transfer of the human beta2 adrenergic receptor cDNA. *J Clin Invest* 101, 337-343.
Gaborit N, Le Bouter S, Szuts V, Varro A, Escande D, Nattel S & Demolombe S. (2007). Regional and tissue specific transcript signatures of ion channel genes in the non-diseased human heart. *J Physiol* 582, 675-693.
Galvez BG, Sampaolesi M, Barbuti A, Crespi A, Covarello D, Brunelli S, Dellavalle A, Crippa S, Balconi G, Cuccovillo I, Molla F, Staszewsky L, Latini R, Difrancesco D & Cossu G. (2008). Cardiac mesoangioblasts are committed, self-renewable progenitors, associated with small vessels of juvenile mouse ventricle. *Cell Death Differ* 15, 1417-1428.
Gepstein L. (2008). Experimental molecular and stem cell therapies in cardiac electrophysiology. *Ann N Y Acad Sci* 1123, 224-231.
Gonzalez D, Gomez-Hernandez JM & Barrio LC. (2007). Molecular basis of voltage dependence of connexin channels: an integrative appraisal. *Prog Biophys Mol Biol* 94, 66-106.
Han W, Bao W, Wang Z & Nattel S. (2002). Comparison of ion-channel subunit expression in canine cardiac Purkinje fibers and ventricular muscle. *Circ Res* 91, 790-797.
He JQ, Ma Y, Lee Y, Thomson JA & Kamp TJ. (2003). Human embryonic stem cells develop into multiple types of cardiac myocytes: action potential characterization. *Circ Res* 93, 32-39.

Herrmann S, Stieber J & Ludwig A. (2007). Pathophysiology of HCN channels. *Pflugers Arch* 454, 517-522.

Hoppe UC & Beuckelmann DJ. (1998). Characterization of the hyperpolarization-activated inward current in isolated human atrial myocytes. *Cardiovasc Res* 38, 788-801.

Hoppe UC, Jansen E, Sudkamp M & Beuckelmann DJ. (1998). Hyperpolarization-activated inward current in ventricular myocytes from normal and failing human hearts. *Circulation* 97, 55-65.

Huang J, Huang A, Zhang Q, Lin YC & Yu HG. (2008). Novel Mechanism for Suppression of Hyperpolarization-activated Cyclic Nucleotide-gated Pacemaker Channels by Receptor-like Tyrosine Phosphatase-{alpha}. *J Biol Chem* 283, 29912-29919.

Kaab S, Nuss HB, Chiamvimonvat N, O'Rourke B, Pak PH, Kass DA, Marban E & Tomaselli GF. (1996). Ionic mechanism of action potential prolongation in ventricular myocytes from dogs with pacing-induced heart failure. *Circ Res* 78, 262-273.

Kashiwakura Y, Cho HC, Barth AS, Azene E & Marban E. (2006). Gene transfer of a synthetic pacemaker channel into the heart: a novel strategy for biological pacing. *Circulation* 114, 1682-1686.

Kehat I, Khimovich L, Caspi O, Gepstein A, Shofti R, Arbel G, Huber I, Satin J, Itskovitz-Eldor J & Gepstein L. (2004). Electromechanical integration of cardiomyocytes derived from human embryonic stem cells. *Nat Biotechnol* 22, 1282-1289.

Kikuchi K, McDonald AD, Sasano T & Donahue JK. (2005). Targeted modification of atrial electrophysiology by homogeneous transmural atrial gene transfer. *Circulation* 111, 264-270.

King WL. (1992). US 5103821.

Lakatta EG. (2010). A paradigm shift for the heart's pacemaker. *Heart Rhythm* 7, 559-564.

Lakatta EG & DiFrancesco D. (2009). What keeps us ticking: a funny current, a calcium clock, or both? *J Mol Cell Cardiol* 47, 157-170.

Lakatta EG, Maltsev VA & Vinogradova TM. (2010). A coupled SYSTEM of intracellular Ca2+ clocks and surface membrane voltage clocks controls the timekeeping mechanism of the heart's pacemaker. *Circ Res* 106, 659-673.

Lakatta EG, Vinogradova TM & Maltsev VA. (2008). The missing link in the mystery of normal automaticity of cardiac pacemaker cells. *Ann N Y Acad Sci* 1123, 41-57.

Leobon B, Garcin I, Menasche P, Vilquin JT, Audinat E & Charpak S. (2003). Myoblasts transplanted into rat infarcted myocardium are functionally isolated from their host. *Proc Natl Acad Sci U S A* 100, 7808-7811.

Lin G, Cai J, Jiang H, Shen H, Jiang X, Yu Q & Song J. (2005). Biological pacemaker created by fetal cardiomyocyte transplantation. *J Biomed Sci* 12, 513-519.

Lin Y-C, Huang J, Kan H, Frisbee JC & Yu H-G. (2009). Rescue of a trafficking defective human pacemaker channel via a novel mechanism: roles of Src, Fyn, Yes tyrosine kinases. *J Biol Chem* 284, 30433-30440.

Lipsius SL & Bers DM. (2003). Cardiac pacemaking: I(f) vs. Ca(2+), is it really that simple? *J Mol Cell Cardiol* 35, 891-893.

Liu YM, Yu H, Li CZ, Cohen IS & Vassalle M. (1998). Cesium effects on i(f) and i(K) in rabbit sinoatrial node myocytes: implications for SA node automaticity. *J Cardiovasc Pharmacol* 32, 783-790.

Marvin WJ, Jr., Chittick VL, Rosenthal JK, Sandra A, Atkins DL & Hermsmeyer K. (1984). The isolated sinoatrial node cell in primary culture from the newborn rat. *Circ Res* 55, 253-260.

Miake J, Marban E & Nuss HB. (2002). Biological pacemaker created by gene transfer. *Nature* 419, 132-133.

Miake J, Marban E & Nuss HB. (2003). Functional role of inward rectifier current in heart probed by Kir2.1 overexpression and dominant-negative suppression. *J Clin Invest* 111, 1529-1536.

Minasi MG, Riminucci M, De Angelis L, Borello U, Berarducci B, Innocenzi A, Caprioli A, Sirabella D, Baiocchi M, De Maria R, Boratto R, Jaffredo T, Broccoli V, Bianco P & Cossu G. (2002). The meso-angioblast: a multipotent, self-renewing cell that originates from the dorsal aorta and differentiates into most mesodermal tissues. *Development* 129, 2773-2783.

Much B, Wahl-Schott C, Zong X, Schneider A, Baumann L, Moosmang S, Ludwig A & Biel M. (2003). Role of subunit heteromerization and N-linked glycosylation in the formation of functional hyperpolarization-activated cyclic nucleotide-gated channels. *J Biol Chem* 278, 43781-43786.

Plotnikov AN, Sosunov EA, Qu J, Shlapakova IN, Anyukhovsky EP, Liu L, Janse MJ, Brink PR, Cohen IS, Robinson RB, Danilo P, Jr. & Rosen MR. (2004). Biological pacemaker implanted in canine left bundle branch provides ventricular escape rhythms that have physiologically acceptable rates. *Circulation* 109, 506-512.

Qu J, Plotnikov AN, Danilo P, Jr., Shlapakova I, Cohen IS, Robinson RB & Rosen MR. (2003). Expression and function of a biological pacemaker in canine heart. *Circulation* 107, 1106-1109.

Qu Y, Whitaker GM, Hove-Madsen L, Tibbits GF & Accili EA. (2008). Hyperpolarization-activated cyclic nucleotide-modulated 'HCN' channels confer regular and faster rhythmicity to beating mouse embryonic stem cells. *J Physiol* 586, 701-716.

Ranjan R, Chiamvimonvat N, Thakor NV, Tomaselli GF & Marban E. (1998). Mechanism of anode break stimulation in the heart. *Biophys J* 74, 1850-1863.

Robinson RB, Brink PR, Cohen IS & Rosen MR. (2006). I(f) and the biological pacemaker. *Pharmacol Res* 53, 407-415.

Robinson RB & Siegelbaum SA. (2003). Hyperpolarization-activated cation currents: from molecules to physiological function. *Annu Rev Physiol* 65, 453-480.

Robinson RB, Yu H, Chang F & Cohen IS. (1997). Developmental change in the voltage-dependence of the pacemaker current, if, in rat ventricle cells. *Pflugers Arch* 433, 533-535.

Rosen MR, Brink PR, Cohen IS & Robinson RB. (2004). Genes, stem cells and biological pacemakers. *Cardiovasc Res* 64, 12-23.

Rosen MR, Brink PR, Cohen IS & Robinson RB. (2008). The utility of mesenchymal stem cells as biological pacemakers. *Congest Heart Fail* 14, 153-156.

Ruhparwar A, Kallenbach K, Klein G, Bara C, Ghodsizad A, Sigg DC, Karck M, Haverich A & Niehaus M. (2010). Adenylate-Cyclase VI Transforms Ventricular Cardiomyocytes into Biological Pacemaker Cells. *Tissue Eng Part A* 16, 1867-1872.

Ruhparwar A, Tebbenjohanns J, Niehaus M, Mengel M, Irtel T, Kofidis T, Pichlmaier AM & Haverich A. (2002). Transplanted fetal cardiomyocytes as cardiac pacemaker. *Eur J Cardiothorac Surg* 21, 853-857.

Saez JC, Berthoud VM, Branes MC, Martinez AD & Beyer EC. (2003). Plasma membrane channels formed by connexins: their regulation and functions. *Physiol Rev* 83, 1359-1400.

Sanders L, Rakovic S, Lowe M, Mattick PA & Terrar DA. (2006). Fundamental importance of Na+-Ca2+ exchange for the pacemaking mechanism in guinea-pig sino-atrial node. *J Physiol* 571, 639-649.

Satin J, Kehat I, Caspi O, Huber I, Arbel G, Itzhaki I, Magyar J, Schroder EA, Perlman I & Gepstein L. (2004). Mechanism of spontaneous excitability in human embryonic stem cell derived cardiomyocytes. *J Physiol* 559, 479-496.

Schweizer PA, Yampolsky P, Malik R, Thomas D, Zehelein J, Katus HA & Koenen M. (2009). Transcription profiling of HCN-channel isotypes throughout mouse cardiac development. *Basic Res Cardiol* 104, 621-629.

Sekar RB, Kizana E, Cho HC, Molitoris JM, Hesketh GG, Eaton BP, Marban E & Tung L. (2009). IK1 heterogeneity affects genesis and stability of spiral waves in cardiac myocyte monolayers. *Circ Res* 104, 355-364.

Severs NJ. (1994). Pathophysiology of gap junctions in heart disease. *J Cardiovasc Electrophysiol* 5, 462-475.

Severs NJ. (2002). Gap junction remodeling in heart failure. *J Card Fail* 8, S293-299.

Severs NJ, Bruce AF, Dupont E & Rothery S. (2008). Remodelling of gap junctions and connexin expression in diseased myocardium. *Cardiovasc Res* 80, 9-19.

Shi W, Wymore R, Yu H, Wu J, Wymore RT, Pan Z, Robinson RB, Dixon JE, McKinnon D & Cohen IS. (1999). Distribution and prevalence of hyperpolarization-activated cation channel (HCN) mRNA expression in cardiac tissues. *Circ Res* 85, e1-6.

Shi W, Yu H, Wu J, Zuckerman J, Wymore R, Dixon JE, Robinson RB, McKinnon D & Cohen IS. (2000). The distribution and prevalence of HCN isoforms in the canine heart and their relation to the voltage dependence of if. . *Biophys J* 78, 353A.

Smits PC, van Geuns RJ, Poldermans D, Bountioukos M, Onderwater EE, Lee CH, Maat AP & Serruys PW. (2003). Catheter-based intramyocardial injection of autologous skeletal myoblasts as a primary treatment of ischemic heart failure: clinical experience with six-month follow-up. *J Am Coll Cardiol* 42, 2063-2069.

Stieber J, Herrmann S, Feil S, Loster J, Feil R, Biel M, Hofmann F & Ludwig A. (2003). The hyperpolarization-activated channel HCN4 is required for the generation of pacemaker action potentials in the embryonic heart. *Proc Natl Acad Sci U S A* 100, 15235-15240.

Stillitano F, Lonardo G, Zicha S, Varro A, Cerbai E, Mugelli A & Nattel S. (2008). Molecular basis of funny current (If) in normal and failing human heart. *J Mol Cell Cardiol* 45, 289-299.

Takahashi K & Yamanaka S. (2006). Induction of pluripotent stem cells from mouse embryonic and adult fibroblast cultures by defined factors. *Cell* 126, 663-676.

Takahashi T, Nagai T, Naito AT, Kanda M, Tokunaga M, Liu M, Ogura T, Lee J-K, Kodama I, Nakaya H & Komuro I. (2009). Abstract 2966: Brown Adipose Tissue Derived-cells Differentiate Into Cardiac Conduction and Pace-maker Cells in vitro and Improve Complete AV Block in vivo. *Circulation* 120, S721-c-.

Tse HF, Xue T, Lau CP, Siu CW, Wang K, Zhang QY, Tomaselli GF, Akar FG & Li RA. (2006). Bioartificial sinus node constructed via in vivo gene transfer of an engineered pacemaker HCN Channel reduces the dependence on electronic pacemaker in a sick-sinus syndrome model. *Circulation* 114, 1000-1011.

Valiunas V, Doronin S, Valiuniene L, Potapova I, Zuckerman J, Walcott B, Robinson RB, Rosen MR, Brink PR & Cohen IS. (2004). Human mesenchymal stem cells make cardiac connexins and form functional gap junctions. *J Physiol* 555, 617-626.

Valiunas V, Kanaporis G, Valiuniene L, Gordon C, Wang HZ, Li L, Robinson RB, Rosen MR, Cohen IS & Brink PR. (2009). Coupling an HCN2-expressing cell to a myocyte creates a two-cell pacing unit. *J Physiol* 587, 5211-5226.

van Rooij E, Marshall WS & Olson EN. (2008). Toward microRNA-based therapeutics for heart disease: the sense in antisense. *Circ Res* 103, 919-928.

Vassalle M. (1995). The pacemaker current (I(f)) does not play an important role in regulating SA node pacemaker activity. *Cardiovasc Res* 30, 309-310.

Vassalle M, Yu H & Cohen IS. (1999). Pacemaker Channels and Cardiac Automaticity. In *Cardiac Electrophysiology: From Cell to Bedside*, third edn, ed. Zipes DP & Jalife J, pp. 94-103. W.B. Saunders Company.

Wainger BJ, DeGennaro M, Santoro B, Siegelbaum SA & Tibbs GR. (2001). Molecular mechanism of cAMP modulation of HCN pacemaker channels. *Nature* 411, 805-810.

Whitaker GM, Angoli D, Nazzari H, Shigemoto R & Accili EA. (2007). HCN2 and HCN4 isoforms self-assemble and co-assemble with equal preference to form functional pacemaker channels. *J Biol Chem* 282, 22900-22909.

Xiao J, Yang B, Lin H, Lu Y, Luo X & Wang Z. (2007). Novel approaches for gene-specific interference via manipulating actions of microRNAs: examination on the pacemaker channel genes HCN2 and HCN4. *J Cell Physiol* 212, 285-292.

Xue T, Cho HC, Akar FG, Tsang SY, Jones SP, Marban E, Tomaselli GF & Li RA. (2005). Functional integration of electrically active cardiac derivatives from genetically engineered human embryonic stem cells with quiescent recipient ventricular cardiomyocytes: insights into the development of cell-based pacemakers. *Circulation* 111, 11-20.

Yang B, Lin H, Xiao J, Lu Y, Luo X, Li B, Zhang Y, Xu C, Bai Y, Wang H, Chen G & Wang Z. (2007). The muscle-specific microRNA miR-1 regulates cardiac arrhythmogenic potential by targeting GJA1 and KCNJ2. *Nat Med* 13, 486-491.

Yeager M. (1998). Structure of cardiac gap junction intercellular channels. *J Struct Biol* 121, 231-245.

Yu H, Chang F & Cohen IS. (1993). Pacemaker current exists in ventricular myocytes. *Circ Res* 72, 232-236.

Yu H, Chang F & Cohen IS. (1995). Pacemaker current i(f) in adult canine cardiac ventricular myocytes. *J Physiol* 485 (Pt 2), 469-483.

Yu X, Chen XW, Zhou P, Yao L, Liu T, Zhang B, Li Y, Zheng H, Zheng LH, Zhang CX, Bruce I, Ge JB, Wang SQ, Hu ZA, Yu HG & Zhou Z. (2007). Calcium influx through If channels in rat ventricular myocytes. *Am J Physiol Cell Physiol* 292, C1147-1155.

Yu X, Duan KL, Shang CF, Yu HG & Zhou Z. (2004). Calcium influx through hyperpolarization-activated cation channels (I(h) channels) contributes to activity-evoked neuronal secretion. *Proc Natl Acad Sci U S A* 101, 1051-1056.

Zhang Q, Huang A, Lin YC & Yu HG. (2009). Associated changes in HCN2 and HCN4 transcripts and I(f) pacemaker current in myocytes. *Biochim Biophys Acta* 1788, 1138-1147.

Zhang YM, Hartzell C, Narlow M & Dudley SC, Jr. (2002). Stem cell-derived cardiomyocytes demonstrate arrhythmic potential. *Circulation* 106, 1294-1299.

Zwi L, Caspi O, Arbel G, Huber I, Gepstein A, Park I-H & Gepstein L. (2009). Cardiomyocyte Differentiation of Human Induced Pluripotent Stem Cells. *Circulation %R 101161/CIRCULATIONAHA109868885* 120, 1513-1523.

31

The Functional Role of Chloride Channels in Cardiac Pacemaker Activity

Zheng Maggie Huang[1,2] and Dayue Darrel Duan[1]

[1]*Department of Pharmacology, School of Medicine, University of Nevada, Reno, NV 89557*

[2]*Center for Translational Medicine, Jefferson Medical College, Thomas Jefferso University, Philadelphia, PA 19107*

USA

1. Introduction

Chloride (Cl^-) channels are transmembrane proteins in biological membranes, which form functional pores and allow the diffusion of negatively-charged Cl^- ions along the electrochemical gradients. These channels can also conduct other anions including I^-, Br^-, NO_3^-, aspartate, glutamate, etc. They are conventionally called Cl^- channels because Cl^- is the most abundant and physiological anions in organisms.

While cation (K^+, Na^+, and Ca^{2+}) channels have received most of attentions in the past 50 years, the role of Cl^- channels in the pacemaker activity of the heart has been largely ignored and understudied (Duan, 2009). The possible contribution of Cl^- currents to spontaneous cardiac action potentials was first described in multicellular preparations of Purkinje fibers by Carmeliet (Carmeliet, 1961) and Hutter & Noble in 1961 (Hutter & Noble, 1961). Later, investigators from several laboratories observed the Cl- dependence of the diastolic depolarization and action potential duration. They characterized a hyperpolarization-activated Cl^- current in multicellular preparations of rabbit sinoatrial node (SAN) (De Mello, 1963;Noma & Irisawa, 1976;Seyama, 1979). Unfortunately, studies in the late 1970s raised serious doubts about the existence and functional role of any type of Cl^- channels in the heart. The potential functional role of the hyperpolarization-activated Cl^- currents in cardiac pacemaker activity has therefore been completely disputed (Hume *et al.*, 2000;Duan *et al.*, 2005).

Recent studies have characterized the functional and molecular expression of several Cl^- channels in cardiac SAN cells from different species (Duan, 2009). These include 1) a hyperpolarization- and cell swelling-activated inwardly rectifying Cl^- current ($I_{Cl.ir}$)(Duan *et al.*, 2000), which may be encoded by ClC-2, a member of the ClC voltage-gated Cl^- channel gene superfamily (Thiemann *et al.*, 1992;Britton *et al.*, 2000;Duan *et al.*, 2000;Britton *et al.*, 2005;Huang *et al.*, 2009); 2) a volume-regulated outwardly-rectifying Cl^- current ($I_{Cl,vol}$)(Hagiwara *et al.*, 1992), which may be encoded by another member of the ClC superfamily, ClC-3 (Duan *et al.*, 1997b;Duan *et al.*, 1999a;Britton *et al.*, 2000); and 3) a Ca^{2+}-activated Cl^- current ($I_{Cl.Ca}$) (Verkerk *et al.*, 2002), which may be encoded by TEME16A (or Ano1) (Schroeder *et al.*, 2008;Caputo *et al.*, 2008;Yang *et al.*, 2008;Hartzell *et al.*, 2009). Therefore, experimental evidence are merging to support the potential role of Cl^- channels in the regulation of cardiac pacemaker activity and these anion channels may represent novel therapeutic targets for arrhythmias. Several recent review articles have summarized the biophysical, pharmacological and molecular properties and the potential functional role of Cl^- channels in the heart (Hiraoka *et al.*, 1998;Hume *et al.*, 2000;Baumgarten & Clemo, 2003;Duan *et al.*, 2005;Duan, 2009). In this chapter, we will highlight the major findings and recent advances in the studies of Cl^- channels in the regulation of cardiac pacemaker activity.

2. Cl^- channels in the heart

The electrophysiological examination of Cl^- channels in the heart can be dated back 50 years ago to the original work of Hutter & Noble (Hutter & Noble, 1961) and Carmeliet (Carmeliet, 1961). However, the existence of any Cl^- channels in cardiovascular system was disputed by a series of studies in the late 1970s (Kenyon & Gibbons, 1979a;Kenyon & Gibbons, 1979b). The discovery of a β-adrenergic receptor activated Cl^- current in rabbit ventricular myocytes (Harvey & Hume, 1989) and a cAMP-activated Cl^- current ($I_{Cl.cAMP}$) in guinea pig heart by Gadsby and colleagues (Bahinski *et al.*, 1989) in 1989 inaugurated the new era of Cl^- channel research in the heart. Patch-clamp studies have now identified at least eight types of Cl^- currents in cardiac cells from different regions of the heart and in different species. The biophysical, pharmacological and molecular properties of these Cl^- channels have been well characterized and are summarized in Table 1 (Hiraoka *et al.*, 1998;Hume *et al.*, 2000;Baumgarten & Clemo, 2003;Duan *et al.*, 2005;Duan, 2009). Several of these Cl^- channels have been found to be expressed in SAN of different species (Table 1).

Current	Activation	Single Channel (pS)	I-V ($[Cl^-]_o \neq [Cl^-]_i$)	I-V ($[Cl^-]_o = [Cl^-]_i$)	Ion selectivity	SAN	Gene
$I_{Cl,PKA}$	Gs-AC-cAMP-PKA	7~13	Outward Rectifying	linear	$Br^- > Cl^- > I^-$	?	CFTR
$I_{Cl,PKC}$	PKC	7~13	Outward Rectifying	linear	$Br^- > Cl^- > I^-$	?	CFTR
$I_{Cl,ATP}$	ATP_o (P_2-receptor)	~12	Outward Rectifying	linear	$Br^- > Cl^- > I^-$	?	CFTR
$I_{Cl,Ca}$	$[Ca^{2+}]_i$	1~2	Outward Rectifying	linear	$I^- > Br^- > Cl^-$	Yes	TMEM 16?
$I_{Cl,swell}$	Cell swelling, membrane stretch	30~60	Outward Rectifying	Outward Rectifying	$I^- > Br^- > Cl^-$	Yes	ClC-3
$I_{Cl,b}$	Basally active	30~60	Outward Rectifying	Outward Rectifying	$I^- > Br^- > Cl^-$	?	ClC-3
$I_{Cl,ir}$	Basally active cell swelling, $[H^+]_o$	1~4	Inward Rectifying	Inward Rectifying	$I^- = Br^- > Cl^-$	Yes	ClC-2
$I_{Cl,acid}$	$[H^+]_o$	?	Outward Rectifying	Outward Rectifying	$Br^- > I^- > Cl^-$	?	?

Table 1. Characteristics of functionally identified Cl^- channels in heart*

* *I-V*, current-voltage relationships; SAN, sino-atrial node; Gs, G-protien; AC, adenylyl cyclase; PKA, protein kinase A; PKC, protein kinase C; CFTR, cystic fibrosis transmembrane conductance regulator; subscripts i and o, intracellular and extracellular, respectively

At the molecular level, all cardiac Cl^- channels described so far may fall into the following Cl^- channel gene families (Figure 1): 1) the cystic fibrosis transmembrane conductance regulator (*CFTR*), which is a member of the adenosine triphosphate-binding cassette (ABC) transporter superfamily and may be responsible for $I_{Cl.cAMP}$, including the Cl^- currents activated by protein kinase A (PKA) ($I_{Cl,PKA}$) (Harvey & Hume, 1989;Bahinski *et al.*, 1989;Nagel *et al.*, 1992), protein kinase C (PKC) ($I_{Cl,PKC}$)(Walsh & Long, 1994;Collier & Hume, 1995), and extracellular ATP ($I_{Cl,ATP}$) (Levesque & Hume, 1995;Duan *et al.*, 1999b;Yamamoto-Mizuma *et al.*, 2004a); 2) *ClC-2,* which may be responsible for $I_{Cl,ir}$(Duan *et al.*, 2000); 3) *ClC-3,* which may be responsible for $I_{Cl,vol}$, including the basally-activated ($I_{Cl,b}$) (Duan *et al.*, 1992;Duan & Nattel, 1994) and swelling activated ($I_{Cl,swell}$) components (Duan & Nattel, 1994;Duan *et al.*, 1995;Duan *et al.*, 1997a;Duan *et al.*, 1997b;Duan *et al.*, 1999a;Duan *et al.*, 2001;Wang *et al.*, 2003;Yamamoto-Mizuma *et al.*, 2004b;Duan, 2010); 4) *CLCA-1,* which was thought to be responsible for the Ca^{2+}-activated Cl^- current ($I_{Cl,Ca}$)(Collier *et al.*, 1996;Xu *et al.*, 2002;Britton *et al.*, 2002); 5) *Bestrophin,* a candidate also for $I_{Cl,Ca}$(Hartzell, 2008); and 6) TMEM16, a novel candidate for $I_{Cl,Ca}$ (Schroeder *et al.*, 2008;Caputo *et al.*, 2008;Yang *et al.*, 2008;Hartzell *et al.*, 2009). A novel Cl^- current activated by extracellular acidosis ($I_{Cl.acid}$) has also been observed in cardiac myocytes but the molecular identity for $I_{Cl.acid}$ is currently not known (Yamamoto & Ehara, 2006).

3. Cl^- channels in cardiac pacemaker activity

The diastolic depolarization of cardiac pacemaker cells in the SAN initiates spontaneous action potentials that propagate to the whole cardiac muscle through specific pathways and drives normal rhythmic contraction of the heart (Liang *et al.*, 2010;DiFrancesco, 2010). The ionic mechanisms of the pacemaker activity have been one of the central research subjects in cardiac electrophysiology (DiFrancesco, 2010). It is generally agreed now that multiple mechanisms such as the hyperpolarization-activated non-selective cationic "funny" current (I_f)(DiFrancesco, 2010),the L-type ($I_{Ca,L}$)(Kurata *et al.*, 2003) and T-type Ca^{2+} currents ($I_{Ca,T}$)(Ono & Iijima, 2010), Na^+/Ca^{2+} exchanger (I_{NCX})(Dobrzynski *et al.*, 2007), and a sustained inward current (I_{st})(Shinagawa *et al.*, 2000), may be involved in the generation and regulation of spontaneous pacemaker activity, although the relative contribution of these individual ionic currents are still under debate.

Early studies using ion-substitution strategies in multicellualr Purkinje fibers and SAN tissues provided initial experimental evidence for the potential physiological role of Cl^- and other anions in the regulation of membrane potentials, the diastolic depolarization and action potential duration of cardiac cells (Carmeliet, 1961;Hutter & Noble, 1961;De Mello, 1963;Noma & Irisawa, 1976). In 1961 Hutter & Noble (Hutter & Noble, 1961) reported that upon the substitution of extracellular Cl^- by impermeant anions the heart rate transiently increased and then eventually decreased to between 40 and 90 % of that found in Cl^- solution. The replacement of Cl^- by permeant anions caused either an arrest or an initial slowing followed by acceleration of the rhythm. These changes were explained by the passive movement of anions during the action potential, assuming that the E_{Cl} was -50 mV (Hutter & Noble, 1961). Later, de Mello (De Mello, 1963) and Noma & Irisawa (Noma & Irisawa, 1976) independently reported the Cl^--dependence of the diastolic depolarization in multicellular preparations of rabbit SAN tissue. Seyama (Seyama, 1977) also reported that 9 % of the total membrane conductance of the resting potential is carried by Cl^-. In 1979,

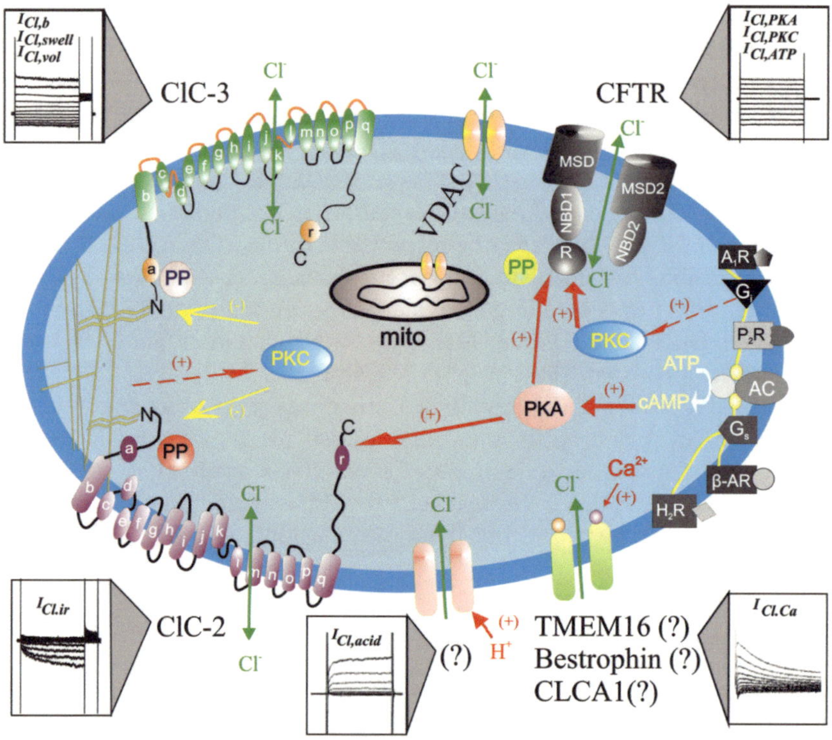

Fig. 1. Schematic representation of Cl- channels in cardiac myocytes. Cl- channels and their corresponding molecular entities or candidates are indicated. ClC-3, a member of voltage-gated ClC Cl- channel family, encodes Cl- channels that are volume-regulated ($I_{Cl,vol}$) and can be activated by cell swelling ($I_{Cl,swell}$) induced by exposure to hypotonic extracellular solutions or possibly membrane stretch. $I_{Cl,b}$ is a basally-activated ClC-3 Cl- current. ClC-2, a member of voltage-gated ClC Cl- channel family, is responsible for a volume-regulated and hyperpolarization-activated inward rectifying Cl- current ($I_{Cl,ir}$). Membrane topology models (α-helices a-r) for ClC-3 and ClC-2 are modified from Dutzler *et al* (Dutzler *et al.*, 2002). $I_{Cl,acid}$ is a Cl- current regulated by extracellular pH and the molecular entity for $I_{Cl,acid}$ is currently unknown. $I_{Cl,Ca}$ is a Cl- current activated by increased intracellular Ca^{2+} concentration ($[Ca^{2+}]_i$); Molecular candidates for $I_{Cl,Ca}$ include CLCA1, a member of a Ca^{2+} -sensitive Cl- channel family (CLCA), bestrophin-2, a member of the Bestrophin gene family, and TMEM16, transmembrane protein 16. CFTR, cystic fibrosis transmembrane conductance regulator, encodes Cl- channels activated by stimulation of cAMP-protein kinase A (PKA) pathway ($I_{Cl,PKA}$), protein kinase C (PKC) ($I_{Cl,PKC}$), or extracellular ATP through purinergic receptors ($I_{Cl,ATP}$). CFTR is composed by two membrane spanning domains (MSD1 and MSD2), two nucleotide binding domains (NBD1 and NBD2) and a regulatory subunit (R). P, phosphorylation sites for PKA and PKC; PP, serine-threonine protein phosphatases; Gi, heterodimeric inhibitory G protein; A_1R, adenosine type 1 receptor; AC, adenylyl cyclase; H_2R, histamine type II receptor; Gs, heterodimeric stimulatory G protein; β-AR, β-adrenergic receptor; P_2R, purinergic type 2 receptor; proposed intracellular signaling pathway for purinergic activation of CFTR. VDAC, voltage-dependent anion channels (porin); mito, mitochondrion. (Duan, 2009)

using the voltage-clamp technique Seyama (Seyama, 1979) identified a time- and voltage-dependent inwardly rectifying Cl^- current in SAN cells of rabbit heart. This inwardly rectifying Cl^- current was only activated by membrane potentials more negative than -60 mV and might contribute to the diastolic depolarization. Eliminating this current component by a replacement of Cl^- with less permeable acetate caused a reduction in frequency of SAN rhythm and an increase in the amplitude of the action potential (Seyama, 1979). Later a similar Cl^- current was reported in frog sinus venosus (Brown *et al.*, 1977). Unfortunately, the biophysical and molecular properties of the hyperpolarization-activated inwardly rectifying Cl^- channels have never been further characterized. Instead, a later study found that substitution of extracellular Cl^- with larger anions including isethionate, glutamate, acetate, and aspartate, reduced the amplitude of I_f without changing the reversal potential and substitution with small anions such as iodide or nitrate supported an intact I_f (Frace *et al.*, 1992). Therefore, the possible important role of the hyperpolarization-activated Cl^- current described in the 1960s and 1970s has been either disputed (Frace *et al.*, 1992) or ignored (Hume *et al.*, 2000;Duan *et al.*, 2005). Very little is known about Cl^- channels and their potential functional role in the heart although recent efforts in the last twenty years have characterized the properties of several Cl^- channels in the heart at the cellular and molecular levels (Duan *et al.*, 2005;Duan, 2009).

3.1 $I_{Cl,ir}$ and ClC-2 Cl^- channels in cardiac pacemaker activity

ClC-2 was cloned originally from rat heart and brain (Thiemann *et al.*, 1992). Later several alternatively spliced forms were cloned from several other tissues and species, including human (Furukawa *et al.*, 1995;Malinowska *et al.*, 1995;Cid *et al.*, 1995;Chu *et al.*, 1996;Chu & Zeitlin, 1997;Furukawa *et al.*, 1998;Cid *et al.*, 2000;Loewen *et al.*, 2000;Furukawa *et al.*, 2002). Expression of ClC-2 cDNA in *Xenopus* oocytes or mammalian cells resulted in hyperpolarization-activated inward-rectifying Cl^- currents which are sensitive to changes in cell volume and extracellular pH (Jordt & Jentsch, 1997;Furukawa *et al.*, 1998;Park *et al.*, 1998;Stroffekova *et al.*, 1998;Cid *et al.*, 2000;Park *et al.*, 2001;Furukawa *et al.*, 2002).

The endogenous $I_{Cl.ir}$ in native cardiac myocytes was identified in guinea pig and mouse hearts for the first time in 2000 (Duan *et al.*, 2000). Under conditions in which cationic inward rectifier channels were blocked, $I_{Cl.ir}$ was activated by membrane hyperpolarization (-40 to -140 mV). Under isotonic conditions, the current activated slowly with a biexponential time course (time constants averaging τ_1=179.76±3.4 and τ_2=2073.66±87.6 ms at -120 mV). Hypotonic cell swelling accelerated the activation (τ_1=97.5±8.5 ms and τ_2=656.4±113.6 ms at -120 mV) and increased the current amplitude whereas hypertonic cell shrinkage inhibited the current (Figure 2). The inwardly rectifying current was carried by Cl^- and had an anion permeability sequence of $Cl^- > I^- >>$aspartate. $I_{Cl.ir}$ was blocked by 9-anthracene-carboxylic acid and cadmium (Cd^{2+}) but not by stilbene disulfonates and tamoxifen (Duan *et al.*, 2000). Subsequently, similar $I_{Cl.ir}$ was found in rat atrial and subepicardial and subendocardial ventricular myocytes (Komukai *et al.*, 2002a;Komukai *et al.*, 2002b). Acidosis (extracellular pH decreased from 7.4 to 6.5) increased $I_{Cl.ir}$, which may underlie the acidosis-induced depolarization of the resting membrane potential (Komukai *et al.*, 2002a;Komukai *et al.*, 2002b). The properties of $I_{Cl.ir}$ in guinea-pig and mouse cardiac myocytes are consistent with currents generated by expression of ClC-2 Cl^- channels.

RT-PCR and Northern blot analysis confirmed transcriptional expression of ClC-2 in both atrial and ventricular tissues and isolated myocytes from mouse and guinea pig hearts

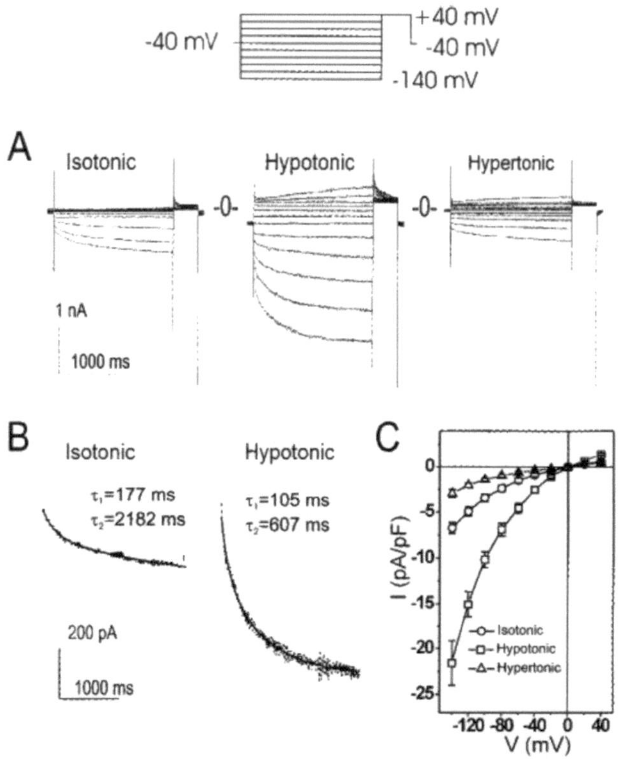

Fig. 2. Hyperpolarization-activated anion current and its sensitivity to cell volume in mouse ventricular myocytes. Currents were recorded using voltage-clamp protocols shown on top. Cells were held at -40 mV, and test potentials were applied from -140 to +40 mV in +20-mV increments for 2 seconds and then to +40 mV for 400 ms before return to the holding potential. The test potentials were applied at an interval of 10 seconds (insert on the top). **A,** Hyperpolarization voltage pulses activated inward currents under isotonic conditions (left panel). Subsequent exposure of the same cell to hypotonic solution (0.79T) caused a further increase in current amplitudes (middle panel). Further exposure of the cell to hypertonic solution caused a decrease in current amplitudes (right panel). **B,** Effects of hypotonic cell swelling on the time course of activation of the inward rectifying current. Representative current recordings from one cell after hyperpolarization to -120 mV under isotonic (left panel) and hypotonic (right panel) conditions, respectively, are shown. The points represent current activation data, and the solid lines are least-square curve fits obtained with the curve fitting program Clampfit (Axon Instruments). The activation process was best fit to a biexponential function with a fast time constant (τ_1) of 177 ms and a slow time constant (τ_2) of 2182 ms under isotonic conditions. Hypotonic cell swelling increased the amplitude of the current and also accelerated the activation kinetics (τ_1=105 ms, τ_2=607 ms). **C,** Mean *I*-V relationship from 5 different cells under isotonic, hypotonic, and hypertonic conditions. Currents were measured at the end of each 2-second test pulse. Mean reversal potentials (E_{rev}) of the currents under isotonic, hypotonic, and hypertonic conditions were 2.0±3.8 mV, 3.3±3.4 mV, and -1.7±3.3 mV (n=5, *P*=NS), respectively, which were very close to the predicted equilibrium potential of Cl^- (E_{Cl}=0 mV) with a symmetrical Cl^- gradient ($[Cl^-]_o$/ $[Cl^-]_i$=118/118 mmol/L).(Duan *et al.*, 2000)

(Duan *et al.*, 2000). The expression of ClC-2 in the heart was further characterized by immunohistochemistry and western blot from several species (Britton *et al.*, 2000). Later studies provided compelling evidence that $I_{Cl.ir}$ is encoded by ClC-2 and its alternatively spliced isoforms in the heart (Britton *et al.*, 2005;Huang *et al.*, 2009).

ClC-2 channels are activated by hyperpolarization, cell swelling, and acidosis and have an inwardly rectifying *I-V* relationship (Duan *et al.*, 2000;Komukai *et al.*, 2002a;Komukai *et al.*, 2002b;Britton *et al.*, 2005;Huang *et al.*, 2009). During the cardiac action potential, therefore, activation of the ClC-2 channels will conduct mainly an inward current as a result of Cl^- efflux at negative membrane potentials and cause a depolarization of the resting membrane potential of cardiac cells. At membrane potentials more positive than the equilibrium potential for Cl^- (E_{Cl}), ClC-2 may conduct a small outward current as a result of Cl^- influx and may accelerate repolarization of the action potential. It is also possible that, in a manner analogous to the role and tissue distribution pattern of the cationic pacemaker channels (I_f) (DiFrancesco, 1984;DiFrancesco, 2006), the hyperpolarization-activated $I_{Cl,ir}$ through ClC-2 channels may normally play a much more prominent role in the sino-atrial (SA) or atrial-ventricular (AV) nodal regions of the heart.

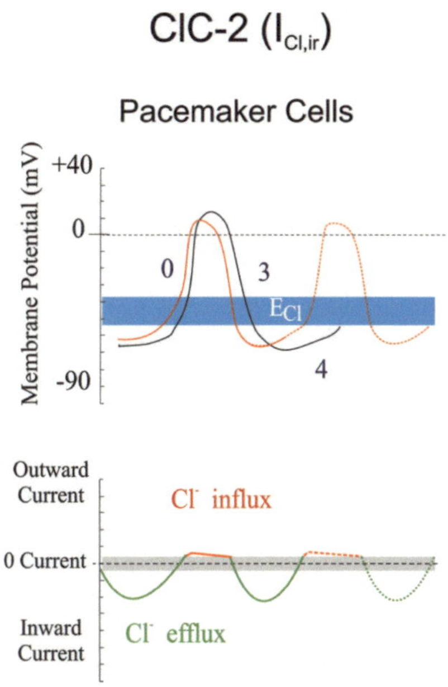

Fig. 3. Modulation of cardiac electrical activity by activation of ClC-2 channels in cardiac pacemaker cells. Changes in action potentials (*top panels*) and membrane currents (*bottom panels*) of cardiac pacemaker cells due to activation of ClC-2 channels are depicted. $I_{Cl.ir}$ is activated by hyperpolarization, cell swelling, and acidosis. *Top panel:* Numbers illustrate conventional phases of a prototype pacemaker action potential under control conditions (black) and after activation of I_{Cl} (red). Range of estimates for normal physiological values for Cl^- equilibrium potential (E_{Cl}) is indicated in blue. *Bottom panel:* Range of zero-current values corresponding to E_{Cl} is shown in grey. Activation of $I_{Cl.ir}$ in pacemaker cells during hyperpolarization causes acceleration of phase 4 depolarization and automaticity, shortening of action potential duration, and decrease in cycle length and action potential amplitude (dashed red line in *top panel*). (Adapted from Duan (Duan, 2009)).

$I_{Cl,ir}$ under basal or isotonic conditions is small, but can be further activated by hypotonic cell swelling (Duan *et al.*, 2000) and acidosis (Komukai *et al.*, 2002a;Komukai *et al.*, 2002b). The volume-sensitivity of the channel also suggests its role in cell volume regulation. The sensitivity of ClC-2 to $[H^+]_o$ and cell volume may be of pathological importance during hypoxia- or ischemia-induced acidosis or cell swelling. Therefore, it may be possible that the significance of $I_{Cl,ir}$ in the heart becomes more prominent under some pathological conditions (ischemia or hypoxia). As a matter of fact, ischemia and acidosis have consistently been shown to depolarize the resting membrane potential of cardiac myocytes, increase automaticity and cause lethal arrhythmias, although the mechanism has remained obscure (Hiraoka *et al.*, 1998;Carmeliet, 1999). It is reasonable to suggest that an increase in ClC-2 conductance could be responsible for these phenomena and be pro-arrhythmic. Drugs targeting ClC-2 channels could be anti-arrhythmic. Therefore, the ClC-2 channels could have important clinical significance for such cardiac diseases as arrhythmias, ischemia and reperfusion, and congestive heart failure. Activation of ClC-2 current should mainly cause a depolarization of the resting membrane potential and it is suggested that the acidosis-induced increase in $I_{Cl,ir}$ might underlie the depolarization of the resting membrane potential during acidosis or hypoxia (Komukai *et al.*, 2002a;Komukai *et al.*, 2002b).

Our recent study found that $I_{Cl,ir}$ was indeed functionally expressed in guinea-pig SAN cells (Huang *et al.*, 2009). $I_{Cl,ir}$ in guinea-pig SAN cells activated upon cell membrane hyperpolarization and hypotonic challenge has a strong inward rectification under symmetrical Cl^- conditions with a reversal potential close to the predicted value of E_{Cl}, and is inhibited by Cd^{2+} (Figure 4). All these properties are identical to those of $I_{Cl,ir}$ in atrial and ventricular myocytes of several species, including guinea-pig (Britton *et al.*, 2005), rat (Duan *et al.*, 2000;Komukai *et al.*, 2002a;Komukai *et al.*, 2002b;Britton *et al.*, 2005), and mouse (Duan *et al.*, 2000). $I_{Cl,ir}$ is neither a part of the I_f nor a result of Cl^- regulation of the I_f activity (Frace *et al.*, 1992) in SAN cells because a) $I_{Cl,ir}$ can be recorded in the presence of a strong I_f blocker (20 mM Cs^+) and in the absence of permeable cations; b) the reversal potential of $I_{Cl,ir}$ is close to the predicted E_{Cl}, suggesting the inward current is carried by Cl^-, not by cations; c) $I_{Cl,ir}$ but not I_f can be inhibited by Cd^{2+}; and d) $I_{Cl,ir}$ but not I_f is specifically inhibited by anti-*ClC-2* Ab. Our data from RT-PCR and immunohistochemistry provided direct evidence for the expression of *ClC-2* in SAN cells. In addition, dialysis of anti-*ClC-2* Ab but not the inactivated pre-absorbed Ab caused an inhibition of $I_{Cl,ir}$ but not I_f, $I_{Ca,L}$, I_{Ks} and $I_{Cl.vol}$. These results further support that *ClC-2* is the gene responsible for the endogenous Cl,ir channels not only in atrial and ventricular myocytes (Britton *et al.*, 2000;Britton *et al.*, 2005) but also in the SAN cells and that the Cl,ir in SAN cells may contribute to the regulation of pacemaker activity of the heart. Interestingly, the prevalence of functional endogenous $I_{Cl,ir}$ in the SAN cells (28/35, 80%) is apparently higher than that in the atrial or ventricular myocytes (Duan *et al.*, 2000). Whether this difference is due to the higher molecular expression or the different activation mechanisms is a legitimate question which may be very difficult to get a clear answer. Immunohistochemistry data reveals no significant difference between the SAN and atrial tissues. Theoretically, a Western blot of membrane fractions would help to quantitatively analyze the differences in the protein expression of ClC-2 in the SAN cells and the atrial myocytes. But, practically, in order to carry out the Western blot analysis on the isolated membrane fractions from SAN cells it would need to collect enough SAN cells from the guinea-pig heart, which means not only a requirement for a pool of tens of hearts but also an isolation and selection of true SAN cells without contamination from the adjacent atrial cells. This is an extremely difficult task to accomplish. Although the confocal images of the SAN cells and atrail or ventricular myocytes would provide information on the subcellular distribution of ClC-2 channels in these cells it would not be able to give quantitative information for a decisive conclusion on the dynamic distribution of the ClC-2 channel protein and the relationship between the distribution and the function of the channels.

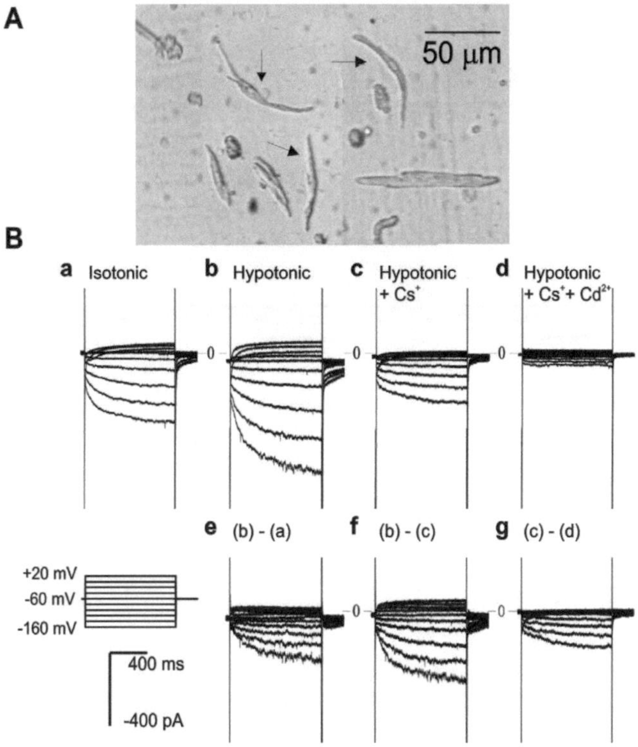

Fig. 4. Whole-cell currents recorded from SAN cells of guinea-pig heart. A. An example of single SAN cells (arrows) isolated from the SAN region of guinea pig heart by enzymatic dispersion. B. Whole-cell currents recorded from SAN cells. When cations (Na^+ and K^+) were included in the extracellular solutions, inward currents were slowly activated upon hyperpolarization under isotonic (a) conditions. Exposure of the same cell to hypotonic extracellular solution caused cell swelling and an increase in the inward current amplitude (b). The difference current caused by hypotonic cell swelling is shown in panel e. Subsequent replacement of 20 mmol/L of NaCl with CsCl caused a significant inhibition of the inward current (c). The Cs^+-sensitive current is shown in panel f. Subsequent addition of 0.2 mmol/L of Cd^{2+} to the hypotonic solution caused an inhibition of the inward current (d). The Cd^{2+}-sensitive currents are shown in panel g. (Huang *et al.*, 2009)

Because the E_{Cl} in cardiac cells under physiological conditions ranges between -65 to -35 mV (Baumgarten & Fozzard, 1981;Vaughan-Jones, 1982), which is very close to the maximum diastolic potential (MDP) of SAN cells, the contribution of $I_{Cl,ir}$ to SAN cell action potential is unique and also more complicated than the activation of I_f and other cation currents (Figure 3). When the membrane potential is negative to E_{Cl}, opening of Cl,ir channel may conduct an

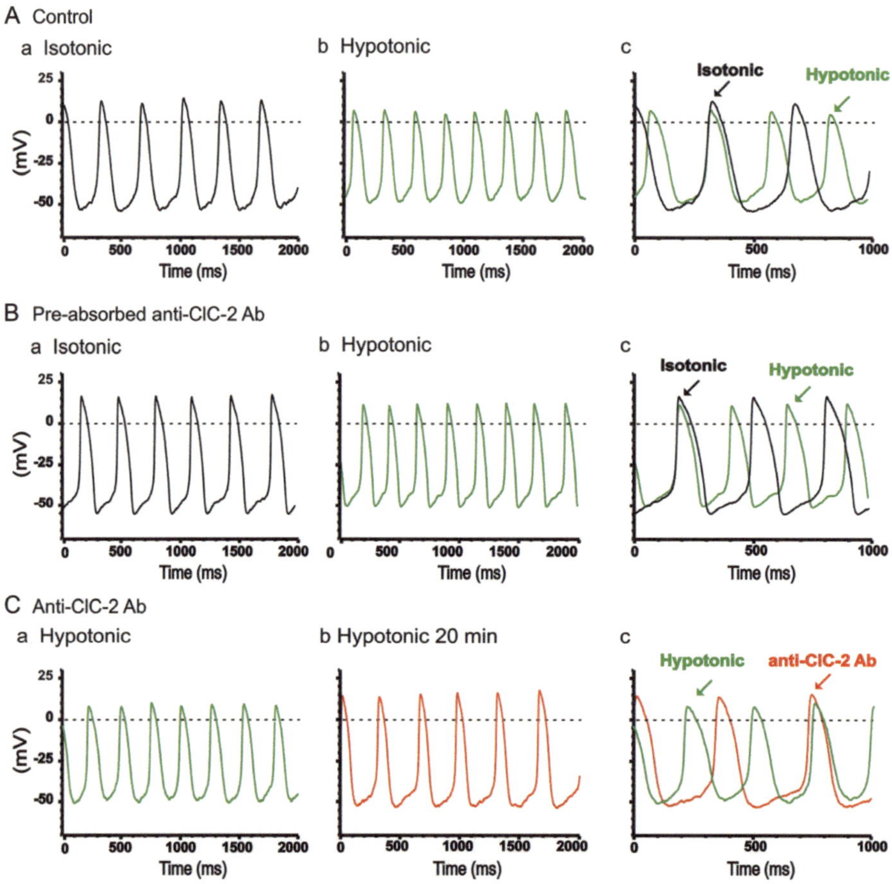

Fig. 5. Effects of Anti-*ClC-2* Ab on pacemaker action potential in SAN cells. A. Representative spontaneous action potentials recorded from an SAN cell by current-clamp (no current injection) with pipette solution containing no anti-ClC-2 Ab under isotonic (a) and hypotonic (b) conditions. For comparison, the action potentials recorded under these conditions were superimposed with an expanded time scale in panel c. The dotted lines indicate zero voltage. **B.** Spontaneous action potentials recorded from a SAN cell by current-clamp using a pipette solution containing pre-absorbed anti-ClC-2 Ab (control) and the cell was exposed to isotonic (a) and hypotonic (b) solutions. For comparison, the action potentials recorded under these conditions were superimposed with an expanded time scale in panel c. **C.** SAN cells were exposed to hypotonic solution for 20 min to fully activate $I_{Cl.ir}$ before whole-cell recordings. Action potentials were recorded immediately after membrane rupture (**a**) and after dialysis of anti-ClC-2 Ab for 20 min (**b**). Panel **c** shows the expanded and superimposed action potentials as shown in panel a and panel b.(Huang *et al.*, 2009)

Inward current (Cl^- efflux), which will depolarize the MDP and increase the diastolic depolarization slope (DDs). At the beginning of diastolic depolarization, the impedance of the cell is very large and activation of a small current may contribute significantly to the depolarization of the action potential (Zhang *et al.*, 2002). Therefore, both the smaller instantaneous $I_{Cl,ir}$ activated at membrane potentials near the MDP and the larger time-dependent $I_{Cl,ir}$ activated at membrane potentials more negative than the MDP may contribute pacemaker current to the phase 4 depolarization of the action potential of SAN cells. When the membrane potential is positive to E_{Cl}, opening of Cl,ir channel may conduct an outward current (Cl^- influx) and make the membrane potential (possibly including the MDP) more negative. But the inward rectification property of Cl,ir may limit the amplitude of the outward current and its contribution to repolarization and APD. Since the MDP may be determined normally by multiple mechanisms (Dobrzynski *et al.*, 2007;Liu *et al.*, 2007) such as I_f, I_{sus}, $I_{Ca,T}$, $I_{Ca,L}$, I_{NCX}, and possibly $I_{Cl,Ca}$ (Verkerk *et al.*, 2002) and $I_{Cl,swell}$ (Hagiwara *et al.*, 1992), the contribution of changes in $I_{Cl,ir}$ to the MDP during hypotonic stress may be further complicated by changes in other ionic currents which may also respond to hypotonic cell swelling such as $I_{Cl,swell}$ (Hagiwara *et al.*, 1992;Duan *et al.*, 2005;Duan, 2009) and I_{Ks} (Rees *et al.*, 1995). In addition, activation of $I_{Cl,ir}$ may also cause a dynamic change in the E_{Cl} (Staley *et al.*, 1996). The analysis of the relationship of the activation of $I_{Cl,ir}$ to the E_{Cl} and the consequent role of this relationship in determining the MDP has been limited by the lack of potent and specific $I_{Cl,ir}$ blocker. The identification of *ClC-2* as the gene responsible for Cl,ir channels in the heart and the availability of specific anti-*ClC-2* Ab provided us specific approach to effectively examine the functional role of Cl,ir in the heart.

In the isolated SAN cells, dialysis of anti-*ClC-2* Ab through the pipette solution for 20 min inhibited $I_{Cl,ir}$ (Figure 5B) and reversed the hypotonic stress-induced increase in DDs and decrease in MDP, APA, APD_{90}, and CL under hypotonic conditions, suggesting that $I_{Cl,ir}$ may play a role in the regulation of diastolic depolarization and the firing rate of spontaneous action potential of SAN cells under stressed conditions. Anti-*ClC-2* Ab, however, did not have significant effect on the hypotonicity-induced shortening of APD_{50} (Huang *et al.*, 2009). This may suggest that the contribution of the $I_{Cl,ir}$ to the repolarization at positive potentials is rather small because of its inward rectification property. These data may provide new mechanistic insight into the tonicity regulation of spontaneous beating rate in guinea-pig SAN reported by Ohba in 1986 (Ohba, 1986). In that study it was found that decreasing the osmolarity by 30% increased the heart rate by 6% and increasing the osmolarity to 130, 150, and 170% decreased the heart rate to 94, 89, and 73%, respectively (Ohba, 1986).

As mentioned above it is possible that the observed anti-*ClC-2* Ab-induced reduction in pacemaker activity under hypotonic conditions may be due to a non-specific block of hypotonic activation of I_{Ks} (Rees *et al.*, 1995) and $I_{Cl.swell}$ (Hagiwara *et al.*, 1992;Duan *et al.*, 2005;Duan, 2009). But we found that anti-*ClC-2* Ab failed to affect I_{Ks} and $I_{Cl,swell}$ under either isotonic or hypotonic conditions. These results are consistent with the observation that anti-*ClC-2* Ab has no effect on APD_{50} and strongly suggest that the activation of ClC-2 channels may play an important role in the diastolic depolarization and firing rate of SAN pacemaker activity but have very little impact on the repolarization at positive potentials during hypotonic stress. In addition, dialysis of pre-absorbed anti-ClC-2 Ab did not cause any changes in the response of the SAN pacemaker activity to hypotonic stress (Figure 5A and B) or in the hypotonic activation of $I_{Cl,ir}$. Therefore, it is highly unlikely that the anti-*ClC-2* Ab-induced reduction in the current amplitude of $I_{Cl,ir}$ and pacemaker activity in the SAN cells under hypotonic conditions are not due to the effects of anti-*ClC-2* Ab but the potential effects of dialysis with pipette solutions *per se*.

In agreement with our findings in the isolated cells, targeted inactivation of ClC-2 channels caused a decrease in HR, especially under exercise stress (Figure 6). The resting HR of the *Clcn2*$^{-/-}$ mice was slower but not significantly different from that of the *Clcn2*$^{+/+}$ and *Clcn2*$^{+/-}$ mice. This may be explained by the fact that $I_{Cl,ir}$ through ClC-2 channels under basal or

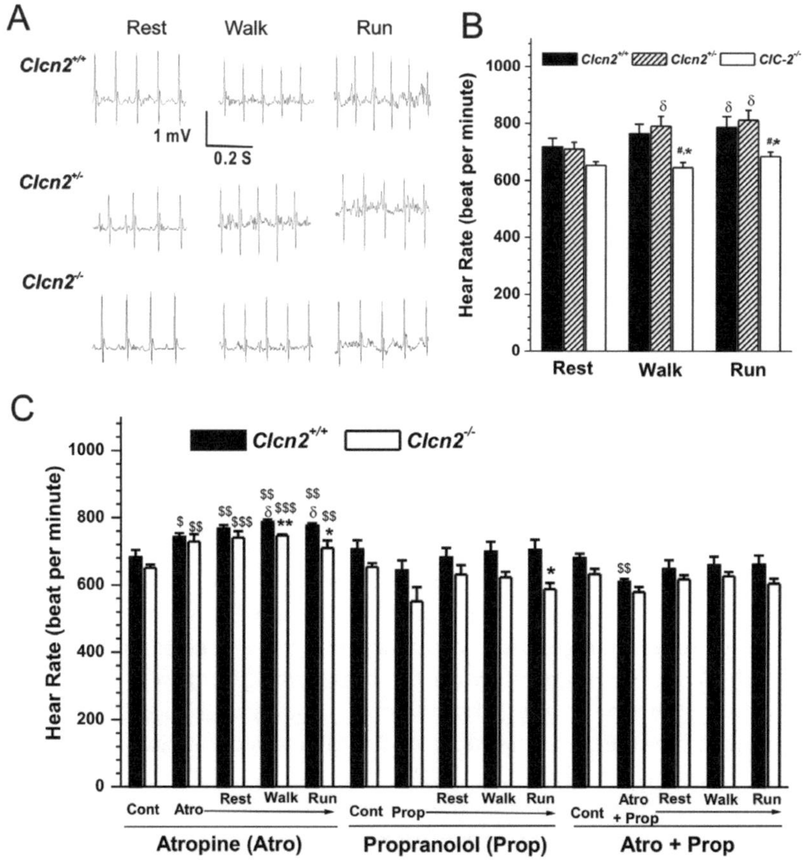

Fig. 6. Telemetry ECG recordings in *Clcn2*$^{-/-}$ mice and their *Clcn2*$^{+/+}$ and *Clcn2*$^{+/-}$ littermates during treadmill exercises. **A.** Representative ECG (Lead II) recordings in *Clcn2*$^{+/+}$, *Clcn2*$^{+/-}$, and *Clcn2*$^{-/-}$ mice while they were subjected to treadmill exercise at a) Rest period: acclimation at 0 m/min, incline 0 ° for 5 min; b) Walk period: walking at 5m/min, incline 0 ° for 5 min; c) Run period: running at 15 m/min, uphill incline 8 ° for 5 min. **B**. Mean heart rate during the last minute of each treadmill exercise segment for the *Clcn2*$^{+/+}$ (n=6), *Clcn2*$^{+/-}$ (n=5), and *Clcn2*$^{-/-}$ (n=7) mice. **C**. Mean heart rate of the *Clcn2*$^{+/+}$ (n=5) and *Clcn2*$^{-/-}$ (n=4) mice before (Control, Cont) and after the intraperitoneal injection of atropine (Atro), propranolol (Prop), or atropine plus propranolol (Atro + Prop) during the last minute of each treadmill exercise segment (Rest, Walk, and Run). * $P < 0.05$, ** $P < 0.01$, *** $P < 0.001$ vs *Clcn2*$^{+/+}$, # $P < 0.05$, ## $P < 0.01$, ### $P < 0.001$ vs *Clcn2*$^{+/-}$; \$ $P < 0.05$, \$\$ $P < 0.01$, \$\$\$ $P < 0.001$ vs control (Cont); □ $P < 0.05$ vs Rest. (Huang *et al.*, 2009)

isotonic conditions is relatively small. It has been known that, however, $I_{Cl,ir}$ is activated in a larger scale by cell swelling (Duan *et al.*, 2000;Britton *et al.*, 2005), acidosis (Komukai *et al.*, 2002a;Komukai *et al.*, 2002b), and PKA phosphorylation (Kajita *et al.*, 2000a;Kajita *et al.*, 2000b;Cuppoletti *et al.*, 2004a;Cuppoletti *et al.*, 2004b;Huang *et al.*, 2008). Indeed, hypoxia, ischemia, and acidosis have consistently been shown to increase automaticity and cause lethal arrhythmias, although the mechanism has remained obscure (Carmeliet, 1999;Duan *et al.*, 2005). Activation of $I_{Cl,ir}$ may explain, at least in part, the increase in automaticity under these stressed or pathological conditions (Komukai *et al.*, 2002a;Komukai *et al.*, 2002b). We found that during acute exercise the maximal HR is lower in *Clcn2*$^{-/-}$ mice than in *Clcn2*$^{+/+}$ and *Clcn2*$^{+/-}$ mice, suggesting that activation of ClC-2 channels in the heart may contribute to the chronotropic response of the mouse to exercise stress. It is possible that activation of ClC-2 channels by β-stimulation induced PKA phosphorylation (Fritsch & Edelman, 1996;Sherry *et al.*, 1997;Kajita *et al.*, 2000a;Kajita *et al.*, 2000b;Cuppoletti *et al.*, 2004a;Cuppoletti *et al.*, 2004b;Huang *et al.*, 2008) may contribute to the regulation of HR during exercise. It has been known that several consensus PKA phosphorylation sites are well conserved in the ClC-2 sequences from different species (Cuppoletti *et al.*, 2004b). These results provide strong evidence for the molecular and functional expression of ClC-2 encoded endogenous Cl,ir channels in the SAN cells. The significance of $I_{Cl,ir}$ in the heart may become more prominent under stressed or pathological conditions. Our results may also shed new light on understanding mechanisms for arrhythmias such as sinus node dysfunction or sick sinus syndrome (Dobrzynski *et al.*, 2007). Cardiac ClC-2 channels may thus represent new therapeutic targets for arrhythmias, congestive heart failure, and ischemic heart diseases.

3.2 $I_{Cl,vol}$ and ClC-3 Cl^- channels in cardiac pacemaker activity

Activation of the volume-regulated outwardly rectifying Cl^- current ($I_{Cl,vol}$) is expected to produce depolarization of the resting membrane potential and significant APD shortening because of its strong outwardly rectifying property (Sorota, 1992;Duan & Nattel, 1994;Du & Sorota, 1997;Duan *et al.*, 1997b;Duan *et al.*, 1999a). Under basal or isotonic conditions $I_{Cl,vol}$ is small (Duan *et al.*, 1992;Sorota, 1992;Duan *et al.*, 1997b;Hume *et al.*, 2000), but can be further activated by stretching of the cell membrane by inflation (Hagiwara *et al.*, 1992;Du & Sorota, 1997) or direct mechanical stretch of membrane β_1-integrin (Browe & Baumgarten, 2003) and/or cell swelling induced by exposure to hypoosmotic solutions (Sorota, 1992;Du & Sorota, 1997;Duan *et al.*, 1997b;Duan *et al.*, 1999a). A strech of the cell membrane by applying positive pressure to inflate the cell activated a Cl^- current with characteristics similar to $I_{Cl,vol}$ in SAN cells isolated from rabbit heart (Hagiwara *et al.*, 1992). Later studies further confirmed the presence of both cell strech- and swelling-activated Cl- currents in SAN cells (Kohl *et al.*, 1994;Arai *et al.*, 1996;Lei & Kohl, 1998). Although it has been suggested that stretch and swelling activate the same anion channel in some non-cardiac cells, further study is needed to determine whether this is true in cardiac myocytes. Baumgarten's laboratory has recently demonstrated that $I_{Cl,swell}$ in ventricular myocytes can be directly activated by mechanical stretch through selectively stretching β1-integrins with mAb-coated magnetic beads (Browe & Baumgarten, 2003;Baumgarten & Clemo, 2003;Browe & Baumgarten, 2004;Browe & Baumgarten, 2006). The stretch-activated Cl^- current may contribute to the pacemaker rhythm under physiological conditions, since the stimulus is almost continuously present in the intact heart (Hagiwara *et al.*, 1992). $I_{Cl,vol}$ may also serve as a mediator of mechanotransduction and volume regulation and play a significant role in the pacemaker function if they act as both the stretch activated channels and cell swelling activated channels in these cells (Hagiwara *et al.*, 1992;Kohl *et al.*, 1994;Arai *et al.*, 1996;Lei & Kohl, 1998;Baumgarten & Clemo, 2003).

The short isoform of ClC-3 (sClC-3), a member of the ClC superfamily of voltage-dependent Cl^- channels, has been proposed to be the molecular correlate of a key component of the native $I_{Cl,vol}$ in cardiac myocytes. (Duan *et al.*, 1997b;Hume *et al.*, 2000;Duan, 2009). A series of recent independent studies from many laboratories further strongly corroborated this hypothesis (please see recent reviews by Duan (Duan, 2009;Duan, 2010) and Hume et al. (Hume *et al.*, 2010)). It has been demonstrated that ClC-3 is widely expressed in cardiac tissues (Britton *et al.*, 2000;Hume *et al.*, 2000). Further studies are needed to answer the questions whether ClC-3 channels are expressed in SAN cells and whether ClC-3 is responsible for both $I_{Cl,vol}$ and the stretch-activated Cl^- channels in these cells.

3.3 Ca^{2+}-activated Cl^- channels and cardiac pacemaker activity

Ca^{2+}-activated chloride channels (CACCs) are widely distributed in cardiac tissues and play important roles in the regulation of cardiac excitability (Verkerk *et al.*, 2003a). Using perforated patch-clamp methodology Verkerk et al. identified a Ca^{2+}-activated Cl^- current ($I_{Cl,Ca}$) in one third of the spontaneously active rabbit SAN cells (Verkerk *et al.*, 2002). It is not known why $I_{Cl,Ca}$ is non-uniformly distributed among SAN cells. But it may be related to the inhomogeneity of function and structure of the SA node (Boyett *et al.*, 2000). $I_{Cl,Ca}$ is activated during the pacemaker cycle. The current is transient outward with a bell-shaped current–voltage relationship. Stimulation of adrenoceptors with noradrenaline doubled the $I_{Cl,Ca}$ density. Action potential clamp measurements demonstrate that $I_{Cl,Ca}$ is activated late during the action potential upstroke. Current clamp experiments show, both in the absence and presence of noradrenaline, that blockade of $I_{Cl,Ca}$ by DIDS (4,4,-diisothiocyanostilbene-2,2,-disulphonic acid) increases the action potential overshoot and duration, measured at 20 % repolarization, but has no effect on intrinsic interbeat interval, upstroke velocity, diastolic depolarization rate and the action potential duration measured at 50 and 90 % repolarization (Verkerk *et al.*, 2002). Therefore, it was suggested that $I_{Cl,Ca}$ may have a limited role in pacemaker synchronization or action potential conduction.

Even though $I_{Cl,Ca}$ is also expected to be outwardly rectifying under physiological conditions the activation of $I_{Cl,Ca}$ will have considerably different effects on cardiac action potential and resting membrane potential from those of ClC-3 channels. This is because the kinetic behavior of $I_{Cl,Ca}$ is significantly determined by the time course of the $[Ca^{2+}]_i$ transient (Zygmunt & Gibbons, 1991). Normally, $I_{Cl,Ca}$ will have insignificant effects on the diastolic membrane potential, as resting $[Ca^{2+}]_i$ is low. When $[Ca^{2+}]_i$ is substantially increased above the physiological resting level, however, $I_{Cl,Ca}$ carries a significant amount of transient outward current. $I_{Cl,Ca}$ will activate early during the action potential in response to an increase in $[Ca^{2+}]_i$ associated with Ca^{2+}-induced Ca^{2+} release (CICR). The time course of decline of the $[Ca^{2+}]_i$ transient will determine the extent to which $I_{Cl,Ca}$ contributes to early phase 1 repolarization. In the rabbit left ventricle, $I_{Cl,Ca}$ contributes to APD shortening in subendocardial myocytes but not in subepicardial myocytes. These differences in functional expression of $I_{Cl,Ca}$ may reduce the electrical heterogeneity in the left ventricle (Verkerk *et al.*, 2004). In Ca^{2+}-overloaded cardiac preparations, $I_{Cl,Ca}$ can contribute to the arrhythmogenic transient inward current (I_{TI}) (Zygmunt, 1994). I_{TI} produces delayed afterdepolarization (DAD) (January & Fozzard, 1988) and induces triggered activity, which is an important mechanism for abnormal impulse formation. In sheep Purkinje and ventricular myocytes, activation of $I_{Cl,Ca}$ was found to induce DAD and plateau transient repolarization (Verkerk *et al.*, 2000). Therefore, blockade of $I_{Cl,Ca}$ may be potentially antiarrhythmogenic by reducing DAD amplitude and triggered activity based on DAD. However, the role of $I_{Cl,Ca}$ in phase 1 repolarization and the generation of EAD and DAD of either normal or failing human heart seem very limited (Verkerk *et al.*, 2003b). Therefore, the clinical relevance of $I_{Cl,Ca}$ blockers remain to be determined.

The molecular identity of CACCs in the heart remains to be determined. CLCA-1 and bestrophins were initially proposed as candidates for CACCs in cardiac tissues(Hartzell *et al.*, 2005;O'Driscoll *et al.*, 2008). It has been demonstrated that at least three members of the murine Bestrophin family, mBest1, mBest2 and mBest3, are expressed in mouse heart. Whole-cell patch clamp experiments with HEK cells transfected with cardiac mBest1 and mBest3 both elicited a calcium sensitive, time independent Cl^- current, suggesting mBest1 and mBest3 may function as pore-forming Cl^- channels that are activated by physiological levels of calcium(O'Driscoll *et al.*, 2008). Very recently, independent studies from three laboratories have identified a new gene, TMEM16 (or Ano1), as a candidate for CACCs (Schroeder *et al.*, 2008;Caputo *et al.*, 2008;Yang *et al.*, 2008). Whether TMEM16 forms the functional endogenous CACCs and how TMEME16 interacts with and the bestrophins in native cardiac myocytes and its functional role in pacemaker activity and electrophysiology remain to be explored.

3.4 Angiotensin II-activated Cl^- channels and cardiac pacemaker activity

An angiotensin-II-activated Cl^- current was found in rabbit SAN cells (Bescond *et al.*, 1994). The current is sensitive to Cl^- channel blockers anthracene-9-carboxylic acid and diphenylamine-2-carboxylic acid and can be totally inhibited by the competitive angiotensin II-receptor 1 (AT1) antagonist losartan and by the presence of intracellular protein kinase C inhibitor. It is suggested that in SAN cells there exist protein kinase-C-sensitive Cl^- channels which may be activated by angiotensin II via the stimulation of the AT1 receptors (Bescond *et al.*, 1994). The molecular mechanism and the exact functional role of these channels, however, have not been further explored.

4. Conclusion

Experimental evidence are merging to support the potential role of several Cl^- channels in the regulation of cardiac pacemaker activity and these anion channels may represent novel therapeutic targets for arrhythmias involving abnormal pacemaker activities.

5. Acknowledgement

Dr. Duan and the research in the Laboratory of Cardiovascular Phenomics, Center of Biomedical Research Excellence and the Department of Pharmacology, University of Nevada, School of Medicine is supported by grants from the National Institutes of Health (R01-HL63914), National Center of Research Resources (NCRR, P20RR15581), and American Diabetes Association Innovation Award (#07-8-IN-08).

6. References

Arai A, Kodama I, & Toyama J (1996). Roles of Cl- channels and Ca2+ mobilization in stretch-induced increase of SA node pacemaker activity. *Am J Physiol* 270, H1726-H1735.

Bahinski A, Nairn AC, Greengard P, & Gadsby DC (1989). Chloride conductance regulated by cyclic AMP-dependent protein kinase in cardiac myocytes. *Nature* 340, 718-721.

Baumgarten CM & Clemo HF (2003). Swelling-activated chloride channels in cardiac physiology and pathophysiology. *Prog Biophys Mol Biol* 82, 25-42.

Baumgarten CM & Fozzard HA (1981). Intracellular chloride activity in mammalian ventricular muscle. *Am J Physiol* 241, C121-C129.

Bescond J, Bois P, Petit-Jacques J, & Lenfant J (1994). Characterization of an angiotensin-II-activated chloride current in rabbit sino-atrial cells. *J Membr Biol* 140, 153-161.

Boyett MR, Honjo H, & Kodama I (2000). The sinoatrial node, a heterogeneous pacemaker structure. *Cardiovasc Res* 47, 658-687.

Britton FC, Hatton WJ, Rossow CF, Duan D, Hume JR, & Horowitz B (2000). Molecular distribution of volume-regulated chloride channels (ClC-2 and ClC-3) in cardiac tissues. *Am J Physiol Heart Circ Physiol* 279, H2225-H2233.

Britton FC, Ohya S, Horowitz B, & Greenwood IA (2002). Comparison of the properties of CLCA1 generated currents and I(Cl(Ca)) in murine portal vein smooth muscle cells. *J Physiol* 539, 107-117.

Britton FC, Wang GL, Huang ZM, Ye L, Horowitz B, Hume JR, & Duan D (2005). Functional characterization of novel alternatively spliced ClC-2 chloride channel variants in the heart. *J Biol Chem* 280, 25871-25880.

Browe DM & Baumgarten CM (2003). Stretch of beta 1 integrin activates an outwardly rectifying chloride current via FAK and Src in rabbit ventricular myocytes. *J Gen Physiol* 122, 689-702.

Browe DM & Baumgarten CM (2004). Angiotensin II (AT1) receptors and NADPH oxidase regulate Cl- current elicited by beta1 integrin stretch in rabbit ventricular myocytes. *J Gen Physiol* 124, 273-287.

Browe DM & Baumgarten CM (2006). EGFR kinase regulates volume-sensitive chloride current elicited by integrin stretch via PI-3K and NADPH oxidase in ventricular myocytes. *J Gen Physiol* 127, 237-251.

Brown HF, Giles W, & Noble SJ (1977). Membrane currents underlying activity in frog sinus venosus. *J Physiol* 271, 783-816.

Caputo A, Caci E, Ferrera L, Pedemonte N, Barsanti C, Sondo E, Pfeffer U, Ravazzolo R, Zegarra-Moran O, & Galietta LJ (2008). TMEM16A, a membrane protein associated with calcium-dependent chloride channel activity. *Science* 322, 590-594.

Carmeliet E (1999). Cardiac ionic currents and acute ischemia: from channels to arrhythmias. *Physiol Rev* 79, 917-1017.

Carmeliet EE (1961). Chloride ions and the membrane potential of Purkinje fibres. *J Physiol* 156, 375-388.

Chu S, Murray CB, Liu MM, & Zeitlin PL (1996). A short ClC-2 mRNA transcript is produced by exon skipping. *Nucl Acids Res* 24, 3453-3457.

Chu S & Zeitlin PL (1997). Alternative mRNA splice variants of the rat ClC-2 chloride channel gene are expressed in lung: genomic sequence and organization of ClC-2. *Nucleic Acids Res* 25, 4153-4159.

Cid LP, Montrose-Rafizadeh C, Smith DI, Guggino WB, & Cutting GR (1995). Cloning of a putative human voltage-gated chloride channel (CIC-2) cDNA widely expressed in human tissues. *Hum Mol Genet* 4, 407-413.

Cid LP, Niemeyer MI, Ramirez A, & Sepulveda FV (2000). Splice variants of a ClC-2 chloride channel with differing functional characteristics. *Am J Physiol Cell Physiol* 279, C1198-C1210.

Collier ML & Hume JR (1995). Unitary chloride channels activated by protein kinase C in guinea pig ventricular myocytes. *Circ Res* 76, 317-324.

Collier ML, Levesque PC, Kenyon JL, & Hume JR (1996). Unitary Cl- channels activated by cytoplasmic Ca2+ in canine ventricular myocytes. *Circ Res* 78, 936-944.

Cuppoletti J, Malinowska DH, Tewari KP, Li QJ, Sherry AM, Patchen ML, & Ueno R (2004a). SPI-0211 activates T84 cell chloride transport and recombinant human ClC-2 chloride currents. *Am J Physiol Cell Physiol* 287, C1173-C1183.

Cuppoletti J, Tewari KP, Sherry AM, Ferrante CJ, & Malinowska DH (2004b). Sites of protein kinase A activation of the human ClC-2 Cl(-) channel. *J Biol Chem* 279, 21849-21856.

De Mello WC (1963). Role of chloride ions in cardiac action and pacemaker potentials. *Am J Physiol* 205, 567-575.

DiFrancesco D (1984). Properties of the cardiac pacemaker (if) current. *Boll Soc Ital Biol Sper* 60 Suppl 4, 29-33.

DiFrancesco D (2006). Funny channels in the control of cardiac rhythm and mode of action of selective blockers. *Pharmacol Res* 53, 399-406.

DiFrancesco D (2010). The role of the funny current in pacemaker activity. *Circ Res* 106, 434-446.

Dobrzynski H, Boyett MR, & Anderson RH (2007). New insights into pacemaker activity: promoting understanding of sick sinus syndrome. *Circulation* 115, 1921-1932.

Du XY & Sorota S (1997). Cardiac swelling-induced chloride current depolarizes canine atrial myocytes. *Am J Physiol* 272, H1904-H1916.

Duan D (2009). Phenomics of cardiac chloride channels: the systematic study of chloride channel function in the heart. *J Physiol* 587, 2163-2177.

Duan D, Cowley S, Horowitz B, & Hume JR (1999a). A serine residue in ClC-3 links phosphorylation-dephosphorylation to chloride channel regulation by cell volume. *J Gen Physiol* 113, 57-70.

Duan D, Fermini B, & Nattel S (1995). Alpha-adrenergic control of volume-regulated Cl-currents in rabbit atrial myocytes. Characterization of a novel ionic regulatory mechanism. *Circ Res* 77, 379-393.

Duan D, Hume JR, & Nattel S (1997a). Evidence that outwardly rectifying Cl- channels underlie volume-regulated Cl- currents in heart. *Circ Res* 80, 103-113.

Duan D & Nattel S (1994). Properties of single outwardly rectifying Cl- channels in heart. *Circ Res* 75, 789-795.

Duan D, Winter C, Cowley S, Hume JR, & Horowitz B (1997b). Molecular identification of a volume-regulated chloride channel. *Nature* 390, 417-421.

Duan D, Ye L, Britton F, Horowitz B, & Hume JR (2000). A novel anionic inward rectifier in native cardiac myocytes. *Circ Res* 86, E63-E71.

Duan D, Ye L, Britton F, Miller LJ, Yamazaki J, Horowitz B, & Hume JR (1999b). Purinoceptor-coupled Cl- channels in mouse heart: a novel, alternative pathway for CFTR regulation. *J Physiol* 521 Pt 1, 43-56.

Duan D, Zhong J, Hermoso M, Satterwhite CM, Rossow CF, Hatton WJ, Yamboliev I, Horowitz B, & Hume JR (2001). Functional inhibition of native volume-sensitive outwardly rectifying anion channels in muscle cells and Xenopus oocytes by anti-ClC-3 antibody. *J Physiol* 531, 437-444.

Duan DD (2010). Volume Matters. Novel Roles of the Volume-Regulated ClC-3 Channels in Hypertension-Induced Cerebrovascular Remodeling. *Hypertension* 56, 346-348.

Duan DY, Fermini B, & Nattel S (1992). Sustained outward current observed after I(to1) inactivation in rabbit atrial myocytes is a novel Cl- current. *Am J Physiol* 263, H1967-H1971.

Duan DY, Liu LL, Bozeat N, Huang ZM, Xiang SY, Wang GL, Ye L, & Hume JR (2005). Functional role of anion channels in cardiac diseases. *Acta Pharmacol Sin* 26, 265-278.

Dutzler R, Campbell EB, Cadene M, Chait BT, & MacKinnon R (2002). X-ray structure of a ClC chloride channel at 3.0 A reveals the molecular basis of anion selectivity. *Nature* 415, 287-294.

Frace AM, Maruoka F, & Noma A (1992). Control of the hyperpolarization-activated cation current by external anions in rabbit sino-atrial node cells. *J Physiol* 453, 307-318.

Fritsch J & Edelman A (1996). Modulation of the hyperpolarization-activated Cl- current in human intestinal T84 epithelial cells by phosphorylation. *J Physiol* 490 (Pt 1), 115-128.

Furukawa T, Horikawa S, Terai T, Ogura T, Katayama Y, & Hiraoka M (1995). Molecular cloning and characterization of a novel truncated from (ClC-2 beta) of ClC-2 alpha (ClC-2G) in rabbit heart. *FEBS Lett* 375, 56-62.

Furukawa T, Ogura T, Katayama Y, & Hiraoka M (1998). Characteristics of rabbit ClC-2 current expressed in Xenopus oocytes and its contribution to volume regulation. *Am J Physiol* 274, C500-C512.

Furukawa T, Ogura T, Zheng YJ, Tsuchiya H, Nakaya H, Katayama Y, & Inagaki N (2002). Phosphorylation and functional regulation of ClC-2 chloride channels expressed in Xenopus oocytes by M cyclin-dependent protein kinase. *J Physiol* 540, 883-893.

Hagiwara N, Masuda H, Shoda M, & Irisawa H (1992). Stretch-activated anion currents of rabbit cardiac myocytes. *J Physiol* 456, 285-302.

Hartzell C, Putzier I, & Arreola J (2005). Calcium-activated chloride channels. *Annu Rev Physiol* 67, 719-758.

Hartzell HC (2008). Physiology. CaCl-ing channels get the last laugh. *Science* 322, 534-535.

Hartzell HC, Yu K, Xiao Q, Chien LT, & Qu Z (2009). Anoctamin/TMEM16 family members are Ca2+-activated Cl- channels. *J Physiol* 587, 2127-2139.

Harvey RD & Hume JR (1989). Autonomic regulation of a chloride current in heart. *Science* 244, 983-985.

Hiraoka M, Kawano S, Hirano Y, & Furukawa T (1998). Role of cardiac chloride currents in changes in action potential characteristics and arrhythmias. *Cardiovasc Res* 40, 23-33.

Huang, Z. M., Britton, F. C., An, C., Yuan, C., Ye, L., Hatton, W. J., and Duan D. (2008). Characterization of ClC-2 channel/PKA interaction in mouse heart. <*[11] Journal*> 22, 721.5.

Huang ZM, Prasad C, Britton FC, Ye LL, Hatton WJ, & Duan D (2009). Functional role of CLC-2 chloride inward rectifier channels in cardiac sinoatrial nodal pacemaker cells. *J Mol Cell Cardiol* 47, 121-132.

Hume JR, Duan D, Collier ML, Yamazaki J, & Horowitz B (2000). Anion transport in heart. *Physiol Rev* 80, 31-81.

Hume JR, Wang GX, Yamazaki J, Ng LC, & Duan D (2010). CLC-3 chloride channels in the pulmonary vasculature. *Adv Exp Med Biol* 661, 237-247.

Hutter O & Noble D (1961). Anion conductance of cardiac muscle. *J Physiol* 157, 335-350.

January CT & Fozzard HA (1988). Delayed afterdepolarizations in heart muscle: mechanisms and relevance. *Pharmacol Rev* 40, 219-227.

Jordt SE & Jentsch TJ (1997). Molecular dissection of gating in the ClC-2 chloride channel. *EMBO J* 16, 1582-1592.

Kajita H, Omori K, & Matsuda H (2000a). The chloride channel ClC-2 contributes to the inwardly rectifying Cl- conductance in cultured porcine choroid plexus epithelial cells. *J Physiol* 523 Pt 2, 313-324.

Kajita H, Whitwell C, & Brown PD (2000b). Properties of the inward-rectifying Cl- channel in rat choroid plexus: regulation by intracellular messengers and inhibition by divalent cations. *Pflugers Arch* 440, 933-940.

Kenyon JL & Gibbons WR (1979a). 4-Aminopyridine and the early outward current of sheep cardiac Purkinje fibers. *J Gen Physiol* 73, 139-157.

Kenyon JL & Gibbons WR (1979b). Influence of chloride, potassium, and tetraethylammonium on the early outward current of sheep cardiac Purkinje fibers. *J Gen Physiol* 73, 117-138.

Kohl P, Kamkin AG, Kiseleva IS, & Noble D (1994). Mechanosensitive fibroblasts in the sino-atrial node region of rat heart: interaction with cardiomyocytes and possible role. *Exp Physiol* 79, 943-956.

Komukai K, Brette F, & Orchard CH (2002a). Electrophysiological response of rat atrial myocytes to acidosis. *Am J Physiol Heart Circ Physiol* 283, H715-H724.

Komukai K, Brette F, Pascarel C, & Orchard CH (2002b). Electrophysiological response of rat ventricular myocytes to acidosis. *Am J Physiol Heart Circ Physiol* 283, H412-H422.

Kurata Y, Hisatome I, Imanishi S, & Shibamoto T (2003). Roles of L-type Ca2+ and delayed-rectifier K+ currents in sinoatrial node pacemaking: insights from stability and bifurcation analyses of a mathematical model. *Am J Physiol Heart Circ Physiol* 285, H2804-H2819.

Lei M & Kohl P (1998). Swelling-induced decrease in spontaneous pacemaker activity of rabbit isolated sino-atrial node cells. *Acta Physiol Scand* 164, 1-12.

Levesque PC & Hume JR (1995). ATPo but not cAMPi activates a chloride conductance in mouse ventricular myocytes. *Cardiovasc Res* 29, 336-343.

Liang H, Halbach M, Hannes T, Fleischmann BK, Tang M, Schunkert H, Hescheler J, & Reppel M (2010). Electrophysiological basis of the first heart beats. *Cell Physiol Biochem* 25, 561-570.

Liu J, Noble PJ, Xiao G, Abdelrahman M, Dobrzynski H, Boyett MR, Lei M, & Noble D (2007). Role of pacemaking current in cardiac nodes: Insights from a comparative study of sinoatrial node and atrioventricular node. *Prog Biophys Mol Biol* 96, 294-304.

Loewen ME, MacDonald DW, Gaspar KJ, & Forsyth GW (2000). Isoform-specific exon skipping in a variant form of ClC-2. *Biochim Biophys Acta* 1493, 284-288.

Malinowska DH, Kupert EY, Bahinski A, Sherry AM, & Cuppoletti J (1995). Cloning, functional expression, and characterization of a PKA-activated gastric Cl- channel. *Am J Physiol* 268, C191-C200.

Nagel G, Hwang TC, Nastiuk KL, Nairn AC, & Gadsby DC (1992). The protein kinase A-regulated cardiac Cl- channel resembles the cystic fibrosis transmembrane conductance regulator. *Nature* 360, 81-84.

Noma A & Irisawa H (1976). Membrane currents in the rabbit sinoatrial node cell as studied by the double microelectrode method. *Pflugers Arch* 364, 45-52.

O'Driscoll KE, Hatton WJ, Burkin HR, Leblanc N, & Britton FC (2008). Expression, localization, and functional properties of Bestrophin 3 channel isolated from mouse heart. *Am J Physiol Cell Physiol* 295, C1610-C1624.

Ohba M (1986). Effects of tonicity on the pacemaker activity of guinea-pig sino-atrial node. *Jpn J Physiol* 36, 1027-1038.

Ono K & Iijima T (2010). Cardiac T-type Ca(2+) channels in the heart. *J Mol Cell Cardiol* 48, 65-70.

Park K, Arreola J, Begenisich T, & Melvin JE (1998). Comparison of voltage-activated Cl-channels in rat parotid acinar cells with ClC-2 in a mammalian expression system. *J Membr Biol* 163, 87-95.

Park K, Begenisich T, & Melvin JE (2001). Protein kinase A activation phosphorylates the rat ClC-2 Cl- channel but does not change activity. *J Membr Biol* 182, 31-37.

Rees SA, Vandenberg JI, Wright AR, Yoshida A, & Powell T (1995). Cell swelling has differential effects on the rapid and slow components of delayed rectifier potassium current in guinea pig cardiac myocytes. *J Gen Physiol* 106, 1151-1170.

Schroeder BC, Cheng T, Jan YN, & Jan LY (2008). Expression cloning of TMEM16A as a calcium-activated chloride channel subunit. *Cell* 134, 1019-1029.

Seyama I (1977). The effect of Na, K and Cl ions on the resting membrane potential of sino-atrial node cell of the rabbit. *Jpn J Physiol* 27, 577-588.

Seyama I (1979). Characteristics of the anion channel in the sino-atrial node cell of the rabbit. *J Physiol* 294, 447-460.

Sherry AM, Stroffekova K, Knapp LM, Kupert EY, Cuppoletti J, & Malinowska DH (1997). Characterization of the human pH- and PKA-activated ClC-2G(2 alpha) Cl-channel. *Am J Physiol* 273, C384-C393.

Shinagawa Y, Satoh H, & Noma A (2000). The sustained inward current and inward rectifier K+ current in pacemaker cells dissociated from rat sinoatrial node. *J Physiol* 523 Pt 3, 593-605.

Sorota S (1992). Swelling-induced chloride-sensitive current in canine atrial cells revealed by whole-cell patch-clamp method. *Circ Res* 70, 679-687.

Staley K, Smith R, Schaack J, Wilcox C, & Jentsch TJ (1996). Alteration of GABAA receptor function following gene transfer of the CLC-2 chloride channel. *Neuron* 17, 543-551.

Stroffekova K, Kupert EY, Malinowska DH, & Cuppoletti J (1998). Identification of the pH sensor and activation by chemical modification of the ClC-2G Cl- channel. *Am J Physiol* 275, C1113-C1123.

Thiemann A, Grunder S, Pusch M, & Jentsch TJ (1992). A chloride channel widely expressed in epithelial and non-epithelial cells. *Nature* 356, 57-60.

Vaughan-Jones RD (1982). Chloride activity and its control in skeletal and cardiac muscle. *Philos Trans R Soc Lond B Biol Sci* 299, 537-548.

Verkerk AO, Tan HL, Kirkels JH, & Ravesloot JH (2003a). Role of Ca2+-activated Cl- current during proarrhythmic early afterdepolarizations in sheep and human ventricular myocytes. *Acta Physiol Scand* 179, 143-148.

Verkerk AO, Tan HL, & Ravesloot JH (2004). Ca2+-activated Cl- current reduces transmural electrical heterogeneity within the rabbit left ventricle. *Acta Physiol Scand* 180, 239-247.

Verkerk AO, Veldkamp MW, Bouman LN, & van Ginneken AC (2000). Calcium-activated Cl(-) current contributes to delayed afterdepolarizations in single Purkinje and ventricular myocytes. *Circulation* 101, 2639-2644.

Verkerk AO, Wilders R, Coronel R, Ravesloot JH, & Verheijck EE (2003b). Ionic remodeling of sinoatrial node cells by heart failure. *Circulation* 108, 760-766.

Verkerk AO, Wilders R, Zegers JG, van Borren MM, Ravesloot JH, & Verheijck EE (2002). Ca(2+)-activated Cl(-) current in rabbit sinoatrial node cells. *J Physiol* 540, 105-117.

Walsh KB & Long KJ (1994). Properties of a protein kinase C-activated chloride current in guinea pig ventricular myocytes. *Circ Res* 74, 121-129.

Wang GX, Hatton WJ, Wang GL, Zhong J, Yamboliev I, Duan D, & Hume JR (2003). Functional effects of novel anti-ClC-3 antibodies on native volume-sensitive osmolyte and anion channels in cardiac and smooth muscle cells. *Am J Physiol Heart Circ Physiol* 285, H1453-H1463.

Xu Y, Dong PH, Zhang Z, Ahmmed GU, & Chiamvimonvat N (2002). Presence of a calcium-activated chloride current in mouse ventricular myocytes. *Am J Physiol Heart Circ Physiol* 283, H302-H314.

Yamamoto S & Ehara T (2006). Acidic extracellular pH-activated outwardly rectifying chloride current in mammalian cardiac myocytes. *Am J Physiol Heart Circ Physiol* 290, H1905-H1914.

Yamamoto-Mizuma S, Wang GX, & Hume JR (2004a). P2Y purinergic receptor regulation of CFTR chloride channels in mouse cardiac myocytes. *J Physiol* 556, 727-737.

Yamamoto-Mizuma S, Wang GX, Liu LL, Schegg K, Hatton WJ, Duan D, Horowitz TL, Lamb FS, & Hume JR (2004b). Altered properties of volume-sensitive osmolyte and anion channels (VSOACs) and membrane protein expression in cardiac and smooth muscle myocytes from Clcn3-/- mice. *J Physiol* 557, 439-456.

Yang YD, Cho H, Koo JY, Tak MH, Cho Y, Shim WS, Park SP, Lee J, Lee B, Kim BM, Raouf R, Shin YK, & Oh U (2008). TMEM16A confers receptor-activated calcium-dependent chloride conductance. *Nature* 455, 1210-1215.

Zhang Z, Xu Y, Song H, Rodriguez J, Tuteja D, Namkung Y, Shin HS, & Chiamvimonvat N (2002). Functional Roles of Cav1.3 ({alpha}1D) Calcium Channel in Sinoatrial Nodes: Insight Gained Using Gene-Targeted Null Mutant Mice. *Circ Res* 90, 981-987.

Zygmunt AC (1994). Intracellular calcium activates a chloride current in canine ventricular myocytes. *Am J Physiol* 267, H1984-H1995.

Zygmunt AC & Gibbons WR (1991). Calcium-activated chloride current in rabbit ventricular myocytes. *Circ Res* 68, 424-437.

32

The Funny Current in Cardiac Non-Pacemaker Cells: Functional Role and Pharmacological Modulation

Laura Sartiani, Elisabetta Cerbai and Alessandro Mugelli
Department of Pharmacology, Center of Molecular Medicine, University of Florence
Italy

1. Introduction

In mammalians, heart rhythm originates in the sinoatrial node, a specialized region of the right atrium with defined anatomical and functional properties. The sinoatrial node acts as primary pacemaker in the heart owing to its unique ability to generate spontaneous action potentials at a rate faster than subsidiary pacemakers (the atrioventricular node and Purkinje fibers) (Vassalle, 1977). Propagation of action potentials from the sinoatrial node is first directed to the atria and then to the ventricles through a specialized conduction system that drives and coordinates the rhythmic contraction of heart chambers (Figure 1).

The pacemaker function of the sinoatrial node derives from a key electrogenic property, the diastolic depolarization phase or pacemaker phase of the action potential. It is a slow, positive increase in voltage across the cell membrane occurring between the end of one action potential and the beginning of the next; it causes the cell membrane to reach the threshold potential required to generate a subsequent action potential (DiFrancesco, 1991; DiFrancesco, 2010). The diastolic depolarization phase is absent in normal atrial and ventricular myocytes that rest at stable membrane potential values at the termination of the action potential.

Investigations aimed at elucidating the ionic mechanisms of pacemaking have proposed different candidates as major contributors responsible for the generation of the diastolic depolarization phase. At present, despite the issue is still a matter of debate, a wealth of information clearly agrees that two major mechanisms, membrane-associated ion currents and calcium release from sarcoplasmic reticulum, contribute to form a coordinated system that drives automaticity of normal cardiac pacemaker cells (Lakatta et al., 2010).

Among the membrane associated currents, the hyperpolarization-activated current or funny current (I_f) is considered a major player in both generation of cardiac spontaneous activity and rate control (DiFrancesco, 1991; DiFrancesco, 2010). I_f is an inward mixed-cation current carried by potassium and sodium, slowly activating on hyperpolarization at voltages comprising the diastolic depolarization phase of sinoatrial node cells (−40/−60 mV); for these reasons it was termed funny current. Accordingly, several loss-of-function mutations (DiFrancesco, 2010), as well as the down-regulation of constitutive subunits of f-channel in pacemaker cells (Zicha et al., 2005) have been demonstrated to cause sinus node dysfunction and rhythm disturbances.

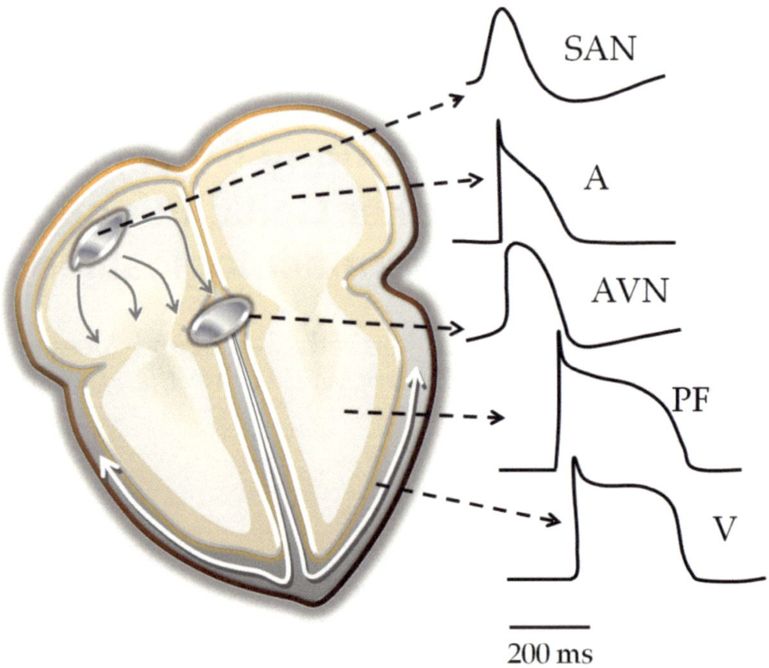

Representative action potentials from different regions of the heart. Displacement in time reflects the temporal sequence of impulse propagation through the heart. Abbreviations: SAN, sinoatrial node; A, atrium; AVN, atrioventricular node; PF, Purkinje fibers; V, ventricle; ms, milliseconds.

Fig. 1. Action potential profiles and propagation in the human heart.

Despite funny current expression has long been considered restricted to the sinus node and other regions of the conducting system, i.e. those cells possessing a diastolic depolarization phase, functional and molecular data collected over the last fifteen years have identified funny channels in non-pacemaker cardiomyocytes of the heart, namely in atrial and ventricular myocytes (Cerbai & Mugelli, 2006; Biel et al., 2009). In this cells, the increased expression of funny current occurring in cardiac diseases (see below), such as in hypertrophy and failure, has been suggested to contribute to ectopic beat formation and enhanced electrical activity.

2. Molecular properties and distribution of funny channels in the normal heart

Funny channel constitutive subunits were cloned starting from the late 1990s (Ludwig et al., 1999; Moosmang et al., 2001; Biel et al., 2009). They belong to the superfamily of the voltage-dependent potassium and cyclic nucleotide regulated channels and represent a gene family comprising four members, termed Hyperpolarization-activated Cyclic Nucleotide-gated (HCN1-4) channels.
The four different subunits assemble in homo-tetramers with distinct biophysical properties, but there is evidence *in vivo* that different subunits may combine in the same protein complex forming hetero-tetramers with specific kinetic and modulatory properties (Figure 2) (Biel et al., 2009). HCN isoforms share a highly conserved transmembrane core sequence, while their N and C termini vary considerably in terms of length and sequence homology.

In the membrane, HCN tetramers form pore-loop channels that arrange around a centrally located pore. Each subunit consists of six α-helical transmembrane segments that include the core sequence, responsible for channel gating properties and ion selectivity, and the intracellular cytosolic C-terminal domain, responsible for channel modulation by cyclic nucleotides.

In the adult heart, a wealth of information documented a robust expression of HCN1, HCN2 and HCN4 isoforms, while very low levels of HCN3 are present (Cerbai & Mugelli, 2006; Biel et al., 2009). In general, there is a strong variation of isoform quantity according to cardiac region, since expression levels of total HCN channels are low in normal atrial and ventricular muscle compared with those detected in the sinoatrial node region and in the conduction system. Moreover, there is also a clear variation of isoform predominance according to species. In the adult sinoatrial node of humans, rabbit, guinea pig, mouse and dog, HCN4 is the dominant isoform, accounting for the majority of the total HCN transcripts. By contrast HCN2 isoform predominates in rat sinoatrial node. The remaining fraction is mainly represented by HCN2 isoform in humans and mouse and HCN1 isoform

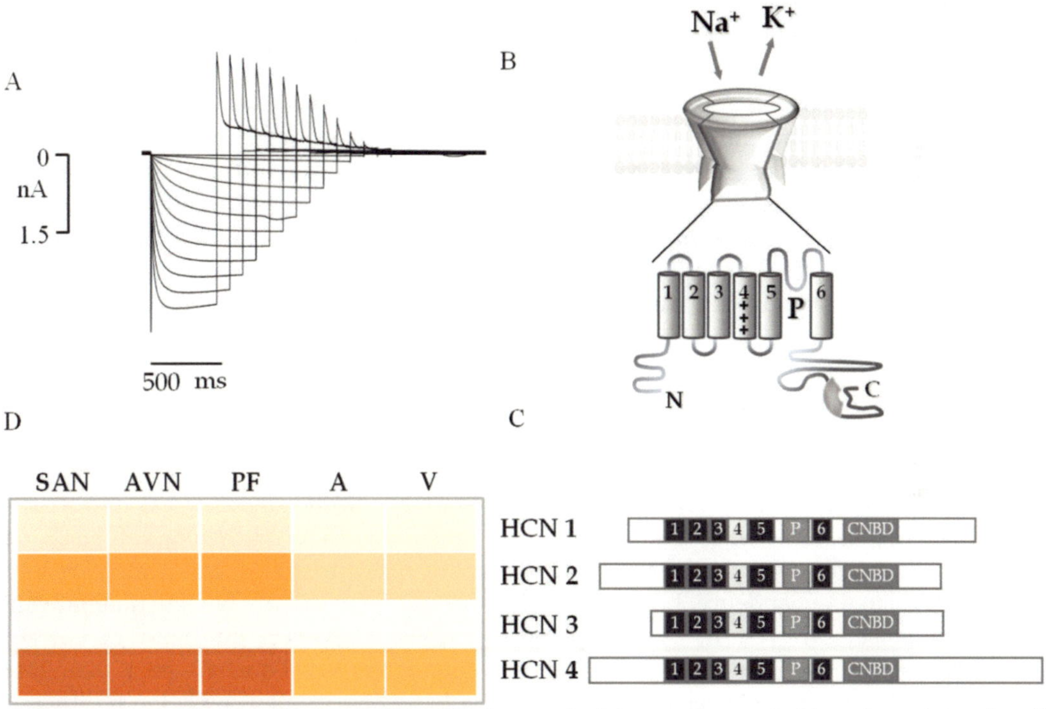

A: Representative family of I_f traces elicited by hyperpolarizing steps recorded in a sinoatrial node cell isolated from guinea-pig. B: Tetrameric structure of HCN channels: each monomer is formed by six trans-membrane segments (1-6), a pore loop (P) between segments 5 and 6, a voltage sensor motif in segment 4 and a cyclic-nucleotide-binding domain (CNBD) in the C-terminal region; C: HCN family formed by four isoforms termed HCN1-4. D: HCN isoform distribution in different regions of the human heart; intensity of colour is an index of isoform expression. Abbreviations: nA, nanoAmpere; ms, milliseconds; SAN, sinoatrial node; A, atrium; AVN, atrioventricular node; PF, Purkinje fibers; V, ventricle.

Fig. 2. Properties, topology and distribution of funny-channels in the heart.

in rabbit. HCN4 is the most abundant isoform in human atrioventricular node and Purkinje fibers, while HCN2 is the most largely expressed isoform in canine Purkinje fibers. Rabbit Purkinje fibers exhibit little I_f which is associated to low levels of HCN4 and HCN1 expressed in equal amount. In the conduction system no expression or only very low expression levels have been reported for HCN3 isoform. Despite the high interspecies variability shown by funny channels in the heart, a number of data point to HCN4 and HCN2 as the most represented isoforms in atrial and ventricular muscle of the majority of mammals, including humans. In these regions low levels of HCN1 and HCN3 have also been detected.

3. Expression and properties of funny channels in ventricular cardiomyocytes

The study of the electrophysiological mechanisms of arrhythmias has characterized the activity of our research group since long time (Vassalle & Mugelli, 1981). In the early 1990s, we were actively studying the electrophysiological alterations occurring in the hypertrophied heart of old spontaneously hypertensive rats. The goal was to get insight into the electrophysiological mechanisms underlying the enhanced arrhythmogenesis occurring in cardiac hypertrophy. We found that action potentials recorded in left ventricular papillary muscles isolated from hypertrophied hearts showed several electrophysiological alterations including an unusual diastolic depolarization phase, which was not present in preparations excised from normal hearts (Barbieri et al., 1994). Interestingly enough, in the same experimental model we documented that the slope of this sort of diastolic depolarization was clearly enhanced upon catecholamine stimulation, similarly to what previously described for the oscillatory current in Purkinje fibers (Vassalle & Mugelli, 1981). We were able to demonstrate that a relevant contribution to the diastolic depolarization phase present in hypertrophied hearts was due to the occurrence of an atypical I_f current that was functionally expressed in ventricular hypertrophic cardiomyoctes, but not in normal cardiomyoctes (Cerbai et al., 1994). Later on we demonstrated that I_f density in the hypertrophied rat hearts was linearly related to the severity of myocardial hypertrophy (Cerbai et al., 1996).

I_f recorded in ventricular rat cardiomyocytes showed electrophysiological properties, responsiveness to autonomic transmitters and sensitivity to pharmacological blockade similar to those observed for I_f expressed in the sinoatrial node (Cerbai et al., 1996). In particular, voltage-dependence, kinetics of activation and ionic selectivity were qualitatively similar to those retrieved in cardiac pacemaker cells. However, threshold of current activation differed substantially, being much more negative (about -70 mV) than that reported for sinoatrial node cells (-40 mV). On the basis of present knowledge on diverse HCN isoform distribution in the heart (see previous paragraph), the observed difference on I_f current activation likely reflects a diverse composition of HCN isoforms contributing to channel complex in the sinoatrial node and in the ventricular tissue. In addition to this, membrane sub-localization with interacting proteins, e.g. caveolin-3, may also contribute to differences in channel voltage activation (Barbuti et al., 2004; Barbuti et al., 2007). Despite the observed properties of funny current in the ventricular cardiomyocytes, a contribution to the diastolic phase of ventricular action potential is possible, since membrane resting potential is also more negative in ventricular cells than in sinoatrial node cells.

Action of catecholamines on the funny current expressed in ventricular myocytes was proved to closely resemble that reported for myocytes from sinoatrial node (Cerbai et al., 1999). In fact, stimulation of β-adrenoceptors shifts the I_f activation curve toward less negative values, with no change in the amplitude of the maximal specific conductance of the current. According to early observations (DiFrancesco & Tortora, 1991; DiFrancesco, 2010), this effect results from a direct binding and positive modulation of channel function exerted by 3'-5'-cyclic adenosine monophosphate nucleotide, whose intracellular levels are greatly enhanced by β-adrenoceptors stimulation. The effect of catecholamines on the funny current expressed in ventricular myocytes is in accordance with the diverse sensitivity to cyclic nucleotide reported for the different channel isoforms. Indeed, HCN2 and HCN4, the most abundant isoforms in the ventricle, are largely modulated by cyclic nucleotides, while HCN1 and HCN3, which are not present or have a very low expression in the ventricle, are weakly affected (Biel et al., 2009).

Subsequent experimental evidence led to the demonstration that I_f over-expression in ventricular cells occurred in other models of cardiac hypertrophy (Stilli et al., 2001) or following myocardial infarction (Sartiani et al., 2006): this suggests the involvement of a common mechanism controlling funny channels expression in cardiac diseases, such as ischemia and pathological hypertrophy. Finally and most importantly, a similar I_f gain-of-function was reported in human cardiac ventricular myocytes isolated from explanted

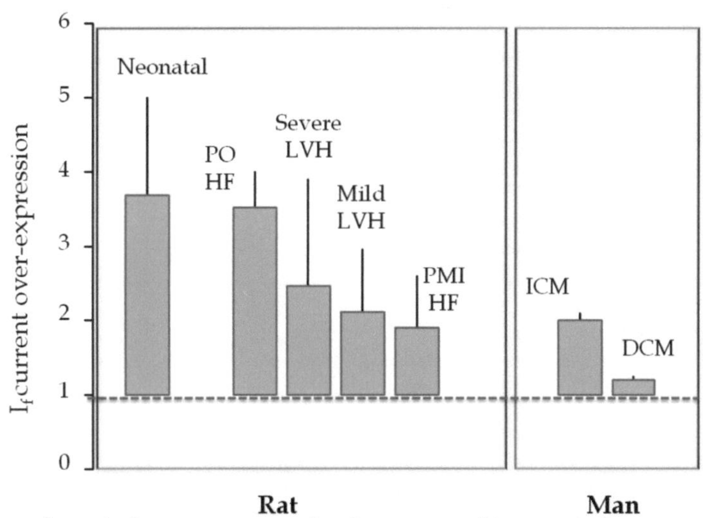

Columns represent the ratio between current density measured in ventricular myocytes from diseased hearts, and respective control; bars are confidence intervals (95%). In newborn rats, values measured at 2 weeks are compared to those at 2 days after birth. LVH-mild, LVH-severe: relative increase of I_f current in rats with mild or severe left ventricular hypertrophy caused by aortic banding or long-lasting pressure overload, respectively. PO-HF, PMI-HF: relative increase of I_f in rats with overt heart failure, resulting from uncompensated hypertrophy due to pressure-overload or following a myocardial infarction due to coronary ligation, respectively. DCM, ICM: relative increase of I_f in patients undergoing cardiac transplantation for terminal dilated or ischemic cardiomyopathy, respectively. For all conditions, the relative increase of I_f density was statistically significant versus controls, that is, normotensive rats, sham-operated rats, or normal donor hearts not transplanted for technical reasons, with the exception of DCM patients.

Fig. 3. I_f over-expression in cardiomyophaties and during cardiac development.

hearts (Cerbai, 1997; Hoppe, 1998). Interestingly enough, in human ventricular myocytes functional over-expression of I_f appeared to be related to the etiology of the disease, since current density is higher in ischemic than in dilated cardiomyopathy (Figure 3) (Cerbai et al., 2001).

Overall, these observations suggested that in the setting of structural and functional myocardial remodeling induced by pathology, I_f gain-of-function may contribute to the increased propensity for arrhythmias, a phenomenon documented both in patients and in experimental animal models. In this context, an over-activation of adrenergic system may increase the arrhythmogenic role played by I_f channels.

In the human healthy ventricle, distribution of HCN isoforms shows a robust expression of HCN2 and HCN4 isoforms. In accordance with the electrophysiological data showing a larger amplitude of funny current in failing human ventricular myocytes, levels of HCN4 and HCN2 isoforms are greatly enhanced both at transcriptional (Figure 4) and protein

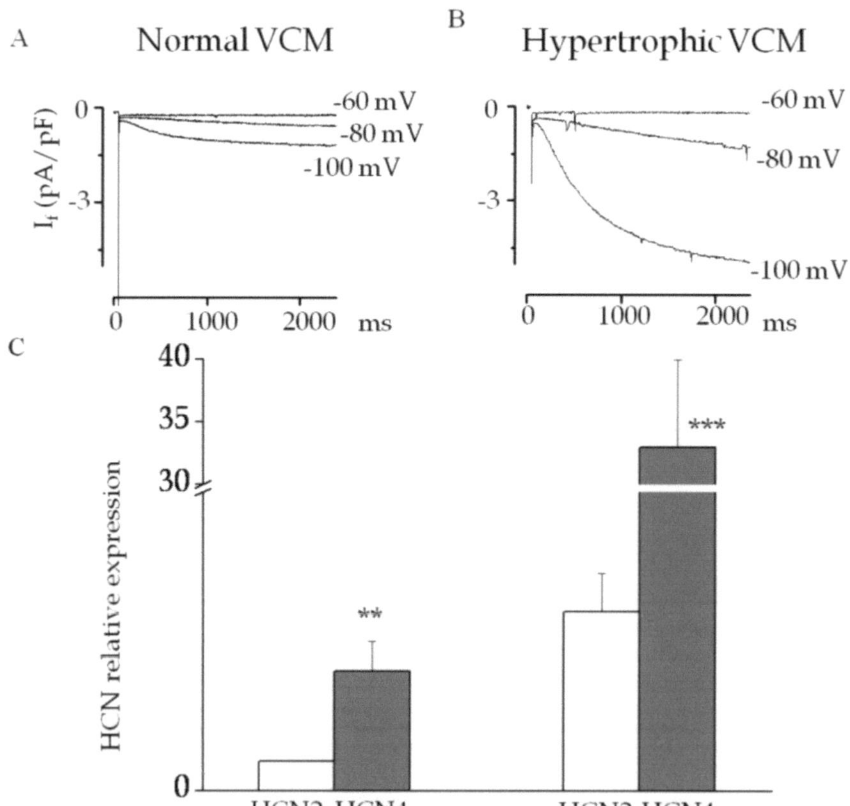

Representative traces of I_f recorded in a normal (A) and a hypertrophic (B) ventricular cardiomyocyte (VCM) isolated from human hearts. C: Quantification of HCN2 and HCN4 mRNA relative to the reference gene Glyceraldehyde-3-Phosphate Dehydrogenase, in human normal and hypertrophic ventricle (Normal V and Hypertrophic V, respectively). Abbreviations: pA, picoAmpere; pF, picoFarad; mV, milliVolts; ms, milliseconds.

Fig. 4. Functional and molecular properties of funny-channel in the human ventricle.

levels (Stillitano et al., 2008). A similar increase of HCN4 and HCN2 has been also documented in animal models of cardiac infarction (Suffredini et al., 2009) and hypertrophy (Fernandez-Velasco et al., 2003) and strongly suggests that cardiac pathology affects funny channel expression in ventricular myocytes. This phenomenon could modify the electrophysiological properties of cardiomyocytes, raising the tendency of the ventricular muscle to develop ectopic action potentials.

In summary, funny channel over-expression in non pacemaker ventricular cells, is a marker of remodeling induced by pathology and is likely to predispose cells to electrical instability. Funny channel over-expression, if associated with particular conditions documented in heart failure -namely a reduced expression of inwardly rectifying potassium current and elevated β-adrenergic stimulation- might contribute to trigger fatal arrhythmias.

3. Expression and properties of funny channels in atrial cardiomyocytes

Existence of funny current in human atrial appendage fibers was documented by Carmeliet on 1984 (Carmeliet, 1984), who first hypothesized the inherent potentiality of this current in human atrial tissue to develop spontaneous activity. The following experimental evidence allowed a thorough description of the properties of the funny current expressed in isolated human atrial myocytes obtained from atrial appendages excised during corrective cardiosurgery (Heidbuchel et al., 1987; Thuringer et al., 1992; Porciatti et al., 1997). On the basis of a number of experimental data it was documented that the funny current in atrial myocytes has a large variability in terms of amplitude and shows an activation voltage more negative than the atrial diastolic potential. These observations led to the general conclusion that the contribution of funny current to atrial electrogenesis is likely to be negligible in normal conditions. Despite this, a clear-cut diastolic depolarization phase is observed in human atrial myocytes, provided that integrity of the intracellular milieu is preserved using the perforated patch technique (Cerbai & Mugelli, 2006).

The physiological role of funny current in normal atrial tissue is still a matter of investigation; however, a contribution to atrial electrogenesis has been suggested in pathological conditions and/or following the activation of specific neurohumoral signals that may amplify current density at physiological potentials (Opthof, 1998; Michels et al., 2005). Among the potentially relevant signals, two are peculiar of the human atrium and have been investigated in our laboratory: serotonin and atrial natriuretic peptide. Serotonin subtype-4 receptors are typically expressed in the human atrium (Kaumann, 1991), where at least four different splicing-variant isoforms have been identified (Blondel et al., 1998; Bach et al., 2001; Lezoualc'h et al., 2007). Serotonin subtype-4 receptors are coupled to Gs proteins that upon stimulation increase intracellular levels of 3'-5'-cyclic adenosine monophosphate (Pindon et al., 2002) that positively modulates the funny current. Atrial natriuretic peptide is synthesized and stored as pro-hormone in granules localized in human atrial myocytes (Venugopal, 2001). Upon atrial distension, the peptide is released and interacts with specific receptors, namely natriuretic peptides receptor A and B. These are membrane-associated receptors coupled to guanylyl cyclase activity that increases intracellular 3'-5'-cyclic guanosine monophosphate nucleotide, which similarly to the adenosine cyclic nucleotide, binds to funny channels and increases the current. Accordingly, both serotonin and atrial natriuretic peptide proved to increase I_f current in human atrial myocytes (Pino et al., 1998; Lonardo et al., 2004). The effect is concentration-dependent and shows an affinity constant (Kd) quite similar to the physiological concentrations of serotonin and atrial natriuretic peptide likely reached upon adequate stimuli, i.e. local release during platelet aggregation or cell stretching, respectively. On the whole, these findings suggest that stimuli most likely involved in atrial arrhythmias are able to cause a gain of function of funny current in human atrial myocytes. Again this phenomenon could influence cell excitability and predispose to the occurrence of atrial arrhythmias.

4. Funny channel over-expression in cardiomyocytes is a marker of regression toward an immature phenotype

The understanding of the mechanisms and factors responsible for the functional over-expression of funny current in cardiac diseases is of great importance. Cardiac remodeling is a well defined phenomenon consisting of modifications in the structural and functional properties of the cardiac tissue (Swynghedauw, 1999), which occurs in several cardiac diseases. We hypothesized that the over-expression of funny channels in the diseased ventricle is likely part of the fetal/embryonic gene pattern that is known to be re-expressed in the heart during remodeling.

Ventricular cardiomyocytes are physiologically quiescent in the adult stage, but their action potentials exhibit a clear-cut diastolic depolarization phase in the immature stage. This property was associated with a robust expression of funny current in both rat fetal and neonatal cardiomyotes (Cerbai et al., 1999; Robinson et al., 1997; Sartiani et al., 2010). Further experimental evidences demonstrated that funny current occurrence and density are maximal in the first week of post-natal life and progressively decrease during maturation, reaching a low steady-state levels at one month of age. A minority of myocytes isolated from the hearts of adult rats express I_f, which, when present, was of small amplitude.

In accordance with data reported in the fetal mouse (Yasui et al., 2001; Mommersteeg et al., 2007; Schweizer et al., 2009), expression analysis in the rat documented that both HCN4 and HCN2 isoforms account for the majority of total HCN transcript in the neonatal ventricle, while HCN1 and HCN3 isoforms are not expressed at detectable levels (Sartiani et al., 2010). Interestingly, HCN4 is down-regulated during rat heart maturation, but in association with HCN2 it undergoes a clear-cut up-regulation after cardiac infarction (Suffredini et al., 2009). This observation confirms the hypothesis that transcriptional regulation in the remodeled heart involves funny channel isoforms typical of the immature ventricle, which are modulated as part of a panel of other key fetal/immature genes.

At variance with experimental animal models, obvious difficulties are encountered to get information on developmental changes of funny current in humans. A useful experimental model to overcome this difficulty is represented by human embryonic stem cells induced to differentiate toward the cardiac phenotype (Sartiani et al., 2007; Bettiol et al., 2007). This model is reported to recapitulate native cardiac embryogenesis and maturation, thus representing a useful tool to study early human cardiac development and growth. Using this model we documented that the funny current is present since the undifferentiated state, where its functional role in association with other ion channels, e.g. delayed rectifier potassium channels, still remains to be elucidated. After induction of cardiac differentiation, funny channels continue to be functionally present both in the early and late stages of cardiac differentiation. During this process the differentiating human cardiomyocytes undergo a number of key changes in terms of excitable properties and molecular phenotype that include modifications of funny channels. In fact, kinetics of I_f activation are markedly slowed-down in late-stage cardiomyocytes compared to the early ones and undifferentiated cells. Changes in kinetics during differentiation and maturation turned out to result from modifications of isoforms contributing to channel complex. In fact, when heterologously re-expressed as homomeric channels, HCN1 shows rapid activation kinetics (tens of milliseconds), whereas HCN2 and HCN4 activate in hundreds of milliseconds. In accordance with functional data, expression analysis of HCN isoform on differentiating cardiomyocytes showed that HCN1 isoform, which has the fastest activation kinetics, is largely expressed in undifferentiated cells and in early-stage cardiomyocytes, but is significantly reduced during maturation. The slower HCN2 isoform is expressed homogeneously throughout the differentiation process while HCN4 results to be dramatically down-regulated. On the whole, these observations suggest that, in accordance with data retrieved in native cardiac tissue (Figure 4), in human cardiomyocytes differentiated from embryonic stem cells HCN2 and HCN4 account for the majority of total HCN transcript and likely contribute to funny channel complex and properties.

In conclusion, funny channels are abundantly expressed in human cardiomyocytes differentiated from embryonic stem cells at all stages of differentiation and thus they represent a marker of immature cardiac phenotype in mammals. During maturation funny channels undergo modifications in terms of current properties and isoform composition. As previously suggested for the rat heart, changes in HCN isoform expression (down-regulation of HCN4) are opposite to those observed in heart hypertrophy and failure (up-regulation of HCN4 and HCN2) where the functional re-expression of funny current likely represent a regression toward an immature cardiac phenotype.

5. Pharmacological modulation of funny channels in the heart

In heart hypertrophy and failure, a complex signaling network contributes to initiate and exacerbate cardiac functional and molecular remodeling. Over the last years, a growing number of experimental evidence has been accumulating and documented the involvement of diverse factors in the patophysiology of the phenomenon. To date only some signalling pathways have been identified and extensively studied. Among the best documented, experimental and clinical evidence points to a central role for the increased levels of systemic and locally released hormonal factors, including norepinephrine, angiotensin II, endothelin I, aldosterone and cytokines (De Mello, 2004; Swynghedauw, 1999).

On the basis of our observation that funny channels are over-expressed in the diseased ventricular tissue, we assessed the involvement of the renin-angiotensin system, that is activated in cardiac hypertrophy/failure, in the regulation of funny channels (Figure 5). Using an experimental model of cardiac hypertrophy, the old spontaneously hypertensive rat, we tested the effect of type-1 angiotensin II receptor antagonists, losartan or irbesartan, orally administered for 8-weeks. The treatment proved to prevent the development of several electrophysiological alterations associated with cardiac hypertrophy, i.e. the action potential prolongation, the transient outward potassium current down-regulation and also the over-expression of funny current (Cerbai et al., 2000; Cerbai et al., 2003).

Recent clinical trials documented that reduction of heart rate with pacing (Rao et al., 2007) or selective bradycardic agents (Swedberg et al., 2010; Böhm et al., 2010) is associated to improved clinical outcomes in heart failure. Studies were performed in animal models to assess whether selective pharmacological intervention able to control heart rate were able to revert and/or ameliorate functional remodeling of ventricular tissue in cardiac diseases. In a rat model of myocardial infarction it was documented that reduction of heart rate with a

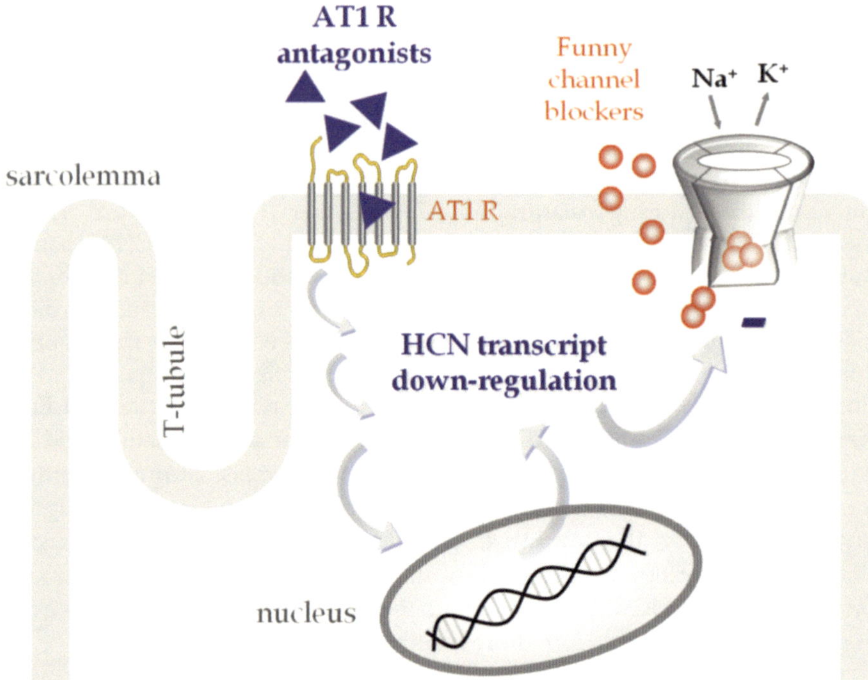

Abbreviations: AT1 R: angiotensin II receptor type 1.

Fig. 5. Schematic representation of pharmacological interventions able to modulate funny channel expression and/or function in cardiomyocytes.

selective bradycardic agent (ivabradine, see below for further details) is able to improve maximal myocardial perfusion and coronary reserve (Dedkov et al., 2007). On the basis of this evidence, we tested whether heart rate reduction with ivabradine in post-infarcted rats could counteract the electrophysiological remodeling of ventricular myocytes. Preliminary results proved that the treatment was able to ameliorate cardiac function as well as ion channels alterations, in particular the down-regulation of transient outward potassium current and the over-expression funny channels occurring in post-infarcted animals (Suffredini et al., 2009; Ceconi et al., 2007). At present, the mechanism(s) responsible for the reduction/reversion of ventricular functional remodeling with heart rate slowing drugs remains unknown and further investigations are necessary.

On the whole, over-expression of funny channels in ventricular cardiomyocytes is promoted by hypertrophic factors whose levels are increased during cardiac hypertrophy and failure. Over-expression of funny channels is inhibited by drugs that revert or prevent many of the electrophysiological alterations described in the remodeled cardiac myocytes.

In the last years, we have explored the pharmacological strategy aimed to modulate directly the cardiac funny channels, identifying novel molecules that act as direct channel blockers. The interest in funny channels direct modulators has emerged due to the approval of ivabradine (a prototype blocker of funny channel with selective bradycardic properties) for the treatment of stable *angina pectoris*. Our experimental approach took advantage of classical medicinal chemistry and electrophysiology and aimed to identify novel derivatives, structurally related to zatebradine (Romanelli et al., 2005), a different prototype blocker of funny channels, whose clinical trials were stopped due to adverse side effects. Moreover, since the most serious side effects of zatebradine are due to unselective blockade of the HCN isoforms present in tissues different from the heart, i.e. retinal rods and nervous system, one additional aim was to develop compounds able to discriminate among the HCN channel isoforms. Our recent results (Melchiorre et al., 2010) have uncovered diverse structural requirements necessary to provide derivative selectivity for the diverse HCN isoforms, which suggest a potential interest of these compounds as novel selective bradycardic agents. Investigations are currently characterizing the pharmacological profile of these novel funny channel blockers especially looking at their isoform selectivity.

6. Summary and conclusion

After their first discovery in the sinoatrial node, funny channels have been identified as key physiological regulators of pacemaker function in the heart. Subsequent studies have documented their expression in the atrial and ventricular muscles, where diverse pathologic conditions, such as cardiac hypertrophy and failure, cause their functional enhancement. This observation and the identification of different signaling pathways able to promote their function in the atria and ventricles has led to the suggestion that the funny current in non pacemaker cardiomyocytes may influence membrane excitability and predispose to the occurrence of arrhythmias. However, this hypothesis remains unproved in both experimental and clinical settings. The recent SHIFT study (Swedberg et al., 2010; Böhm et al., 2010) showed that ivabradine improves clinical outcomes in chronic heart failure, pointing to the reduction of heart rate as fundamental mechanism of drug action. However, the accompanying editorial (Teerlink, 2010) hypothesized that other mechanisms such us blockade of funny channels in the ventricle may contribute to the beneficial effects of ivabradine. Despite the progresses made, numerous key questions still remains unanswered and deserve a thorough investigation in the future. Among the most important, some of the unknown issues relate to:

i. the relevance and the specific role of funny channels in non pacemaker cells in different cardiac diseases.
1. the factors and signalling pathways controlling the expression, the cellular processing, and the sub-cellular compartmentation of funny channels in the normal and diseased heart.
2. the identifications of proteins and/or other (bio)molecules able to interact and modulate funny channels function in physiological and pathological conditions.

7. Acknowledgments

This work was supported by grants from Ministero dell'Istruzione, dell'Universita` e della Ricerca, Rome (Programmi di Ricerca di Interesse Nazionale 2008838SN9) and from European Union (STREP Project "NORMACOR", 6th European Framework Program, contract LSH M/CT/2006/018676).

8. References

Bach, T.; Syversveen, T.; Kvingedal, A.M.; Krobert, K.A.; Brattelid, T.; Kaumann, A.J. & Levy, F.O. (2001). 5HT4(a) and 5-HT4(b) receptors have nearly identical pharmacology and are both expressed in human atrium and ventricle. *Naunyn-Schmiedeberg's archives of pharmacology*, 363, 146-160, pISSN: 0028-1298.

Barbieri, M.; Varani, K.; Cerbai, E.; Guerra, L.; Li, Q.; Borea, P.A. & Mugelli, A. (1994). Electrophysiological basis for the enhanced cardiac arrhythmogenic effect of isoprenaline in aged spontaneously hypertensive rats. *Journal of Molecular and Cellular Cardiology*, 26, 7, 849-860, pISSN: 0022-2828.

Barbuti, A.; Gravante, B.; Riolfo, M.; Milanesi, R.; Terragni, B. and DiFrancesco, D. (2004). Localization of pacemaker channels in lipid rafts regulates channel kinetics. *Circulation Research*, 94, 10, 1325-1331, pISSN: 0009-7330.

Barbuti, A.; Terragni, B.; Brioschi, C. & DiFrancesco, D. (2007). Localization of f-channels to caveolae mediates specific beta2-adrenergic receptor modulation of rate in sinoatrial myocytes. *Journal of Molecular and Cellular Cardiology*, 42, 1, 71-78, pISSN: 0022-2828.

Bettiol, E.; Sartiani, L.; Chicha, L.; Krause, K.H.; Cerbai, E. & Jaconi, M.E. (2007). Fetal bovine serum enables cardiac differentiation of human embryonic stem cells. *Differentiation; research in biological diversity*, 75, 8, 669-681, pISSN: 0301 -4681.

Biel, M.; Wahl-Schott, C.; Michalakis, S. & Zong, X. (2009). Hyperpolarization-activated cation channels: from genes to function. *Physiological Reviews*, 89, 3, 847-885, pISSN: 0031-9333.

Blondel, O.; Gastineau, M.; Dahmoune, Y.; Langlois, M. & Fischmeister, R. (1998). Cloning, expression, and pharmacology of four human 5-hydroxytryptamine 4 receptor isoforms produced by alternative splicing in the carboxyl terminus. *Journal of Neurochemistry*, 70, 2252-2261, pISSN: 0022-3042.

Böhm, M.; Swedberg, K.; Komajda, M.; Borer, J.S.; Ford, I.; Dubost-Brama, A.; Lerebours, G.; Tavazzi, L.; SHIFT Investigators. (2010) Heart rate as a risk factor in chronic heart failure (SHIFT): the association between heart rate and outcomes in a randomised placebo-controlled trial. *Lancet*, 376 (9744), 886-94, pISSN: 0140-6736.

Carmeliet, E. (1984). Existence of pacemaker current I_f in human atrial appendage fibres. *The Journal of physiology*, 357, 125P, abstract, pISSN: 0022-3751.

Ceconi, C.; Comini, L.; Suffredini, E.; Cerbai, E.; Ferrari, R.; Bouly, M. & Mugelli, A. (2007). Structural and electrophysiological effects on cardiac remodeling by ivabradine. *European heart journal supplements: journal of the European Society of Cardiology*, 28, 42, abstract, ISSN: 1520-765X.

Cerbai, E. & Mugelli, A. (2006). I(f) in non-pacemaker cells: role and pharmacological implications. *Pharmacological research:the official journal of the Italian Pharmacological Society*, 53, 5, 416-423, pISSN: 1043-6618.

Cerbai, E.; Pino, R.; Rodriguez, M.L. & Mugelli, A. (1999). Modulation of the pacemaker current I_f by beta-adrenoceptor subtypes in ventricular myocytes isolated from hypertensive and normotensive rats. *Cardiovascular Research*, 42, 1, 121-129, pISSN: 0008-6363.

Cerbai, E.; Barbieri, M. & Mugelli, A. (1994). Characterization of the hyperpolarization-activated current, I_f, in ventricular myocytes isolated from hypertensive rats. *The Journal of physiology*, 481, 585-591, pISSN: 0022-3751.

Cerbai, E.; Barbieri, M. & Mugelli, A. (1996). Occurrence and properties of the hyperpolarization-activated current I_f in ventricular myocytes from normotensive and hypertensive rats during aging. *Circulation*, 94, 1674-1681, pISSN: 0009-7322.

Cerbai, E.; Crucitti, A.; Sartiani, L.; De Paoli, P.; Pino, R., Rodriguez, M.L.; Gensini, G. & Mugelli, A. (2000). Long-term treatment of spontaneously hypertensive rats with losartan and electrophysiological remodeling of cardiac myocytes. *Cardiovascular Research*, 45, 2, 388-396, pISSN: 0008-6363.

Cerbai, E.; De Paoli, P.; Sartiani, L.; Lonardo, G. & Mugelli, A. (2003). Treatment with irbesartan counteracts the functional remodeling of ventricular myocytes from hypertensive rats. *Journal of Cardiovascular Pharmacology*, 41, 5, 804-812, pISSN: 0160-2446.

Cerbai, E.; Pino, R.; Porciatti, F.; Sani, G.; Toscano, M.; Maccherini, M.; Giunti, G. & Mugelli, A. (1997). Characterization of the hyperpolarization-activated current, I_f, in ventricular myocytes from human failing heart. *Circulation*, 95, 568-571, pISSN: 0009-7322.

Cerbai, E.; Pino, R.; Sartiani, L. & Mugelli, A. (1999). Influence of postnatal development on I_f occurrence and properties in neonatal rat ventricular myocytes. *Cardiovascular Research*, 42, 416–423, pISSN: 0008-6363.

Cerbai, E.; Sartiani, L.; De Paoli, P.; Pino, R.; Maccherini, M.; Bizzarri, F.; DiCiolla, F.; Davoli, G.; Sani, G. & Mugelli, A. (2001). The properties of the pacemaker current I_f in human ventricular myocytes are modulated by cardiac disease. *Journal of Molecular and Cellular Cardiology*, 33, 441-448, pISSN: 0022-2828.

De Mello, W.C. (2004). Heart failure: how important is cellular sequestration? The role of the renin-angiotensin-aldosterone system. *Journal of Molecular and Cellular Cardiology*, 37, 2, 431-438, pISSN: 0022-2828.

Dedkov, E. I.; Zheng, W.; Christensen, L. P.; Weiss, R. M.; Mahlberg-Gaudin, F. & Tomanek, R. J. (2007). Preservation of coronary reserve by ivabradine-induced reduction in heart rate in infarcted rats is associated with decrease in perivascular collagen. *American Journal of Physiology. Heart and Circulatory Physiology*, 293, 1, H590-H598, pISSN: 0363-6135.

DiFrancesco, D. & Tortora, P. (1991). Direct activation of cardiac pacemaker channels by intracellular cyclic AMP. *Nature*, 351, 6322, 145-147, pISSN: 0028-0836.

DiFrancesco, D. (1991). The contribution of the 'pacemaker' current (I_f) to generation of spontaneous activity in rabbit sino-atrial node myocytes. *The Journal of Physiology*, 434, 23-40, pISSN: 0022-3751.

DiFrancesco, D. (2010). The role of the funny current in pacemaker activity. *Circulation Research*, 106, 3, 434-446, pISSN: 0009-7330.

Fernandez-Velasco, M.; Goren, N.; Benito, G.; Blanco-Rivero, J.; Boscá, L. & Delgado, C. (2003). Regional distribution of hyperpolarization-activated current I_f and hyperpolarization-activated cyclic nucleotide-gated channel mRNA expression in ventricular cells from control and hypertrophied rat hearts. *The Journal of Physiology*, 553, 395–405, pISSN: 0022-3751.

Heidbuchel, H.; Vereecke, J. & Carmeliet, E. (1987). The electrophysiological effects of acetylcholine in single human atrial cells. *Journal of Molecular and Cellular Cardiology*, 19, 1207-1219, pISSN: 0022-2828.

Hoppe, U.C.; Jansen, E.; Sudkamp, M. & Beuckelmann, D.J. (1998). Hyperpolarization-activated inward current in ventricular myocytes from normal and failing human hearts. *Circulation,* 97, 55-65, pISSN: 0009-7322.

Kaumann, A.J. (1991). 5-HT4-like receptors in mammalian atria. *Journal of neural transmission. Supplementum,* 34, 195-201.

Lakatta, E.G.; Maltsev, V.A. & Vinogradova, T.M. (2010). A coupled SYSTEM of intracellular Ca^{2+} clocks and surface membrane voltage clocks controls the timekeeping mechanism of the heart's pacemaker. *Circulation Reseach,* 106, 4, 659-73, pISSN: 0009-7330.

Lezoualc'h, F.; Steplewski, K.; Sartiani, L.; Mugelli, A.; Fischmeister, R. & Bril, A. (2007). Quantitative mRNA analysis of serotonin 5-HT4 receptor isoforms, calcium handling proteins and ion channels in human atrial fibrillation. *Biochemical and Biophysical Research Communication,* 357, 1, 218-224, pISSN: 0006-291X.

Lonardo, G.; Cerbai, E.; Casini, S.; Giunti, G.; Bonacchi, M.; Battaglia, F.; Fiorani, B.; Stefano P.L.; Sani, G. & Mugelli, A. (2004). Atrial natriuretic peptide modulates the hyperpolarization-activated current (I_f) in human atrial myocytes. *Cardiovascular Research,* 63, 528-536, pISSN: 0008-6363.

Lonardo, G.; Cerbai, E.; Casini, S.; Giunti, G.; Bonacchi, M.; Battaglia, F.; Fiorani, B.; Stefano, P.L.; Sani, G. & Mugelli, A. (2004). Atrial natriuretic peptide modulates the hyperpolarization-activated current (I_f) in human atrial myocytes. *Cardiovascular Research,* 63, 528-536, pISSN: 0008-6363.

Ludwig, A.; Zong, X.; Stieber, J.; Hullin, R.; Hofmann, F. & Biel, M. (1999). Two pacemaker channels from human heart with profoundly different activation kinetics. *The EMBO Journal,* 18, 9, 2323-2329, *p*ISSN: 0261-4189.

Melchiorre, M.; Del Lungo, M.; Guandalini, L.; Martini, E; Dei, S.; Manetti, D.; Scapecchi, S.; Teodori, E.; Sartiani, L.; Mugelli, A.; Cerbai, E. & Romanelli, M. N. (2010). Design, synthesis, and preliminary biological evaluation of new isoform-selective f-current blockers. *Journal of Medicinal Chemistry,* Aug 26 [Epub ahead of print], pISSN: 0022-2623.

Michels, G.; Er, F.; Khan, I.; Sudkamp, M.; Herzig, S. & Hoppe, U.C. (2005). Single-channel properties support a potential contribution of hyperpolarization-activated cyclic nucleotide-gated channels and I_f to cardiac arrhythmias. *Circulation,* 111, 399-404, pISSN: 0009-7322.

Mommersteeg, M.T.; Hoogaars, W.M.; Prall, O.W.; de Gier-de Vries, C.; Wiese, C.; Clout, D.E.; Papaioannou, V.E.; Brown, N.A.; Harvey, R.P.; Moorman, A.F. & Christoffels, V.M. (2007). Molecular pathway for the localized formation of the sinoatrial node. *Circulation Research,* 100, 354-362, pISSN: 0009-7330.

Moosmang, S.; Stieber, J.; Zong, X.; Biel, M.; Hofmann, F. & Ludwig, A. (2001). Cellular expression and functional characterization of four hyperpolarization-activated pacemaker channels in cardiac and neuronal tissues. *European journal of Biochemistry/FEBS,* 268, 6, 1646-1652, pISSN: 0014-2956.

Opthof, T. (1998). The membrane current (I_f) in human atrial cells: implications for atrial arrhythmias. *Cardiovascular Research,* 38, 537-540, pISSN: 0008-6363.

Pindon, A.; van Hecke, G.; van Gompel, P.; Lesage, A.S.; Leysen, J.E. & Jurzak, M. (2002). Differences in signal transduction of two 5-HT_4 receptor splice variants: compound specificity and dual coupling with Galpha s- and Galpha i/o-proteins. *Molecular Pharmacology,* 61, 85-96, pISSN: 0026-895X.

Pino, R.; Cerbai, E., Calamai, G.; Alajmo, F.; Borgioli, A.; Braconi, L.; Cassai, M.; Montesi, G.F. & Mugelli, A. (1998). Effect of 5-HT4 receptor stimulation on the pacemaker current I_f in human isolated atrial myocytes. *Cardiovascular Research,* 40, 516-522, pISSN: 0008-6363.

Porciatti, F.; Pelzmann, B.; Cerbai, E.; Schaffer, P.; Pino, R.; Bernhart, E.; Koidl , B. & Mugelli, A. (1997). The pacemaker current I_f in single human atrial myocytes and the effect of beta-adrenoceptor and A1-adenosine receptor stimulation. *British Journal of Pharmacology,* 122, 5, 963-969, pISSN: 0007-1188.

Rao, K.; Fisher, M.L.; Robinson, S.; Shorofsky, S. & Gottlieb, S. (2007). Effect of chronic changes in heart rate on congestive heart failure. *Journal of Cardiac Failure,* 13, 4, 269-274, pISSN: 1071-9164.

Robinson, R.B.; Yu, H.; Chang, F. & Cohen, I.S. (1977). Developmental change in the voltage-dependence of the pacemaker current, I_f, in rat ventricle cells. *Pflügers Archiv: European Journal of Physiology,* 433, 533–535, pISSN: 0031-6768.

Romanelli, M.N.; Cerbai, E.; Dei, S.; Guandalini, L; Martelli, C.; Martini, E.; Scapecchi, S.; Teodori, E. & Mugelli, A. (2005). Design, synthesis and preliminary biological evaluation of zatebradine analogues as potential blockers of the hyperpolarization-activated current. *Bioorganic & medicinal chemistry,* 13, 4, 1211-1220, pISSN: 0968-0896.

Sartiani, L.; Stillitano, F.; Luceri, C.; Suffredini, S.; Toti, S.; De Filippo, C.; Cuomo, V.; Tattoli, M.; Dolara, P.; Mugelli, A. & Cerbai, E. (2010). Prenatal exposure to carbon monoxide delays postnatal cardiac maturation. *Laboratory Investigation; a journal of technical methods and pathology,* Jul 19 [Epub ahead of print], pISSN: 0023-6837.

Sartiani, L.; Bettiol, E.; Stillitano, F.; Mugelli, A.; Cerbai, E. & Jaconi, M. E. (2007). Developmental changes in cardiomyocytes differentiated from human embryonic stem cells: a molecular and electrophysiological approach. *Stem Cells,* 25, 5, 1136-1144, pISSN: 0250-6793.

Sartiani, L.; De Paoli, P.; Stillitano, F.; Aimond, F.; Vassort, G.; Mugelli, A. & Cerbai, E. (2006). Functional remodeling in post-myocardial infarcted rats: focus on beta-adrenoceptor subtypes. *Journal of Molecular and Cellular Cardiology,* 40, 2, 258-266, pISSN: 0022-2828.

Schweizer, P.; Yampolsky, P. & Malik, R. (2009). Transcription profiling of HCN-channel isotypes throughout mouse cardiac development. *Basic Research in Cardiology,* 104, 621-629, pISSN: 0300-8428.

Stilli, D.; Sgoifo, A.; Macchi, E.; Zaniboni, M.; De Iasio, S.; Cerbai, E.; Mugelli, A.; Lagrasta, C.; Olivetti, G. & Musso, E. (2001). Myocardial remodeling and arrhythmogenesis in moderate cardiac hypertrophy in rats. *American Journal of Physiology. Heart and Circulatory Physiology,* 280, 1, H142-H150, pISSN: 0363-6135.

Stillitano, F.; Lonardo, G.; Zicha, S.; Varro, A.; Cerbai, E.; Mugelli, A. & Nattel S. (2008). Molecular basis of funny current (I_f) in normal and failing human heart. *Journal of Molecular and Cellular Cardiology,* 45, 2, 289-299, pISSN: 0022-2828.

Suffredini, S.; Stillitano, F.; Brogioni, S.; Comini, L.; Ceconi, C.; Sartiani, L.; Bouly, M.; Ferrari, R.; Mugelli, A. & Cerbai E. (2009). Electrophysiological remodeling in post-myocardial infarcted rats: focus on f-current and heart rate. *European heart journal supplements: journal of the European Society of Cardiology*, 30, 868, abstract, ISSN: 1520-765X.

Swedberg, K.; Komajda, M.; Böhm, M.; Borer, J.S.; Ford, I.; Dubost-Brama, A.; Lerebours, G.; Tavazzi, L; SHIFT Investigators. (2010). Ivabradine and outcomes in chronic heart failure (SHIFT): a randomised placebo-controlled study. *Lancet*, 376 (9744), 875-85, pISSN: 0140-6736.

Swynghedauw, B. (1999). Molecular mechanism of myocardial remodeling. *Physiological Reviews*, 79, 215-262, pISSN: 0031-9333.

Teerlink, JR. (2010). Ivabradine in heart failure—no paradigm SHIFT···yet. *Lancet*, 376 (9744), 847-49, pISSN: 0140-6736.

Thuringer, D.; Lauribe, P. & Escande, D. (1992). A hyperpolarization-activated inward current in human myocardial cells. *Journal of Molecular and Cellular Cardiology*, 24, 451-455, pISSN: 0022-2828.

Vassalle, M. (1977). The relationship among cardiac pacemakers. Overdrive suppression. *Circulation Research*, 41, 269-277, pISSN: 0009-7330.

Vassalle, M. & Mugelli, A. An oscillatory current in sheep cardiac Purkinje fibers. *Circulation Research*, 48, 5, 618-631, pISSN: 0009-7330.

Venugopal, J. (2001). Cardiac natriuretic peptides - hope or hype? *Journal of Clinical Pharmacy and Therapeutics*, 26, 1, 15-31, pISSN: 0269-4727.

Yasui, K.; Liu, W.; Opthof, T.; Kada, K.; Lee, JK.; Kamiya, K. & Kodama, I. (2001). I(f) current and spontaneous activity in mouse embryonic ventricular myocytes. *Circulation Research*, 88, 536-542, pISSN: 0009-7330.

Zicha, S.; Fernández-Velasco, M.; Lonardo, G.; L'Heureux, N. & Nattel, S. (2005). Sinus node dysfunction and hyperpolarization-activated (HCN) channel subunit remodeling in a canine heart failure model. *Cardiovascular Research*, 66, 3, 472-81, pISSN: 0008-6363.